Harper's Handbook of Therapeutic Pharmacology

Harper's Handbook of Therapeutic Pharmacology

R. Marilyn Schmidt, B.S.
Federal Regulatory Affairs
Consultant and
Technical Writer

Solomon Margolin, Ph.D.
President
AMR Biological Research, Inc.
Princeton, N.J.

HARPER & ROW, PUBLISHERS
PHILADELPHIA

Cambridge
Hagerstown
New York
San Francisco

London
Mexico City
São Paulo
Sydney

1817

3 5 6 4 2

Library of Congress Cataloging in Publication Data

Schmidt, R Marilyn.
    Harper's handbook of therapeutic pharmacology.

    Bibliography
    Includes index.
    1. Drugs.   2. Pharmacology. I. Margolin, Solomon, joint author.   II. Title.   III. Title: Handbook of therapeutic pharmacology.   [DNLM: 1. Drug therapy— Handbooks.   2. Pharmacology—Handbooks.   QV4.3 H295]
RM300.S275   615'.7   79-27049
ISBN 0-397-54264-X

The authors and publisher have exerted every effort to ensure that drug selection and dosage set forth in this text are in accord with current recommendations and practice at the time of publication. However, in view of ongoing research, changes in government regulations, and the constant flow of information relating to drug therapy and drug reactions, the reader is urged to check the package insert for each drug for any change in indications and dosage and for added warnings and precautions. This is particularly important when the recommended agent is a new or infrequently employed drug.

Contents

viii   **Contents**

Preface

The authors have endeavored to orient the reader quickly and concisely to the vast array of pharmaceutical products available for therapeutic and diagnostic uses. The numerous drugs are arranged primarily according to their major effects on a specific organ system. Combination products, for the most part, are not included unless they are unique or serve a unique therapeutic use.

The information for each drug or group of drugs is presented in a standardized format to simplify comparisons and interrelationships. The organ system arrangement is used since patients are customarily segregated in this manner in hospitals and by health care specialists. For example, patients with cardiovascular diseases are usually located in one section of a hospital and are cared for primarily by the cardiologist or internist and coronary care nurses. Consequently, we have attempted to segregate drugs affecting the cardiovascular system into the antiarrhythmic agents, anti-infectives, or vasoconstrictors which are used primarily by those professionals working within this specialty. A similar pattern is followed for adverse effects.

Health professionals and the pharmaceutical industry have become increasingly aware of special dosage variations and considerations in treating the various age groups of patients, particularly the pediatric and geriatric populations. In this book we have attempted to include information pertinent to these age groups, in addition to the usual adult dosage and maximal recommended daily dosage, if available.

Among the many important responsibilities of the health professional is the administration of drugs prescribed by the physician and the observation of drug therapeutic effects, interactions, and adverse effects. In addition, it is frequently the re-

ix

sponsibility of the nurse to counsel and instruct the patient in the use of drugs during their illness. The nurse is often the first line observer of drug effects since she/he has more frequent contact with the patient than does the physician. Consequently, the nurse plays a vital role in the use of drugs and the treatment of the patient.

To facilitate use of this book, the authors have included several specialty sections. Because of variations in definitions and traditional usage, a "Glossary" defines the terms as used in this book. In the text, each drug is identified not only by the generic name but also by select trade or brand names. A "Drug Directory" located before the "Index," lists by both generic and representative trade names of all drugs discussed in this book.

Within each group of drugs, the specific therapeutic classification is presented.

For example, "Psychotherapeutic Agents" is divided into four therapeutic classes: antipsychotic agents, antianxiety agents, antidepressants, and psychostimulants. For each class, information is arranged as follows: general clinical uses, specific products and dosages, pharmacology, special precautions, adverse effects, and clinical guidelines. Since the nurse plays an increasingly important role in drug therapy, the guidelines contain information pertaining to administration, effects, drug interactions, and overdosage/antidotes.

A chapter titled, "Drug Overdosage, Intoxication, Abuse," discusses separately the drugs useful in these conditions since information of this type often is difficult to find when needed. Throughout the text, whenever possible, information is presented on specific antidotes for each drug substance and also for treatment of overdosage.

R. Marilyn Schmidt, B.S., and
Solomon Margolin, Ph.D.

Instructions for use

HARPER'S HANDBOOK OF THER-APEUTIC PHARMACOLOGY is designed to facilitate your search for information about a drug or group of drugs. Information is arranged by the organ system which mimics that of hospital and medical specialty organization.

If one is looking for information about a specific drug, regardless of its use, consult the Drug Directory. Generic names and the most commonly used trade or brand names are included. Trade names are consistently distinguished throughout the book text and are identified by capital letters. When a series of page numbers is cited, it denotes that information about a drug is located in more than one section because of the various uses of that specific drug. For example, gentamicin is included in Chapter 2, Anti-Infective Agents, also Chapter 7, Drugs Affecting The Urinary Tract, and Chapter 11, Drugs Affecting The Eye.

To locate the complete information about a group of drugs such as the analgesic agents, consult the Index. The location of the principal information and also specific use information will be cited.

To determine if a drug is available as a generic drug, consult the Drug Directory. A dagger (†) appearing after the generic name designates that this drug is available generically.

Certain drugs are restricted in their use by inclusion in the list of Federal Controlled Substances. Each drug restricted in use by the Controlled Substances Act is designated with a "C" followed by a I, II, III, IV, or V, further designating the extent of control as is explained in Chapter 1, Principles of Therapeutic Pharmacology, Controlled Drugs.

Drugs in each group (and also in the Drug Directory), which are combination products—that is, which contain more than one active drug substance—are designated in the footnotes.

Before attempting to find information about any group of drugs it is advisable to consult the Table of Contents so that the organization of this reference text is clear. If difficulty is encountered in locating information about any drug or group of drugs, the authors would appreciate being notified.

About the factual content of this reference

The authors and editors of this book have expended considerable time and effort to ensure that the facts and opinions offered in the text and tables of this book are in accordance with official standards and with the consensus of foremost authorities at the time of publication.

However, drug therapy is a very dynamic branch of medicine, marked by the continual marketing of new drugs and the discontinuation and withdrawal (often without notice) of older drug products. In addition, the Food and Drug Administration constantly orders changes in the labeling of even well-established drug products, on the basis of ongoing studies of their safety and efficacy. For this reason, no claims are made that statements made here concerning the current status of these drugs will continue to reflect the stated view or that the data presented in tabular form are, or will remain, complete and correct in every detail.

The most important aspect of this problem lies in the area of dosage recommendations. Every effort has been made to check that statements made in the tables are, within the limits of space, precisely correct. However, dosage schedules are frequently ordered changed in accordance with accumulating clinical experiences.

For this reason, we urge that, *before administering any drug, you check the manufacturer's latest dosage recommendations* as presented in the package insert which accompanies each unit of every drug product.

Principles of therapeutic pharmacology

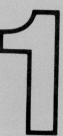

DRUG NAMES

The name by which a drug is most commonly known today is the trade name, a name coined by the manufacturer and exclusively his to use. An example is LIBRIUM Capsules, the trade name of Roche Laboratories for chlordiazepoxide. The trade name is also called the "brand" or "unofficial" name. Since it is unique and the property of the manufacturer, it is usually protected by registration as a trademark. This name is the one emphasized in advertisements and promotional literature to the physician. However, each time it is displayed prominently in an advertisement, by Federal Food, Drug, and Cosmetic regulation, it must be accompanied by the generic or official name.

The generic name of a drug, also referred to as the "official" or "nonproprietary" name, is a word related to the chemical name or structure of a drug. This name must be approved by the Council of Drugs of the American Medical Association and the Federal Food and Drug Administration before use in labeling and advertisements.

Trade names are usually designed so that they are easy to use and remember. Most prescriptions have been written by the trade name, not the generic name. Consequently, most physicians continue to prescribe by trade name long after the patent has expired on a drug and after other firms are marketing the product, frequently at a lower price than the original manufacturer.

When new drugs are developed, the chemical compound (the active ingredient), its uses, and the processes for synthesis are usually protected by patents. Life of a patent in the United States at present is 17 years. Therefore, during this 17-year period, a new drug is protected from being made or sold by other firms unless an agreement exits for appropriate compensation to the firm developing the drug. An example is chlordiazepoxide hydrochloride (generic name), a drug developed by Roche Laboratories and sold as LIBRIUM Capsules (registered trade name). When the patent expired in 1976, several other films also began manufacturing and selling chlordiazepoxide hydrochloride, with FDA approval. One firm, Smith Kline French Laboratories, now sells their brand of chlordiazepoxide hydrochloride as SK-LYGEN Capsules; other firms sell this drug by the generic name, chlordiazepoxide.

In recent years, the Federal Food and Drug Administration actions have sought comparable quality of generic and brand name drugs by requiring bioavailability and bioequivalence studies of these drugs. These requirements assure that the percentage of a drug contained in a drug product that enters the systemic circulation in an unchanged form after administration is comparable for the various marketed products.

Generic drugs often have lower prices than trade name or brand name drugs. The controversy concerning quality of the two groups of drugs continues regardless of the assurances offered by the regulatory agencies. Since third party payment, that is, payment by government agencies, for example, primarily requires the use of the lower priced drugs, it appears that in the near future the use of generic name drugs will increase.

All drugs in this text are listed by generic name and cross-referenced to the trade (brand) names. Because of space requirements, it is impossible to list all trade names.

DRUG ACTIONS AND INTERACTIONS

A drug is defined as any chemical or biological agent affecting the living cell. It may be administered to aid in diagnosis, for prophylaxis, or for therapy. Each drug may have both favorable and unfavorable actions. In addition, two or more drugs administered concurrently may interact. Drug interactions may produce an additional, or enhanced, effect, or may counteract or prevent the expected drug response.

To produce the desired effect, a drug must achieve an adequate concentration at its site of action. The concentration depends on the amount of drug administered, extent and rate of absorption, distribution, binding or localization in tissues, inactivation, and excretion. After a drug is administered, a latent period usually occurs between administration and onset of effects. The duration of this latent period is influenced by the route of administration and penetration of drug to the site of action. The duration of drug effects is determined largely by the rate of absorption, inactivation or binding, and excretion of the drug. However, redistribution and accumulation in storage depots may also be influencing factors.

In order for a drug to be effective, it must be absorbed and become biologically available. Drugs administered orally in solution are generally absorbed more rapidly than those administered in solid form such as tablets or capsules. For drugs administered in solid form, the onset of action depends on the rate and extent of dissolution. Absorption depends on several factors: local conditions at the site of absorption; the concentration of the drug; circulation to the site of absorption; the area of the absorbing surface. The rate of absorption is most importantly determined by the route of administration, as well as the physicochemical characteristics of the drug and its pharmaceutical formulation.

Oral administration is generally the safest, most convenient, and most economical route of administration. However, with oral administration, emesis may result from irritation to the gastric mucosa; absorption also may be impeded by gastric or intestinal contents. Absorption of drugs from the intestinal tract depends on diffusion and specialized active processes. The intestinal epithelium does not adequately absorb ionized forms of drugs. Some drugs are particularly useful because they are absorbed minimally and act within the intestinal or gastric lumen.

Other factors which influence absorption from the gastrointestinal tract include gastric emptying, pH, solubility of drug in gastrointestinal fluids, and concentration; formulation of the drug may be such as to delay or prolong the dissolution, and consequently, the action of a drug. These formulations are referred to as sustained action or prolonged action products.

Parenteral administration, i.e., intravenous, intramuscular, subcutaneous, results in more rapid and predictable drug absorption and action than oral administration. However, parenteral administration is more expensive and less safe than oral administration. Subcutaneous administration is rarely employed and is limited to those drugs not irritating to tissue.

The most widely used route of parenteral administration is the intramuscular. Formulations for intramuscular administration consist of aqueous vehicles, which allow the drug to be absorbed rapidly and oil vehicles, which allow the drug to be absorbed more slowly and at an even rate. Substances which are irritating when administered subcutaneously can frequently be administered intramuscularly with only minimal if any irritation.

Intravenous administration is limited to aqueous solutions; drugs in oily vehicles or those that precipitate blood constituents or hemolyze erythrocytes should not be administered by this route. The action of the drug, in most cases, is manifested without delay; this may be of utmost importance in emergency situations. Certain irritating and hypertonic solutions can be given only in this manner since the blood vessel walls are relatively insensitive and the drug, if administered slowly, is greatly diluted by the blood. Many dangers attend intravenous administration; unfavorable reactions are more prone to occur than with any other route of administration. Repeated administration is limited by the patency of the veins. The danger of drug interactions due to drug incompatibilities is particularly prominent when patients are given more than one drug by the intravenous route.

Pulmonary administration is used for gases and volatile drugs which may be inhaled; they are absorbed through the pulmonary alveolar endothelium or mucous membranes of the respiratory tract thereby gaining rapid access to the circulation. Solutions of drugs which can be vaporized (atomized) and the fine droplets in air (aerosol) inhaled may present certain advantages. There is almost instant absorption of the drug into the blood and in the case of lung disease, the drug is applied locally to the site of pathology. The disadvantages are the difficulty in regulating the dosage, and the irritating effect of many gaseous and volatile drugs on the pulmonary bronchiolar epithelium and alveolar endothelium.

Dermal administration is limited by the fact that few drugs readily penetrate intact skin. However, absorption may be enhanced by suspending the drug in an appropriate base formula and rubbing the preparation on the skin (inunction). Since most drugs applied to the skin come in contact with epithelial surfaces which are damaged, drug absorption may be considerable and systemic effects can take place.

Absorption occurs readily through mucous membranes. The mucous membranes of the oropharynx, nose, conjunctiva, rectum, vagina, and urethra are accessible to local treatment. In addition, with certain drugs, systemic effects may also be obtained. Absorption from the oral (buccal) mucosa may be extremely rapid and a higher blood concentration may be achieved than by intestinal tract absorption because the drug is not subjected to possible destructive action of intestinal enzymes or complex formation with the intestinal contents. Also, metabolic inactivation of drugs as a result of passage through the liver is avoided.

Absorption from the rectal mucosa is useful when vomiting is present or when the patient is unconscious or uncooperative. An advantage is that the absorbed drug does not pass through the liver where it may be partially inactivated before entering the systemic circulation. Absorption by this route may be irregular and incomplete, and certain drugs cause irritation of the rectal mucosa.

Following the absorption or injection of a drug into the circulatory system, it may pass through the various body fluid compartments, namely, plasma, interstitial fluid, transcellular fluids, and cellular fluids. Certain drugs cannot pass cell membanes and, therefore, are restricted in their distribution and potential effects; some pass through the cell membranes and are distributed throughout all fluid compartments. Some drugs accumulate in various tissues and organs.

Placental transfer of drugs may occur. Nonionized drugs or those with high fat solubility, including barbiturates, salicylates, anesthetic gases, certain alkaloids, sulfonamides, and alcohol, readily enter the fetal circulation from the maternal circulation. Transfer is least with certain quaternary ammonium ions, various glucuronides, and other drugs with high dissociation and/or low lipid solubility.

The effect of a drug is usually ended by biotransformation and excretion, and to a lesser extent from redistribution of the drug from its site of action into other tissues. Metabolic breakdown of drugs, usually resulting in drug inactivation, occurs mainly in the liver but also takes place in plasma, kidney, and other tissues. Many factors effect drug metabolism, namely, administration of another drug or drugs, route of administration, age, body temperature, nutritional status, and pathological states.

Drugs are excreted primarily through the kidneys, but also in the feces and during lactation, in the milk. Pulmonary excretion is used for elimination of anesthetic gases and vapors. Drugs can be excreted unchanged or as metabolites. Any degree of renal impairment will interfere with the excretion of certain drugs. Plasma concentrations may increase to toxic levels if renal or hepatic functions are inadequate. Metabolites of drugs formed in the liver are excreted by way of the bile into the intestinal tract. The metabolites may be excreted into feces or reabsorbed into the blood and ultimately excreted in the urine. Any impairment of liver function may interfere with excretion in the bile. Drugs excreted into the milk present problems if the mother is nursing. Certain drugs or their metabolites, which may be active or inactive, may be passed to the infant and cause adverse effects.

Drug actions in certain patients must be monitored with particular care. In general, since most drugs are metabolized in the liver and excreted by the kidney, any patient with impaired renal or hepatic function may require dosage adjustment to avoid drug accumulation and possible toxicity. Patients with cardiovascular abnormalities or suicidal tendencies also require particular attention to drug actions, interactions, and dosage, as do children. Elderly and debilitated patients usually require smaller-than-normal doses. Body weight should be considered in dosage determination. In certain instances, therapy should be initiated with a small dose which is then increased gradually, depending on the response of the patient. Because of the sedative actions of drugs such as the central nervous system depressants (barbiturates, other sedative agents, tranquilizers, psychotherapeutic agents) patients should be cautioned against engaging in hazardous occupations requiring mental alertness, such as operating machinery or driving a motor vehicle.

DRUG INTERACTIONS

Drug interactions, essentially, the modification of the effects of one drug by another administered earlier, later, or at the same time, may be therapeutically useful or possibly harmful to the patient. A therapeutically useful effect is illustrated by the effect of probenecid on penicillin excretion; the probenecid prevents the excretion of penicillin by its renal tubular blocking action, thereby resulting in elevated serum levels. An unfavorable or adverse drug interaction is illustrated by the enhancement of sedative (CNS depressant) drugs such as meprobamate, chlordiazepoxide, diazepam, and barbiturates by ethyl alcohol; the action of the sedative drugs is prolonged and enhanced in most cases.

Although many drug interactions are clinically obvious, others are reflected in laboratory tests. An example is the inhibitory effect of phenobarbital on some anticoagulants; when the patient is removed from phenobarbital therapy, the extra anticoagulant effect may result in hemorrhage. Some drug interactions reflected in clinical laboratory data may be interpreted as disease effects rather than drug interaction effects.

When used in reference to drug interactions, the term "enhancement" means potentiation or increasing the actions of another drug, whereas "inhibition" means antagonism or decrease in the action of another drug.

Drug actions or interactions are of particular significance in certain groups of patients, namely, the pregnant, lactating, hypersensitive, elderly, debilitated, and young. Usage of drugs in pregnancy has received much attention in both the lay and professional literature as a result of the thalidomide tragedy. The safety of the majority of drugs for use during pregnancy or lactation has not been established; therefore any drug should be used in pregnant patients or in women of childbearing potential only when, in the judgment of the physician, it is essential to the welfare of the patient. It is advisable to avoid all drug use during the first three months of pregnancy if medically possible.

Another condition in which it is imperative that special precautions be taken is that of hypersensitivity. Any patient with a history of allergies, urticaria, hay fever, or other allergic symptoms or idiosyncratic reactions to drugs should be treated with care and proper precautions taken to treat any serious allergic reactions which might occur. Any drug known to cause allergic (hypersensitivity) reactions in a patient is contraindicated in that patient. Allergic reactions to chemically similar compounds should be noted and any related drug used with extreme caution if at all.

ABBREVIATIONS AND CALCULATIONS

morning	am	cubic centimeter	cc	syrup	syr
evening	pm	milliliter	ml	tablet	tab
every hour	qh	liter	l	by mouth	po
every 2 hr	q2h	ounce	oz	by rectum	pr
four times/day	qid	gram	gm	intramuscular	im
three times/day	tid	tablespoon	tbs	intraperitoneal	ip
twice/day	bid	teaspoon	tsp	intravenous	iv
every day	qd	grain	gr	subcutaneous	sc
once daily	od	ampoule	amp	hypodermically	hypo
at bedtime	hs	capsule	cap	of each	aa
when required	prn	elixir	elix	right eye	OD
before meals	ac	solution	sol	left eye	OS
after meals	pc	suppository	supp	immediately	stat

DOSAGE UNITS COMMONLY USED AND DOSE EQUIVALENTS

Dose equivalents adopted by the United States Pharmacopeia (USP XVI) are also approved by the Federal Food and Drug Administration. These conversions are not acceptable for compounding or in converting a pharmaceutical formula; in these instances "exact" equivalents must be used.

Metric Weight		Approximate Apothecary Equivalent	
30	gm	1	oz
15	gm	4	dr
1	gm	15	gr
0.3	gm	5	gr
60	mg	1	gr
10	mg	1/6	gr
0.1	mg	1/600	gr
1000	ml	1	qt
250	ml	8	fl oz
30	ml	1	fl oz
4	ml	1	fl dr
1	ml	15	min
0.6	ml	10	min

Common measures used by both medical staff and patients at home should be known:

1 teaspoon	= 5 ml or 1/6 fl oz
1 tablespoon	= 15 ml or 1/2 fl oz
1 wine glass	= 60 ml or 2 fl oz
1 teacup	= 120 ml or 4 fl oz
1 tumbler	= 240 ml or 8 fl oz

CONVERSION GUIDES

Rough guides which may be used for conversion and comparison of metric and apothecary systems of measurement are as follows:

$$\text{pounds} \div 2 \text{ (or 2.2)} = \text{kg}$$
$$\text{grains/pound} \div 7 = \text{gm/kg}$$

For converting °F to °C, the formula is 5/9 °F minus 32 = °C

For converting °C to °F, the formula is 9/5 °C plus 32 = °F

CALCULATION OF DOSAGES

FOR TABLETS OR CAPSULES: The number of tablets or capsules to be administered is calculated by dividing the desired dose by the strength of the tablet or capsule available.

EXAMPLE: Desired dose is 250 mg; each capsule contains 125 mg; therefore 2 capsules should be administered. Divide dose to be administered by contents of each capsule.

IF DOSAGE IS IN MG AND TABLET IS IN GRAINS: If the dose ordered is 1 tablet codeine sulfate 60 mg and the only drug available is a tablet containing codeine sulfate gr 1/2; how much should be administered to obtain the 60 mg dose?

EXAMPLE: 1 gr = 60 mg; if the tablet contains gr 1/2, it is then equivalent to 1/2 of 60 or 30 mg. To substitute the tablet gr 1/2 for the 60 mg dose, two gr 1/2 tablets would be required.

FOR SOLUTIONS: To make a given quantity of a solution, pure drug (100%) in dry crystalline form is usually used. For example, to prepare 1000 ml of a solution of sodium chloride 5%, the following example may be followed:

$$\text{EXAMPLE: a 5\% solution} = \frac{5 \text{ gm}}{100 \text{ ml}}$$

To prepare 1000 ml of a 5% solution using a 20% salt solution, the following example may be followed;

$$\text{EXAMPLE:} \quad \frac{5\%}{20\%} = \frac{x}{1000 \text{ ml}}$$
$$20x = 5000$$
$$x = 250 \text{ ml}$$

Therefore, use 250 ml of a 20% solution and qs to 1000 ml.

CONTROLLED DRUGS—THE FEDERAL COMPREHENSIVE DRUG ABUSE PREVENTION AND CONTROL ACT OF 1970

Physicians and nurses who handle drugs must guard against contributing to drug abuse through acquiescence to demands of some patients and through careless handling of drugs. Certain drugs likely to be abused are subject to the Federal Comprehensive Drug Abuse Prevention and Control Act of 1970. This act, promulgated by the Food and Drug Administration, requires that any drug listed as a controlled substance in certain categories must be labelled as follows: "Caution: Federal Law prohibits the transfer of this drug to any person other than the patient for whom it was prescribed." Each drug or substance controlled is listed in one of five schedules depending upon the drug's potential for abuse, its medical usefulness, and the degree of dependence if abused. Schedule II, III, and IV drugs require the above warning.

The five schedules and examples of drugs included are as follows:

SCHEDULE I DRUGS:

Drugs and other substances having a high potential for abuse and no current accepted medical usefulness.

Included are certain opiates and derivatives, hallucinogenic substances and depressants.

EXAMPLES: dextrophan, furethidine, properidine, acodeine methylbromide, heroin, lysergic acid diethylamide (LSD), marihuana, peyote, psilocybin

SCHEDULE II DRUGS:

Drugs having a high potential for abuse and accepted medical usefulness.

Included are opium and opiates, and opium derivatives such as salts and other derivatives; excluded are naloxone and its salts.

EXAMPLES: raw opium, apomorphine, codeine, hydrocodone, morphine, cocaine, anileridine, levomethorphan, methadone, amphetamine and its salts and isomers, phenmetrazine and its salts, methylphenidate, methaqualone.

SCHEDULE III DRUGS:

Drugs having a lesser degree of abuse potential and accepted medical usefulness. Abuse of these drugs leads to moderate dependence problems.

Included in this schedule are certain stimulant and depressant drugs and their salts.

EXAMPLES: benzphetamine, chlorphentermine, mazindol, phendimetrazine, amobarbital, secobarbital, pentobarbital, glutethimide, phencyclidine, dihydrocodeinone, ethylmorphine

SCHEDULE IV DRUGS:

Drugs in this group have a low abuse potential, accepted medical usefulness; abuse leads to moderate dependence problems.

Included in this group are both stimulants and certain depressants not included in other groups.

EXAMPLES: barbital, chlordiazepoxide, chloral hydrate, diazepam, mebutamate, meprobamate, oxazepam, paraldehyde, phenobarbital, diethylpropion, phentermine, pemoline, fenfluramine

SCHEDULE V DRUGS:

Drugs in this group have a low abuse potential, accepted medical usefulness, and limited dependence factors.

Included in Schedule V are preparations containing narcotic and nonnarcotic drugs. Narcotics included conform to certain limited quantities.

EXAMPLES:
1. Not more than 200 mg codeine/100 ml or /100 gm
2. Not more than 100 mg dihydrocodeine/100 ml or /100 gm
3. Not more than 100 mg of ethylmorphine/100 ml or /100 gm
4. Not more than 2.5 mg diphenoxylate or not less than 25 μg atropine sulfate per dosage unit
5. Not more than 100 mg or opium/100 ml or /100 gm

It is mandatory that accurate records be maintained of all drugs classified as "controlled." Prescriptions for drugs listed in Schedule II may not be refilled, and emergency telephone prescriptions for these drugs may be dispensed if the physician furnishes a written, signed prescription to the pharmacy within 72 hours. Prescriptions for drugs listed in Schedules III and IV may be refilled up to five times within 6 months after the date of issue if authorized by the physician. Prescriptions for Schedule V drugs may be refilled only as expressly authorized by the prescribing practitioner on prescription.

In addition to the federal control of drugs with abuse potential, many states have additional controlled substances acts. Because of the variations among the states, it is essential that all personnel handling these drugs are familiar with the regulations. For additional information concerning federal regulations, "Manual for the Medical Practitioner" may be obtained from the Drug Enforcement Administration, U.S. Department of Justice, Washington, D.C. 20537.

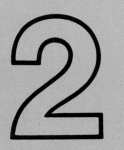

Anti-infective agents

INTRODUCTION

The anti-infective agents include those natural and synthetic products which are either suppressive or lethal to pathogenic bacteria, fungi, yeasts, viruses, protozoans, worms, and other parasites. The anti-infective agents act directly or indirectly on the infecting organism to "cure" the disease produced. Administration of the anti-infective agent may be oral, parenteral, or topical, depending upon the infecting organism, the toxicity and pharmacology of the anti-infective agent, and the condition of the patient.

SPECIFIC THERAPEUTIC CLASSIFICATION

The anti-infective agents have been divided into groups based primarily on the type of infection to be treated. Formulations specific for an organ system are discussed in detail in that section and are also mentioned here. Cross referral has been necessitated by the multiplicity of uses for some drugs.

The anti-infective agents are grouped as follows: amebicides, anthelmin- tic agents, antibacterial agents, antifungal/ anticandidal agents, antileprosy agents, an- timalarial agents, antiparasitic agents, antitoxoplasmosis agents, antituberculosis agents, antiviral agents, and trichomon- acides.

Amebicides

GENERAL CLINICAL USES

Amebiasis, caused by *Entameba histolytica*, may be eradicated by three therapeutic approaches, each acting on the parasite in a different location:

1. Drugs acting within the intestinal lumen but ineffective in the tissue forms of the disease: carbasone, paromomycin.

2. Drugs acting indirectly in the intestinal lumen by modifying intestinal bacteria necessary for survival of the amebae: tetracyclines, erythromycins.

3. Drugs acting against amebae in the intestinal wall, liver, or other tis- sues: emetine hydrochloride, chloroquine, metronidazole.

SPECIFIC PRODUCTS AND DOSAGES

GENERIC NAME	TRADE NAME	ROUTE OF ADMIN.	USUAL DAILY DOSAGE
carbarsone	(G)*	po	**Adults:** 250 mg bid or tid **Children:** dosage varies with age
chloroquine hydrochloride	ARALEN	im	**Adults:** 160–200 mg chloroquine base daily **Children:** up to 5 mg base/kg
chloroquine phosphate	ARALEN Phosphate	po	**Adults:** 1 gm (600 mg base) daily for 2 days; 500 mg (300 mg base) daily for 2–3 weeks
emetine hydrochloride	(G)	im/sc	**Adults:** up to 65 mg/day divided in 2 equal doses **Children:** 10–20 mg/day

*(G) Designates availability as a generic product.

(continued overleaf)

GENERIC NAME	TRADE NAME	ROUTE OF ADMIN.	USUAL DAILY DOSAGE
erythromycin/ erythromycin stearate	(G)* E-MYCIN ERYTHROCIN ILOTYCIN ROBIMYCIN	po	**Adults:** 250–500 mg qid or 500 mg bid **Children:** 30–50 mg/kg/day divided in 3 or 4 doses
metronidazole	FLAGYL	po	**Adults:** 500–750 mg tid **Children:** 35–50 mg/kg/day divided in 3 equal doses
oxytetracycline hydrochloride	TERRAMYCIN	po	**Adults:** 1–2 gm divided in 2 or 4 equal doses **Children:** 25–50 mg/kg/day divided in 4 equal doses
paromomycin sulfate	HUMATIN	po	**Adults and children:** 25–35 mg/kg/day divided in 3 equal doses
tetracycline	(G) ACHROMYCIN PANMYCIN SUMYCIN TETRACYN	po	**Adults:** 1–2 gm daily divided in 2 or 4 equal doses **Children:** 25–50 mg/kg/day divided in 2 or 4 equal doses

*(G) Designates availability as a generic product.

Carbarsone

PHARMACOLOGY

Carbarsone, an arsenic derivative, is effective against the trophozite form of *Entamoeba histolytica* within the lumen of the colon. It is directly amebicidal, probably by inactivating–SH groups. Carbarsone is absorbed from the gastrointestinal tract and excreted slowly by the kidneys.

SPECIAL PRECAUTIONS
• Do not administer to patients with liver or kidney disease or in the presence of contracted visual or color fields.
• Do not administer to patients with a history of hypersensitivity to organic or inorganic arsenicals.

ADVERSE EFFECTS
CNS EFFECTS: neuritis, hemorrhagic encephalitis
GASTROINTESTINAL EFFECTS: nausea, vomiting, diarrhea, abdominal pain, cramps
METABOLIC AND ENDOCRINE EFFECTS: edema, splenomegaly
HEPATIC EFFECTS: icterus, hepatitis, liver necrosis
ALLERGIC EFFECTS: pruritus
DERMATOLOGIC EFFECTS: skin eruptions, exfoliative dermatitis
OPHTHALMIC EFFECTS: visual disturbances, papilledema, retinal edema

CLINICAL GUIDELINES
ADMINISTRATION
• Repeatedly examine vision and skin for adverse effects.
EFFECTS:
• Arsenic intolerance may be characterized by skin eruption, pruritus, gastrointestinal irritation, renal disturbances, and visual disturbances.

OVERDOSAGE/ANTIDOTE:
• Symptoms of overdosage include nausea, vomiting, abdominal pain, diarrhea, shock, coma, convulsions, ulcerations of mucous membranes and skin, kidney damage.
• Untoward reactions may be treated with dimercaprol (BAL in Oil), an antiarsenical compound, 3 mg/kg qid for 2 days, then bid for a total of 10 days. For further information about dimercaprol, see Chapter 20, *Drug Overdosage, Intoxication, Abuse,* page 692.

Chloroquine Hydrochloride/ Chloroquine Phosphate

For detailed information, see *Antimalarial Agents,* pages 78 and 80.

Emetine Hydrochloride

PHARMACOLOGY
Emetine hydrochloride, an amebicidal agent, is highly effective against vegatative forms of *Entamoeba histolytica.* It acts by inhibiting protein synthesis. When administered orally, emetine hydrochloride is a local irritant to the stomach and produces vomiting. Parenteral administration is necessary for systemic effects, as needed in amebiasis. The drug is distributed widely in the tissues after parenteral administration.

SPECIAL PRECAUTIONS
• Do not administer to patients with organic disease of the heart or kidneys unless the patient has amebic hepatitis.
• Use cautiously in aged or debilitated patients.
• Safe use in pregnancy has not been established.
• Do not use in patients who have a history of hypersensitivity to emetine hydrochloride or related compounds.

ADVERSE EFFECTS
CNS EFFECTS: weakness, depression, headache
RESPIRATORY EFFECTS: dyspnea
CARDIOVASCULAR EFFECTS: hypotension, precordial pain, tachycardia, reversible ECG changes appearing about day 7
GASTROINTESTINAL EFFECTS: nausea, vomiting, diarrhea
LOCAL EFFECTS: irritation at site of injection

CLINICAL GUIDELINES
ADMINISTRATION:
• Patient should be at absolute bed rest during therapy and several days thereafter.
• Monitor cardiovascular system bid to tid.
EFFECTS:
• Precordial pain caused by emetine may resemble that of coronary thrombosis.
• Dyspnea may persist until the drug is stopped.
OVERDOSAGE/ANTIDOTE:
• Emetine hydrochloride overdosage (1.25 gm total dose) may cause cardiovascular abnormalities resulting in death. This alkaloid persists in the body and toxicity is cumulative.
• There is no specific antidote. Treat supportively.

Erythromycin/Erythromycin Stearate

For detailed information, see *Antibacterial Agents—Erythromycins,* page 39.

Metronidazole

For detailed information, see *Trichomonacidal Agents,* page 97.

Paromomycin Sulfate

PHARMACOLOGY

Paromomycin closely parallels neomycin in *in vivo* and *in vitro* antibacterial action. It is poorly absorbed from the gastrointestinal tract. The action is local within the gastrointestinal tract. Paromomycin is effective in treating infections of *Entamoeba histolytica*, *Shigella*, *Salmonella*, and *Candida albicans* in the gastrointestinal tract. It is also indicated in the management of hepatic coma, as an adjunctive therapy.

SPECIAL PRECAUTIONS

- Do not administer to patients with a history of hypersensitivity to paromomycin.
- Do not administer to patients with intestinal obstruction.
- Overgrowth of nonsusceptible bacteria or fungi may occur.
- Use cautiously in patients with ulcerative lesions of the bowel to avoid renal toxicity through inadvertent absorption.

ADVERSE EFFECTS

GASTROINTESTINAL EFFECTS: nausea, abdominal cramps, diarrhea

CLINICAL GUIDELINES

ADMINISTRATION:
- Administer at meal times to minimize gastric effects.

EFFECTS:
- Prolonged exposure does not result in overgrowth of staphylococci or *Candida*.

DRUG INTERACTIONS:
- Exhibits cross resistance with neomycin and streptomycin.

Tetracycline/Oxytetracycline

For detailed information, see *Antibacterial Agents—Tetracyclines*, page 61.

Anthelmintic Agents

GENERAL CLINICAL USES

The intestinal worms most common in humans are listed below with the anthelmintic drugs which are relatively specific for each infection.

Roundworm: *Ascaris lumbricoides*—piperazine, pyrantel pamoate, thiabendazole, hexylresorcinol, mebendazole, dithiazanine iodide

Hookworm: *Necator americanus*, *Ancylostoma duodenale*—hexylresorcinol, tetrachloroethylene, mebendazole

Threadworms: *Strongyloides stercoralis*—thiabendazole, dithiazanine iodide

Pinworms: *Enterobius vermicularis*—oxytetracycline, piperazine, pyrvinium pamoate, hexylresorcinol, mebendazole, pyrantel pamoate

Tapeworm: *Taenia saginata*, *Taenia solium*, *Diphyllobothrium latum*, *Hymenolepsis nana*—hexylresorcinol

Whipworms: *Trichuris trichiura*—mebendazole, hexylresorcinol, dithiazanine iodide

Trichina worms: *Trichella spiralis*—thiabendazole

SPECIFIC PRODUCTS AND DOSAGES

GENERIC NAME	TRADE NAME	ROUTE OF ADMIN.	USUAL DAILY DOSAGE
dithiazanine iodide	(G)*	po	**Children:** 50 mg/10 lb in divided doses initially, then 10 mg/10 lb **Adults:** 100 mg tid for 1 day, then 200 mg tid for 4 days; may be repeated in 2 weeks
hexylresorcinol	(G) JAYNE'S P–W VERMIFUGE	po	**Infants and children to 6 yrs:** 0.1 gm for each year **Children 6–8 yrs:** 0.6 gm **Children 8–12 yrs:** 0.8 gm **Adults and children over 12 yrs:** 1 gm
mebendazole	VERMOX	po	**Children:** 100 mg tid for 3 days **Adults:** 100 mg tid for 3 days
oxytetracycline	(G) TERRAMYCIN	po	**Children:** 25–50 mg/kg divided in 4 equal doses **Adults:** 1–2 divided in 4 equal doses. See *Tetracyclines* for additional information
piperazine	(G) ANTEPAR ANTHECOLE PIPIZAN	po	**Children:** 75 mg/kg/day **Adults:** 3.5 gm for 2 consecutive doses; maximum: 2.5 gm/day × 7 days
pyrantel pamoate	ANTIMINTH	po	**Adults and children:** 11 mg pyrantel base/kg; maximum total dose 1 gm
pyrvinium pamoate	POVAN NEMA	po	**Adults and children:** 5 mg pyrvinium base/kg; maximum: 350 mg
tetrachloroethylene	(G)	po	0.12 ml/kg; maximum 5 ml
thiabendazole	MINTEZOL	po	22 mg/kg bid for 1–2 days; maximum daily dose 3 gm

*(G) Designates availability as a generic product.

Dithiazanine Iodide

PHARMACOLOGY

Dithiazanine iodide is effective in treating trichuriasis, strongyloidiasis, ascariasis, and enterobiasis. It acts by interfering with the respiratory enzyme system in the infecting organisms. After oral administration, it is absorbed from the normal gastrointestinal tract in minute amounts; absorption is increased in the presence of inflammation.

GENERAL PRECAUTIONS

• Do not use in patients with renal disease.

• In patients developing persistant vomiting or diarrhea, dosage reduction or cessation may be required.

• Use cautiously in dehydrated patients or in those with electrolyte depletion.

• In acutely ill patients, supportive measures may be required prior to treatment.

ADVERSE EFFECTS

URINARY TRACT EFFECTS: transient albuminuria

GASTROINTESTINAL EFFECTS: anorexia, nausea, vomiting, abdominal cramps, and diarrhea

ALLERGIC EFFECTS: urticaria, fever, and edema

CLINICAL GUIDELINES

ADMINISTRATION:

• Administer after meals to minimize gastrointestinal irritation.

EFFECTS:

• Absorption of the drug has resulted in blue discoloration of the skin and sclera which disappears several days after medication is stopped.

• Discontinue therapy if urine or sclerae become bluish green in color.

DRUG INTERACTIONS:

• Do not administer potentially nephrotoxic drugs concomitantly.

OVERDOSAGE/ANTIDOTE:

• Deaths associated with use of dithiazanine iodide have occurred following administration of as little as 100 mg. All deaths were preceded by gastrointestinal symptoms, hypotension, acidosis, and coma.

• There is no specific antidote.

Hexylresorcinol

PHARMACOLOGY

Hexylresorcinol has a wide range of antihelmintic actions including activity against roundworm, whipworm, hookworm, pinworm, and tapeworm (dwarf). After oral administration approximately one third is absorbed from the gastrointestinal tract; the absorbed drug is excreted by the kidneys and the unabsorbed drug is excreted in the feces. Hexylresorcinol, a phenol, exerts a direct antihelmintic effect.

SPECIAL PRECAUTIONS

• Do not administer to patients with acute intestinal obstruction or perforation, peptic ulcer, appendicitis, or profound toxemia.

• Safe use in pregnancy has not been established.

• Do not administer to patients with a history of hypersensitivity to hexylresorcinol.

ADVERSE EFFECTS

GASTROINTESTINAL EFFECTS: irritation, epigastric distress, ulceration of mucous membrane, swelling and itching of buccal mucosa

CLINICAL GUIDELINES

ADMINISTRATION:

• In the evening prior to dosing, only a light meal of soft food should be eaten.

• Two hours after dosing, a saline cathartic is given to cleanse the bowel of affected worms.

• Food may be eaten after 5 hours.

EFFECTS:

• If the drug contacts the oral mucosa, painful ulceration may occur.

OVERDOSAGE/ANTIDOTE:
- Overdosage is characterized by an exaggeration of the adverse effects.
- There is no specific antidote.

Mebendazole

PHARMACOLOGY
Mebendazole exerts its antihelmintic activity against roundworm, hookworm, pinworm, and whipworm by blocking glucose uptake in the susceptible helminth. After oral administration an insignificant amount of mebendazole which is absorbed is excreted in the urine.

SPECIAL PRECAUTIONS
- Do not use in patients with a history of hypersensitivity to mebendazole.
- Safe use in pregnancy or in children under 2 years has not been established.

ADVERSE EFFECTS
GASTROINTESTINAL EFFECTS: diarrhea, abdominal pain

CLINICAL GUIDELINES
ADMINISTRATION:
- No fasting or purging is necessary.
EFFECTS:
- If patient is not cured, treatment may be repeated.

Oxytetracycline

PHARMACOLOGY
Oxytetracycline is used as adjunctive therapy to amebicides in amebiasis and also in treating pinworm infestations. In amebiasis the tetracyclines act indirectly by modifying the intestinal flora necessary for ameba survival.

SPECIAL PRECAUTIONS, ADVERSE EFFECTS, CLINICAL GUIDELINES
See *Antibacterial Agents—Tetracyclines,* page 61.

Piperazine

PHARMACOLOGY
Piperazine is used to treat pinworm (*Enterobius vermicularis*) and roundworm (*Ascaris lumbricoides*) infestations. Piperazine appears to paralyze the muscle that results in expulsion of the worm by peristalsis.

Piperazine is readily absorbed from the gastrointestinal tract. The drug is excreted in the urine primarily. Orally administered piperazine is essentially devoid of pharmacological activity.

SPECIAL PRECAUTIONS
- Do not administer to patients with impaired renal or hepatic function, convulsive disorders, or a history of hypersensitivity to piperazine.
- Avoid prolonged or repeated treatment of children because of the potential neurotoxicity.
- Safe use in pregnancy has not been established.
- Administer cautiously to patients with severe malnutrition or anemia.

ADVERSE EFFECTS
CNS EFFECTS: headache, vertigo, ataxia, tremors, choreiform movements, muscle weakness, hyporeflexia, paresthesia, convulsions, EEG abnormalities, sense of detachment, memory defect
GASTROINTESTINAL EFFECTS: nausea, vomiting, abdominal cramps, diarrhea

ALLERGIC EFFECTS: urticaria, erythema multiforme, purpura, fever, arthralgia
OPHTHALMIC EFFECTS: blurring of vision, paralytic strabismus

CLINICAL GUIDELINES

ADMINISTRATION:
• Prior fasting, cathartics, or enemas are unnecessary.
• To prevent reinfection, practice of personal and environmental hygiene should be recommended.

EFFECTS:
• Watch for signs of partial intestinal obstruction; if present discontinue therapy.
• Discontinue drug if CNS, significant gastrointestinal, or hypersensitivity reactions occur.

DRUG INTERACTIONS:
• Do not administer other potentially nephrotoxic or hepatotoxic drugs concomitantly.

OVERDOSAGE/ANTIDOTE:
• Overdosage is characterized by an exaggeration of the adverse effects.
• There is no specific antidote. Treat supportively.

Pyrantel Pamoate

PHARMACOLOGY

The anthelmintic activity (*Enterobius vermicularis* and *Ascaris lumbricoides*) is probably due to the neuromuscular blocking property of the drug. After oral administration, pyrantel pamoate is partially absorbed. Peak plasma levels are reached in 1 to 3 hours. Over 50% of the drug is excreted in the feces in unchanged form; small amounts, approximately 7%, are excreted in the urine.

SPECIAL PRECAUTIONS

• Safe use in pregnancy has not been established.

• Use cautiously in patients with pre-existing liver dysfunction; minor transient elevations of SGOT may occur.
• Do not use in patients with a history of hypersensitivity to pyrantel pamoate.

ADVERSE EFFECTS

CNS EFFECTS: headache, dizziness, drowsiness, insomnia, tenesmus
GASTROINTESTINAL EFFECTS: anorexia, nausea, vomiting, gastralgia, abdominal cramps, diarrhea
DERMATOLOGIC EFFECTS: rash

CLINICAL GUIDELINES

ADMINISTRATION:
• Monitor liver function periodically.

EFFECTS:
• If changes in hepatic function tests occur or if signs of sensitization occur, discontinue therapy.

Pyrvinium Pamoate

PHARMACOLOGY

Pyrvinium pamoate is useful in treating enterobiasis (pinworm infestation). The anthelmintic effect is due to interference with the carbohydrate metabolism of the parasite. Pyrvinium pamoate is not absorbed from the gastrointestinal tract in appreciable quantities. The action is local within the gastrointestinal tract.

SPECIAL PRECAUTIONS

• Safe use in pregnancy has not been established.
• Do not use in patients with a history of hypersensitivity to pyrvinium pamoate.

ADVERSE EFFECTS

GASTROINTESTINAL EFFECTS: nausea, vomiting, cramps, diarrhea
ALLERGIC EFFECTS: photosensitization, hypersensitivity reactions

ADMINISTRATION:
- Administer before or after meals.
- Advise patients to swallow tablets to avoid staining the teeth.
- Advise patients in hygienic practices to avoid reinfection.

EFFECTS:
- Caution patients that the stool will be colored bright red.
- If vomiting occurs, the vomitus will probably be colored red and will stain most materials.

Tetrachloroethylene

PHARMACOLOGY
Tetrachloroethylene is useful in treating infestations of hookworm. After oral administration, it is not absorbed appreciably from the gastrointestinal tract. The mechanism of action in removing hookworms apparently is through paralysis of the worms resulting in release of their attachment from the intestinal wall. The worms are then expelled by purgation before they can reattach themselves to the intestinal wall. The drug is ineffective against *Ascaris*.

SPECIAL PRECAUTIONS
- Use cautiously in severely anemic patients; they may collapse during therapy. Collapse is less likely to occur if purgation is omitted.
- Safe use in pregnancy has not been established.
- Do not use in patients with a history of hypersensitivity to tetrachloroethylene.

ADVERSE EFFECTS
CNS EFFECTS: headache, vertigo, inebriation, rarely loss of consciousness, central nervous system depression, giddiness
CARDIOVASCULAR EFFECTS: collapse
GASTROINTESTINAL EFFECTS: burning in stomach, abdominal cramps, nausea, vomiting

ADMINISTRATION:
- Advise patients to consume a light meal with low fat content the evening prior to treatment.
- The drug is to be ingested on an empty stomach.
- A saline purgative may or may not be administered 2 hours after the drug is administered to facilitate expulsion of worm and eliminate drug.

EFFECTS:
- Watch patient for signs of collapse if purgation is used.

OVERDOSAGE/ANTIDOTE:
- Overdosage is characterized by an exaggeration of the adverse effects, particularly the central nervous system effects.
- There is no specific antidote. Treat supportively.

Thiabendazole

PHARMACOLOGY
Thiabendazole is effective in the eradication of threadworm (*Strongyloides sterocoralis*), trichinosis (*Trichinella spiralis*), and roundworm. Thiabendazole is administered orally. It acts by interference of the metabolic pathways in the helminths.

SPECIAL PRECAUTIONS
- Do not use in patients with a history of hypersensitivity to thiabendazole or related compounds.
- Safe use in pregnancy has not been established.
- Use cautiously in patients with impaired renal and hepatic function.

ADVERSE EFFECTS
CNS EFFECTS: vertigo, headache, weakness, dizziness

URINARY TRACT EFFECTS: crystalluria

AUTONOMIC EFFECTS: flushing and chills

GASTROINTESTINAL EFFECTS: nausea, vomiting, and diarrhea

METABOLIC AND ENDOCRINE EFFECTS: hyperglycemia and angioedema

HEMATOLOGIC EFFECTS: leukopenia

ALLERGIC EFFECTS: pruritus

DERMATOLOGIC EFFECTS: rash and xanthopsia

OTIC EFFECTS: tinnitus

CLINICAL GUIDELINES

ADMINISTRATION:
- Patient requires no special diet or purgation.
- Advise patient not to engage in physical activities for several hours after receiving the drug.
- Patient may be incapacitated for several hours after receiving the drug.

EFFECTS:
- Urine may have an unusual odor from thiabendazole.

Antibacterial Agents

The antibacterial agents are classified according to chemical similarity into the following groups:

Aminoglycosides

Cephalosporins

Chloramphenicol

Clindamycin and lincomycin

Erythromycins

Miscellaneous antibacterial agents

Nitrofurans

Penicillins

Polymyxins

Sulfonamides

Tetracyclines

Aminoglycosides

Although the aminoglycoside antibiotics share many pharmacological and toxicological properties, their antibacterial spectra and clinical uses are unique. Consequently, each product will be discussed individually.

SPECIFIC PRODUCTS AND DOSAGES

Appropriate susceptibility and identification studies should be performed. Specimens should be collected for laboratory testing, however, before therapy is initiated; therapy may be initiated on an empiric basis while awaiting the laboratory results.

GENERIC NAME	TRADE NAME	ROUTE OF ADMIN.	USUAL DAILY DOSAGE	
			ADULTS	**INFANTS AND CHILDREN**
amikacin sulfate	AMIKIN	im	15 mg/kg/day divided in 2–3 equal doses	**Children:** 15 mg/kg/day divided in 2–3 equal doses **Newborns:** 10 mg/kg initially; 7.5 mg/kg bid thereafter
			Do NOT exceed 1.5 gm/day	
	AMIKIN	iv	Use im dose but add to 200 ml vial of sterile diluent; admin. over 30–60 min.	**Children:** use im dose but add to 200 ml vial of sterile diluent infuse over 30–60 min. **Infants:** infuse over 1–2 hr.
gentamicin sulfate	GARAMYCIN Inj.	im/iv	3–5 mg/kg/day in 3 equal doses	5–7.5 mg/kg/day in 3–4 equal doses
	GARAMYCIN Pediatric Inj.	im/iv	Not recommended	**Children:** 2.0–2.5 mg/kg tid **Infants and neonates:** 2.5 mg/kg tid **Premature or fullterm neonates 1 week of age or less:** 2.5 mg/kg bid
	GARAMYCIN Cream	topical	See Chapter 9, *Drugs Affecting the Skin,* page 418.	
	GARAMYCIN Oint.	topical	See Chapter 9, *Drugs Affecting the Skin,* page 418.	
	GARAMYCIN Ophth. Soln. Ophth. Oint.	ophthalmic	See Chapter 11, *Drugs Affecting the Eye,* page 443.	
kanamycin sulfate	KANTREX Cap.	po	4–12 gm/day in divided doses	Not established
	KANTREX Inj.	im/iv	7.5–15 mg/kg/day in divided doses; maximum 1.5 gm/day	Same as adults
	KANTREX Pediatric Inj.	im/iv	——	7.5–13 mg/kg/day in divided doses
	KANTREX Inj.	ip	0.5 gm	Not established
	KANTREX Inj.	inhalation	250 mg bid to qid	Not established
neomycin sulfate	MYCIFRADIN MYCIGUENT NEOBIOTIC*	po	40–100 mg/kg/day divided in 4 to 6 doses	50 mg/kg/day divided in 4 doses
	MYCIFRADIN Sulfate	im	15 mg/kg/day divided in 4 equal doses	7.5–15 mg/kg/day divided in 4 doses
		topical	See Chapter 9, *Drugs Affecting the Skin,* page 418.	
		otic	See Chapter 12, *Drugs Affecting the Ear,* page 464.	
		ophthalmic	See Chapter 11, *Drugs Affecting the Eye,* page 443.	
streptomycin sulfate	(G)†	im	1–4 gm/day in divided doses	20–40 mg/kg/day in divided doses
tobramycin sulfate	NEBCIN	im/iv	3–5 mg/kg/day divided in 3 equal doses	Including neonates, up to 4 mg/kg/day divided in 2 equal doses
viomycin sulfate	VIOCIN Sulfate	im	1 gm bid	Not established

*Contains more than one active ingredient.
†(G) Designates availability as a generic product.

Amikacin Sulfate

GENERAL CLINICAL USES

Amikacin sulfate is indicated in the short-term treatment of serious infections due to susceptible strains of gram-negative bacteria, including *Pseudomonas* species, *Escherichia coli*, species of indole-positive and indole-negative *Proteus, Providencia* species, *Klebsiella-Enterobacter-Serratia* species, and *Aerobacter* (*Mima-Herellea*) species.

Amikacin sulfate has been effective in bacteremia and septicemia (including neonatal sepsis); in serious infections of the respiratory tract, bones and joints, central nervous system, and skin and soft tissues; intra-abdominal infections including peritonitis; and in burns and postoperative infections.

It may be considered initial therapy in suspected gram-negative infections.

PHARMACOLOGY

Amikacin sulfate is absorbed rapidly after intramuscular administration. The peak serum level occurs about 1 hour after administration. The drug is excreted unchanged in the urine. Amikacin has been found in the cerebrospinal fluid, pleural fluid, and peritoneal cavity following parenteral administration.

SPECIAL PRECAUTIONS

• Since nephrotoxicity and ototoxicity (both auditory and vestibular) have occurred, it is essential to monitor patients closely.
• Do not use in patients with a history of hypersensitivity to amikacin.
• Amikacin is potentially nephrotoxic, ototoxic, and neurotoxic; avoid concurrent or serial systemic or topical use of other ototoxic or nephrotoxic agents because of potential for additive effects.
• Assess kidney function prior to starting therapy and daily during the course of treatment.
• If signs of renal dysfunction such as decreased creatinine clearance, decreased urine specific gravity, increased BUN, creatinine, or oliguria occur, consider dosage reduction.
• Cross allergenicity among aminoglycosides has been demonstrated.
• Overgrowth of nonsusceptible organisms may occur.
• Safe use in pregnancy has not been established.

ADVERSE EFFECTS

CNS EFFECTS: fever, headache, paresthesia, tremor
CARDIOVASCULAR EFFECTS: hypertension
URINARY TRACT EFFECTS: albuminuria, presence of red and white cells and casts in urine, azotemia
GASTROINTESTINAL EFFECTS: nausea, and vomiting
HEMATOLOGIC EFFECTS: eosinophilia, and anemia
DERMATOLOGIC EFFECTS: rash
MUSCULOSKELETAL EFFECTS: arthralgia

CLINICAL GUIDELINES

ADMINISTRATION:
• Patients should be well hydrated to minimize chemical irritation of the renal tubules; if signs of renal irritation appear (casts, white or red cells, or albumin), hydration should be increased.
EFFECTS:
• Amikacin has been effective in infections caused by gentamicin- and/or tobramycin-resistant strains of gram-negative organisms, particularly *Proteus rettgeri*, *Providencia stuartii*, *Serratia marcescens*, and *Pseudomonas aeruginosa*.
DRUG INTERACTIONS:
• Do not give concurrently with potent diuretics (ethacrynic acid, furosemide,

meralluride sodium, sodium mercaptomerin, or mannitol); amikacin (and also other aminoglycosides) toxicity may be enhanced by altering antibiotic concentrations in serum and tissue.

• Do not use (systemic or topical) concurrently or serially with other drugs with ototoxic or nephrotoxic potential, such as kanamycin, gentamicin, tobramycin, neomycin, streptomycin, cephaloridine, paromomycin, viomycin, polymyxin B, colistin, and vancomycin.

• Consider possibility of neuromuscular blockage and respiratory paralysis when amikacin is administered concomitantly with anesthetic or neuromuscular blocking drugs; if blockage occurs, calcium salts may reverse in this phenomenon.

OVERDOSAGE/ANTIDOTE:

• Overdosage is characterized by an exaggeration of the adverse effects.

• Peritoneal dialysis or hemodialysis will aid in removal of amikacin from the blood. There is no specific antidote.

Gentamicin Sulfate

GENERAL CLINICAL USES

Gentamicin sulfate is effective in treating infections caused by susceptible strains of gram-negative bacteria including *Pseudomonas aeruginosa*, *Proteus* species (indole-positive and indole-negative), *Escherichia coli*, *Klebsiella-Enterobacter-Serratia* species, *Citrobacter* species, and *Staphylococcus* species (coagulase-positive and coagulase-negative).

When administered parenterally, use of gentamicin should be restricted to treatment of serious infections including neonatal sepsis.

Topically applied gentamicin sulfate is usually limited to serious gram-negative infections in burn patients and to infected dermatitides. It may also be used in treating infections of the eye. For additional information, see Chapter 9, *Drugs Affecting the Skin*, and Chapter 11, *Drugs Affecting the Eye*.

PHARMACOLOGY

Gentamicin sulfate is a wide-spectrum bactericidal agent administered parenterally and topically; it is not administered orally because of poor absorption from the gastrointestinal tract. Following parenteral administration gentamicin sulfate is excreted unchanged in the urine. The renal clearance is similar to that of endogenous creatinine.

SPECIAL PRECAUTIONS

• Dosage must be adjusted in patients, adult and pediatric, with impaired renal function. Consult package insert for detailed information.

• Monitor renal function during treatment with gentamicin or other aminoglycosides.

• The aminoglycoside antibiotics, including gentamicin sulfate, are potentially nephrotoxic and neurotoxic.

• If other ototoxic drugs or rapidly acting diuretic agents are administered concomitantly, the potential for ototoxicity of these drugs may be enhanced.

• Neurotoxic and nephrotoxic antibiotics may be absorbed from body surfaces after local irrigation or application.

• Increased nephrotoxicity has been reported following concomitant administration of aminoglycoside antibiotics and cephalothin.

• Neuromuscular blockade and respiratory paralysis have been reported in animals, and consequently, may occur in humans, particularly if other neuromuscular blocking agents such as succinylcholine or tubocurarine are given concomitantly.

• Use cautiously in premature infants or neonates because of their renal immaturity.
• Cross allergenicity among aminoglycosides has been established.
• Do not administer to patients with a history of hypersensitivity to gentamicin sulfate or any other aminoglycoside.
• Safe use in pregnancy has not been established.
• If tinnitus, dizziness, or vertigo occurs, discontinue therapy.
• Monitor serum concentrations when feasible and during prolonged use.

ADVERSE EFFECTS

CNS EFFECTS: fever, lethargy, confusion, depression, dizziness, headache, pseudotumor cerebri

RESPIRATORY EFFECTS: pulmonary fibrosis, respiratory depression, laryngeal edema

CARDIOVASCULAR EFFECTS: hypotension, hypertension

URINARY TRACT EFFECTS: increased BUN, NPN, serum creatinine; oliguria, casts or protein in urine

GASTROINTESTINAL EFFECTS: nausea, vomiting, depressed appetite, increased salivation, stomatitis

METABOLIC AND ENDOCRINE EFFECTS: decreased serum albumin, weight loss

HEPATIC EFFECTS: increased SGOT and SGPT, increased unbound serum bilirubin, transient hepatomegaly

HEMATOLOGIC EFFECTS: anemia, leukopenia, increased and decreased reticulocyte counts, agranulocytosis, thrombocytopenia, splenomegaly

ALLERGIC EFFECTS: urticaria, anaphylactoid reactions

DERMATOLOGIC EFFECTS: purpura, skin tingling, numbness, rash, itching, burning alopecia

OPHTHALMIC EFFECTS: visual disturbances

MUSCULOSKELETAL EFFECTS: arthralgia, muscle twitching

OTIC EFFECTS: hearing loss, tinnitus, and vertigo

LOCAL EFFECTS: pain, subcutaneous atrophy, fat necrosis with intramuscular administration; erythema, pruritus, possible photosensitization with topical administration

CLINICAL GUIDELINES

ADMINISTRATION:
• Assure patient's urine is alkaline when treating urinary tract infections; this antibiotic is more active in alkaline than acid medium.
• In patients with impaired renal function, dosage must be adjusted to maintain specified serum concentrations.
• Assure that patient is adequately hydrated.

EFFECTS:
• Occurrence of tinnitus, roaring in ears, or hearing loss is a sign of ototoxicity; inform physician immediately.
• When applied topically, antimicrobial activity is reduced in presence of serum.

DRUG INTERACTIONS:
• Gentamicin sulfate is incompatible with heparin; a precipitate forms.
• Gentamicin sulfate is inactivated when mixed with carbenicillin and allowed to stand.
• The neuromuscular blocking effect of the aminoglycosides may enhance similar action of general anesthetics, parenterally administered magnesium, or other compounds with muscle relaxant properties.

OVERDOSAGE/ANTIDOTE:
• Overdosage is characterized by exaggeration of the adverse effects.
• There is no specific antidote. Peritoneal dialysis and hemodialysis will aid in removal of gentamicin sulfate from the blood.

Kanamycin Sulfate

GENERAL CLINICAL USES

Kanamycin sulfate, administered parenterally, is used for short-term treatment of infections caused by penicillin-resistant staphylococci, coliform organisms, *Salmonella*, and *Shigella*; it is also effective in treating infections caused by susceptible strains of *Staphylococcus aureus*, *Staphylococcus epidermidis*, *Neisseria gonorrhoeae*, *Hemophilus influenzae*, *Escherichia coli*, *Enterobacter aerogenes*, *Shigella*, *Salmonella*, *Klebsiella pneumoniae*, *Serratia marcescens*, *Mima-Herellea*, and strains of *Proteus*. Strains of *Mycobacterium* may possibly be susceptible.

When administered orally, kanamycin sulfate is indicated when suppression of intestinal bacteria is desirable such as prior to surgery. It also may be used adjunctively in hepatic coma to reduce the ammonia-forming bacteria in the intestinal tract.

PHARMACOLOGY

Kanamycin sulfate is a bactericidal antibiotic which may be administered orally for a topical effect within the gastrointestinal tract, parenterally (intramuscularly or intravenously) for systemic effects, or as an aerosol in respiratory tract infections. It is absorbed from the gastrointestinal tract to a very slight degree and is excreted unchanged in the feces. Following intramuscular administration it reaches peak serum levels within one hour. It diffuses rapidly into most body fluids including synovial and peritoneal fluids, and also bile. Significant concentrations are reached in cord blood and amniotic fluid following intramuscular administration in pregnant patients, and also in spinal fluid of infants. The drug is excreted rapidly in the urine.

SPECIAL PRECAUTIONS

- Contraindicated in the presence of intestinal obstruction and in individuals with a history of hypersensitivity to the drug or related drugs.
- The aminoglycoside antibiotics, including kanamycin sulfate, are nephrotoxic and neurotoxic.
- If other ototoxic drugs or rapidly acting diuretic agents are administered concomitantly, the potential for ototoxicity of these drugs may be enhanced.
- Neuromuscular blockage and respiratory paralysis have been reported in animals, and consequently may occur in humans, particularly if neuromuscular blocking agents such as succinylcholine or tubocurarine are also given.
- Use cautiously in premature infants or neonates because of their renal immaturity.
- Cross allergenicity among the aminoglycosides has been established.
- Overgrowth of nonsusceptible organisms may occur.
- Safe use in pregnancy has not been established.
- Monitor serum concentrations when feasible and during prolonged use.
- Following oral administration, kanamycin sulfate may be absorbed from denuded or ulcerated areas of the intestinal tract.
- If signs of renal irritation appear such as casts, white or red cells, and albumin, hydration should be increased and a reduction in dosage may be desirable.

ADVERSE EFFECTS

CNS EFFECTS: headache, paresthesias, and fever

URINARY TRACT EFFECTS: albuminuria; presence of RBC, WBC, and granular casts in urine; azotemia, oliguria

GASTROINTESTINAL EFFECTS: stomatitis, diarrhea, vomiting, nausea; with oral administration, malabsorption syndrome characterized by increased fecal fat decreased serum carotene, and fall in xylose absorption

METABOLIC AND ENDOCRINE EFFECTS: proctitis

DERMATOLOGIC EFFECTS: rash

OTIC EFFECTS: tinnitus, vertigo, deafness

LOCAL EFFECTS: irritation, pain

CLINICAL GUIDELINES

ADMINISTRATION:

• Assure patient's urine is alkaline when treating urinary tract infections; kanamycin sulfate is more active in alkaline than acid medium.

• In patients with impaired renal function, dosage must be adjusted to maintain specific serum concentrations.

EFFECTS:

• Occurrence of dizziness, vertigo, tinnitus, roaring in ears, or hearing loss are signs of ototoxicity; inform physician immediately.

DRUG INTERACTIONS:

• When administered intraperitoneally and concomitantly with anesthesia and muscle-relaxing drugs (ether, tubocurarine, succinylcholine, decamethonium, sodium citrate) neuromuscular paralysis with respiratory depression may occur.

• Avoid concurrent systemic administration of other ototoxic and/or nephrotoxic drugs, particularly streptomycin, polymyxin B, colistin, neomycin, gentamicin, and viomycin.

• Irreversible deafness may result from concurrent use of rapidly acting diuretic agents, e.g., ethacrynic acid, furosemide, sodium mercaptomerin, and mannitol.

• For intravenous use, it may be diluted with normal saline or dextrose 5% in water. Do not mix with other antibacterial agents.

Neomycin Sulfate

GENERAL CLINICAL USES

Neomycin sulfate is administered orally to suppress the bacteria in the intestines which in turn decrease the ammonia produced and also to eliminate most pathogenic bacteria from the gastrointestinal tract prior to surgery, and to treat diarrhea due to enteropathogenic *Escherichia coli.*

Topically administered neomycin, neomycin sulfate, and neomycin palmitate are commonly used to treat superficial infections caused by susceptible organisms. For detailed information see Chapter 9, *Drugs Affecting the Skin.*

Intramuscular sulfate may be useful in urinary tract infections caused by susceptible organisms when other antibacterial agents are ineffective.

PHARMACOLOGY

Neomycin is a bactericidal antibiotic which is poorly absorbed from the gastrointestinal tract; the small amounts which are absorbed are excreted in the urine; the unabsorbed portion is excreted in the feces. Since neomycin is absorbed from both the peritoneum and pleura, it should not be used for irrigation of these membranes. Neomycin and its salts are absorbed minimally from the skin.

SPECIAL PRECAUTIONS

• Contraindicated in the presence of intestinal obstruction and in individuals hypersensitive to neomycin and related drugs.

• The aminoglycoside antibiotics are potentially nephrotoxic and neurotoxic.

• If other nephrotoxic or neurotoxic drugs or rapidly acting diuretic agents are administered concomitantly, the potential for toxicity may be enhanced.

• Neuromuscular blockade and respirato-

ry paralysis have been reported in animals, and consequently may occur in humans, particularly if neuromuscular blocking agents such as succinylcholine or tubocurarine are also given.
- Patients with renal insufficiency may develop toxic blood levels.
- Cross allergenicity among the aminoglycosides has been established.
- Safe use in pregnancy has not been established.
- Overgrowth of nonsusceptible organisms may occur.

ADVERSE EFFECTS

URINARY TRACT EFFECTS: casts, red and white cells in urine
GASTROINTESTINAL EFFECTS: nausea, diarrhea, malabsorption, vomiting
ALLERGIC EFFECTS: hypersensitivity, skin rash
OTIC EFFECTS: deafness, tinnitus
LOCAL EFFECTS: hypersensitivity reactions, primarily rashes

CLINICAL GUIDELINES

ADMINISTRATION:
- Assure patient's urine is alkaline when treating urinary tract infections; the aminoglycoside antibiotics are more active in alkaline than acid medium.
- In patients with impaired renal function, dosage must be adjusted to maintain specified serum concentrations.
- Contact dermatitis may occur with neomycin sulfate solutions.
- When treating hepatic coma, withdraw protein from the diet and avoid use of diuretic agents.
EFFECTS:
- Occurrence of tinnitus or hearing loss is a sign of ototoxicity; inform physician immediately.
DRUG INTERACTIONS:
- The neuromuscular blocking effect of

the aminoglycosides may enhance similar action of general anesthetics, parenterally administered magnesium, or other compounds with neuromuscular blocking activity such as succinylcholine or tubocurarine.
- Enhanced toxicity may result from concurrent administration of other ototoxic and/or nephrotoxic drugs, e.g., streptomycin, kanamycin, polymyxin B, colistin, viomycin, gentamicin, and cephaloridine, and also potent diuretics such as ethacrynic acid, furosemide, urea, and mannitol.
OVERDOSAGE/ANTIDOTE:
- Overdosage is characterized by an exaggeration of the adverse effects.
- There is no specific antidote. Peritoneal dialysis may be helpful.

Streptomycin Sulfate

GENERAL CLINICAL USES

Streptomycin sulfate is limited in use because of the availability of more effective and safer antibiotics; it is used primarily to treat infections such as tuberculosis, tularemia, and bubonic plague, and also in combination with other antibiotics to treat enterococcal endocarditis.

Streptomycin may be used to treat infections caused by susceptible strains of *Mycobacterium tuberculosis, Yersinia pestis, Francisella tularensis, Brucella, Donovanosis, Hemophilus ducreyi, Neisseria gonorrhoeae, Hemophilus influenzae, Klebsiella pneumoniae, Escherichia coli, Proteus* species, *Enterobacter aerogenes, Klebsiella pneumoniae, Streptococcus faecalis, Streptococcus* species, and gram-negative bacilli.

PHARMACOLOGY

Streptomycin sulfate is a bactericidal antibiotic usually administered intramuscularly. A peak serum level is reached within one hour. Streptomycin sulfate passes through the placenta; it is excreted in small amounts in milk, saliva, and sweat. Appreciable amounts are found in all organ tissues except the brain. Significant amounts have been found in pleural fluid and tuberculous cavities.

SPECIAL PRECAUTIONS

- Streptomycin sulfate is potentially nephrotoxic and neurotoxic.
- If other ototoxic drugs or rapidly acting diuretic agents are administered concomitantly, the potential for ototoxicity of these drugs may be enhanced.
- Neuromuscular blockage and respiratory paralysis have been reported in animals, and consequently may occur in humans, particularly if neuromuscular blocking agents such as succinylcholine or tubocurarine are also given.
- Use cautiously in premature infants or neonates because of their renal immaturity.
- The risk of severe neurotoxic reactions is sharply increased in patients with impaired kidney function or prerenal azotemia.
- Cross allergenicity among aminoglycosides has been established.
- Do not administer to patients with a history of hypersensitivity to streptomycin sulfate or any of the aminoglycosides.
- Safe use in pregnancy has not been established.
- Overgrowth of nonsusceptible organisms may occur.

ADVERSE EFFECTS

CNS EFFECTS: peripheral neuritis, dizziness, fever, circumoral or perioral paresthesias
CARDIOVASCULAR EFFECTS: myocarditis
URINARY TRACT EFFECTS: azotemia, renal damage
GASTROINTESTINAL EFFECTS: nausea, vomiting
HEPATIC EFFECTS: hepatic necrosis

HEMATOLOGIC EFFECTS: leukopenia, neutropenia, agranulocytosis, hemolytic anemia, pancytopenia, eosinophilia, thrombocytopenic purpura rarely
ALLERGIC EFFECTS: anaphylactic shock, urticaria
DERMATOLOGIC EFFECTS: rash, angioneurotic edema, exfoliative dermatitis
OTIC EFFECTS: vertigo, deafness, tinnitus
OPHTHALMIC EFFECTS: amblyopia
MUSCULOSKELETAL EFFECTS: muscular weakness
LOCAL EFFECTS: with intramuscular injection, pain; sterile abscesses with superficial injection

CLINICAL GUIDELINES

ADMINISTRATION:
- Assure patient's urine is alkaline when treating urinary tract infections; these antibiotics are more active in alkaline than acid medium.
- In patients with impaired renal function, dosage must be adjusted to maintain specified serum concentrations.
- Intramuscular injection should be deep into the muscle.
- Monitor serum concentrations when feasible and during prolonged use.

EFFECTS:
- Occurrence of tinnitus or hearing loss is a sign of ototoxicity; inform physician immediately.

DRUG INTERACTIONS:
- The neuromuscular blocking effect of the aminoglycosides may enhance similar action of general anesthetics, parenterally administered magnesium, or other compounds with neuromuscular blocking properties.
- Avoid concurrent use of other neurotoxic and/or nephrotoxic antibiotics particularly neomycin, kanamycin, gentamicin, and cephaloridine; also paromomycin, viomycin, polymyxin B, colistin, vancomycin, and tobramycin.

OVERDOSAGE/ANTIDOTE:
- Overdosage is characterized by an exaggeration of the adverse effects.
- There is no specific antidote. Peritoneal dialysis may be helpful.

Tobramycin Sulfate

GENERAL CLINICAL USES

Tobramycin sulfate is used to treat serious infections caused by susceptible strains of the following organisms: *Pseudomonas aeruginosa, Escherichia coli, Proteus* species (indole-positive and indole-negative), *Providencia, Klebsiella-Enterobacter-Serratia* group, *Citrobacter* species, group D streptococci, and staphylococci including *Staphylococcus aureus* (coagulase-positive and coagulase-negative). Infections treated include septicemia, CNS infections including meningitis, neonatal sepsis, serious lower respiratory tract infections, gastrointestinal tract infections including peritonitis, skin, bone, and soft tissue infections including burns; serious complicated and recurrent urinary tract infections.

PHARMACOLOGY

Tobramycin sulfate administered intramuscularly reaches a peak concentration in approximately 1 hour. Intravenous infusion of tobramycin sulfate for 30 minutes results in serum concentrations similar to those obtained by intramuscular administration. Tobramycin sulfate is eliminated by glomerular filtration with renal clearance similar to that of endogenous creatinine. Following parenteral administration, tobramycin may be detected in tissues and body fluids; also in bile and stool which suggests minimal biliary excretion. Small quantities have been detected in cerebrospinal fluid, sputum, peritoneal fluid, and abscess fluids. It crosses the placental membranes.

SPECIAL PRECAUTIONS
- The aminoglycoside antibiotics are potentially nephrotoxic and neurotoxic; monitor serum concentrations.
- If other ototoxic drugs or rapidly acting diuretic agents are administered concomitantly, the potential for ototoxicity of these drugs may be enhanced.
- Neuromuscular blockade and respiratory paralysis have been reported in animals, and consequently may occur in humans, particularly if neuromuscular blocking agents such as succinylcholine or tubocurarine are also given.
- Use cautiously in premature infants or neonates because of their renal immaturity.
- Cross allergenicity among aminoglycosides has been established.
- Do not administer to patients with a history of hypersensitivity to tobramycin sulfate or to any aminoglycoside.
- Safe use in pregnancy has not been established.

ADVERSE EFFECTS
CNS EFFECTS: headache, fever, lethargy
URINARY TRACT EFFECTS: increased BUN, NPN, and serum creatinine; oliguria, cylindruria, increased proteinuria
GASTROINTESTINAL EFFECTS: nausea, and vomiting
HEPATIC EFFECTS: increased SGOT and SGPT, increased serum bilirubin
HEMATOLOGIC EFFECTS: anemia, granulocytopenia, thrombocytopenia
ALLERGIC EFFECTS: urticaria
DERMATOLOGIC EFFECTS: rash, itching
OTIC EFFECTS: dizziness, vertigo, tinnitus, hearing loss

CLINICAL GUIDELINES
ADMINISTRATION:
- Assure patient's urine is alkaline when treating urinary tract infections; these antibiotics are more active in alkaline than acid medium.

• In patients with impaired renal function, dosage must be reduced to maintain specified serum concentrations.

• Monitor serum concentrations when feasible and during prolonged use.

EFFECTS:

• Occurrence of tinnitus or hearing loss is a sign of ototoxicity; inform physician immediately.

DRUG INTERACTIONS:

• The neuromuscular blocking effect of the aminoglycosides may enhance similar action of general anesthetics, parenterally administered magnesium, or other compounds with muscular relaxant properties.

• Concurrent and sequential use of other neurotoxic and/or nephrotoxic antibiotics, particularly streptomycin, neomycin, kanamycin, gentamicin, cephaloridine, paromomycin, viomycin, polymyxin B, colistin, and vancomycin should be avoided.

• Do not administer concurrently with potent diuretics; antibiotic serum concentration may be increased and toxicity also incurred.

Viomycin Sulfate

GENERAL CLINICAL USES

Viomycin sulfate should be restricted for use in patients with pulmonary tuberculosis unable to tolerate other drug therapy such as streptomycin, isoniazid, and/or aminosalicylic acid. Viomycin sulfate is useful as adjunctive therapy when treatment with the primary drug has failed or in patients with demonstrated intolerance of hypersensitivity to primary antituberculous drugs.

PHARMACOLOGY

Viomycin sulfate, administered intramuscularly, is absorbed readily. Small amounts diffuse into the spinal fluid and body cavities. Excretion is primarily by the kidneys.

SPECIAL PRECAUTIONS

• Administer only when patient can be closely observed and laboratory facilities are available.

• Do not administer to any patient with a history of hypersensitivity to viomycin sulfate.

• Patients should be monitored (renal, hepatic, hematologic, audiometric, and caloric tests) closely with appropriate laboratory tests.

• In patients with renal impairment, serious toxic reactions may occur with dosages other patients could tolerate.

• Do not administer viomycin sulfate with other ototoxic drugs.

• Administer with great caution with other drugs having neuromuscular blocking activity (curariform effects).

ADVERSE EFFECTS

CARDIOVASCULAR EFFECTS: ECG changes

URINARY TRACT EFFECTS: hematuria, proteinuria, cylindruria, nitrogen retention, decreased creatinine clearance, renal loss of K, Cl, and Ca.

ALLERGIC EFFECTS: eosinophilia, rash, fever, laryngeal edema

OTIC EFFECTS: vertigo, tinnitus, hearing loss

MUSCULOSKELETAL EFFECTS: muscle weakness, tetany, edema

CLINICAL GUIDELINES

ADMINISTRATION:

• Inject well into the body of a relatively large muscle; alternate injection sites, and administer slowly.

• Supplemental potassium and calcium may be necessary when viomycin sulfate is given daily.

EFFECTS:
- If renal insufficiency occurs, discontinue therapy.

DRUG INTERACTIONS:
- Do not administer viomycin, streptomycin, or other ototoxic drugs concomitantly.
- Viomycin is most effective when used in combination with other antituberculous agents.

OVERDOSAGE/ANTIDOTE:
- Overdosage is characterized by an exaggeration of the adverse effects.
- There is no specific antidote.

Cephalosporins

The cephalosporins are cefadroxil monohydrate, cefamandole nafate, cefazolin sodium, cefoxitin sodium, cephalexin, cephaloglycin, cephaloridine, cephalothin sodium, cephapirin sodium, and cephradine.

SPECIFIC PRODUCTS AND DOSAGES

GENERIC NAME	TRADE NAME	ROUTE OF ADMIN.	USUAL DAILY DOSAGE	
			ADULTS	**INFANTS AND CHILDREN**
cefadroxil monohydrate	DURICEF	po	0.5–1 gm bid	Not established
cefamandole nafate	MANDOL	im/iv	3–12 gm/day in divided doses	50–150 mg/kg/day in equally divided doses
cefazolin sodium	ANCEF KEFZOL	im/iv	0.5–2 gm/day administered in 3–4 equal doses or by infusion over 3–5 min/day; daily doses of 6–12 gm have been administered	25–50 mg/kg/day divided in 3 or 4 doses may be increased to 100 mg/kg/day
cefoxitin sodium	MEFOXIN	im/iv	3–12 gm/day in 3–4 divided doses	Not established
cephalexin	KEFLEX	po	1–4 gm/day in divided doses	25–100 mg/kg/day divided in 4 doses
cephaloglycin	KAFOCIN	po	250–500 mg qid	25–50 mg/kg/day divided in 4 doses
cephaloridine	LORIDINE	im	0.5–1 gm tid to qid	30–50 mg/kg/day in divided doses
		iv	0.5–1 gm tid to qid	30–50 mg/kg/day
cephalothin sodium	KEFLIN neutral	im/iv	0.5–1.0 gm every 4–6 hr.	80–160 mg/kg/day in divided doses

(continued overleaf)

GENERIC NAME	TRADE NAME	ROUTE OF ADMIN.	USUAL DAILY DOSAGE	
			ADULTS	INFANTS AND CHILDREN
cephalothin sodium, cont.		ip	6 mg/100 ml in dialysis fluid; 0.1–4% in saline	Not established
cephapirin sodium	CEFADYL	im/iv	0.5–1.0 gm tid or qid; daily doses up to 12 gm have been used	40–80 mg/kg/day divided in 4 doses
cephradine	ANSPOR VELOSEF	im/iv	0.5–1 gm qid	50–100 mg/kg divided in 4 doses
	ANSPOR VELOSEF	po	250–1000 mg qid	25–100 mg/kg/day in equally divided doses

GENERAL CLINICAL USES

The cephalosporins, cephaloridine, cefazolin, cephalexin, cefamandole nafate, cefoxitin sodium, cephradine, cephapirin, and cephalothin, are indicated for infections of the lower respiratory tract, soft tissue, and genitourinary tract. Parenterally administered forms are also useful for treating septicemias, meningitis, and bone and joint infections.

Cephaloglycin and cefadroxil are indicated specifically for treating infections of the urinary tract.

PHARMACOLOGY

The cephalosporins are structurally and pharmacologically related to the penicillins. Cephalexin, cephaloglycin, cefadroxil, and cephradine, formulated for oral administration, are well absorbed from the gastrointestinal tract, and cephradine, cephapirin, cephalothin, cefazolin, cephaloridine, cefamandole, and cefoxitin are effective following either intramuscular or intravenous administration.

Cephalosporins are widely distributed in body fluids and most tissues. They do not pass the blood-brain barrier even when meninges are inflamed, but readily cross the placental barrier. The cephalosporins are excreted in the urine. Maximal concentrations are reached in the urine. However, cephaloglycin does not achieve adequate antibacterial blood levels, and consequently is used only to treat urinary tract infections.

In general, the cephalosporins are active against the following organisms in vitro: beta hemolytic streptococci, staphylococci, Strep. pneumoniae, H. influenzae, Klebsiella species, Proteus mirabilis, and E. coli. Cefamandole and cefoxitin are unique in that they have an extended spectrum of antibacterial activity to include anaerobes: Clostridium and Bacteriodes. Cefamandole is not effective against Bacteroides fragilis.

SPECIAL PRECAUTIONS

- All cephalosporins should be administered cautiously to penicillin-sensitive patients.
- Evaluation of renal function prior to therapy and at appropriate intervals is suggested; reduce dosage accordingly.
- Cephaloridine is nephrotoxic.
- Superinfections may occur; Pseudomonas is commonly the causative organism.

• Administer cautiously when administering concurrently with other antibiotics having nephrotoxic potential (gentamicin, kanamycin, polymyxin B, and colistin). However cephamandole nafate may be used concomitantly with an aminoglycoside.

• There is some clinical and laboratory evidence of partial cross allergenicity of the penicillins and cephalosporins; patients have had severe reactions (including anaphylaxis) to both drugs.

• Any patient who has demonstrated some form of allergy, particularly to drugs, should receive these antibiotics cautiously and only when absolutely necessary.

• The use of cephaloglycin in premature infants and in infants under one year is not recommended.

• Prolonged use may result in overgrowth of nonsusceptible organisms.

• Do not administer to patients hypersensitive to any of the cephalosporin group of antibiotics.

• Safe use in infants and in pregnant and lactating women has not been established.

ADVERSE EFFECTS

CNS EFFECTS: malaise, dizziness, fatigue, chills, headache, vertigo, paresthesias

RESPIRATORY EFFECTS: with cephradine, dyspnea

URINARY TRACT EFFECTS: increased BUN, decreased creatinine clearance; with cephaloridine, severe, acute renal failure, in some cases terminating in death

GASTROINTESTINAL EFFECTS: nausea, vomiting, diarrhea, abdominal pain, dyspepsia, bloating, glossitis; oral candidiasis; with cephaloglycin, gastrointestinal bleeding and severe enterocolitis

HEPATIC EFFECTS: transient increases in SGOT, SGPT, alkaline phosphatase, bilirubin, and LDH

HEMATOLOGIC EFFECTS: eosinophilia, neutropenia, thrombocytopenia, hemolytic anemia, leukopenia, positive Coombs' test

ALLERGIC EFFECTS: drug fever, maculopapular rash, exfoliative dermatitis, urticaria, reactions resembling serum sickness, anaphylaxis, edema, pruritus, joint pain

LOCAL EFFECTS: pain, induration, tenderness, elevation of skin temperature; and with intravenous administration, thrombophlebitis

CLINICAL GUIDELINES

ADMINISTRATION:

• Before initiating therapy with any of the cephalosporin antibiotics, inquire carefully concerning previous hypersensitivity reactions to both cephalosporins and penicillins.

• When administering cephalothin sodium, use small intravenous needles in the larger veins to reduce the risk of thrombophlebitis.

• Administer by deep intramuscular injection; following accidental subcutaneous administration sterile abscesses have been reported.

• Before administering any antibiotic with intravenous solutions, check the current official labeling to confirm compatibility of solutions; consider fluid and electrolyte status of patient.

• Oral forms should be taken with a full glass of water.

EFFECTS:

• A false positive reaction for glucose in the urine may occur with CLINITEST tablets but not with TES-TAPE test tape.

• Positive direct Coombs' tests have been reported in patients receiving cephalosporins.

• Addition of 10 to 25 mg hydrocortisone to intravenous solutions of cephalothin sodium may reduce the incidence of thrombophlebitis.

- Monilial vaginitis may occur.

DRUG INTERACTIONS:

- Cephradine is physically compatible with most commonly used intravenous fluids and electrolyte solutions (such as 5% dextrose injection, sodium chloride injection, or M/5 sodium lactate).
- Cephradine is NOT compatible with lactated Ringer's injection because of the incompatibility between calcium ions and the sodium carbonate present in cephradine.
- A false positive reaction for glucose in the urine may occur with CLINITEST tablets, Fehling's solution, or Benedicts' solution, but not with CLINISTIX and TESTAPE.

OVERDOSAGE/ANTIDOTE:

- Overdosage is characterized by an exaggeration of the adverse effects.
- There is no specific antidote.

Chloramphenicol and Its Salts

GENERAL CLINICAL USES

Chloramphenicol and its salts should be reserved for use in serious infections caused by susceptible organisms including a wide range of gram-positive and gram-negative bacteria, *Salmonella typhi* and other Salmonella species, *Hemophilus influenzae*, *Rickettsia* and lymphogranuloma-psittacosis group.

Chloramphenicol is the drug of choice in many ophthalmic infections. For specific products and information see Chapter 11, page 442.

SPECIFIC PRODUCTS AND DOSAGES

GENERIC NAME	TRADE NAME	ROUTE OF ADMIN.	USUAL DAILY DOSAGE	
			ADULTS	CHILDREN
chloramphenicol	(G)* CHLOROMYCETIN	po/iv	50–100 mg/kg in divided doses at 6-hr. intervals	50–100 mg/kg in divided doses at 6-hr. intervals
	CHLOROMYCETIN Cream	topical	See Chapter 9, page 418.	
	ANTIBIOPTO Ophth. Soln. and Oint.	ophth.	See Chapter 11, page 443.	
	CHLOROMYCETIN Ophth. Oint.			
	CHLOROPTIC Soln.			
	CHLOROPTIC S.O.P. Oint.			
	OPHTHOCHLOR Soln.			
	ECONOCHLOR Ophth. Soln. and Oint.			

*(G) Designates availability as a generic product.

PHARMACOLOGY

Chloramphenicol administered orally is absorbed rapidly from the gastrointestinal tract. Peak serum levels are reached in 1 hour. The drug is inactivated primarily in the liver. Excretion is by the kidneys in an unchanged form and as a conjugate with glucuronic acid. Chloramphenicol passes the blood-brain barrier and is also detected in milk, ascitic fluid, and serum. It crosses the placental barrier in low concentrations.

Chloramphenicol penetrates the eye and is, consequently, the drug of choice in many ophthalmic infections caused by bacteria susceptible to this drug. When applied topically, it is not absorbed unless the skin surface is abraded.

SPECIAL PRECAUTIONS
* Since serious and fatal blood dyscrasias have occurred, monitor hematologic parameters frequently during therapy; baseline values should be available.
* Do not administer to any patients with a history of hypersensitivity to chloramphenicol.
* Repeated courses are not recommended nor is prolonged treatment.
* Avoid concurrent administration with other drugs depressing the bone marrow.
* Safe use in pregnancy has not been established.
* Overgrowth of nonsusceptible organisms, including fungi, may occur.
* Newborn infants are unable to conjugate to glucuronide; severe overdosage can occur.

ADVERSE EFFECTS
CNS EFFECTS: headache, mild depression, mental confusion, delirium, optic and peripheral neuritis
GASTROINTESTINAL EFFECTS: nausea, vomiting, glossitis, stomatitis, diarrhea, enterocolitis
HEMATOLOGIC EFFECTS: aplastic anemia, hypoplastic anemia, leukemia, thrombocytopenia, granulocytopenia, pancytopenia, paroxsymal nocturnal hemoglobinemia
ALLERGIC EFFECTS: fever, macular and vesicular rashes, angioedema, urticaria, anaphylaxis, Herxheimer reactions
EFFECTS IN NEWBORN AND PREMATURE INFANTS: Gray syndrome characterized by abdominal distention with or without emesis, progressive pallid cyanosis, vasomotor collapse, death
LOCAL EFFECTS: itching, burning

CLINICAL GUIDELINES
ADMINISTRATION:
* Assure that baseline and frequent hematologic (WBC and differential) parameters are evaluated.
EFFECTS:
* If any hematologic abnormalities occur, the drug should be discontinued.
* Adults or children with impaired renal or hepatic function may have reduced ability to metabolize and excrete chloramphenicol; dosage should be adjusted accordingly to maintain desired blood concentration.
DRUG INTERACTIONS:
* Do not administer concurrently with other bone marrow depressing drugs.
OVERDOSAGE/ANTIDOTE:
* Overdosage is characterized by an exaggeration of the adverse effects.
* There is no specific antidote. Treat supportively.

Clindamycin and Lincomycin

GENERAL CLINICAL USES
Clindamycin and lincomycin should be reserved for serious infections of the respiratory tract, skin and soft tissues, blood, peritoneum, and genital tract

when less toxic antimicrobial agents are inappropriate. Clindamycin and lincomycin are used to treat infections due to susceptible strains of streptococci, pneumococci, and staphylococci; clindamycin is also useful in infections due to susceptible strains of anaerobic bacteria.

Clindamycin and lincomycin should be used for penicillin-allergic patients or other appropriate patients based on the judgment of the physician.

SPECIFIC PRODUCTS AND DOSAGES

Susceptibility testing should be performed before and at appropriate intervals during therapy. Dosage may be individualized for each patient based on the severity of the infection, the infecting organism, and the patient's response.

GENERIC NAME	TRADE NAME	ROUTE OF ADMIN.	USUAL DAILY DOSAGE	
			ADULTS	CHILDREN
clindamycin hydrochloride hydrate	CLEOCIN Hydrochloride	po	150–450 mg tid or qid	8–25 mg/kg/day divided into 3 or 4 doses
clindamycin phosphate	CLEOCIN Phosphate	im/iv	600–2700 mg/day in 2, 3, or 4 doses	15–40 mg/kg/day in 3 or 4 equal doses
clindamycin palmitate hydrochloride	CLEOCIN Pediatric	po	———	8–25 mg/kg/day divided in 3 or 4 equal doses
lincomycin hydrochloride	LINCOCIN	po	500 mg tid to qid	30–60 mg/kg/day divided into 3 or 4 doses
	LINCOCIN	im	600 mg od to bid	10 mg/kg/day od or bid
	LINCOCIN	iv	600 mg–1 gm bid to tid; 8 gm daily has been given	10–20 mg/kg/day
	LINCOCIN	subconjunctival	See Chapter 11, *Drugs Affecting the Eye,* page 443.	

Clindamycin

PHARMACOLOGY

Clindamycin administered orally is rapidly absorbed; peak serum levels are reached in 1/2 to 1 hour. Clindamycin palmitate, also for oral administration, converts *in vivo* by hydrolysis to active clindamycin. Clindamycin phosphate, a water-soluble ester, is suitable for intravenous and intramuscular administration; it is converted to active clindamycin. After intramuscular administration, peak levels are reached within 3 hours in adults and 1 hour in children. Clindamycin is excreted primarily by the kidneys. It has been reported in breast milk.

SPECIAL PRECAUTIONS

• Can cause severe colitis which may end fatally; discontinue if significant diarrhea occurs.

- Use with caution in patients with a history of gastrointestinal disease, particularly colitis.
- Antiperistaltic agents (opiates, diphenoxylate with atropine) may prolong and/or worsen the condition.
- Do not administer to patients with a history of hypersensitivity to clindamycin or lincomycin, or to patients with a history of asthma or significant allergies.
- Overgrowth of nonsusceptible organisms, particularly yeasts, may occur.
- Use very cautiously in patients with impaired renal and hepatic function.
- With prolonged therapy, monitor renal, hepatic, and hematopoietic functions initially and at appropriate intervals.
- Cross resistance exists between lincomycin and clindamycin.

ADVERSE EFFECTS

CNS EFFECTS: vertigo
GASTROINTESTINAL EFFECTS: glossitis, stomatitis, nausea, vomiting, pruritus ani, severe persistant diarrhea, severe abdominal cramps, passage of blood and mucus, perimembranous colitis
HEPATIC EFFECTS: jaundice, increased SGOT and SGPT
HEMATOLOGIC EFFECTS: transient neutropenia, eosinophilia, agranulocytosis, thrombocytopenic purpura rarely
ALLERGIC EFFECTS: maculopapular rash, urticaria, anaphylaxis, erythema multiforme rarely
DERMATOLOGIC EFFECTS: morbilliform rash
LOCAL EFFECTS: pain, induration, sterile abscess, thrombophlebitis

CLINICAL GUIDELINES

ADMINISTRATION:
- Older patients may tolerate therapy less well than young patients.
- Administer by deep intramuscular injection; avoid prolonged use of indwelling catheters to minimize the risk of sterile abscess and thrombophlebitis.
- Take capsules with a full glass of water to avoid esophageal irritation.
- Do not inject undiluted drug as a bolus; infuse over at least 10 to 60 minutes.

DRUG INTERACTIONS:
- The neuromuscular blocking properties may enhance similar properties in other medications.
- Antagonism has been demonstrated with erythromycin *in vitro*; do not administer concurrently because of the possible clinical significance.
- No inactivation or incompatibility has occurred with clindamycin phosphate in intravenous solutions containing sodium chloride, glucose, calcium or potassium, and solutions containing vitamin B complex in concentrations usually used clinically.
- No incompatibility has been demonstrated with cephalothin, kanamycin, gentamicin, penicillin, or carbenicillin.
- The following drugs are physically incompatible with clindamycin phosphate: ampicillin, diphenylhydantoin (phenytoin), barbiturates, aminophylline, calcium gluconate, and magnesium sulfate.
- Antiperistaltic agents such as opiates and diphenoxylate with atropine (LOMOTIL) may prolong or worsen the diarrhea which may occur.

OVERDOSAGE/ANTIDOTE:
- Overdosage may result in vomiting, nausea, cramps, and diarrhea.
- There is no specific antidote. Hemodialysis and peritoneal dialysis do not effectively remove clindamycin from the serum.

Lincomycin Hydrochloride

PHARMACOLOGY
Lincomycin hydrochloride may be either bactericidal or bacteriostatic de-

pending upon the organism and the concentration of antibiotic. Following oral administration lincomycin hydrochloride is absorbed rapidly from the gastrointestinal tract. Peak levels are reached in 2 to 4 hours. It is excreted in the bile and urine. Intramuscular administration results in peak levels in 30 minutes. Lincomycin hydrochloride has been reported in breast milk. Lincomycin does not share antigenicity with the penicillins; some cross resistance has been reported with use of erythromycin.

SPECIAL PRECAUTIONS

- Lincomycin can cause severe colitis which may end fatally; discontinue if significant diarrhea occurs.
- Antiperistaltic agents such as opiates or diphenoxylate with atropine may prolong and/or worsen the condition.
- Use with caution in patients with a history of gastrointestinal disease, particularly colitis, and with a history of asthma or significant allergies.
- Do not administer to patients with a history of hypersensitivity to lincomycin or clindamycin.
- Safe use in pregnancy has not been established.
- Overgrowth of nonsusceptible organisms may occur.
- Note that lincomycin has neuromuscular blocking properties and may enhance similar properties of other agents.
- Not recommended for children less than one month of age.
- If lincomycin therapy is required in patients with renal impairment, administer dosage 25 to 30 percent of that recommended to patients with normal renal function.
- With prolonged therapy, monitor renal, hepatic, and hematopoietic functions initially and at appropriate intervals.

- Cross resistance exists between lincomycin and clindamycin.

ADVERSE EFFECTS

CNS EFFECTS: vertigo
CARDIOVASCULAR EFFECTS: hypotension following parenteral administration; cardiopulmonary arrest after rapid intravenous administration
GASTROINTESTINAL EFFECTS: glossitis, stomatitis, nausea, vomiting, pruritus ani, severe persistent diarrhea, severe abdominal cramps, passage of blood and mucus, pseudomembranous colitis
HEPATIC EFFECTS: jaundice, increased SGOT and SGPT
HEMATOLOGIC EFFECTS: neutropenia, leukopenia, agranulocytosis, thrombocytopenic purpura, aplastic anemia; pancytopenia rarely
ALLERGIC EFFECTS: angioneurotic edema, serum sickness, anaphylaxis, erythema multiforme rarely
DERMATOLOGIC EFFECTS: rash, urticaria, vaginitis, vestibulobullous dermatitis
OTIC EFFECTS: tinnitus
LOCAL EFFECTS: pain infrequently

CLINICAL GUIDELINES

ADMINISTRATION:
- For optimal absorption, administer nothing by mouth except water 1 to 2 hours before and after oral administration.
- Rapid intravenous administration has resulted in cardiopulmonary arrest.
- Older patients may tolerate therapy less well than young patients.

DRUG INTERACTIONS:
- Cross resistance has *not* been demonstrated between lincomycin hydrochloride and penicillin, chloramphenicol, ampicillin, cephalosporins, or the tetracyclines.
- Physically incompatible with novobiocin and kanamycin.

• Physically compatible with these antibiotics in infusion solution: penicillin G sodium (for 4 hours), cephalothin, tetracycline hydrochloride, cephaloridine, colistimethate (for 4 hours), ampicillin, methicillin, chloramphenicol, polymyxin B sulfate.
• Physically compatible with these infusion solutions: dextrose in water 5% and 10%; dextrose in saline 5% and 10%; Ringer's Solution; Sodium lactate 1/6 molar; Travert 10%; Electrolyte No. 1; Dextran in Saline 6% w/v; B complex; B complex with ascorbic acid.
• With cyclamate-containing beverages and kaopectate, absorption is markedly reduced.

Erythromycins

GENERAL CLINICAL USES

The erythromycins may be used to treat infections caused by susceptible strains of the following organisms: gram-positive bacteria (*Streptococcus* and *Staphylococcus*), *Listeria monocytogenes, Neisseria, Bordatella, Brucella, Pasteurella, Hemophilus, Mycoplasma pneumoniae* (*PPLO*), *Actinomyces, Treponema* species, *Entamoeba histolytica*, and *Corynebacterium diphtheriae*. Gram-negative organisms are not sensitive to the erythromycins.

Infections of the upper and lower respiratory tract, skin and soft tissue, and pharynx may be successfully treated; in addition, endocarditis, primary syphilis, and intestinal amebiasis have been treated. The erythromycins may be used topically for dermal infections, usually in combination with other agents.

SPECIFIC PRODUCTS AND DOSAGES

GENERIC NAME	TRADE NAME	ROUTE OF ADMIN.	USUAL DAILY DOSAGE	
			ADULTS	CHILDREN
erythromycin	(G)* ERYTHROCIN E-MYCIN ILOTYCIN ROBIMYCIN ROMYCIN	po	0.25–4 gm/day in divided doses	30–100 mg/kg/day in divided doses
			also see *Amebicides*, page 11.	
	ERYTHROCIN Oint. ILOTYCIN Oint.	topical	See Chapter 9, *Drugs Affecting the Skin*, page 418.	
erythromycin estolate	ILOSONE	po	0.25–1 gm qid	30–100 mg/kg/day in divided doses

*(G) designates availability as a generic product.

(continued overleaf)

GENERIC NAME	TRADE NAME	ROUTE OF ADMIN.	USUAL DAILY DOSAGE	
			ADULTS	CHILDREN
erythromycin ethylsuccinate	PEDIAMYCIN	po	0.4–1 gm qid	200–400 mg qid
erythromycin gluceptate	ILOTYCIN Gluceptate	iv	15–20 mg/kg/day in divided doses	Same as adult
erythromycin lactobionate	ERYTHROCIN Lactobionate	iv	15–20 mg/kg/day by infusion	Same as adult
erythromycin stearate	(G)* ERYTHROCIN Stearate ETHRIL QID MYCIN	po	0.25–1 gm qid	30–100 mg/kg/day divided in 3–4 doses

*(G) Designates availability as a generic product.

PHARMACOLOGY

Erythromycin exerts its antibacterial action by inhibiting bacterial protein synthesis. When administered orally, erythromycin is rapidly absorbed, particularly is the stomach is empty. Erythromycin is partially inactivated by the gastric juice and consequently should be administered before meals or in one of the acid-resistant forms such as erythromycin estolate. The drug passes the blood-brain barrier in low concentrations unless inflammation is present. Following oral administration, peak plasma levels are reached in 1 to 4 hours; erythromycin is concentrated in the liver and excreted in the bile and feces. Less than 5 percent is excreted in the urine. Erythromycin crosses the placental barrier but fetal plasma levels are low.

Several salts of erythromycin are available. Erythromycin succinate is formulated as a liquid for use primarily in children. Erythromycin gluceptate and erythromycin lactobionate are for intravenous use, particularly when oral or rectal administration is not possible or if high serum levels are required.

SPECIAL PRECAUTIONS

• Do not administer to patients with known hypersensitivity to erythromycin or erythromycin salts.
• Since erythromycin is excreted primarily by the liver, it should be administered cautiously to patients with impaired hepatic function.
• Erythromycin estolate therapy has resulted in cholestatic hepatitis infrequently; this hepatitis is characterized by abnormal hepatic function, peripheral eosinophilia, and leukocytosis. Symptoms include malaise, nausea, vomiting, abdominal cramps, and fever. Jaundice may or may not be present. Severe abdominal pain may simulate biliary colic, pancreatitis, perforated ulcer, or an acute abdomen.
• With prolonged administration, overgrowth of nonsusceptible bacteria or fungi may occur.
• Safe use in pregnancy has not been established.

ADVERSE EFFECTS

GASTROINTESTINAL EFFECTS: abdominal cramping and discomfort, nausea, vomit-

ing, diarrhea, severe abdominal pain simulating abdominal surgical emergency
HEPATIC EFFECTS: cholestatic hepatitis characterized by abnormal hepatic function, nausea, vomiting, abdominal cramps, fever; jaundice with erythromycin estolate
HEMATOLOGIC EFFECTS: eosinophilia
ALLERGIC EFFECTS: urticaria, rash, anaphylaxis

CLINICAL GUIDELINES
ADMINISTRATION:
• Administer to patients with empty stomach for maximal absorption.
• Intramuscular administration is not recommended in small children because they have inadequate muscle mass for deep placement of injection.
• Erythromycin lactobionate solution is stable for 2 weeks if refrigerated.
EFFECTS:
• Severe abdominal pain simulating biliary colic, pancreatitis, perforated ulcer, or an acute abdomen is related to hepatic toxicity.
DRUG INTERACTIONS:
• Erythromycin lactobionate solution should not be mixed with solutions containing inorganic salts or saline since precipitation may occur.
• When administered with urinary alkalizers, the antibacterial activity is enhanced (when the urine is alkaline).
OVERDOSAGE/ANTIDOTE:
• Overdosage is characterized by an exaggeration of the adverse effects.
• There is no specific antidote; treat supportively.

Miscellaneous Antibacterial Agents

SPECIFIC PRODUCTS AND DOSAGES

GENERIC NAME	TRADE NAME	ROUTE OF ADMIN.	USUAL DAILY DOSAGE	
			ADULTS	CHILDREN
bacitracin, zinc bacitracin	(G)*	im	——	**Under 2500 gm:** 900 units/ kg/day divided in 2–3 doses **Over 2500 gm:** 1000 units/ kg/day divided in 2–3 doses
	NEO-POLYCIN† cream, Oint., Aerosol POLYSPORIN† Oint. CORTISPORIN	topical	See Chapter 9, *Drugs Affecting the Skin,* page 418.	
	NEO-POLYCIN† NEOSPORIN POLYSPORIN	ophth.	See Chapter 11, *Drugs Affecting the Eye,* page 442.	

*(G) Designates availability as a generic product.
†Contains more than one active ingredient.

(continued overleaf)

GENERIC NAME	TRADE NAME	ROUTE OF ADMIN.	USUAL DAILY DOSAGE	
			ADULTS	CHILDREN
gramicidin	MYCOLOG† NEOSPORIN-G† SPECTROCIN†	topical	See Chapter 9, *Drugs Affecting the Skin,* page 418.	
novobiocin calcium	ALBAMYCIN Calcium	po	250–500 mg qid	15–45 mg/kg/day in divided doses
novobiocin sodium	ALBAMYCIN Sodium	po	250–500 mg qid	15–45 mg/kg/day divided in 2 doses
		iv/im	500 mg bid	15–30 mg/kg/day divided in 2 doses
troleandomycin	TAO	po	250–500 mg qid	125–250 mg (6.6–11 mg/kg) qid
vancomycin hydrochloride	VANCOCIN Hydrochloride	iv	500 mg qid or 1 gm bid	20 mg/lb/day in divided doses
	VANCOCIN	po	500 mg qid or 1 gm bid	20 mg/lb/day in divided doses

*(G) Designates availability as a generic product.
†Contains more than one active ingredient.

Bacitracin/Zinc Bacitracin

GENERAL CLINICAL USES

Bacitracin, administered intramuscularly, is limited in use to treating infants with staphylococcal pneumonia and empyema caused by susceptible strains of *Staphylococcus aureus.*

Bacitracin is useful, in combination with other antimicrobial agents, in preventing or treating superficial bacterial infections of the skin. Please refer to Chapter 9, *Drugs Affecting the Skin,* page 417, for additional information. Bacitracin is also useful in ophthalmic preparations. For detailed information see Chapter 11, *Drugs Affecting the Eye,* page 442.

PHARMACOLOGY

Bacitracin administered intramuscularly is rapidly and completely absorbed. The mechanism of its antibacterial activity is unknown. It is excreted slowly by glomerular filtration and is distributed widely in all organs, pleural fluids, and ascitic fluids. When applied topically it is not absorbed from intact skin.

SPECIAL PRECAUTIONS
- Do not administer to patients with a history of hypersensitivity to bacitracin or related compounds.
- Overgrowth of nonsusceptible organisms, including fungi, may occur.
- Renal toxicity has been associated with intramuscular administration.
- Safe use in pregnancy has not been established.

ADVERSE EFFECTS
URINARY TRACT EFFECTS: albuminuria, cylindruria, azotemia
GASTROINTESTINAL EFFECTS: nausea, vomiting

DERMATOLOGIC EFFECTS: rash
LOCAL EFFECTS: transient pain at injection site

CLINICAL GUIDELINES

ADMINISTRATION:
• Inject into the upper outer quadrant of the buttock, alternating right and left sides to avoid multiple injections in the same region.
• Assure that patients receiving bacitracin intramuscularly maintain an adequate fluid intake.

EFFECTS:
• Signs of nephrotoxicity include albuminuria, cylindruria, and azotemia.

DRUG INTERACTIONS:
• Avoid concurrent administration of other nephrotoxic drugs such as streptomycin, kanamycin, polymyxin B, colistin, neomycin, and viomycin.

OVERDOSAGE/ANTIDOTE:
• Overdosage is characterized by an exaggeration of the adverse effects.
• There is no specific antidote.

Gramicidin

PHARMACOLOGY
Gramicidin is bacteriostatic against certain gram-positive bacteria. It is usually formulated in combination with other antibiotics to provide a wide range of antibacterial activities for dermal and ophthalmologic use.

SPECIAL PRECAUTIONS
• Do not use in patients with a history of hypersensitivity to gramicidin or other components of the formulation.
• Do not use in the eyes or external ear canal if the ear drum is perforated.
• Prolonged use may result in overgrowth of nonsusceptible organisms, including fungi.

CLINICAL GUIDELINES
ADMINISTRATION:
• Cleanse wound thoroughly before application.

DRUG INTERACTIONS:
• Gramicidin is usually formulated in combination with polymyxin B, neomycin, and bacitracin to provide a wide antibacterial spectrum.

Novobiocin Calcium
Novobiocin Sodium

GENERAL CLINICAL USES
Novobiocin is a narrow-spectrum antibiotic effective against most gram-positive pathogens such as staphylococci. However, staphylococci develop resistance rapidly. Some strains of *Proteus* and *Pseudomonas pseudomaleolli* are susceptible.

PHARMACOLOGY
Novobiocin, administered orally, is rapidly absorbed from the gastrointestinal tract. It may also be administered intramuscularly as the sodium salt. The incidence of adverse effects is high and superinfections occur. Novobiocin is limited in use because of the availability of superior antimicrobial agents.

SPECIAL PRECAUTIONS
• A metabolite may produce yellowish discoloration of the skin and sclerae 24 hours after administration.
• Do not administer to newborn and premature infants because it interferes with metabolism of bilirubin.
• Safe use in pregnancy has not been established.
• Do not use in patients with a history of hypersensitivity to novobiocin and related compounds.

ADVERSE EFFECTS

CNS EFFECTS: fever
RESPIRATORY EFFECTS: pneumonitis
CARDIOVASCULAR EFFECTS: myocarditis
GASTROINTESTINAL EFFECTS: nausea, vomiting, diarrhea
HEMATOLOGIC EFFECTS: blood dyscrasias
DERMATOLOGIC EFFECTS: rash, discoloration of skin and sclerae
LOCAL EFFECTS: pain with parenteral administration

CLINICAL GUIDELINES

OVERDOSAGE/ANTIDOTE:
- Overdosage is characterized by an exaggeration of the adverse effects of the drug novobiocin.
- There is no specific antidote.

Troleandomycin

GENERAL CLINICAL USES

Troleandomycin is useful in treating respiratory tract infections caused by susceptible strains of *Streptococcus pyogenes* and *Diplococcus pneumoniae.*

PHARMACOLOGY

Troleandomycin, a water-soluble and acid-resistant antibacterial agent, is absorbed from the gastrointestinal tract following oral administration; it is excreted principally by the liver.

SPECIAL PRECAUTIONS

- Do not administer to patients with a history of hypersensitivity to troleandomycin.
- Safe use in pregnancy has not been established.
- Administer cautiously to patients with impaired hepatic function; monitor hepatic function with appropriate clinical laboratory tests because of the potential for hepatic toxicity.

ADVERSE EFFECTS

GASTROINTESTINAL EFFECTS: abdominal cramping and discomfort, nausea, vomiting, diarrhea
HEPATIC EFFECTS: allergic-type cholestatic hepatitis with or without jaundice, eosinophilia, leukocytosis, upper right quadrant pain
ALLERGIC EFFECTS: urticaria, rash, anaphylaxis

CLINICAL GUIDELINES

ADMINISTRATION:
- Be aware that an allergic type of cholestatic hepatitis has occurred with this drug.
EFFECTS:
- Some patients have experienced jaundice accompanied by right upper quadrant pain, fever, nausea, vomiting, eosinophilia, and leukocytosis 2 weeks or more after therapy was initiated.
OVERDOSAGE/ANTIDOTE:
- Overdosage is characterized by an exaggeration of the adverse effects.
- There is no specific antidote.

Vancomycin

GENERAL CLINICAL USES

Vancomycin is useful in life-threatening infections caused by susceptible strains of organisms which cannot be treated with another effective, less toxic antimicrobial agent such as the penicillins or cephalosporins. Severe infections caused by susceptible strains of staphylococci are treated beneficially.

Vancomycin is also indicated for the treatment of staphylococcal enteritis.

PHARMACOLOGY

Vancomycin is poorly absorbed following oral administration. Consequently it is administered intravenously for systemic effects. Oral administration results in topical activity within the gastrointestinal lumen. Following parenteral administration it penetrates into the cerebrospinal fluid only when the meninges are inflamed. Since vancomycin is excreted primarily by the kidneys, impaired renal function may delay excretion.

SPECIAL PRECAUTIONS
- Use cautiously in patients with impaired renal function.
- Do not administer to patients with a history of hypersensitivity to vancomycin.
- Safe use in pregnancy has not been established.
- Ototoxicity and renal toxicity have been associated with vancomycin.
- Avoid use in patients with impaired hearing.
- Elderly patients are more susceptible to hearing loss than young patients.
- Avoid concurrent or sequential use of other neurotoxic and/or nephrotoxic drugs.
- Monitor renal, hepatic, and hematologic parameters periodically.
- Administer intravenously only; intramuscular administration is very irritating to tissues and should not be used.

- Overgrowth of nonsusceptible organisms including fungi may occur.

ADVERSE EFFECTS
CNS EFFECTS: chills, fever
GASTROINTESTINAL EFFECTS: nausea
ALLERGIC EFFECTS: urticaria, eosinophilia, anaphylactoid reactions

CLINICAL GUIDELINES
ADMINISTRATION:
- Administer vancomycin intravenously in a volume of 200 ml glucose or saline to minimize thrombophlebitis.

EFFECTS:
- Tinnitus may precede hearing loss.

DRUG INTERACTIONS:
- Concurrent or sequential administration of drugs with neurotoxic and/or nephrotoxic potential such as streptomycin, neomycin, kanamycin, gentamicin, polymyxin B, colistin, cephaloridine, paromomycin, viomycin, or tobramycin may result in enhanced toxicity.

OVERDOSAGE/ANTIDOTE:
- Overdosage may be characterized by an exaggeration of the adverse effects.
- There is no specific antidote.

Nitrofurans

GENERAL CLINICAL USES
The nitrofurans, furazolidone, nitrofurantoin and nitrofurazone have activity against gram-positive and gram-negative bacteria, and also protozoans.

Furazolidone is useful in treating bacterial or protozoal diarrhea and enteritis caused by susceptible organisms including *Escherichia coli*, staphylococci, *Salmonella*, *Shigella*, *Proteus*, *Aerobacter aerogenes*, *Vibrio cholerae*, *Giardia lamblia*. It has also been administered topically for treatment of vaginal infections caused by trichomonads.

Nitrofurantoin is used in treating urinary tract infections such as pyelonephritis, pyelitis, and cystitis caused by susceptible strains of *Escherichia coli*, enterococci, *Staphyloccus aureus*, *Klebsiella-Aerobacter*, *Proteus*, and *Pseudomonas*.

Nitrofurazone is indicated for adjunctive therapy of patients with second and third degree burns when bacterial resistance to other agents is a problem. It is also indicated in skin grafting where bacterial contamination may cause graft rejection and/or donor site infection, particularly in hospitals with historical resistant-bacteria epidemics. It is also used in urethral inserts in urinary tract infections.

SPECIFIC PRODUCTS AND DOSAGES

GENERIC NAME	TRADE NAME	ROUTE OF ADMIN.	USUAL DAILY DOSAGE	
			ADULTS	CHILDREN
furazolidone	FUROXONE TRICOFURON*	po intravag.	100 mg qid See Chapter 14, page 515.	**5 yrs. and over:** 25–50 mg qid
nitrofurantoin, macrocrystals	(G)† CYANTIN FURADANTIN MACRODANTIN N-TOIN TRANTOIN	po	50–100 mg qid	**1–4 yrs.:** 12–25 mg qid **Over 3 mos.:** 5–7 mg/kg/ day divided in 4 equal doses
nitrofurazone	(G) FURAZYME NISEPT NITROFURASTAN	topical	See Chapter 9, page 418.	

*Contains more than one active ingredient.
†(G) Designates availability as a generic product.

Furazolidone

PHARMACOLOGY

Furazolidone, an antimicrobial agent, is not absorbed after oral administration. It acts on pathogens within the intestinal lumen but does not significantly alter the normal bowel flora nor result in fungal overgrowth. The mechanism of bacteriostatic and/or bactericidal action is unknown but is presumed to be an interference with bacterial growth.

SPECIAL PRECAUTIONS

• Do not administer to patients with a history of hypersensitivity to furazolidone or related drugs.

• Safe use in pregnancy has not been established.
• When administered intravaginally, sensitization may occur.
• Do not use in infants under 1 month.

ADVERSE EFFECTS

CNS EFFECTS: fever, headache, malaise
CARDIOVASCULAR EFFECTS: orthostatic hypotension
GASTROINTESTINAL EFFECTS: nausea, vomiting
METABOLIC AND ENDOCRINE EFFECTS: hypoglycemia
HEMATOLOGIC EFFECTS: mild reversible intravascular hemolysis

ALLERGIC EFFECTS: urticaria, vesicular morbilliform rash
MUSCULOSKELETAL EFFECTS: arthralgia
LOCAL EFFECTS: sensitization reactions, contact dermatitis

CLINICAL GUIDELINES
DRUG INTERACTIONS:
• Administer sedatives, antihistamines, tranquilizers, oral narcotics concurrently in reduced dosages and with caution.
• Do not administer MAO-inhibiting drugs, tyramine-containing foods, or indirectly acting sympathomimetic amines (phenylephrine, ephedrine) and anorectics (amphetamines) concurrently with furazolidone.
• An ANTABUSE-like effect may occur in some patients ingesting ethyl alcohol during and within 4 days after therapy.
OVERDOSAGE/ANTIDOTE:
• Overdosage is characterized by an exaggeration of the adverse effects.
• There is no specific antidote.

Nitrofurantoin

PHARMACOLOGY
The mechanism of bacteriostatic and/or bactericidal action is unknown but is presumed to be an interference with bacterial multiplication. Nitrofurantoin is rapidly and completely absorbed from the gastrointestinal tract following oral administration. The macrocrystals are absorbed more slowly and excretion is somewhat less than regular nitrofurantoin. Nitrofurantoin is tightly bound to serum protein but is rapidly excreted by the kidneys resulting in high urine concentrations.

SPECIAL PRECAUTIONS
• Do not administer to patients with anuria, oliguria, or significant impairment of renal function.
• Hemolytic anemia of the primaquine-

sensitivity type has been induced.
• Superinfections may occur; the organism most commonly implicated is *Pseudomonas*.
• Peripheral neuropathy may occur; predisposing conditions include renal impairment, anemia, diabetes, electrolyte imbalance, vitamin B deficiency, debilitating disease.
• Pulmonary reactions progressing to diffuse interstitial pneumonitis or pulmonary fibrosis have occurred.
• Do not use in pregnant patients at term or infants less than 1 month of age because of the possibility of hemolytic anemia due to immature enzyme systems.
• Do not administer to patients with a history of hypersensitivity to this drug or related drugs.
• Safe use in pregnancy and lactation has not been established.

ADVERSE EFFECTS
CNS EFFECTS: peripheral neuropathy, headache, dizziness, drowsiness
GASTROINTESTINAL EFFECTS: anorexia, nausea, vomiting, abdominal pain, diarrhea
HEPATIC EFFECTS: hepatitis rarely, cholestatic jaundice
HEMATOLOGIC EFFECTS: hemolytic anemia, granulocytopenia, leukopenia, eosinophilia, megaloblastic anemia
ALLERGIC EFFECTS: pulmonary sensitivity reactions manifested by fever, chills, cough, chest pain, dyspnea, pulmonary infiltration with pleural effusion; may progress to malaise, dyspnea on exertion, cough, altered pulmonary function, diffuse interstitial pneumonitis or fibrosis; asthmatic attack; anaphylaxis, urticaria
OPHTHALMIC EFFECTS: nystagmus
MUSCULOSKELETAL EFFECTS: arthralgia

CLINICAL GUIDELINES
ADMINISTRATION:
• Administer with milk or food to minimize gastrointestinal upset.

EFFECTS:
- May impart a brown color to the urine; warn patients.

DRUG INTERACTIONS:
- May result in an ANTABUSE-like reaction in sensitive individuals when combined with alcohol.
- Probenecid (BENEMID) may delay elimination from the body and therefore increase the effects of nitrofurantoin.
- Phenobarbital may reduce its absorption and hasten its elimination from the body.
- Nalidixic acid (NEGGRAM) may reduce its antimicrobial action and impair effectiveness.

Nitrofurazone

PHARMACOLOGY
Nitrofurazone, a broad-spectrum antibacterial agent, is bactericidal against most bacteria commonly causing surface infections, including many that have become antibiotic resistant. It acts by inhibiting enzymes necessary for carbonydrate metabolism in bacteria. When administered topically it is without appreciable toxicity to human cells.

SPECIAL PRECAUTIONS
- Do not use in patients with a history of hypersensitivity to nitrofurazone or related compounds.
- Safe use in pregnancy has not been established.
- Overgrowth of nonsusceptible organisms including fungi may occur.

ADVERSE EFFECTS
ALLERGIC EFFECTS: sensitization reactions

Penicillins

GENERAL CLINICAL USES
The penicillins have been used to successfully treat infections caused by penicillin-sensitive organisms such as staphylococci (NOT penicillinase-producing strains unless so indicated), streptococci *(Groups A, C, G, H, L, M)*, Pneumococci, *Corynebacterium diphtheriae, Bacillus anthracis, Clostridia, Actinomyces bovis, Streptobacillus moniformis, Listeria monocytogenes, Leptospira, Neisseria gonorrhoeae, Treponema pallidum*.

The penicillins have been effective in prophylaxis of streptococcal infections which may lead to bacterial endocarditis and recurrence of rheumatic fever.

Of the more recently developed penicillins, three, ampicillin, carbenicillin, and amoxicillin, are effective against a somewhat wider range of organisms. Ampicillin is useful in infections due to susceptible strains of gram-negative bacteria including *Shigella, Salmonella, Neisseria gonorrhoeae, N. meningitidis, Escherichia coli, Hemophilus influenzae, Proteus mirabilis*, and also gram-positive bacteria including beta hemolytic streptococci, nonpenicillinase-producing staphylococci, and *Diplococcus pneumoniae*.

Carbenicillin also is bactericidal against both gram-negative and gram-positive organisms including *Staphylococcus aureus* (nonpenicillinase-producing), *Staphylococcus albus, Diplococcus pneumoniae*, beta hemolytic streptococci, *Streptococcus faecalis, Hemophilus influenzae, Neisseria* species,

Escherichia coli, Salmonella species, *Pseudomonas aeruginosa, Proteus mirabilis, Proteus morganii, Proteus rettgeri, Proteus vulgaris,* and *Enterobacter* species.

Amoxicillin is indicated for the treatment of infections caused by gram-negative organisms including *H. influenzae, E. coli, P. mirabilis,* and *N. gonorrhoeae*; gram-positive organisms including streptococci (including *Streptococcus faecalis*), *D. pneumoniae,* and nonpenicillinase–producing staphylococci.

SPECIFIC PRODUCTS AND DOSAGES
The dosage for each patient should be individualized, based on the severity of the infection and the infecting organism. Susceptibility testing should be performed at appropriate intervals during therapy.

GENERIC NAME	TRADE NAME	ROUTE OF ADMIN.	USUAL DAILY DOSAGE	
			ADULTS	CHILDREN UNDER 12 YRS.
amoxicillin	AMOXIL LAROTID POLYMOX	po	250–500 mg tid	20–40 mg/kg/day in equally divided doses every 8 hr.
ampicillin/ampicillin trihydrate	ALPEN AMCILL OMNIPEN PENBRITIN PRINCIPEN TOTACILLIN	po	250–500 mg qid	50–100 mg/kg/day in equally divided doses every 6–8 hr.
ampicillin sodium	AMCILL–S OMNIPEN–N POLYCILLIN N PRINCIPEN N TOTACILLIN–N	im/iv	250–500 mg bid to qid	25–100 mg/kg/day in equally divided doses every 6–8 hr.
carbenicillin disodium	GEOPEN PYOPEN	im/iv	200 mg/kg/day in divided doses or contin. drip; maximum: 40 gm/day; maximum im: 2 gm/day	100–500 mg/kg/day in equally divided doses
carbenicillin indanyl sodium	GEOCILLIN	po	382–764 mg qid	Not established
cloxacillin sodium	TEGOPEN	po	250–500 mg qid	50–100 mg/kg/day in 4 equally divided doses
dicloxacillin sodium	DYNAPEN PATHOCIL VERACILLIN	po	125–500 mg qid	12.5–25 mg/kg/day in 4 equally divided doses
hetacillin	VERSAPEN	po	225–450 mg qid	22.5–45.0 mg/kg/day in equally divided doses

(continued overleaf)

GENERIC NAME	TRADE NAME	ROUTE OF ADMIN.	USUAL DAILY DOSAGE	
			ADULTS	CHILDREN UNDER 12 YRS.
hetacillin potassium	VERSAPEN–K	po	225–450 mg qid	——————
methicillin sodium	AZAPEN CELBENIN STAPHCILLIN	im	1 gm every 4–6 hr.	25 mg/kg every 6 hr.
	AZAPEN CELBENIN STAPHCILLIN	iv	1 gm every 6 hr.	Not established
nafcillin sodium	NAFCIL UNIPEN	iv	0.5–1 gm every 4 hr.	Not established
	NAFCIL UNIPEN	im	500 mg every 4–6 hr.	10–25 mg/kg/day divided in 2 doses
	UNIPEN	po	250–1000 mg every 4–6 hr.	50 mg/kg/day divided in 4 equal doses
oxacillin sodium	BACTOCILL	po	0.5–1 gm every 4–6 hr.	50–100 mg/kg/day in 4–6 equally divided doses
	BACTOCILL PROSTAPHLIN	im/iv	250 mg–1 gm every 4–6 hr.	50–100 mg/kg/day in 4 equally divided doses
penicillin G	(G)* PFIZERPEN G	po	200,000–500,000 units every 6–8 hrs.	25,000–90,000 units/kg/day in 3–6 divided doses
penicillin G benzathine	BICILLIN L–A BICILLIN C–R†	im/iv	1,200,000 units single dose; for syphilis: 2.4 mill. units	300,000–900,000 units single dose
penicillin G procaine	(G) CRYSTICILLIN DURACILLIN A–S WYCILLIN	im	600,000–1,200,000 units/day; for gonorrhea: 4,800,000/day	10,000 units/kg/day
penicillin V potassium (potassium phenoxymethyl penicillin)	(G) BETAPEN–VK COMPOCILLIN–VK LEDERCILLIN–VK ROBICILLIN VK V–CILLIN K	po	125–500 mg bid to qid (200,000–800,000 units)	15–62.5 mg divided in 3–6 equal doses

*(G) Designates availability as a generic product.
†Contains more than one active ingredient.

PHARMACOLOGY

The penicillins, both natural and semisynthetic, are broad-spectrum bactericidal antibiotics. They exert their bactericidal activity by interfering with the formation and integrity of the bacterial cell wall. Following oral or parenteral administration small amounts are found in all body tissues and cerebrospinal fluid. The drug is excreted in the urine.

Ampicillin, ampicillin sodium, and ampicillin trihydrate are similar to penicillin G in their activity following oral administration. The ampicillins are inactivated by penicillinase but are acid stable and well absorbed from the gastrointestinal tract.

Amoxicillin, a semisynthetic penicillin, is an analog of ampicillin with similar activity. It is stable in gastric juice and diffuses into most body tissues and fluids.

Carbenicillin disodium, a semisynthetic injectable penicillin, is a benzyl penicillin derivative. Carbenicillin disodium is not absorbed from the gastrointestinal tract and consequently must be administered intramuscularly or intravenously. For oral administration carbenicillin indanyl sodium is available; it is acid stable and well absorbed following oral administration.

Cloxacillin sodium, a synthetic penicillin, is resistant to acidic destruction and is well absorbed following oral administration. It is distributed throughout the body but the highest concentrations occur in the kidney and liver. Significant amounts are also excreted in the bile.

Dicloxacillin sodium also resists destruction by penicillinase and gastric acid. It is well absorbed from the gastrointestinal tract following oral administration. Blood levels achieved are higher than those obtained with the other available orally administered penicillins.

Hetacillin and hetacillin sodium are acid stable and well absorbed following oral administration. They are converted *in vivo* to ampicillin, which is similar in activity to benzyl penicillin.

Methicillin sodium, another semisynthetic injectable penicillin, resists inactivation by staphylococcal penicillinase. It is equally active against penicillin-sensitive and penicillinase-producing strains of *Staphylococcus aureus*. The antimicrobial spectrums of methicillin sodium and penicillin G are similar qualitatively, but a higher concentration of drug is needed for bactericidal activity against streptococci and pneumococci than with penicillin G. Methicillin sodium is not acid resistant nor is it absorbed after oral administration. Administration must be intramuscular or intravenous.

Nafcillin sodium, a semisynthetic penicillin, is readily soluble and is resistant to inactivation by staphylococcal penicillinase. It acts similarly to methicillin.

Oxacillin sodium is a penicillinase-resistant, and acid-resistant semisynthetic penicillin. Its resistance to gastric acid is greater than that of penicillin G. In the presence of inflammation of the meninges, effective antibacterial levels may be achieved in the central nervous system.

Penicillin G, the most commonly used penicillin, may be administered intravenously, intramuscularly, or orally. If administered orally, it is to a large extent inactivated by gastric juice.

Penicillin G benzathine, administered intramuscularly, is absorbed very slowly and converted by hydrolysis to penicillin G. Penicillin G procaine also acts similarly.

Penicillin V potassium when administered orally is more acid stable than penicillin G and is better absorbed. Higher blood levels are produced than with penicillin G. This product is not a substitute for parenterally administered penicillin.

SPECIAL PRECAUTIONS
• Do not use penicillin administered orally as adjunctive anti-infective prophylaxis prior to genitourinary tract instrumentation or surgery, lower intestinal tract surgery, sigmoidoscopy, or childbirth.
• Do not use in patients with a history of hypersensitivity to any of the penicillins. Anaphylactoid reactions have occurred. These reactions are more frequent after parenteral than oral therapy.
• Patients with a history of sensitivity to multiple allergens or cephalosporins are more likely to experience hypersensitivity reactions to the penicillins.
• Do not rely on oral administration in patients with serious illnesses, or with nausea, vomiting, gastric dilatation, cardiospasm, or intestinal hypermotility.
• In streptococcal infections, therapy must be continued for a minimum of 10 days to eliminate the organisms.
• Prolonged therapy may promote over-

growth of nonsusceptible organism, including fungi; superinfections may occur.
• Use with caution in patients with impaired renal function.
• Methicillin cannot be excreted in infants because of their poorly developed renal function.
• Safe use in pregnancy has not been established.
• In cardiac patients receiving disodium carbenicillin, monitor cardiac function and electrolyte levels periodically because of the sodium content of disodium carbenicillin.

ADVERSE EFFECTS

CNS EFFECTS: convulsions
URINARY TRACT EFFECTS: hematuria, casts, azotemia, oliguria, albuminuria, cylinduria
GASTROINTESTINAL EFFECTS: nausea, vomiting, epigastric distress, diarrhea, black hairy tongue, glossitis, stomatitis
HEPATIC EFFECTS: elevated SGOT and SGPT with semisynthetic penicillins including oxacillin sodium, cloxacillin sodium, dicloxacillin sodium, and carbenicillin disodium.
HEMATOLOGIC EFFECTS: eosinophilia, hemolytic anemia, leukopenia, thrombocytopenia; in uremic patients, carbenicillium disodium has produced hemorrhagic manifestations associated with abnormalities of prothrombin and clotting times.
ALLERGIC EFFECTS: skin eruptions (masculopapular to exfoliative dermatitis), urticaria, serum sickness, laryngeal edema, anaphylaxis, fever, arthralgia, prostration.
LOCAL EFFECTS: pain, phlebitis, thrombophlebitis with intravenous injection

CLINICAL GUIDELINES

ADMINISTRATION:
• Caution patient to watch for itching, rash, red spots; these are sign of allergy to the penicillins.
• To obtain high blood levels with oral administration, administer on an empty stomach.
• Confirm that patient has had no hypersensitivity reactions to any of the penicillins prior to administration.
• Discard any reconstituted material for intravenous administration after 24 hours.
• Rapid intravenous administration of ampicillin or any penicillin may result in convulsions.

EFFECTS:
• Anaphylactoid reactions require immediate emergency treatment. Administer epinephrine, oxygen, intravenous steroids, and airway management including intubation, as needed.

DRUG INTERACTIONS:
• Methicillin sodium should not be mixed with other antibiotics; administer each separately.
• Carbenicillin for intramuscular injection ONLY may be diluted with 0.5% lidocaine hydrochloride (without epinephrine) or Bacteriostatic Water containing 0.9% Benzyl Alcohol.
• Cloxacillin activity may be decreased by concurrent use of antacids, chloramphenicol, erythromycin, paromomycin, tetracyclines, and troleandomycin.

OVERDOSAGE/ANTIDOTE:
• Overdosage may be characterized by nausea, vomiting, and/or diarrhea.
• There is no specific antidote; treat supportively.

Polymyxins

The polymyxins include three products: colistimethate sodium, colistin sulfate, and polymyxin B sulfate. Each product will be discussed separately because each has specific uses.

SPECIFIC PRODUCTS AND DOSAGES

GENERIC NAME	TRADE NAME	ROUTE OF ADMIN.	USUAL DAILY DOSAGE	
			ADULTS AND CHILDREN	INFANTS
colistimethate sodium	COLY-MYCIN M	im/iv	2.5–5 mg/kg/day divided in 2 or 4 doses; do not exceed 5 mg/kg/day	2.5–5 mg/kg/day divided in 2 or 4 doses
colistin sulfate	COLY-MYCIN S	po	3–5 mg/kg/day divided in 3 doses	3–5 mg/kg/day divided in 3 doses
		otic	See Chapter 12, *Drugs Affecting the Ear*, page 464.	
		ophth.	See Chapter 11, *Drugs Affecting the Eye*, page 443.	
polymyxin B sulfate	AEROSPORIN	iv	15,000–25,000 units/kg/day	Up to 40,000 units/kg/day
		im	25,000–30,000 units/kg/day	Up to 40,000–45,000 units/kg/day
		intrathecal	50,000 units/day	20,000–50,000 units/day
	NEO-POLYCIN* STATROL*	ophth.	See Chapter 11, *Drugs Affecting the Eye*, page 443.	
	NEO-POLYCIN*	topical	See Chapter 9, *Drugs Affecting the Skin*, page 418.	
	AEROSPORIN*	otic	See Chapter 12, *Drugs Affecting the Ear,* page 464.	

*Contains more than one active ingredient.

Colistimethate Sodium

GENERAL CLINICAL USES

Colistimethate sodium is used primarily in infections caused by gram-negative bacteria, namely, *Pseudomonas aeruginosa, Aerobacter aerogenes, Escherichia coli*, and *Klebsiella pneumoniae*. It is also useful in treating infections such as bacteremia, meningitis, peritonitis, and especially, urinary tract infections.

PHARMACOLOGY

Colistimethate sodium is a bactericidal antibiotic, administered intravenously or intramuscularly, active against gram-negative bacilli. Following intramuscular or intravenous administration blood levels de-cline with a half-life reached in 2 to 3 hours. Colistimethate sodium passes the placental barrier. It is excreted primarily in the urine.

SPECIAL PRECAUTIONS

• Hospitalize patients so that they can be supervised constantly.

• Monitor renal function closely, particularly in patients with pre-existing renal damage; decline in renal function with advanced age should be considered.

• Discontinue therapy if BUN increases and urine output diminishes.

• Do not administer concurrently with other nephrotoxic and neurotoxic drugs such as kanamycin, streptomycin, neomycin, gentamicin, and viomycin or other members of the polymyxin group.

• Do not administer to patients with a history of hypersensitivity reactions to colistimethate sulfate or related drugs.
• Overgrowth of nonsusceptible organisms may occur.
• Safe use in pregnancy has not been established.

ADVERSE EFFECTS

CNS EFFECTS: vertigo, slurring of speech, circumoral paresthesias or numbness, tingling or formication of the extremities, dizziness, tingling of the tongue
RESPIRATORY EFFECTS: respiratory arrest following intramuscular administration
URINARY TRACT EFFECTS: decreased urine output, an increased BUN and serum creatinine
GASTROINTESTINAL EFFECTS: gastrointestinal disturbances
ALLERGIC EFFECTS: drug fever
DERMATOLOGIC EFFECTS: generalized pruritus

CLINICAL GUIDELINES

ADMINISTRATION:
• Baseline renal function values should be obtained prior to therapy and monitored frequently throughout therapy with any of the polymyxins.
• Advise patients not to drive vehicles or use hazardous machinery while on therapy.
DRUG INTERACTIONS:
• Do not administer curariform muscle relaxants (tubocurarine, succinylcholine, gallamine, decamethonium), sodium citrate, and other neurotoxic drugs, such as ether, concurrently because of possible respiratory depression.
• Do not administer colistimethate sodium concurrently with kanamycin, streptomycin, or polymyxin B sulfate because of the neuromuscular blocking effect.

• For infusion, may be mixed with 5% dextrose in water, 5% dextrose with normal saline; 5% dextrose with 0.45% sodium chloride; 5% dextrose with 0.225% sodium chloride; lactated Ringer's solution, or invert sugar solution 10%.
OVERDOSAGE/ANTIDOTE:
• Overdosage may result in renal insufficiency, muscle weakness, and apnea.
• There is no specific antidote. If apnea occurs, it may be treated with assisted respiration, oxygen, and calcium chloride injection.

Colistin Sulfate

GENERAL CLINICAL USES
Colistin sulfate is used primarily in infants and children to treat diarrhea caused by susceptible gram–negative bacilli. It is also used to treat gastroenteritis caused by *Shigella* and other susceptible bacteria when these species are refractory to other agents.

PHARMACOLOGY
Colistin sulfate is bactericidal against most gram-negative enteric pathogens including *Pseudomonas aeruginosa*; most strains of *Proteus* are resistant. Colistin sulfate administered orally is absorbed in very small quantities.

SPECIAL PRECAUTIONS
• Hospitalize patients so that they can be supervised constantly.
• Monitor renal function closely, particularly in patients with pre-existing renal damage.
• Discontinue therapy if BUN increases and urine output diminishes.
• Do not administer concurrently with other nephrotoxic and neurotoxic drugs

such as kanamycin, streptomycin, neomycin, gentamicin, and viomycin or other members of the polymyxin group.

• Do not administer to patients with a history of hypersensitivity reactions to colistin sulfate or related compounds.

ADVERSE EFFECTS

• None reported.

CLINICAL GUIDELINES

ADMINISTRATION:

• Baseline renal function values should be obtained prior to therapy and monitored frequently throughout therapy with any of the polymyxins.

EFFECTS:

• Suppression of bacterial flora may occur with prolonged use.

DRUG INTERACTIONS:

• Do not administer concurrently with kanamycin, streptomycin, polymyxin B sulfate, or bleomycin because of the neuromuscular blocking effect.

• Cross resistance to polymyxin B does exist.

Polymyxin B Sulfate

GENERAL CLINICAL USES

Polymyxin B sulfate is valuable for treating infections caused by *Pseudomonas* species, in particular meningitis in which instance it may be administered intrathecally. It is also useful for treating infections caused by susceptible strains of *Hemophilus influenzae, Escherichia coli, Aerobacter aerogenes, Klebsiella pneumoniae.*

PHARMACOLOGY

Polymyxin B sulfate is bactericidal against almost all gram-negative bacilli except the *Proteus* group. All gram-positive bacteria, fungi, and gram negative cocci

are resistant. Polymyxin B sulfate is not absorbed from the normal alimentary tract and it loses one half of its activity in the presence of serum. It is usually administered intramuscularly or intravenously; excretion is slow by way of the kidneys. Polymyxin B sulfate does not pass the normal blood-brain barrier and tissue diffusion is poor. Development of resistant strains of bacteria is infrequent. Polymyxin B sulfate when applied topically is poorly absorbed particularly from the surface of large burns and similar skin conditions.

SPECIAL PRECAUTIONS

• Hospitalize patients so that they can be supervised constantly.

• Monitor renal function closely, particularly in patients with pre-existing renal damage.

• Discontinue therapy if BUN increases and urine output diminishes.

• Neurotoxicity is characterized by transient neurological disturbances such as circumoral or perioral paresthesias, tingling or formication of the extremities, generalized pruritus, vertigo, ataxia, dizziness, slurring of speech, blurring of vision.

• Do not administer to patients with a history of sensitivity reactions to polymyxins.

• Respiratory paralysis from neuromuscular blockade can occur, particularly if administered soon after anesthesia and/or muscle relaxants.

• Safe use in pregnancy has not been established.

• Overgrowth of nonsusceptible organisms may occur.

ADVERSE EFFECTS

CNS EFFECTS: facial flushing, dizziness progressing to ataxia, drowsiness, irritability, perioral paresthesias, numbness of the extremities, signs of meningeal irritation with intrathecal administration (fever, headache, stiff neck, increased cell count, protein in cerebrospinal fluid)

RESPIRATORY EFFECTS: apnea

URINARY TRACT EFFECTS: albuminuria, cellular casts, azotemia, diminished urine output, increased BUN

ALLERGIC EFFECTS: fever, urticarial rash

OPHTHALMIC EFFECTS: blurring of vision

LOCAL EFFECTS: pain (severe) at intramuscular injection site; thrombophlebitis at intravenous injection site

CLINICAL GUIDELINES

ADMINISTRATION:

• Parenteral solutions of polymyxin B sulfate should be refrigerated and any unused portion discarded after 72 hours.

• Do not store in alkaline solutions.

• Baseline renal function values should be obtained prior to therapy and monitored frequently throughout therapy with any of the polymyxins.

• Do not apply more than 200 mg daily in cases of denuded surfaces or open wounds.

EFFECTS:

• Watch patients receiving the polymyxins for signs of superinfection.

• Diminished urine output and rising BUN are indications for terminating therapy with this drug.

DRUG INTERACTIONS:

• Do not administer curariform muscle relaxants (tubocurarine, succinylcholine, gallamine, and decamethonium), sodium citrate, and other neurotoxic drugs, such as ether, concurrently because of possible respiratory depression.

• Concurrent administration of other nephrotoxic and neurotoxic drugs, particularly kanamycin, streptomycin, colistin, neomycin, gentamicin, and viomycin, should be avoided.

OVERDOSAGE/ANTIDOTE:

• Symptoms of overdosage include renal insufficiency, muscle weakness, and apnea.

• There is no specific antidote.

Sulfonamides

GENERAL CLINICAL USES

The sulfonamides are useful in infections caused by susceptible strains of *Escherichia coli, Klebsiella-Aerobacter, Staphylococcus aureus, Proteus mirabilis*, and less frequently *Proteus vulgaris;* also *Neisseria meningitides, Shigella, Salmonella*, and *Hemophilus influenzae*. The sulfonamides have been useful as adjunctive therapy in the treatment of toxoplasmosis, malaria (*Plasmodium falciparum*), meningococcal meningitis, chancroid, trachoma, inclusion conjunctivitis, actinomycosis, and nocardiosis. The sulfonamides are used to control bacillary dysentery caused by susceptible strains of *Shigella*.

Although most sulfonamides are of little value in treating topical infections, mafenide acetate applied topically is indicated for adjunctive therapy of patients with second and third degree burns.

The sulfonamides are also of value in the treatment of eye infections. For additional information see Chapter 11, *Drugs Affecting the Eye*, page 442.

SPECIFIC PRODUCTS AND DOSAGES

GENERIC NAME	TRADE NAME	ROUTE OF ADMIN.	USUAL DAILY DOSAGE	
			ADULTS	INFANTS AND CHILDREN
mafenide	SULFAMYLON Cream	topical	See Chapter 9, *Drugs Affecting the Skin,* page 418.	
phthalysulfathiazole	SULFATHALIDINE	po	**Initial:** 50–100 mg/kg/ day divided in 3–6 doses; maximum: 8 gm/day	Not established
sulfabenzamide	SULTRIN* Vag. Cream; Tablets	intravag.	See Chapter 14, *Drugs Affecting the Reproductive Tract,* page 516.	
sulfacetamide sodium	SULTRIN* Vag. Cream; Tablets SEBIZON Lotion (G)† BLEPH–10 or –30 BLEPHAMIDE* S.O.P. CETAMIDE Oint. ISOPTO CETAMIDE Soln. METIMYD* Oint. OPTIMYD* Soln. SULF–10	intravag. topical ophth.	See Chapter 14, *Drugs Affecting the Reproductive Tract,* page 516. See Chapter 9, *Drugs Affecting the Skin,* page 418. See Chapter 11, *Drugs Affecting the Eye,* page 443.	
sulfachlorpyridazine	SONILYN	po	**Initial:** 2–4 gm/day **Maintenance:** 2–4 gm/ day divided in 3–6 doses	**Initial:** 75 mg/kg/day **Maintenance:** 150 mg/kg/ day divided in 4–6 doses; maximum: 6 gm/day
sulfacytine	RENOQUID	po	**Initial:** 500 mg, then 250 mg qid	Not recommended in children under 14 yrs.
sulfadiazine	(G)† COCO-DIAZINE CREMODIAZINE SULADYNE*	po	**Initial:** 2–4 gm **Maintenance:** 1 gm every 4–6 hrs.	**Initial:** 75 mg/kg/day **Maintenance:** 150 mg/kg/ day in 4–6 doses; maximum: 6 gm/day
sulfameter	SULLA	po	**Initial:** 500 mg tid **Maintenance:** 500 mg. od	Not established

*Contains more than one active ingredient.
†(G) Designates availability as a generic product.

(continued overleaf)

GENERIC NAME	TRADE NAME	ROUTE OF ADMIN.	USUAL DAILY DOSAGE	
			ADULTS	INFANTS AND CHILDREN
sulfamethizole	THIOSULFIL FORTE	po	0.5–1 gm tid or qid	30–45 mg/kg/day divided in 4 doses
sulfamethoxazole	AZO GANTANOL* BACTRIM* GANTANOL SEPTRA*	po	**Initial:** 2 gm/day **Maintenance:** 2 gm/ day divided in 2 doses	**Initial:** 50–60 mg/kg/day **Maintenance:** 50–60 mg/ kg/day divided in 2 doses
sulfamethoxypyridazine	MIDICEL	po	**Initial:** 1 gm/day **Maintenance:** 0.5 gm/day	**Initial:** 30 mg/kg/day **Maintenance:** 15 mg/kg/ day in divided doses
sulfanilamide	(G)† SULFAMAL* VAGITROL Cr., Supp.	intravag.	See Chapter 14, *Drugs Affecting the Reproductive Tract,* page 512.	
sulfasalazine	AZULFIDINE S.A.S.–500 SULCOLON	po	2–4 gm/day in evenly divided doses	30–60 mg/kg/day divided in 3–6 doses
sulfathiazole	SULTRIN* Vag Cream Tab TRIPLE SULFA Cream	intravag.	See Chapter 14, *Drugs Affecting the Reproductive Tract,* page 516.	
sulfinpyrazone	ANTURANE	po	See Chapter 13, *Drugs Affecting the Musculoskeletal System,* page 485.	
sulfisoxazole	(G)† AZO-GANTRISIN* GANTRISIN SK-SOXAZOLE SODIZOLE SOXOMIDE	po	**Initial:** 2–4 gm 1st dose **Maintenance:** 4–8 gm/day divided in 3–6 doses	**Initial:** 75 mg/kg/day **Maintenance:** 150 mg/ kg/day divided in 4–6 doses
	VAGILIA Vag. Cream	intravag.	See Chapter 14, *Drugs Affecting the Reproductive Tract,* page 516.	
sulfisoxazole acetyl	GANTRISIN	po/iv/im	Same as sulfixoxazole	
sulfisoxazole diolamine	GANTRISIN	sc	**Initial:** 50 mg/kg 1st dose **Maintenance:** 100 mg/ kg/day divided in 3–4 doses	Not established

*Contains more than one active ingredient.
†(G) Designates availability as a generic product.

(continued facing page)

GENERIC NAME	TRADE NAME	ROUTE OF ADMIN.	USUAL DAILY DOSAGE	
			ADULTS	INFANTS AND CHILDREN
sulfisoxazole diolamine, continued	GANTRISIN	iv	**Initial:** 50 mg/kg/day **Maintenance:** 100 mg/ kg/day divided in 4 doses	Not established
	GANTRISIN	im	**Initial:** 50 mg/kg/day **Maintenance:** 100 mg/ kg/day divided in 2 or 3 doses	Not established
	GANTRISIN	ophth.	See Chapter 11, *Drugs Affecting the Eye,* page 444.	

PHARMACOLOGY

The sulfonamides exert bacteriostatic activity by preventing growth and multiplication of susceptible bacteria. When used for treating urinary tract infections, the sulfonamides may be bactericidal because of the high concentration achieved in the urine.

The sulfonamides, unless designed for local effects within the gastrointestinal tract, are rapidly absorbed, usually in the small intestine, following oral administration. They are inactivated by the liver by acetylation or conjugation. Excretion is primarily by the kidneys. Small amounts are excreted also in the feces, bile, milk, and other secretions. They are distributed throughout tissues in the body.

Certain bacteria develop resistance to the sulfonamides and cross resistance can then occur with other sulfonamides.

For treating urinary tract infections, a sulfonamide such as sulfisoxazole, which is excreted in the active rather than the acetylated form, should be used. For treating infections within the gastrointestinal tract certain sulfonamides such as phthalysulfathiazole and succinylsulfathiazole, which are poorly absorbed, are indicated.

In general, when applied topically sulfonamides are of little value since pus and cellular debris usually inhibit their action. However, mafenide acetate, which is bacteriostatic against both gram-negative and gram-positive organisms, including *Pseudomonas aeruginosa* and certain strains of anaerobes, diffuses through devascularized areas of tissue and is particularly useful in treating second and third degree burns. Changes in the acidity of the environment by pus and serum do not interfere with the activity of mafenide.

The sulfonamides are of value in treating certain infections of the eye and also certain forms of vaginitis. For additional information, see Chapter 11, *Drugs Affecting the Eye*, page 444, and Chapter 14, *Drugs Affecting the Reproductive Tract*, page 515.

SPECIAL PRECAUTIONS

• Since the sulfonamides can pass into the fetus and into the milk of lactating mothers, do not use in nursing mothers; kernicterus may develop in the infant.

• Note that *in vitro* sensitivity tests are not always reliable. When the patient is already taking sulfonamides, follow-up cultures should have aminobenzoic added to the culture media.

• May cause photosensitivity.

• Cross sensitization can occur between any of the thiazides including those used for hypertension, diuresis, hyperglycemia, or carbonic anhydrase inhibition.

• Use with extreme caution in patients with renal impairment.

• Safe use in pregnancy has not been established.

• Do not administer to patients with intestinal or urinary tract obstruction.

ADVERSE EFFECTS

CNS EFFECTS: malaise, headache, lassitude, dizziness, mental depression, psychoses, peripheral neuritis, insomnia

CARDIOVASCULAR EFFECTS: periarteritis, nodosalike vascular lesions, vasculitis

URINARY TRACT EFFECTS: toxic nephrosis with oliguria, anuria, crystalluria, gross or microscopic hematuria

GASTROINTESTINAL EFFECTS: nausea, vomiting, abdominal pain, anorexia, stomatitis, pancreatitis

METABOLIC AND ENDOCRINE EFFECTS: hypoglycemia, goiter production rarely

HEPATIC EFFECTS: hepatitis with focal or diffuse necrosis, cholestatic jaundice

HEMATOLOGIC EFFECTS: leukopenia, granulocytopenia, agranulocytopenia, aplastic anemia, thrombopenia, hypoprothrombinemia, methemoglobinemia, periarteritis nodosa, LE phenomenon

ALLERGIC EFFECTS: urticaria, purpura, rash, serum-sicknesslike syndrome, erythema multiforme, exfoliative dermatitis, anaphylactoid reactions, allergic myocarditis

DERMATOLOGIC EFFECTS: photosensitivity, erythema nodosum, exfoliative dermatitis, cyanosis

OTIC EFFECTS: tinnitus

LOCAL EFFECTS: pain, burning sensation

CLINICAL GUIDELINES

ADMINISTRATION:

• Fluids are restricted only to obtain a high urine concentration of drug in urinary tract infections. The daily fluid intake should be between 3000 and 4000 ml for the average adult.

• If the urine is acidic, give alkalinizing agents such as sodium bicarbonate concomitantly.

• Administer drugs immediately after eating to minimize gastrointestinal disturbances.

• Wounds should be cleansed and debrided prior to application; use sterile technique.

EFFECTS:

• If a rash develops, terminate therapy immediately.

• In patients with impaired renal function, adjust dose accordingly.

• Sulfonamides may enhance hypoglycemia caused by tolbutamide.

• Urine may be discolored brown or orange-yellow.

• Occasionally white fabrics in contact with sulfacetamide sodium lotion may become discolored (yellowish), but this discoloration can be removed by ordinary laundering.

DRUG INTERACTIONS:

• Do not mix sulfisoxazole diolamine with parenteral fluids; precipitation may occur.

• May increase the effects of oral anticoagulants, oral antidiabetic preparations, methotrexate, phenytoin; dosage adjustment may be necessary.

• Sulfisoxazole may decrease the effects of penicillin.

• Local anesthetics related to PABA may antagonize the action of the sulfonamides (applied topically).

OVERDOSAGE/ANTIDOTE:

• Overdosage consists of an exaggeration

of the adverse effects, primarily, nausea and vomiting; also abdominal pain, and possibly diarrhea; blood may be noted in the urine; reduced urine formation.
• There is no specific antidote. Treat supportively.

• Excessive topical application of mafenide may result in acidosis because of carbonic anhydrase inhibition. Accidental ingestion has resulted in diarrhea.
• There is no specific antidote. Treat acidosis by restoring acid-base balance.

Tetracyclines

GENERAL CLINICAL USES
The tetracyclines are broad-spectrum antibiotics useful in infections caused by susceptible strains of *Escherichia coli, Enterobacter aerogenes, Shigella* species, *Mima* species and *Herellea* species, *Hemophilus influenzae, Klebsiella* species, streptococci, *Diplococcus pneumoniae, Staphylococcus aureus, Neisseria gonorrhoeae, Treponema pallidum* and *Treponema pertenue, Listeria monocytogenes, Clostridium* species, *Bacillus anthracis, Fusobacterium fusiforme, Actinomyces* species, rickettsiae, *Mycoplasma pneumoniae*; agents of psittacosis, ornithosis, lymphogranuloma venereum and granuloma inguinale; *Borrelia recurrentis, Hemophilus ducreyi, Bartonella bacilliformis, Pasteurella pestis, Pasteurella tularensis, Bacteroides species, Vibrio coma, Vibrio fetus, Brucella* species; adjunctive to amebicides in acute intestinal amebiasis; in severe acne.

Applied topically, tetracycline hydrochloride is useful in treating acne vulgaris.

SPECIFIC PRODUCTS AND DOSAGES
Appropriate susceptibility and identification studies should be performed. However, therapy may be initiated while awaiting the laboratory results. Dosage adjustment may be necessary, depending upon the infecting organism and the severity of the infection.

GENERIC NAME	TRADE NAME	ROUTE OF ADMIN.	USUAL DAILY DOSAGE	
			ADULTS	**CHILDREN**
demeclocycline hydrochloride	DECLOMYCIN	po	150 mg qid or 300 mg bid	3–6 mg/lb/day divided in 2 or 4 doses
doxycycline hyclate	VIBRAMYCIN Hyclate	iv	**Initial:** 200 mg/day then 200 mg/day divided in 2 doses	Not recommended in children under 8 yrs; children weighing 100 lb or less: 1–2 mg/lb

(continued overleaf)

GENERIC NAME	TRADE NAME	ROUTE OF ADMIN.	USUAL DAILY DOSAGE	
			ADULTS	**CHILDREN**
doxycycline hyclate	VIBRAMYCIN Hyclate	po	**Initial:** 100 mg bid	Under 100 lbs.: **Initial:** 2 mg/lb/day divided in 2 equal doses
	DOXY-II		**Maintenance:** 50–100 mg/bid	**Maintenance:** 1 mg/lb/day as a single dose or divided in 2 doses
doxycycline calcium	(G)† VIBRAMYCIN Calcium	po	See *Doxycycline hyclate*	
doxycycline monohydrate	VIBRAMYCIN Monohydrate	po	See *Doxycycline hyclate*	
methacycline hydrochloride	RONDOMYCIN	po	600 mg/day in 2–4 doses	3–6 mg/lb/day divided in 2–4 doses
minocycline hydrochloride	MINOCIN VECTRIN	po	**Initial:** 200 mg/day **Maintenance:** 100 mg bid	**Initial:** 4 mg/kg/day **Maintenance:** 2 mg/kg bid
		iv	**Initial:** 200 mg/day **Maintenance:** 100 mg bid; maximum: 400 mg per 24 hrs.	**Initial:** 4 mg/kg/day **Maintenance:** 2 mg/kg bid
oxytetracycline	(G)† TERRAMYCIN TERRASTATIN*	po	1–2 gm/day divided in 4 equal doses	25–50 mg/kg/day divided in 4 equal doses
	TERRAMYCIN IM	im	250 mg/day	15–25 mg/kg/day
	TERRAMYCIN IV	iv	250–500 mg every 12 hrs; max. 500 mg every 6 hr	12 mg/kg/day divided in 2 doses
	TERRA-CORTRIL*	topical	See Chapter 9, *Drugs Affecting the Skin,* page 418.	
	TERRA-CORTRIL*	ophth.	See Chapter 11, *Drugs Affecting the Eye,* page 443.	
	TERRA-MYCIN* with Polymixin B	vaginal	See Chapter 14, *Drugs Affecting the Reproductive Tract,* page 516.	
oxytetracycline calcium	TERRAMYCIN Calcium	po	See *Oxytetracycline* above	
oxytetracycline hydrochloride	TERRAMYCIN OXY-KESSO OXY-TETRACHELLE	po	See *Oxytetracycline* above	
tetracycline/ tetracycline hydrochloride	(G)† PANMYCIN SUMYCIN TETRACYN SK-TETRACYCLINE ACHROMYCIN	po	1–2 gm/day divided in 2–4 equal doses	25–50 mg/kg/day in 2–4 equal doses
	ACHROMYCIN IM	im	250 mg/day or 300 mg divided in 2 or 3 doses	15–25 mg/kg divided in 2 or 3 doses; maximum: 250 mg/day
	ACHROMYCIN IV	iv	250–500 mg bid do not exceed 500 mg/6 hr	12 mg/kg/day divided in 2 doses; 10–20 mg/kg may be given
	ACHROMYCIN Ophth. Soln., Oint.	ophth.	See Chapter 11, *Drugs Affecting the Eye,* page 444.	
	TOPICYCLINE	topical	See Chapter 9, *Drugs Affecting the Skin,* page 418.	
tetracycline phosphate complex	TETREX	po	250 mg qid	25 mg/kg/day divided in 4 equal doses

*Contains more than one active ingredient.
†(G) Designates availability as a generic product.

PHARMACOLOGY

The tetracyclines, primarily bacteriostatic agents, exert their effect by inhibiting protein synthesis. Following oral administration, the tetracyclines are absorbed rapidly but incompletely. Consequently, they alter the intestinal flora. They are concentrated by the liver and excreted in the urine by glomerular filtration and also the feces in a biologically active form. The tetracyclines diffuse into the brain, saliva, pleural fluid, semen, and prostatic fluid; they are also found in the milk of lactating mothers. Cross resistance among the tetracyclines is common.

The phosphate complex of tetracycline is absorbed more rapidly and more completely from the gastrointestinal tract than the free base or its salt; higher blood levels are produced by the phosphate complex than other forms. Doxycycline hydrochloride, due to its virtually complete absorption, causes fewer side effects of the lower bowel, particularly diarrhea, than the other tetracyclines.

When the tetracyclines are applied topically, absorption is mimimal from the skin.

SPECIAL PRECAUTIONS
• In patients with renal dysfunction, doses over 2 grams daily administered intravenously have been associated with liver failure.
• Monitor patients for renal and hepatic dysfunction, particularly pregnant patients and those with pyelonephritis.
• Administration during the last half of pregnancy and in children up to 8 years may cause permanent discoloration (yellow-gray-brown) of teeth; enamel hypoplasia has also been reported.
• An increase in BUN may occur because of the antimetabolic action of the tetracyclines; this is no problem in patients with normal renal function but in patients with significantly impaired renal function, azotemia, hyperphosphatemia, and acidosis may occur.
• Reduce dosage in patients with renal impairment.
• Overgrowth of nonsusceptible organisms including fungi may occur; discontinue therapy and reinstitute appropriate therapy.
• Do not use in patients with a history of hypersensitivity to any of the tetracyclines or related compounds.
• All tetracyclines form a stable calcium complex in bone-forming tissue. A reversible decrease in fibula growth rate has been observed in premature infants given tetracyclines.
• Cross sensitization among the tetracyclines is very common.
• Photosensitivity manifested by an exaggerated sunburn reaction has been observed in some individuals taking tetracyclines. Patients who are apt to be exposed to direct sunlight or ultraviolet light should be advised that this reaction can occur. This reaction has not occurred with minocycline hydrochloride.
• Safe use in pregnancy has not been established.

ADVERSE EFFECTS
CNS EFFECTS: dizziness, headache, lightheadedness
URINARY TRACT EFFECTS: increased BUN
GASTROINTESTINAL EFFECTS: anorexia, nausea, vomiting, diarrhea, glossitis, dysphagia, enterocolitis, inflammatory lesions with monilial overgrowth in the anogenital region
METABOLIC AND ENDOCRINE EFFECTS: brown-black microscopic discoloration of the thyroid gland without alteration of thyroid function results with prolonged administration
HEPATIC EFFECTS: hepatic cholestasis usually associated with high dosages

HEMATOLOGIC EFFECTS: hemolytic anemia, thrombocytopenia, neutropenia, eosinophilia

ALLERGIC EFFECTS: urticaria, angioneurotic edema, anaphylaxis, anaphylactoid purpura, pericarditis, exacerbation of systemic lupus erythematosus; bulging fontanels in young infants

DERMATOLOGIC EFFECTS: maculopapular and erythematous rashes, exfoliative dermatitis, photosensitivity resembling a severe sunburn

LOCAL EFFECTS: irritation and pain after intramuscular injection; thrombophlebitis with intravenous administration; allergic reactions occasionally severe dermatitis, stinging, burning, slight yellowing of skin with topical administration

CLINICAL GUIDELINES

ADMINISTRATION:
• Administer oral preparations at least 1 hour before meals or 2 hours after meals.
• Do not give pediatric oral dosage with milk formula.
• Inadvertent subcutaneous injection may cause pain and induration which may be relieved by applying an ice pack.
• Warn patients that photosensitivity manifested as an exaggerated sunburn reaction may occur, particularly if patients are exposed to direct sunlight or ultraviolet light.

EFFECTS:
• With doxycycline hydrochloride fewer gastrointestinal side effects occur, particularly diarrhea, because of the complete absorption of the drug.

DRUG INTERACTIONS:
• Since tetracyclines depress prothrombin activity, patients receiving anticoagulants may require lower doses of the anticoagulant.
• Avoid administering tetracycline in conjunction with penicillin since the bacteriostatic drug may interfere with the bactericidal action of penicillin.
• Antacids containing aluminum, calcium, or magnesium, and also some foods and dairy products, impair absorption and should not be given to patients taking tetracyclines.
• When administering tetracyclines intravenously, avoid use of calcium-containing solutions since these tend to form precipitates especially in neutral or alkaline solutions.

OVERDOSAGE/ANTIDOTE:
• Overdosage is characterized by an exaggeration of the adverse effects.
• There is no specific antidote. Tetracyclines can be removed slowly by dialysis using the artificial kidney; chlortetracycline is not removed by this technique.

Antifungal/Anticandidal Agents

GENERAL CLINICAL USES
Infections caused by fungi are divided into three groups based on the type of infection and the infecting organism.

I. *Systemic fungal infections*, which include histoplasmosis, coccidioidomycosis, North American blastomycosis, paracoccidioidomycosis (South American blastomycosis), sporotrichosis, cryptococcosis, penicilliosis, aspergillosis, mucormycosis, and chromoblastomycosis. Amphotericin B, hydroxystilbamidine isethionate, and flucytosine are used for infections by susceptible strains of organisms causing these infections.

II. *Dermatophytic infections* are caused primarily by species of *Epidermophyton*, *Trichophyton*, *Microsporum*, and also *Malassezia furfur*. Therapy for infections caused by these organisms may be systemic or topical. Effective agents include griseofulvin, tolnaftate, haloprogin, iodochlorhydroxyquin, acrisorcin, undecylenic acid and salts, selenium sulfide, amphotericin B, clotrimazole, and miconazole nitrate. Prior to therapy the infecting organism should be identified by microscopic examination or culture. Medication should be continued until the infecting organism is eradicated.

III. *Candidiasis (moniliasis)* caused by *Candida albicans, C. krusei, C. tropicalis*, and *C. pseudotropicalis* is treated primarily by the topical route but parenteral medication is available for systemic infections. Drugs used in the treatment of candidiasis include amphotericin B, flucytosine, nystatin, candicidin, and gentian violet.

SPECIFIC PRODUCTS AND DOSAGES: SYSTEMIC FUNGAL INFECTIONS

GENERIC NAME	TRADE NAME	ROUTE OF ADMIN.	USUAL DOSAGE
amphotericin B	FUNGIZONE	iv	Administer by slow iv infusion over 6 hr., 0.1 mg/ml; 0.25 mg/kg/day and increase as tolerance permits to 1.0 mg/kg/day; do not exceed 1.5 mg/kg/day
	FUNGIZONE	topical	See Chapter 9, page 409.
	FUNGIZONE	ophth.	See Chapter 11, page 439.
flucytosine	ANCOBON	po	50–150 mg/kg/day qid
hydroxystilbamidine isethionate	(G)*	iv	Infuse 225 mg in 200 ml 5% dextrose injection or sodium chloride injection over 24 hrs.; total course is 5–25 gm

*(G) Designates availability as a generic product.

Amphotericin B

PHARMACOLOGY

Amphotericin B is used primarily for treatment of patients with progressive and potentially fatal fungal infections. Amphotericin B is fungistatic rather than fungicidal in the concentrations obtained in body fluids following intravenous administration. The drug is not absorbed when administered orally. Amphotericin B is excreted slowly by the kidneys. It acts by inhibiting the permeability of the cell membrane.

Amphotericin B is also effective when applied topically for monilial vulvovaginitis and other mucocutaneous infections due to *Candida* species. For information concerning topical application see *Candidiasis* and also Chapter 9, *Drugs Affecting the Skin*, page 419.

SPECIAL PRECAUTIONS

• Do not use in patients with a history of hypersensitivity unless in the opinion of the physician, the condition requiring treatment is life-threatening and amenable only to amphotericin B therapy.
• Safe use in pregnancy has not been established.
• Administer intravenously only in hospitalized patients or those under close clinical observation because adverse effects are potentially dangerous.
• Monitor BUN and serum creatinine at least weekly during therapy; it may be necessary to reduce dosage until renal function improves.
• Weekly determinations of blood picture and serum potassium levels should be made.
• Use with caution, if at all, in patients with impaired renal function.

ADVERSE EFFECTS

CNS EFFECTS: fever, shaking chills, headache, malaise, peripheral neuropathy, convulsions
CARDIOVASCULAR EFFECTS: phlebitis, local venous pain at injection site, thrombophlebitis, ventricular fibrillation, cardiac arrest, hypertension, hypotension
URINARY TRACT EFFECTS: anuria, oliguria, azotemia
GASTROINTESTINAL EFFECTS: anorexia, vomiting, nausea, dyspepsia, cramping epigastric pain, diarrhea, malaise, hemorrhagic gastroenteritis
METABOLIC AND ENDOCRINE EFFECTS: weight loss, hypokalemia
HEPATIC EFFECTS: acute liver failure
HEMATOLOGIC EFFECTS: normochromic, normocytic anemia; leukopenia, agranulocytosis, eosinophilia, leukocytosis
ALLERGIC EFFECTS: anaphylactoid reactions
DERMATOLOGIC EFFECTS: maculopapular rash, pruritus
OPHTHALMIC EFFECTS: blurred vision, and diplopia
OTIC EFFECTS: hearing loss, tinnitus, transient vertigo
MUSCULOSKELETAL EFFECTS: muscle and joint pain
LOCAL EFFECTS: drying, erythema, pruritus, burning sensation

CLINICAL GUIDELINES

ADMINISTRATION:
• Administer slowly.
• Extravasation may cause irritation.
• Amphotericin B is heat labile and sensitive to light; protect from light during administration.
• Cream may discolor the skin minimally; the lotion and ointment may stain nail lesions.
EFFECTS:
• Adding a small amount of heparin to the infusion may lessen the incidence of thrombophlebitis.
• Aspirin or antihistamines may modify the severity of adverse effects.
• Discoloration of fabrics by the ointment may be removed by applying a standard cleaning fluid. Discoloration by cream may be removed with soap and water.
DRUG INTERACTIONS:
• Do not administer corticosteroids con-

comitantly unless they are necessary to control drug reactions.
- Administer only with great caution other nephrotoxic antibiotics and antineoplastic agents concomitantly.
- Do not mix with antibiotics or sodium chloride; precipitation may occur.

OVERDOSAGE/ANTIDOTE:
- Overdosage is characterized by an exaggeration of the adverse effects.
- There is no specific antidote. Treat symptomatically.

Flucytosine

PHARMACOLOGY

Flucytosine is effective in infections caused by *Candida* and/or *Cryptococcus*. Most strains of *Cryptococcus* have responded whereas 40 to 50 percent of *Candida* clinical isolates have been resistant. Susceptibility studies should be performed early and repeated at appropriate intervals during therapy. The mode of action of flucytosine is unknown. Flucytosine is administered orally, absorbed from the gastrointestinal tract, and excreted primarily by the kidneys.

SPECIAL PRECAUTIONS

- Do not use in patients with a history of hypersensitivity to flucytosine or related compounds.
- Use with extreme caution in patients with impaired renal function and with bone marrow depression.
- Monitoring of renal, hepatic, and hematologic parameters before and during therapy is essential.
- Safe use in pregnancy has not been established.

ADVERSE EFFECTS

CNS EFFECTS: confusion, hallucinations, headache, sedation, vertigo

URINARY TRACT EFFECTS: increased BUN, increased serum creatinine

GASTROINTESTINAL EFFECTS: nausea, vomiting, diarrhea

HEPATIC EFFECTS: elevation of hepatic enzymes (SGOT, SGPT, alkaline phosphatase)

HEMATOLOGIC EFFECTS: anemia, leukopenia, thrombocytopenia

DERMATOLOGIC EFFECTS: rash

CLINICAL GUIDELINES

ADMINISTRATION:
- Nausea and vomiting may be reduced or avoided if capsules are given a few at a time over a 15-minute period.
- If the patient has impaired renal function, the initial dose should be at the lower level.

DRUG INTERACTIONS:
- Do not administer concomitantly other drugs with neurotoxic or nephrotoxic effects such as gentamicin, kanamycin, and other aminoglycosides.

OVERDOSAGE/ANTIDOTE:
- Overdosage is characterized by an exaggeration of the adverse effects.
- There is no specific antidote. Treat supportively.

Hydroxystilbamidine Isethionate

PHARMACOLOGY

Hydroxystilbamidine isethionate is not absorbed from the gastrointestinal tract; therefore, it is administered parenterally only. The mechanism of action may be through inhibition of enzymes. Hydroxystilbamidine isethionate is excreted slowly in the bile and urine; tissue concentrations, particularly liver and kidneys, remain high for a period of time after treatment.

SPECIAL PRECAUTIONS

- Use cautiously in patients with impaired renal and hepatic function.

- Advise patients to avoid excessive or direct sunlight.
- Safe use in pregnancy has not been established.
- Do not administer to patients with a history of hypersensitivity to hydroxystilbamidine isethionate and related compounds.

ADVERSE EFFECTS
CNS EFFECTS: dizziness, headache, flushing, syncope, paresthesias, degenerative changes, trigeminal neuralgia
RESPIRATORY EFFECTS: dyspnea
CARDIOVASCULAR EFFECTS: hypotension, tachycardia, circulatory collapse
URINARY TRACT EFFECTS: incontinence, renal insufficiency
AUTONOMIC EFFECTS: sweating
GASTROINTESTINAL EFFECTS: nausea, vomiting, fecal incontinence
METABOLIC AND ENDOCRINE EFFECTS: hypoglycemia, salivation, edema of face and eyelids.
HEPATIC EFFECTS: hepatitis

DERMATOLOGIC EFFECTS: formication
OPHTHALMIC EFFECTS: light sensitivity

CLINICAL GUIDELINES
ADMINISTRATION:
- Protect freshly prepared solutions from light and heat.
- Infuse slowly over a period of at least 30 minutes, preferably 60 minutes.
- Monitor renal and hepatic functions frequently.
EFFECTS:
- Exposure to sunlight (excessive) may result in severe erythema.
- This drug is a tissue irritant; patient may have pain at site of injection, cold applications may be indicated.
DRUG INTERACTIONS:
- Heparin and hydroxystilbamidine isethionate are compatible in solution.
OVERDOSAGE/ANTIDOTE:
- Overdosage is characterized by an exaggeration of the adverse effects.
- There is no specific antidote. Treat supportively.

SPECIFIC PRODUCTS AND DOSAGES: DERMATOPHYTIC INFECTIONS

GENERIC NAME	TRADE NAME	ROUTE OF ADMIN.	USUAL DOSAGE
acrisorcin	AKRINOL	topical	Apply small quantity to affected area bid
clotrimazole	LOTRIMIN MYCELEX	topical	Apply bid
	GYNE-LOTRIMIN	intravag.	See Chapter 14, *Drugs Affecting the Reproductive Tract*, page 515.
griseofulvin, ultramicrosize	GRIS-PEG	po	**Adults:** 250–500 mg/day in single or divided doses **Children:** 2.5 mg/lb/day
griseofulvin, microsize	GRISACTIN GRIFULVIN V FULVICIN U/V	po	**Adults:** 0.5–1.0 gm/day in single or divided doses **Children:** 5 mg/lb/day
haloprogin	HALOTEX	topical	Apply liberally bid

(continued facing page)

GENERIC NAME	TRADE NAME	ROUTE OF ADMIN.	USUAL DOSAGE
iodochlorhydroxyquin	(G)† HYSONE* NYSTAFORM* RACET* VIOFORM*	topical	bid or tid; continue 1 week after symptoms abate
miconazole nitrate	MICATIN MICATIN MONISTAT 7	topical intravag.	Cover affected area bid See Chapter 14, *Drugs Affecting the Reproductive Tract*, page 516.
selenium sulfide	EXSEL SELSUN	topical	Cover affected area and lather; rinse after 5–10 min; once daily
sodium thiosulfate	TINVER Lotion	topical	See Chapter 9, *Drugs Affecting the Skin*, page 419.
tolnaftate	TINACTIN	topical	Apply liberally bid
undecylenic acid	(G) DESENEX	topical	Apply liberally bid
undecylenate calcium	CRUEX Powder	topical	Apply liberally bid
undecylenate zinc	CRUEX Cream	topical	Apply liberally bid

*Contains more than one active ingredient.
†(G) Designates availability as a generic product.

Acrisorcin

PHARMACOLOGY

Acrisorcin is useful in treating tinea versicolor caused by *Malassezia furfur*. Following topical application, absorption does not occur.

SPECIAL PRECAUTIONS
• Do not use in any patient with a history of hypersensitivity to acrisorcin.
• Do not use around the eyes.

ADVERSE EFFECTS
LOCAL EFFECTS: blisters, erythematous vesicular eruptions, hives, pruritus; burning in patients with eczema

CLINICAL GUIDELINES
ADMINISTRATION:
• Warn patients that pruritus may occur after exposure to ultraviolet light.
• Advise patients to take a daily soapy bath and use a stiff brush on the lesions. Remove all soap, dry, then apply acrisorcin.
• Towels and all clothing in contact with the lesions must be laundered after each use.
EFFECTS:
• If irritation or sensitization occurs, discontinue therapy immediately.
• Eczema may become slightly worse after treatment with acrisorcin.

Clotrimazole

PHARMACOLOGY
Clotrimazole is a broad-spectrum topically applied fungicidal agent which inhibits the growth of *Malassezia furfur*,

Trichophyton rubrum, T. mentagrophytes, Epidermophyton floccosum, Microsporum canis, and *Candida albicans*. No single-step or multiple-step resistance has developed during successive passages of *Candida albicans* and *T. mentagrophytes*. Small quantities of clotrimazole are absorbed following topical application.

SPECIAL PRECAUTIONS
• Do not use in patients with a history of hypersensitivity to clotrimazole.
• Safe use in pregnancy has not been established.
• If irritation or sensitivity develops, discontinue.

ADVERSE EFFECTS
LOCAL EFFECTS: erythema, stinging, blistering, peeling, edema, pruritus, urticaria, general irritation

CLINICAL GUIDELINES
ADMINISTRATION:
• Advise patient in hygienic practices.
• Relief of pruritus usually occurs within the first week of treatment.
EFFECTS:
• If no clinical improvement is noted after 4 weeks, review diagnosis.

Griseofulvin, Ultramicrosize
Griseofulvin, Microsize

PHARMACOLOGY
Griseofulvin, a fungistatic agent, is useful in treating infections caused by *Trichophyton rubrum, T. tonsurans, T. mentagrophytes, T. interdigitales, T. verracosum,* *T. megnini, T. gallinae, T. crateriform, T. sulfureum, T. schoenleini, Microsporum audouini, M. canis, M. gypseum, Epidermophyton floccosum*. It is not effective in bacterial infections, candidiasis, histoplasmosis, actinomycosis, sporotrichosis, chronoblastomycosis, coccidioidomycosis, North American blastomycosis, cryptococcosis, tinea versicolor, and nocardiosis.

After oral administration, griseofulvin is absorbed from the gastrointestinal tract and excreted rapidly in the urine. The drug is tightly bound to new keratin which becomes highly resistant to fungal invasions. Griseofulvin has a greater affinity for diseased than new tissues.

SPECIAL PRECAUTIONS
• Do not administer to patients with porphyria, hepatocellular failure, and to patients with a history of hypersensitivity to griseofulvin.
• Safe use in pregnancy has not been established.
• Monitor renal, hepatic, and hematopoietic systems periodically.
• The possibility of cross sensitivity between penicillin and griseofulvin exists.

ADVERSE EFFECTS
CNS EFFECTS: paresthesias of the hands, feet; headache, fatigue, dizziness, isomnia, mental confusion, impairment of performance of routine activities.
URINARY TRACT EFFECTS: proteinuria occurs rarely
GASTROINTESTINAL EFFECTS: oral thrush, nausea, vomiting, epigastric distress, and diarrhea
HEMATOLOGIC EFFECTS: leukopenia rarely; granulocytopenia
ALLERGIC EFFECTS: skin rash, urticaria, angioneurotic edema rarely

ADMINISTRATION:
- Caution patients to avoid exposure to intense natural or artificial sunlight since photosensitivity reactions may occur; lupus erythematosus may be aggravated.
- Advise patients in proper hygienic procedures.
- Griseofulvin is absorbed more rapidly when taken with a fat meal.

EFFECTS:
- Symptomatic relief should be obtained in 48 to 96 hours.
- An oral dose of 125 mg griseofulvin, ultramicrosize, is biologically equivalent to 250 mg griseofulvin, microsize.

DRUG INTERACTIONS:
- Griseofulvin decreases the activity of warfarin-type anticoagulants; dosage adjustment may be necessary.
- Barbiturates usually depress griseofulvin activity.

OVERDOSAGE/ANTIDOTE:
- Overdosage is characterized by an exaggeration of the adverse effects.
- There is no specific antidote.

Haloprogin

PHARMACOLOGY
Haloprogin is an antifungal agent useful in infections caused by *Trichophyton rubrum, T. tonsurans, T. mentagrophytes, Microsporum canis, Epidermophyton floccosum,* and *Malassazia furfur.* When applied topically, absorption is minimal.

SPECIAL PRECAUTIONS
- Safe use in pregnancy has not been established.
- Do not use in patients with a history of hypersensitivity to haloprogin or related compounds.
- In mixed or nonsusceptible fungal infections, supplemental systemic medication may be required.
- Keep out of the eyes.

ADVERSE EFFECTS
LOCAL EFFECTS: irritation, burning sensation, vesicle formation, increased maceration, pruritus, exacerbation of pre-existing lesions.

CLINICAL GUIDELINES
ADMINISTRATION:
- Advise patient in hygienic practices.
- Cleanse skin thoroughly before application.

EFFECTS:
- If no improvement occurs in 4 weeks, discontinue therapy.
- If sensitization or irritation occurs, discontinue and institute appropriate therapy if necessary.

Iodochlorhydroxyquin

PHARMACOLOGY
Iodochlorhydroxyquin is available commercially in combination with hydrocortisone and nystatin for topical administration. Idochlorhydroxyquin is an antifungal and antibacterial agent which may be absorbed through the skin.

SPECIAL PRECAUTIONS
- Safe use in pregnancy has not been established.
- Do not use in patients with a history of hypersensitivity to iodine compounds.
- Keep out of the eyes.
- If irritation or sensitization develops, discontinue use.

ADVERSE EFFECTS
LOCAL EFFECTS: irritation, rash, burning, pruritus, hypersensitivity

CLINICAL GUIDELINES

ADMINISTRATION:

• Advise patients that skin, hair, or fabrics may be stained. Advise patients in hygienic practices.

DRUG INTERACTIONS:

• If thyroid tests are contemplated, wait at least 1 month after discontinuance of therapy to perform these tests.

• The ferric chloride test for phenylketonuria (PKU) can yield a positive result if iodochlorhydroxyquin is present.

Miconazole Nitrate

PHARMACOLOGY

Miconazole nitrate, an antifungal agent, is effective in the topical treatment of tinea pedis, tinea cruris, and tinea corporis caused by *Trichophyton mentagrophytes, T. rubrum, Epidermophyton floccosum,* and also cutaneous infections caused by *Candida albicans,* and tinea versicolor due to *Malassezia furfur.* Miconazole nitrate inhibits the growth of the common dermatophytes.

SPECIAL PRECAUTIONS

• Discontinue medication if a reaction suggesting sensitivity or chemical irritation occurs.

• Avoid introduction into the eyes.

ADVERSE EFFECTS

LOCAL EFFECTS: irritation, burning, maceration

CLINICAL GUIDELINES

EFFECTS:

• Pruritus may be relieved in 1 week.

• If no improvement is seen after a month of treatment, redetermine diagnosis.

Selenium Sulfide

PHARMACOLOGY

Selenium sulfide, a topically applied antifungal agent, is usually formulated as a detergent suspension. It is effective in treating tinea versicolor caused by *Malassezia furfur;* also in treating suborrheic dermatitis of the scalp, including dermatides.

SPECIAL PRECAUTIONS

• Avoid contact with the eyes and genital area.

ADVERSE EFFECTS

LOCAL EFFECTS: diffuse hair loss, sensitization reactions, discoloration of the hair; oiliness of the hair and scalp may increase

CLINICAL GUIDELINES

ADMINISTRATION:

• Do not use in patients with a history of hypersensitivity to selenium sulfide.

• Absorption may occur if applied to inflamed or damaged epithelium.

• Safe use in infants has not been established.

EFFECTS:

• Gray hair may become tinted orange.

OVERDOSAGE/ANTIDOTE:

• If taken orally, selenium sulfide is readily absorbed and is toxic. Nausea and vomiting usually occur after oral ingestion. Toxicity is characterized by fatty infiltration (reversible) of the liver and renal tubular injury.

• There is no specific antidote. Induce vomiting or perform lavage. Use general supportive measures as required. Administer a purgative to hasten elimination.

Sodium Thiosulfate

PHARMACOLOGY

Sodium thiosulfate is an antifungal agent effective in most fungal infections of the skin. The action may be due to the slow release of sulfur; an acidic environment promotes the decomposition to sulfur and improves the antifungal action.

SPECIAL PRECAUTIONS

- Discontinue use if irritation or sensitivity develops.
- Do not use in or about the eyes.

Tolnaftate

PHARMACOLOGY

Tolnaftate, a fungicidal agent, is applied topically as a cream, lotion, or powder. It is effective in infections caused by *Trichophyton rubrum*, *T. mentagrophytes*, *T. tonsurans*, *Microsporum canis*, *M. audouini*, *Epidermophyton floccosum*, and tinea versicolor due to *Malassezia furfur*. It is not effective against bacteria or *Candida* species. Tolnaftate applied topically is not absorbed in any significant amount.

SPECIAL PRECAUTIONS

- If signs of sensitization or irritation occur, discontinue treatment.
- If a patient does not improve after 4 weeks treatment, the diagnosis should be reviewed.
- If infection is mixed, that is, non-susceptible fungi and bacteria, supplemental topical or systemic therapy may be necessary.
- Do not put in the eyes.

ADVERSE EFFECTS

LOCAL EFFECTS: sensitization, irritation

CLINICAL GUIDELINES

ADMINISTRATION:
- Advise patients that daily bathing will control perspiration in tinea pedis; a foot powder in the shoes and hose will help odor.
- In tinea cruris and corporis, wet compresses promote healing of exudative lesions and do not interfere with fungicidal activity.

Undecylenic Acid
Calcium Undecylenate
Zinc Undecylenate

PHARMACOLOGY

Undecylenic acid, calcium undecylenate, and zinc undecylenate are used in the treatment of athlete's foot and ringworm of the body but not of the nails and hairy area.

SPECIAL PRECAUTIONS

- Do not use near the eyes or mucous membranes.
- Do not use if the skin is broken or pustular.

ADVERSE EFFECTS

LOCAL EFFECTS: irritation rarely

CLINICAL GUIDELINES

ADMINISTRATION:
- When used in the skin, the concentration should not exceed 10 percent.
- Advise patient in hygienic procedures.

EFFECTS:
- These agents may or may not control tinea pedis and tinea capitis.

SPECIFIC PRODUCTS AND DOSAGES: CANDIDIASIS (VAGINAL, CUTANEOUS, ORAL)

GENERIC NAME	TRADE NAME	ROUTE OF ADMIN.	USUAL DAILY DOSAGE
amphotericin B	FUNGIZONE	topical	Apply liberally to lesions bid or qid; see Chapter 9, *Drugs Affecting the Skin*, page 419.
candicidin	CANDEPTIN VANOBID	intravag.	Apply bid
clotrimazole	LOTRIMIN GYNE-LOTRIMIN	topical intravag.	Apply bid Once daily at bedtime
flucytosine	ANCOBON	po	50–150 mg/kg/day divided in 4 doses
gentian violet	HYVA Vaginal Tab.	intravag.	Once daily at night
miconazole nitrate	MONISTAT 7 MICATIN	intravag. topical	Apply once daily at bedtime Apply bid
nifuroxime	MICOFUR TRICOFURON*	intravag.	Apply once or twice daily
nystatin	MYCOSTATIN NILSTAT NYSTAFORM*	po	**Infants:** 200,000 units qid **Children and adults:** 400,000-600,000 units qid
	NILSTAT Cream, Oint. MYCOSTATIN Cream Oint. Powder Vag Tabs	topical topical topical	Apply liberally od or bid; see Chapter 9, *Drugs Affecting the Skin*, page 419. Apply bid

*Contains more than one active ingredient.

Amphotericin B

For detailed information, see *Systemic Fungal Infections*, page 65.

Candicidin

PHARMACOLOGY
Candicidin has antimonilial activity against *Candida albicans* and also other candidal species. Absorption is minimal following topical administration.

SPECIAL PRECAUTIONS
• Do not use in patients with a history of hypersensitivity to candicidin. Patients should be advised to refrain from coitus or the partner should use a condom during treatment.
• Refrigerate candicidin to assure potency.

ADVERSE EFFECTS
LOCAL EFFECTS: irritation, sensitization

CLINICAL GUIDELINES
ADMINISTRATION:
- During pregnancy, insert manually rather than by ointment applicator or tablet inserter.

Clotrimazole

For detailed information, see *Dermatophytic Infections*, pages 68 and 69.

Flucytosine

For detailed information, see *Systemic Fungal Infections*, pages 65 and 67.

Gentian Violet (Methylrosaniline Chloride)

PHARMACOLOGY
Gentian violet is an effective candicidal agent and also an effective antibacterial agent for gram-positive bacteria. It is anthelmintic for *Strongyloides* and *Oxyuris*.

SPECIAL PRECAUTIONS
- Do not use in patients with a history of hypersensitivity to gentian violet.

ADVERSE EFFECTS
LOCAL EFFECTS: chemical vulvovaginitis, staining of skin

CLINICAL GUIDELINES
ADMINISTRATION:
- Advise patients that staining may occur; use a sanitary pad.
- Advise patients to refrain from coitus or partner should use a condom.

Miconazole Nitrate

PHARMACOLOGY
Miconazole nitrate is effective against *Monilia albicans* and other monilial species. The mode of action is unknown. Small amounts are absorbed from the human vagina.

SPECIAL PRECAUTIONS
- Do not use in patients with a history of hypersensitivity to miconazole nitrate.
- Do not use in first trimester of pregnancy unless the physician considers it essential to the welfare of the patient.

ADVERSE EFFECTS
LOCAL EFFECTS: vulvovaginal burning, itching, irritation
SYSTEMIC EFFECTS: headache, pelvic cramps, hives, skin rash

Nifuroxime

PHARMACOLOGY
Nifuroxime, a nitrofuran, is fungicidal. It acts by disrupting the enzymatic metabolism of the microbial cell without appreciable toxicity to human tissue.

SPECIAL PRECAUTIONS
- Do not use in patients with a history of hypersensitivity to nifuroxime.

ADVERSE EFFECTS
LOCAL EFFECTS: sensitization, irritation, burning, pruritus, erythema

Nystatin

PHARMACOLOGY
Nystatin may be administered topically, including intravaginally, or systemi-

cally. Topical or intravaginal administration is useful in treating vulvovaginal candidiasis whereas systemic administration is useful in treating intestinal infections caused by *Candida albicans* and other candidal species. Systemic administration is also useful in treating candidal infections of the oral cavity (thrush).

Nystatin is both fungistatic and fungicidal. It acts by binding sterols in the cell membrane of the fungus. It has no appreciable antibacterial activity. No detectable blood levels have been measured after intravaginal, topical, or systemic administration. Most of the unabsorbed nystatin passes through the gastrointestinal tract unchanged in the faces after oral administration.

SPECIAL PRECAUTIONS
• Do not use in patients with a history of hypersensitivity to nystatin, with viral diseases of the skin such as vaccinia and varicella, fungal diseases of the skin except candidiasis.

ADVERSE EFFECTS
LOCAL EFFECTS: irritation, hypersensitivity
GASTROINTESTINAL EFFECTS: diarrhea, gastrointestinal distress, nausea, vomiting

CLINICAL GUIDELINES
ADMINISTRATION:
• Relief should occur 24 to 72 hours after initiation of treatment.
• Advise patient in hygienic practices.

Antileprosy Agents

GENERAL CLINICAL USES
Leprosy is caused by *Mycobacterium leprae*, which is susceptible to the following agents: acetosulfone sodium, dapsone, rifampin, and sulfoxone sodium. However, dapsone is the only drug approved by the U.S. regulatory authorities.

SPECIFIC PRODUCTS AND DOSAGES

GENERIC NAME	TRADE NAME	ROUTE OF ADMIN.	USUAL DAILY DOSAGE	
			ADULTS	CHILDREN
acetosulfone sodium	PROMACETIN	po	0.5–4 gm/day in divided doses	7.1 mg/kg/day
dapsone	AVLOSULFON	po	6–10 mg/kg/wk in divided doses	1/4 to 1/2 adult dose

(continued facing page)

GENERIC NAME	TRADE NAME	ROUTE OF ADMIN.	USUAL DAILY DOSAGE	
			ADULTS	CHILDREN
rifampin	RIFADIN RIMACTANE	po	300–600 mg/day in divided doses	Not established
sulfoxone sodium	DIASONE Sodium	po	330 mg twice weekly to 6 times/week	4.7 mg/kg/day twice weekly to 6 times/week

Acetosulfone Sodium
Dapsone
Sulfoxone Sodium

PHARMACOLOGY

These agents, the sulfones, are bacteriostatic against *Mycobacterium leprae*. The mechanism of action is probably similar to that of the sulfonamides. The sulfones are absorbed slowly but nearly completely from the gastrointestinal tract and are distributed throughout all the tissues. Excretion is by way of the kidneys. The sulfones have been detected in human milk, bile, and pleural fluid.

GENERAL PRECAUTIONS

• Safe use in pregnancy has not been established.
• Do not use in patients with a history of hypersensitivity to the sulfones or related compounds.

ADVERSE EFFECTS

CNS EFFECTS: headache, nervousness, insomnia, paresthesia, reversible psychosis
URINARY TRACT EFFECTS: hematuria
GASTROINTESTINAL EFFECTS: anorexia, nausea, vomiting
HEMATOLOGIC EFFECTS: hemolysis, methemoglobinemia, hemolytic anemia, infectious-mononucleosislike syndrome, leukopenia, agranulocytosis
ALLERGIC EFFECTS: drug fever, pruritus, allergic dermatitis
DERMATOLOGIC EFFECTS: rash, cyanosis, pallor
OPHTHALMIC EFFECTS: blurred vision
MUSCULOSKELETAL EFFECTS: peripheral neuritis

CLINICAL GUIDELINES

ADMINISTRATION:
• To minimize gastrointestinal complaints, administer with meals.
• Monitor hemoglobin level periodically.
EFFECTS:
• Hemolysis occurs usually in all patients receiving sulfones; if hypoxia is manifest, inform physician immediately.
• Methemoglobinemia may occur; mucous membranes will be a brownish hue and the patient cyanotic.
DRUG INTERACTIONS:
• The sulfones and streptomycin appear to act additively.
OVERDOSAGE/ANTIDOTE:
• Overdosage is characterized by an exaggeration of the adverse effects.
• There is no specific antidote.

Rifampin

For detailed information, see *Antituberculosis Agents*, pages 85 and 93. Rifampin has been found effective in clinical experience in treating leprosy but to date is not approved by the U.S. regulatory authorities.

Antimalarial Agents

GENERAL CLINICAL USES

Malarial infections are caused by four species of protozoans: *Plasmodium fal-ciparum, P. vivax, P. malariae,* and *P. ovale.* The clinical symptoms produced by these organisms are similar. The disease is transmitted by a bite from an infected mosquito which injects sporozoites to man.

The therapy of malaria is divided into two phases: (1) drugs preventing erythrocyte invasion, also known as causal prophylactic agents; (2) suppressive drugs, which destroy the blood schizonts, including amodiaquine hydrochloride, chloroquine hydrochloride, chloroquine phosphate, hydroxychloroquine sulfate, quinine, quinine hydrochloride, quinine sulfate, and amodiaquine.

SPECIFIC PRODUCTS AND DOSAGES

GENERIC NAME	TRADE NAME	ROUTE OF ADMIN.	USUAL DOSAGE
amodiaquine hydrochloride	CAMOQUIN	po	**Acute attack:** **Adults:** 600 mg initially; 300 mg in 3 hrs.; 400 mg in 12 hrs.; 400 mg in 24 hrs. **Children:** 10 mg/kg in 3 divided doses every 12 hrs. **Suppression:** **Adults:** 300–600 mg/wk. **Children:** 5 mg/kg/wk.
chloroguanide hydrochloride	PALUDRINE GUANATROL	po	**Prophylaxis and suppression:** **Adults:** 100 mg/day **Children less than 1 yr.:** 25–50 mg/day; **1–4 yrs.:** 50 mg/day; **5–8 yrs.:** 75 mg/day
chloroquine hydrochloride	ARALEN Hydrochloride	im	**Acute Attack:** **Adults:** 200–300 mg/day; may repeat in 6 hr; do not exceed 800 mg base in 24 hr. **Children:** 5 mg base/kg; may repeat in 6 hrs; maximum: 10 mg base/kg in 24 hrs.

(continued facing page)

GENERIC NAME	TRADE NAME	ROUTE OF ADMIN.	USUAL DOSAGE
chloroquine phosphate	(G)* ARALEN Phosphate	po	**Acute Attack:** **Adults:** 1 gm (600 mg base); 500 mg (300 mg base) in 6 hrs; then 500 mg (300 mg base)/day × 2 days **Children:** 10 mg/kg base; then 5 mg/kg base in 6 hrs; and 5 mg/kg base daily × 2 days **Suppression:** **Adults:** 300 mg base/wk. **Children:** 5 mg base/kg/wk.
hydroxychloroquine sulfate	PLAQUENIL	po	**Suppression:** **Adults:** 400 mg/wk. **Infants and children:** 5 mg base/kg/ week
primaquine phosphate	(G)	po	**Adults:** 15–45 mg base/day **Children:** 1.75 mg/14.5 kg/day
pyrimethamine	DARAPRIM	po	**Adults:** 25 mg/week **Children 4–10 yrs.:** 12.5 mg/wk. **Infants to 4 yrs.:** 6.25 mg/wk.
quinine/quinine dihydrochloride/ quinine sulfate	(G)	po	**Adults:** 1 gm tid for 3 doses; then 600 mg tid **Children:** 10 mg/kg tid for 7 days

*(G) Designates availability as a generic product.

Chloroguanide Hydrochloride

PHARMACOLOGY

Chloroguanide hydrochloride exerts both causal prophylactic and suppressive activities by interference with porphyrin metabolism of plasmodia. Chloroguanide hydrochloride is absorbed slowly but adequately from the gastrointestinal tract. Peak plasma levels are attained in 2 to 4 hours. Chronic administration does not result in accumulation; the drum accumulates slightly in tissues, with the liver containing a greater amount than other tissues. Chloroguanide is excreted in the urine primarily but also in the feces.

SPECIAL PRECAUTIONS
• Safe use in pregnancy has not been established.
• Do not administer to patients with a history of hypersensitivity to chloroguanide or related compounds.

ADVERSE EFFECTS
URINARY TRACT EFFECTS: hematuria, epithelial cells and casts in urine
GASTROINTESTINAL EFFECTS: vomiting, abdominal pain, diarrhea
HEMATOLOGIC EFFECTS: myelocytes

CLINICAL GUIDELINES

ADMINISTRATION:
• Advise patient to take medication after meals or with a glass of milk to avoid gastric irritation.

EFFECTS:
• Appetite may be suppressed because of gastric irritation.

DRUG INTERACTIONS:
• When administered with pentaquine, and quinine, no synergism occurs.

OVERDOSAGE/ANTIDOTE:
• Overdosage, whether deliberate or accidental, with amounts as large as 14.5 grams, have been followed by complete recovery.
• There is no specific antidote; use supportive therapy.

Amodiaquine Hydrochloride
Chloroquine Hydrochloride
Chloroquine Phosphate
Hydroxychloroquine Sulfate

PHARMACOLOGY

Chloroquine phosphate and hydroxychloroquine sulfate are malarial suppressive agents. They are useful in extraintestinal amebiasis. They are absorbed very rapidly after oral administration but excretion by way of the kidneys is slow. Chloroquine hydrochloride, also a suppressive agent, is administered intramuscularly. Chloroquine accumulates in the liver, splenic leukocytes, and parasitized erythrocytes. It also has anti-inflammatory properties. The exact mechanism of its malarial suppressive effect is unknown.

SPECIAL PRECAUTIONS

• Use cautiously in patients with hepatic disease because of accumulation in the liver; use cautiously in alcoholic patients.

• Do not use in patients with severe gastrointestinal, neurological, or hematologic disorders; psoriasis; or porphyria.
• Safe use in pregnancy has not been established.
• Do not use in patients with retinal or visual field changes.
• Do not administer to patients with a history of hypersensitivity to chloroquine or related compounds.

ADVERSE EFFECTS

CNS EFFECTS: headache, psychic stimulation, psychotic episodes, convulsions, neuromyopathy
CARDIOVASCULAR EFFECTS: inversion or depression of T waves in ECG, widening of QRS complex in ECG; hypotension
GASTROINTESTINAL EFFECTS: anorexia, nausea, vomiting, diarrhea, abdominal cramps
DERMATOLOGIC EFFECTS: pruritus, lichenoid skin eruptions, bleaching of hair and skin, mucosal pigmentary changes, lichenplanuslike eruptions
OPHTHALMIC EFFECTS: blurring of vision, difficulty in accomodation, diplopia, irreversible retinal damage
OTIC EFFECTS: nerve-type deafness, tinnitus, reduced hearing

CLINICAL GUIDELINES

ADMINISTRATION:
• Patients should have ophthalmic evaluation prior to therapy.
• Periodic complete blood counts should be performed.

EFFECTS:
• Question and test patients periodically for knee and ankle reflexes to detect muscle weakness; if weakness occurs, discontinue drug.
• May cause irreversible visual changes.

- May precipitate a severe attack of psoriasis; porphyria may be exacerbated.
- Parasites may become resistant to chloroquine.

DRUG INTERACTIONS:
- Do not administer concomitantly with gold or phenylbutazone; all drugs produce dermatitis.

OVERDOSAGE/ANTIDOTE:
- With intramuscular administration, inadvertent overdosage or toxic doses may produce respiratory depression or shock with hypotension.
- Respiratory depression is treated with artificial respiration and administration of oxygen. In cases of shock with hypotension, a potent vasopressor such as NEO-SYN-EPHRINE Hydrochloride (phenylephrine hydrochloride) should be given intramuscularly in doses of 2 to 5 mg.
- After ingestion, chloroquine is very rapidly and completely absorbed. Toxic symptoms occur within 30 minutes. These consist of headache, drowsiness, visual disturbances, cardiovascular collapse, and convulsions followed by sudden and early respiratory and cardiac arrest. The ECG may reveal atrial standstill, nodal rhythm, prolonged intraventricular conduction time, and progressive bradycardia leading to ventricular fibrillation and/or arrest.
- Treatment is symptomatic and must be prompt with immediate evacuation of the stomach by emesis or gastric lavage until the stomach is completely emptied. Activated charcoal, at least five times the estimated dose of chloroquine ingested, may be administered by stomach tube after lavage to inhibit further intestinal absorption.
- Fluids may be forced and sufficient ammonium chloride (8 gm daily in divided doses for adults) may be administered for a few days to acidify the urine to help promote urinary excretion.

Primaquine Phosphate

PHARMACOLOGY
Primaquine phosphate, a suppressive agent, is readily absorbed after oral administration. Maximal plasma concentrations are reached in about 6 hours but the concentration falls rapidly thereafter. The mechanism of antimalarial action is unknown. Primaquine phosphate is usually administered in combination with the agent chloroquine for prophylaxis of all types of malaria.

SPECIAL PRECAUTIONS
- Toxic in Negroes, Sardinians, Sephardic Jews, Greeks, and Iranians.
- Do not use in patients with a tendency to develop granulocytopenia such as patients with active forms of rheumatoid arthritis and lupus erythematosus.
- Safe use in pregnancy has not been established.
- Do not use in patients with a history of hypersensitivity to primaquine phosphate or related compounds.

ADVERSE EFFECTS
GASTROINTESTINAL EFFECTS: abdominal cramps, epigastric distress
HEMATOLOGIC EFFECTS: mild anemia, methemoglobinemia, leukocytosis, cyanosis, leukopenia, granulocytopenia, agranulocytosis

CLINICAL GUIDELINES
ADMINISTRATION:
- To avoid gastric distress administer at mealtime or with antacids.
EFFECTS:
- Watch for hemolysis which may occur due to primaquine sensitivity; may darken urine, or hemoglobin may decrease suddenly.

DRUG INTERACTIONS:
- Do not administer concurrently with drugs affecting hemoglobin picture or producing hemolysis (sulfonamides, nitrofurans, antipyretics, analgesics, sulfones).

OVERDOSAGE/ANTIDOTE:
- Granulocytopenia or agranulocytosis may be signs of overdosage.
- There is no specific antidote.

Pyrimethamine

PHARMACOLOGY

Pyrimethamine, a folic acid antagonist, is highly selective against plasmodia and *Toxoplasma gondii*. The antimalarial action is similar to chloroquine but the potency is greater. After oral administration, pyrimethamine is absorbed slowly, distributed widely in the tissues, and localized in erythrocytes, leukocytes, kidneys, and liver. Pyrimethamine is excreted slowly by the kidneys. It has been detected in the milk of nursing mothers.

SPECIAL PRECAUTIONS
- Safe use in pregnancy has not been established.
- Do not administer to patients with a history of hypersensitivity to pyrimethamine or related compounds.

ADVERSE EFFECTS
GASTROINTESTINAL EFFECTS: anorexia, vomiting, atrophic glossitis
HEMATOLOGIC EFFECTS: with large doses, megaloblastic anemia, leukopenia, thrombocytopenia, pancytopenia.

CLINICAL GUIDELINES
ADMINISTRATION:
- Administer with meals to minimize vomiting.

- Perform blood counts including platelet counts at appropriate intervals.

EFFECTS:
- Assure that drug is taken continuously for approximately 10 weeks to lessen the possibility of emergence of insensitive or resistant strains.

DRUG INTERACTIONS:
- Concurrent administration of folinic acid may reduce adverse effects.

OVERDOSAGE/ANTIDOTE:
- Symptoms of overdosage are central nervous central nervous system stimulation including convulsions.
- No specific antidote is known. A parenteral barbiturate may be used followed by folinic acid (LEUCOVORIN).

Quinine and Congeners: Quinine, Quinine Dihydrochloride, Quinine Sulfate

PHARMACOLOGY

Quinacrine and its congeners are suppressive drugs and thereby control overt clinical attacks of malaria. The primary action is schizontocidal and there is no lethal effect on sporozoites or pre-erythrocytic tissue forms. These drugs also have analgesic and antipyretic activities. After oral administration they are readily absorbed and distributed in the tissues including the liver. Peak plasma levels occur 1 to 3 hours after oral administration. No accumulation occurs with continued administration. Excretion is primarily in the urine but small amounts have been detected in the feces, gastric juice, bile, and saliva.

SPECIAL PRECAUTIONS
- Safe use in pregnancy has not been established.
- Do not use in patients with a history of

hypersensitivity to quinine or its congeners.

• Do not administer to patients with tinnitus or optic neuritis.

ADVERSE EFFECTS

CNS EFFECTS: vertigo, fever, headache, apprehension, excitement, confusion, delirium, syncope

RESPIRATORY EFFECTS: asthma; with overdosage stimulation rather than depression

CARDIOVASCULAR EFFECTS: flushing of skin, ventricular tachycardia rarely with overdosage

URINARY TRACT EFFECTS: anuria, uremia

GASTROINTESTINAL EFFECTS: nausea, vomiting, abdominal pain, diarrhea

HEMATOLOGIC EFFECTS: hypoprothrombinemia, agranulocytosis, purpura rarely

DERMATOLOGIC EFFECTS: skin hot, flushed, sweating; papular scarlatiniform or urticarial rash; angioedema of face

OPHTHALMIC EFFECTS: disturbed color perception, blurred vision, photophobia, diplopia, night blindness, scotomata, constricted visual fields

OTIC EFFECTS: tinnitus, decreased auditory acuity

CLINICAL GUIDELINES

ADMINISTRATION:

• Renal excretion is twice as rapid when urine is acidic as when it is alkaline.

EFFECTS:

• Watch for signs of hemolytic reactions —dark urine or sudden decrease in hemoglobin.

OVERDOSAGE/ANTIDOTE:

• The fatal overdose in adults is approximately 8 gm. Overdosage is characterized by an exaggeration of the adverse effects; cardiac depression may occur.

• There is no specific antidote. Alkaloid precipitants may be used. The longer the patient survives, the better the prognosis since quinine is rapidly destroyed in the body.

Antiparasitic Agents (Scabicides/Pediculicides)

GENERAL CLINICAL USES

The parasitic infections of man include scabies (*Sarcoptes scabiei var. hominis*), head louse (*Pediculus capitis*), body louse (*Pediculus corporis*), crab louse (*Phthirus pubis*), and mite causing rosacea (*Demodex folliculorum*). The antiparasitic agents useful in treating infestations by these organisms include crotamiton and gamma benzene hexachloride. Crotamiton is useful in treating scabies, whereas gamma benzene hexachloride is useful in treating scabies, head lice, body lice, crab lice, and also their nits.

SPECIFIC PRODUCTS AND DOSAGES

GENERIC NAME	TRADE NAME	ROUTE OF ADMIN.	USUAL DAILY DOSAGE
crotamiton	EURAX	topical	Massage into skin of entire body; repeat in 24 hrs.
gamma benzene hexachloride	KWELL GAMENE	topical	Apply to entire body; leave on for 24 hrs.; wash thoroughly. Second or third application may be made at weekly intervals.

Crotamiton

PHARMACOLOGY
Crotamiton is an effective scabicide. It is applied topically and skin absorption is minimal.

SPECIAL PRECAUTIONS
• Do not use in patients with a history of hypersensitivity to crotamiton, or in those in whom it causes irritation.
• Do not apply to acutely inflamed skin, raw, weeping surfaces, or in the eyes and mouth.
• Safe use in pregnancy has not been established.

ADVERSE EFFECTS
LOCAL EFFECTS: irritation, sensitization

CLINICAL GUIDELINES
ADMINISTRATION:
• Clothing and bed linen should be changed daily; a cleansing bath should be taken 48 hours after the last application of medication.
EFFECTS:
• May cause irritation or rash; discontinue therapy if rash occurs.

Gamma Benzene Hexachloride

PHARMACOLOGY
Gamma benzene hexachloride is an ectoparasiticide. Lipoid solvents enhance percutaneous absorption of gamma benzene hexachloride. It is used topically and is not readily absorbed into the skin.

SPECIAL PRECAUTIONS
• Do not use in patients with a history of hypersensitivity to or irritation from gamma benzene hexachloride.
• Safe use in pregnancy has not been established.

ADVERSE EFFECTS
DERMATOLOGIC EFFECTS: eczematous eruptions

CLINICAL GUIDELINES
ADMINISTRATION:
• Clothing and bed linen should be changed daily; a cleansing bath should be taken 48 hours after the last application of medication.
EFFECTS:
• May cause irritation or rash; discontinue if rash occurs.
OVERDOSAGE/ANTIDOTE:
• Overdosage is characterized by CNS manifestations (depression) which can be

antagonized by the administration of pentobarbital or phenobarbital.
• Overdosage may be treated with calcium gluconate administered intravenously in combination with the barbiturates. Epinephrine should not be used because ventricular fibrillation may result. There is no specific antidote.

Antitoxoplasmosis Agent

GENERAL CLINICAL USES
Pyrimethamine is usually used in combination with a sulfonamide to treat toxoplasmosis. Pyrimethamine is synergistic with the sulfonamides and may be administered either orally or ophthalmically. It is also effective in the treatment of malaria.

SPECIFIC PRODUCTS AND DOSAGES

GENERIC NAME	TRADE NAME	ROUTE OF ADMIN.	USUAL DAILY DOSAGE
pyrimethamine	DARAPRIM	po	**Adults:** 50–75 mg/day for 1–3 weeks; reduce dosage **Children:** 1 mg/kg/day divided in 2 equal doses for 2–4 days; reduce dosage
		ophth.	See Chapter 11, *Drugs Affecting the Eye*, page 444.

PHARMACOLOGY
See *Antimalarial Agents*, pages 78 and 81.

SPECIAL PRECAUTIONS
• The dosage required to treat toxoplasmosis is 10 to 20 times the recommended antimalarial dosage and approaches the toxic level. If signs of folic or folinic acid deficiency develop, reduce dosage or discontinue the drug.
• Perform semiweekly blood counts including platelet counts.
• Safe use in pregnancy has not been established.

• Do not use in patients with a history of hypersensitivity to pyrimethamine or related compounds.

ADVERSE EFFECTS
GASTROINTESTINAL EFFECTS: anorexia, vomiting, atrophic glossitis
HEMATOLOGIC EFFECTS: with large doses, megaloblastic anemia, leukopenia, thrombocytopenia, pancytopenia

CLINICAL GUIDELINES
See *Antimalarial Agents*, pages 78 and 81.

Antituberculosis Agents

GENERAL CLINICAL USES

The selection of an antituberculosis agent depends upon bacterial resistance, the development of untoward effects, and the possible presence of atypical mycobacteria. Of the drugs available for the treatment of tuberculosis, resistance may occur to one or more.

The antituberculosis drugs are divided into two groups: primary and secondary therapies. The primary therapy includes aminosalicylic acid, ethambutol, isoniazid, rifampin, and streptomycin sulfate. The secondary therapies include capreomycin sulfate, cycloserine, ethionamide, kanamycin sulfate, pyrazinamide, and viomycin.

SPECIFIC PRODUCTS AND DOSAGES

Conduct periodically appropriate bacterial susceptibility tests to determine if bacterial resistance has developed.

GENERIC NAME	TRADE NAME	ROUTE OF ADMIN.	USUAL DAILY DOSAGE	
			ADULTS	CHILDREN
aminosalicylic acid	PAS	po	10–12 gm/day divided in 2–3 doses	200–300 mg/kg/day divided in 3–4 doses
aminosalicylic acid resin	REZIPAS	po	20–24 gm/day divided in 2–3 doses	400–600 mg/kg/day divided in 3 or 4 doses
capreomycin sulfate	CAPASTAT Sulfate	im	Up to 20 mg/kg/day	Not recommended
cycloserine	SEROMYCIN	po	0.5–1 gm/day in divided doses	Not established
ethambutol hydrochloride	MYAMBUTOL	po	15–25 mg/kg/day as a single dose	Not recommended
ethionamide	TRECATOR-SC	po	0.5–1 gm daily in divided doses	Not established
isoniazid	(G)† INH Tablets NYDRAZID	po	5–20 mg/kg/day in single divided doses; maximum: 300 mg/day	10–30 mg/kg/day as single or divided doses; maximum: 500 mg/day
kanamycin sulfate	KANTREX	im	15 mg/kg/day in divided doses. Do not exceed 1.5 gm/day	Not recommended

(continued facing page)

GENERIC NAME	TRADE NAME	ROUTE OF ADMIN.	USUAL DAILY DOSAGE	
			ADULTS	CHILDREN
pyrazinamide	PZA	po	20–35 mg/kg/day divided in 3–4 doses	Not established
rifampin	RIFADIN RIFAMATE* RIMACTANE RIMACTAZID*	po	600 mg as a single dose	10–20 mg/kg/day in a single dose; do not exceed 600 mg/day
streptomycin sulfate	(G)†	im	0.25–1 gm/day as a single dose	20 mg/kg/day as a single dose
viomycin	VIOCIN Sulfate	im	1 gm bid every other day	Not established

*Contains more than one active ingredient.
†Designates availability as a generic product.

Aminosalicylic Acid
Aminosalicylic Acid Resin

PHARMACOLOGY

Aminosalicylic acid and aminosalicylic acid resin should not be used as the sole therapeutic agents for tuberculosis since they are bacteriostatic against *Mycobacterium tuberculosis*. They should be administered with other antituberculosis agents such as streptomycin, isoniazid, or both. Aminosalicylic acid delays the development of bacterial resistance to streptomycin and isoniazid.

Aminosalicylic acid is absorbed rapidly after oral ingestion and approximately 85 percent is excreted in the urine.

SPECIAL PRECAUTIONS

• Do not administer to patients with a history of hypersensitivity to aminosalicylic acid or related compounds.
• Immediately terminate therapy if signs of hypersensitivity occur.
• Use cautiously in patients with impaired renal or hepatic function and with gastric ulcer.
• Safe use in pregnancy has not been established.

ADVERSE EFFECTS

CNS EFFECTS: encephalopathy
RESPIRATORY EFFECTS: Loffler's syndrome
CARDIOVASCULAR EFFECTS: vasculitis
GASTROINTESTINAL EFFECTS: nausea, vomiting, diarrhea, abdominal pain
METABOLIC AND ENDOCRINE EFFECTS: goiter with or without myxedema, hypokalemia, acidosis
HEPATIC EFFECTS: jaundice, hepatitis
HEMATOLOGIC EFFECTS: leukopenia, agranulocytosis, thrombocytopenia, hemolytic anemia
ALLERGIC EFFECTS: fever, skin eruptions, infectious-mononucleosislike syndrome

CLINICAL GUIDELINES

ADMINISTRATION:
• Administer with meals to minimize gastric irritation.
• Maintain patients urine at alkaline or neutral pH to avoid aminosalicylic acid stones.

EFFECTS:
• Aminosalicylic acid is neither antipyretic nor analgesic.

DRUG INTERACTIONS:
• Patients who are being treated with anticoagulants may require an adjustment of the anticoagulant dosage.
• Do not administer concurrently with probenecid because of possible inhibition of renal excretion.
• The effects of diphenylhydantoin and isoniazid may be potentiated.

OVERDOSAGE/ANTIDOTE:
• Overdosage is characterized by an exaggeration of the adverse effects.
• There is no specific antidote.

Capreomycin Sulfate

PHARMACOLOGY
Capreomycin sulfate is to be used concomitantly with other antituberculosis agents. It is administered parenterally since absorption from the gastrointestinal tract is insignificant. Following intramuscular administration, peak serum concentrations are reached in 1 to 2 hours. Administration daily for 30 days did not result in significant accumulation in subjects with normal renal function. Capreomycin sulfate is excreted in the urine in an essentially unaltered form.

SPECIAL PRECAUTIONS
• Use with great caution in patients with renal insufficiency or pre-existing auditory impairment.
• Simultaneous administration of other parenteral drugs which also have ototoxic or nephrotoxic potential should be undertaken with great caution. These drugs are streptomycin, viomycin, polymyxin, colistin sulfate, gentamicin, tobramycin, vancomycin, kanamycin, and neomycin.
• Safe use in pregnancy and in infants and children has not been established.
• Assess vestibular and auditory function prior to initiation of therapy and at regular intervals during treatment.
• Assess renal function throughout the period of treatment; dosage reduction may be required in patients with known or suspected renal impairment.
• Assess serum potassium levels frequently because hypokalemia may occur.
• Partial neuromuscular blockage was demonstrated; this action was enhanced by ether anesthesia.
• Use with caution in patients with a history of hypersensitivity to this and related drugs.

ADVERSE EFFECTS
URINARY TRACT EFFECTS: tubular necrosis, elevation of BUN or NPN, casts, erythrocytes and leukocytes in urine sediment; depression of PSP excretion
METABOLIC AND ENDOCRINE EFFECTS: hypokalemia
HEPATIC EFFECTS: decreased BSP excretion
HEMATOLOGIC EFFECTS: leukocytosis, leukopenia, eosinophilia
ALLERGIC EFFECTS: urticaria
DERMATOLOGIC EFFECTS: maculopapular skin rash
OTIC EFFECTS: subclinical and clinical auditory loss, tinnitus, vertigo
LOCAL EFFECTS: pain, induration, and excessive bleeding at injection sites; sterile abscess

CLINICAL GUIDELINES
ADMINISTRATION:
• Assure complete dissolution before administration.
• May acquire a pale straw color and darken in time; this is not associated with loss of potency or development of toxicity.
• Administer by deep intramuscular injection into a large muscle mass.

EFFECTS:
• Superficial injection may be associated

with increased pain and development of sterile abscess.
- Watch for changes in hearing acuity.

DRUG INTERACTIONS:
- Cross resistance has been reported between capreomycin and viomycin; also between capreomycin, kanamycin, and neomycin.
- No cross resistance has been reported between capreomycin and isoniazid, aminosalicylic acid, cycloserine, streptomycin, ethionamide, or ethambutol.
- Partial neuromuscular blockage demonstrated with capreomycin was enhanced by ether anesthesia.

OVERDOSAGE/ANTIDOTE:
- Overdosage is characterized by an exaggeration of the adverse effects.
- There is no specific antidote. Treat supportively.

Cycloserine

PHARMACOLOGY
Cycloserine is not used as a sole therapeutic agent but in conjunction with other effective tuberculocidal agents. It is a broad spectrum antibiotic which inhibits cell wall synthesis in susceptible organisms. After oral administration it is absorbed rapidly with peak blood levels occurring in 3 to 4 hours. Cycloserine diffuses throughout the body fluids and tissues including across the blood-brain barrier. The drug is excreted in the urine in an active form.

SPECIAL PRECAUTIONS
- Do not administer to patients with epilepsy, depression, severe anxiety, psychosis, or severe renal insufficiency.
- Do not administer to patients with a history of hypersensitivity to cycloserine and related drugs.
- Discontinue or reduce dosage if patient develops allergic dermatitis, symptoms of CNS toxicity such as convulsions, psychosis,

somnolence, depression, confusion, hyperreflxia, headache, tremor, vertigo, paresis, or dysarthria.
- Toxicity is closely related to excessive blood levels.
- Safe use in pregnancy or children has not been established.

ADVERSE EFFECTS
CNS EFFECTS: convulsions, drowsiness, somnolence, headache, tremor, dysarthria, vertigo, confusion and disorientation with loss of memory, psychosis, paresis, hyperreflexia, paresthesias, clonic seizures
HEPATIC EFFECTS: elevated serum transaminase
HEMATOLOGIC EFFECTS: megaloblastic anemia, sideroblastic anemia, anemia
ALLERGIC EFFECTS: rash

CLINICAL GUIDELINES
ADMINISTRATION:
- Administer after meals for best effects.
- Monitor hematologic, renal, and hepatic parameters periodically. Determine blood levels weekly.

EFFECTS:
- If patient develops dermatitis, discontinue drug immediately.
- The risk of convulsions is increased in alcoholic patients.

DRUG INTERACTIONS:
- Advise patient not to use alcoholic beverages excessively.
- Can and should be administered concurrently with streptomycin, aminosalicylic acid, and/or isoniazid.

OVERDOSAGE/ANTIDOTE:
- Symptoms of overdosage include CNS depression with drowsiness, somnolence, dizziness, hyperreflexia, mental confusion, convulsions, and allergic dermatitis.
- There is no specific antidote. Pyridoxine (vitamin B^6) 300 mg or more daily and anticonvulsants may be given to relieve convulsions.

Ethambutol Hydrochloride

PHARMACOLOGY

Ethambutol hydrochloride is not to be used as a sole agent but always in combination with one or more antituberculosis drugs such as isoniazid or streptomycin. Ethambutol hydrochloride is specifically effective against mycobacteria when growing actively; it appears to interfere with cell metabolism. After oral administration peak plasma levels are attained in 2 to 4 hours. Excretion is primarily renal but drug is also detected in the feces. No drug accumulation has been noted in patients with normal renal function but it has occurred in patients with renal insufficiency.

SPECIAL PRECAUTIONS

- Do not administer to patients with a history of hypersensitivity to ethambutol hydrochloride or related compounds.
- Safe use in pregnancy has not been established.
- Do not administer to patients with optic neuritis.
- In patients with decreased renal function, dosage must be reduced as determined by serum levels.
- Complete ophthalmoscopic examination should be conducted prior to therapy and periodically during therapy.
- Patients with pre-existing ophthalmologic abnormalities should be informed of possible adverse optic effects.
- Renal, hepatic, and hematologic parameters should be evaluated periodically during long-term therapy.

ADVERSE EFFECTS

CNS EFFECTS: fever, malaise, headache, dizziness, mental confusion, disorientation, hallucinations
GASTROINTESTINAL EFFECTS: anorexia, abdominal pain, nausea, vomiting
METABOLIC AND ENDOCRINE EFFECTS: elevated serum uric acid, precipitation of gout

HEPATIC EFFECTS: abnormal liver function tests
ALLERGIC EFFECTS: anaphylactoid reactions
DERMATOLOGIC EFFECTS: dermatitis, and pruritus
OPHTHALMIC EFFECTS: decrease in visual acuity, optic neuritis, reversible visual disturbances
MUSCULOSKELETAL EFFECTS: joint pain, tingling and numbness of extremities due to peripheral neuritis

CLINICAL GUIDELINES

ADMINISTRATION:
- Administration with food does not interfere with absorption.
- Patients should have monthly eye examinations; loss of vision has occurred.

EFFECTS:
- Watch for signs of decrease in visual acuity.

DRUG INTERACTIONS:
- Isoniazid, cycloserine, ethionamide, pyrazonamide, viomycin, and aminosalicylic acid have been administered concomitantly.

OVERDOSAGE/ANTIDOTE:
- Overdosage is characterized by an exaggeration of the adverse effects.
- There is no specific antidote.

Ethionamide

PHARMACOLOGY

Ethionamide suppresses multiplication of strains of *Mycobacterium tuberculosis.* Organisms resistant to streptomycin, aminosalicylic acid, isoniazid, viomycin, and cycloserine are sensitive to ethionamide. To treat tuberculosis, ethionamide is not used alone but in combination with isoniazid, aminosalicylic acid, streptomycin, or cycloserine.

Administered orally, ethionamide reaches peak plasma levels in about 3 hours and is widely distributed in the organs and tissues. It is metabolized slowly. A small amount is excreted in active form in the urine.

SPECIAL PRECAUTIONS
• Safe use in pregnancy has not been established.
• Do not use in patients with a history of hypersensitivity to ethionamide or related compounds.
• Do not use in patients with severe hepatic damage.

ADVERSE EFFECTS
CNS EFFECTS: mental depression, drowsiness, asthenia, convulsions, peripheral neuritis
CARDIOVASCULAR EFFECTS: postural hypotension
GASTROINTESTINAL EFFECTS: anorexia, nausea, vomiting, stomatitis
METABOLIC AND ENDOCRINE EFFECTS: gynecomastia, impotence, menorrhagia
HEPATIC EFFECTS: jaundice and/or hepatitis, elevated SGOT and SGPT
ALLERGIC EFFECTS: rash, purpura
OPTHALMIC EFFECTS: optic neuritis

CLINICAL GUIDELINES
ADMINISTRATION:
• Administer with meals to minimize gastric irritation.
• Monitor hepatic, renal, and hematologic parameters frequently; determine SGOT or SGPT prior to and every 2 to 4 weeks during therapy.
EFFECTS:
• Difficulty in the management of diabetes mellitus may become a problem in patients receiving ethionamide.
DRUG INTERACTIONS:
• Isoniazid, aminosalicylic acid, streptomycin, and cycloserine have been administered concurrently.
OVERDOSAGE/ANTIDOTE:
• Overdosage is characterized by an exag-

geration of the adverse effects.
• There is no specific antidote.

Isoniazid

PHARMACOLOGY
Isoniazid is a slow acting but potent tuberculostatic agent. The mechanism of action is unknown. Susceptible strains of bacteria take up the drug, which may inhibit synthesis of an essential component of the cell. Isoniazid is absorbed readily after oral administration. Peak plasma levels develop within 1 to 2 hours after ingestion. Isoniazid diffuses into all body fluids, pleural and ascitic fluids, saliva, milk, feces, and cerebrospinal fluid. The skin acts as a storage depot. Isoniazid is excreted in the urine unchanged and as acetylisoniazid, isonicotinic acid, and as an isonicotinic acid conjugate.

SPECIAL PRECAUTIONS
• Do not use in patients with a history of hypersensitivity to isoniazid; terminate therapy at first signs of hypersensitivity.
• Severe and sometimes fatal hepatitis has been reported; monitor hepatic function at monthly intervals.
• Defer preventive treatment in individuals with acute hepatic disease.
• Safe use in pregnancy has not been established.
• Ophthalmologic examinations should be performed before and periodically after isoniazid therapy is initiated.
• Use cautiously in patients with convulsive disorders, pre-existing hepatic disorders, and severe renal dysfunction.

ADVERSE EFFECTS
CNS EFFECTS: peripheral neuropathy, paresthesias, convulsions, toxic encephalopathy, optic neuritis and atrophy, toxic psychosis
GASTROINTESTINAL EFFECTS: nausea, vom-

iting, epigastric distress

METABOLIC AND ENDOCRINE EFFECTS: pyridoxine deficiency, pellagra, hyperglycemia, metabolic acidosis, gynecomastia

HEPATIC EFFECTS: elevated SGOT and SGPT, bilirubinemia, hepatitis (with and without jaundice) sometimes fatal

HEMATOLOGIC EFFECTS: agranulocytosis, hemolytic or aplastic anemia, thrombocytopenia, eosinophilia

ALLERGIC EFFECTS: fever, skin eruptions (morbilliform, maculopapular, pruritic, or exfoliative), lymphadenopathy, vasculitis

MUSCULOSKELETAL EFFECTS: rheumatic syndrome, systematic lupus-erythematosuslike syndrome

CLINICAL GUIDELINES

ADMINISTRATION:
- Instruct patients to report immediately any of the prodromal symptoms of hepatitis such as fatigue, weakness, anorexia, and malaise.

EFFECTS:
- Large doses (40 to 50 mg/kg) may increase the potential for seizures in patients with a history of seizures by sensitizing the nervous system to auditory and also visual stimuli.

DRUG INTERACTIONS:
- Pyridoxine does not lower plasma levels of isoniazid; however, it may partially prevent adverse neurological effects.
- Concomitant administration of aminosalicylic acid produces higher concentrations of active isoniazid.
- May increase the effects of phenytoin, disulfiram, oral anticoagulants, oral antidiabetic drugs, antihypertensive drugs, atropinelike drugs, sedatives and narcotics, and stimulant drugs; dosage adjustment may be necessary.

OVERDOSAGE/ANTIDOTE:
- Symptoms of overdosage occur within 30 minutes and include nausea, vomiting, dizziness, slurring of speech, blurring of vision, and visual hallucinations. Respiratory distress and CNS depression, progressing rapidly from stupor to profound coma, may occur; severe intractable seizures also have occurred. Metabolic acidosis, acetonuria, and hyperglycemia are typical laboratory findings.
- There is no specific antidote. Rapid control of metabolic acidosis is fundamental to management. Administer sodium bicarbonate intravenously at once and repeat as needed. Forced osmotic diuresis must be started early and should be continued for some hours after clinical improvement. Hemodialysis is advised for severe cases.

Kanamycin Sulfate

For detailed information, see *Aminoglycosides,* pages 20 and 25.

Pyrazinamide

PHARMACOLOGY

Pyrazinamide should be administered with another tuberculostatic agent such as viomycin or isoniazid since it is a tuberculostatic agent. Pyrazinamide is well absorbed from the gastrointestinal tract. Peak plasma levels are reached in about 2 hours. It is excreted primarily by the kidneys.

SPECIAL PRECAUTIONS
- Patients should be hospitalized.
- Safe use in pregnancy has not been established.
- Do not use in patients with a history of hypersensitivity to pyrazinamide or related compounds.

ADVERSE EFFECTS

CNS EFFECTS: malaise, fever

URINARY TRACT EFFECTS: dysuria

GASTROINTESTINAL EFFECTS: anorexia, nausea, vomiting

METABOLIC AND ENDOCRINE EFFECTS: elevated plasma uric acid levels, attacks of acute gouty arthritis; diabetes mellitus may be difficult to control

HEPATIC EFFECTS: jaundice, hepatic necrosis, elevated SGOT and SGPT, decreased plasma prothrombin, elevated plasma fibrinogen, reduced plasma albumin and globulin, elevation of plasma protein bound iodine

MUSCULOSKELETAL EFFECTS: arthralgia

CLINICAL GUIDELINES

ADMINISTRATION:
• Administer with meals to minimize gastric irritation.
• Monitor liver function prior to and at appropriate intervals during therapy.

EFFECTS:
• Watch for signs of hepatic dysfunction; if they occur, discontinue therapy.

DRUG INTERACTIONS:
• Viomycin and isoniazid have been administered concurrently.

OVERDOSAGE/ANTIDOTE:
• Overdosage is characterized by an exaggeration of the adverse effects.
• There is no specific antidote.

Rifampin

PHARMACOLOGY

Rifampin may be used in conjunction with at least one other antituberculosis drug such as isoniazid or ethambutol. Rifampin acts by interference with bacterial metabolism. It is absorbed readily following oral administration. It crosses the placental barrier. Rifampin is eliminated mainly through the bile and to a much lesser extent, the urine.

SPECIAL PRECAUTIONS
• Do not administer to patients with a history of hypersensitivity to rifampin.
• Since rifampin has produced liver dysfunction including jaundice, monitor liver function periodically, particularly in patients with pre-existing liver dysfunction.
• Do not administer concurrently with other hepatotoxic drugs.
• Meningococci may rapidly become resistant.
• Safe use in pregnancy has not been established.

ADVERSE EFFECTS

CNS EFFECTS: headache, drowsiness, fatigue, ataxia, dizziness, inability to concentrate, mental confusion

URINARY TRACT EFFECTS: hemoglobinuria, hematuria, renal insufficiency, acute renal failure

GASTROINTESTINAL EFFECTS: heartburn, epigastric distress, anorexia, nausea, vomiting, gas, cramps, diarrhea

METABOLIC AND ENDOCRINE EFFECTS: menstrual disturbances, elevation of BUN and serum uric acid

HEPATIC EFFECTS: hepatitis, shocklike syndrome with hepatic involvement, abnormal liver function tests including elevations in serum bilirubin, BSP, alkaline phosphatase, serum transaminase

HEMATOLOGIC EFFECTS: eosinophilia, thrombocytopenia, transient leukopenia, hemolytic anemia, decreased hemoglobin

ALLERGIC EFFECTS: hypersensitivity reactions including pruritus, urticaria, rash, sore mouth and tongue

OPHTHALMIC EFFECTS: visual disturbances

MUSCULOSKELETAL EFFECTS: muscle weakness, pain in extremities, generalized numbness

CLINICAL GUIDELINES

ADMINISTRATION:
• Warn patients that feces, urine, saliva, sputum, sweat, and tears may be colored red-orange by rifampin and its metabolites.
• Reliability of oral contraceptives may be diminished in some patients being treated for tuberculosis.

DRUG INTERACTIONS:

• Isoniazid and ethambutol have been administered concurrently with rifampin.

• Rifampin increases the requirement for anticoagulant drugs of the coumarin type.

OVERDOSAGE/ANTIDOTE:

• Symptoms of overdosage include nausea, vomiting, and increasing lethargy which are noted soon after ingestion. Unconsciousness may occur with severe hepatic involvement. Brownish-red or orange discoloration of urine, sweat, saliva, tears, and feces is proportional to the amount of rifampin ingested.

• There is no specific antidote. Activated charcoal slurry following evacuation of the stomach may be useful. Active diuresis will help to promote excretion of the drug. Extracorporeal hemodialysis may be required.

Streptomycin Sulfate

For detailed information, see *Aminoglycosides*, pages 20 and 27.

Viomycin Sulfate

For detailed information, see *Aminoglycosides*, pages 20 and 30.

Antiviral Agents

GENERAL CLINICAL USES

At present the antiviral agents marketed in the United States are amantadine hydrochloride, idoxuridine, and vidarabine monohydrate. Amantadine hydrochloride, administered orally, has been found useful in preventing infections of the respiratory tract in persons exposed to confirmed A_2 strains of influenza virus; it is not virucidal. It has been used concurrently with vaccine for prophylaxis. Idoxuridine, a virucidal agent administered topically, is used to treat herpes simplex keratitis of the eyelids, conjunctiva, and also the cornea.

Vidarabine monohydrate administered topically is useful in acute keratoconjunctivitis and recurrent epithelial keratitis due to herpes simplex.

Vidarabine for intravenous infusion is indicated in the treatment of herpes simplex virus encephalitis.

SPECIFIC PRODUCTS AND DOSAGES

GENERIC NAME	TRADE NAME	ROUTE OF ADMIN.	USUAL DAILY DOSAGE
amantadine hydrochloride	SYMMETREL	po	**Adults:** 200 mg/day divided in 2 doses or as a single dose

(continued facing page)

GENERIC NAME	TRADE NAME	ROUTE OF ADMIN.	USUAL DAILY DOSAGE
amantadine hydrochloride (continued)	SYMMETREL	po	**Children 1–9 yrs.:** 2–4 mg/lb/day divided in 2 or 3 equal doses **Children 9–12 yrs.:** 200 mg/day divided in 2 doses
idoxuridine	STOXIL DENDRID HERPLEX	ophth.	See Chapter 11, page 444.
vidarabine monohydrate	VIRA-A	ophth.	See Chapter 11, page 444.
vidarabine	VIRA-A	iv infusion	15 mg/kg/day

Amantadine Hydrochloride

PHARMACOLOGY

Amantadine hydrochloride impedes penetration of influenza A_2 virus into the host cell. The exact mechanism of action is unknown. Following oral administration it is readily absorbed and excreted unchanged in the urine. Amantadine hydrochloride is excreted in breast milk.

SPECIAL PRECAUTIONS

• Do not administer to patients with a history of hypersensitivity to amantadine hydrochloride.
• Patients with a history of epilepsy or other seizures may have increased seizure activity.
• Patients with a history of congestive heart failure or peripheral edema may develop congestive failure while receiving amantadine hydrochloride.
• Safe use in pregnancy and lactation has not been established.
• Use with caution in patients with impaired renal function.
• Administer cautiously in patients with liver disease, psychotic patients or severely psychoneurotic patients or patients receiving concurrently CNS stimulants.

ADVERSE EFFECTS

CNS EFFECTS: irritability, tremor, slurred speech, ataxia anxiety, mental depression, insomnia, lethargy, dizziness, psychosis, convulsions, hallucinations, weakness
RESPIRATORY EFFECTS: dyspnea
CARDIOVASCULAR EFFECTS: congestive heart failure, orthostatic hypotension, peripheral edema, livedo recticularis
URINARY TRACT EFFECTS: retention
GASTROINTESTINAL EFFECTS: nausea, anorexia, vomiting, constipation, dry mouth
HEMATOLOGIC EFFECTS: leukopenia, neutropenia
DERMATOLOGIC EFFECTS: rash, eczematous dermatitis rarely
OPHTHALMIC EFFECTS: oculogyric episodes, blurring of vision

CLINICAL GUIDELINES

ADMINISTRATION:
• Monitor renal, hepatic, and hematopoietic parameters.
• Watch patient for signs of psychiatric disturbances and cardiovascular changes.
• Adjust dosage in patients with renal impairment, congestive heart failure, peripheral edema, or orthostatic hypotension.
DRUG INTERACTIONS:
• The dose of anticholinergic drugs or of

amantadine hydrochloride should be reduced if atropinelike effects appear when these drugs are used concurrently.

• Amantadine and levodopa administered concurrently result in rapid therapeutic benefits.

OVERDOSAGE/ANTIDOTE:

• Symptoms of overdosage include hyperactivity, convulsions, possibly arrhythmias and hypotension.

• There is no known antidote. Acidification of the urine facilitates renal excretion.

Idoxuridine

For detailed information, see *Drugs Affecting the Eye,* page 445.

Vidarabine/Vidarabine Monohydrate

PHARMACOLOGY

Vidarabine administered intravenously is rapidly deaminated into arabinosylhypoxanthine (Ara-Hx) which is promptly distributed through the tissues. The mean half-life is 3.3 hours. Excretion is primarily by the kidneys. In patients with impaired renal function, Ara-Hx accumulation may occur.

Vidarabine monohydrate is formulated for ophthalmic administration in a sterile inert base.

Vidarabine/vidarabine monohydrate has *in vitro* and *in vivo* antiviral activity. Virus multiplication is inhibited.

SPECIAL PRECAUTIONS

• Do not administer to patients with a history of hypersensitivity to vidarabine.

• Do not administer intramuscularly or subcutaneously.

• Use special care in administering to patients susceptible to fluid overloading or cerebral edema.

• Use with caution during pregnancy; a safe dose for the embryo or fetus has not been established.

ADVERSE EFFECTS

CNS EFFECTS: tremor, dizziness, hallucinations, confusion, psychosis, ataxia

GASTROINTESTINAL EFFECTS: anorexia, nausea, vomiting, diarrhea, hematemesis

HEMATOLOGIC EFFECTS: decrease in hemoglobin or hematocrit, white cell count, and platelet counts; SGOT elevation; decrease in reticulocyte count; elevated total bilirubin

METABOLIC EFFECTS: weight loss, malaise

DERMATOLOGIC EFFECTS: rash, pruritus

OPHTHALMIC EFFECTS: after ophthalmic administration, lacrimation, foreign body sensation, conjunctival injection, irritation, superficial punctate keratitis, pain, photophobia, punctal occlusions, sensitivity

LOCAL EFFECTS: pain at injection site

CLINICAL GUIDELINES

ADMINISTRATION:

• Monitor renal, hepatic, and hematologic parameters.

• Do not administer by intramuscular or subcutaneous routes because of low solubility and poor absorption.

• Any appropriate intravenous solution is suitable for use as a diluent.

• Use aseptic technique in preparing drug.

EFFECTS:

• In eye infections, if no signs of improvement occur after 7 days, or complete re-epithelialization has not occurred in 21 days, other forms of therapy should be considered. Some severe cases may require longer treatment.

• After re-epithelialization has occurred, treat for an additional 7 days at a reduced dosage (such as twice daily) in order to prevent recurrence.

OVERDOSAGE/ANTIDOTE:
• An acute massive overdosage of the intravenous form produced no serious evidence of adverse effects. Doses over 20 mg/kg/day can produce bone marrow depression with concomitant thrombocytopenia and leukopenia.
• Acute massive oral overdosage is not expected to be toxic because drug absorption from the gastrointestinal tract is minimal. The oral LD_{50} is greater than 5,020 mg/kg in the mouse and rat.
• Overdosage by ocular administration is unlikely because any excess should be expelled quickly from the conjunctival sac.

Trichomonacides

GENERAL CLINICAL USES
Trichomoniasis, a venereal infection caused by *Trichomonas vaginalis*, may be treated with systemic and/or topical medications. Topical therapy is not usually the sole therapy. For systemic treatment, metronidazole has been useful in treating both male and female patients with trichomoniasis; it is also effective in treating infections caused by *Entamoeba histolytica* (see *Amebicides*, page 11. For topical therapy, furazolidone, metronidazole, and povidone-iodine preparations are available.

SPECIFIC PRODUCTS AND DOSAGES

GENERIC NAME	TRADE NAME	ROUTE OF ADMIN.	USUAL DAILY DOSAGE
furazolidone	TRICOFURON* FUROXONE	vaginal po	1 suppository bid **Adults:** 100 mg qid **Children 5 yrs. and older:** 25–50 mg qid **1–4 yrs:** 17–25 mg qid **1 month–1 yr:** 8–17 mg qid
metronidazole	FLAGYL	po	**Female:** 250 mg tid **Male:** 250 mg tid
povidone-iodine	BETADINE ISODINE	douche	2 tablespoonfuls in 1 quart water once daily

*Contains more than one active ingredient.

Furazolidone

For detailed information, see *Nitrofurans*, page 45.

Metronidazole

PHARMACOLOGY

Metronidazole is directly trichonomacidal and amebicidal. Following oral administration it is well absorbed with a peak serum level reached in about 1 hour. It is excreted in the urine. However, pharmacologically, metronidazole appears inert in that it has no effect on the cardiovascular or respiratory systems. Metronidazole crosses the placental barrier and has been found in breast milk.

SPECIAL PRECAUTIONS

• Do not use in patients with evidenced or history of blood dyscrasias, hypersensitivity to metronidazole, or with central nervous system organic disease.
• Monitor leukocyte count before and after therapy, since a mild leukopenia has been reported.

ADVERSE EFFECTS

CNS EFFECTS: headache, dizziness, vertigo, rarely incoordination and ataxia, irritability, depression, insomnia, weakness, numbness, paresthesias, confusion
RESPIRATORY EFFECTS: nasal congestion
CARDIOVASCULAR EFFECTS: flattening of T wave in ECG
URINARY TRACT EFFECTS: dysuria, cystitis, pelvic pressure, polyuria, incontinence, pyuria
GASTROINTESTINAL EFFECTS: nausea, anorexia, vomiting, diarrhea, epigastric distress, abdominal cramps, constipation, a metallic taste, furry tongue, dry mouth, glossitis, stomatitis, proctitis
METABOLIC AND ENDOCRINE EFFECTS: decreased libido
HEMATOLOGIC EFFECTS: leukopenia
ALLERGIC EFFECTS: urticaria, pruritus
DERMATOLOGIC EFFECTS: mild erythematous eruption
MUSCULOSKELETAL EFFECTS: fleeting joint pains

CLINICAL GUIDELINES

EFFECTS:
• Urine may be darkened.
• Proliferation of *Candida* may occur in the mouth and/or vagina.
• Discontinue if abnormal neurological signs occur.
DRUG INTERACTIONS:
• Do not administer with any beverage or drug containing ethyl alcohol since an ANTABUSE-like effect may occur.
OVERDOSAGE/ANTIDOTE:
• Overdosage is characterized by an exaggeration of the adverse effects, namely, weakness, gastric irritation, nausea, and vomiting. Disorientation and confusion may occur.

Povidone-Iodine

For detailed information, see Chapter 9, *Drugs Affecting the Skin*, page 424.

Psychotherapeutic agents

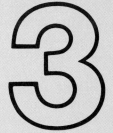

INTRODUCTION

The term psychotherapeutic, introduced only in recent years, is used for drugs which cause a pronounced effect on, and alteration or reversal of, the symptoms characterizing psychiatric disorders. The psychotherapeutic drugs, available since the 1950's, have resulted in the reduction of the number of patients hospitalized and also have reduced the duration of hospitalization. In addition, patients who once required hospitalization can now be treated as outpatients. The hazards to the patients receiving drug therapy are much less than those encountered with prior therapies such as electrical or drug-induced convulsive treatments, insulin coma, sleep therapy, or prefrontal lobotomy.

SPECIFIC THERAPEUTIC
CLASSIFICATION

The psychotherapeutic agents have been divided into four groups, each group representing a general classification according to clinical indications:

1. *Antianxiety agents* (minor tranquilizers): The chief uses are in mild emotional disorders such as anxiety, tension, and agitation, occurring alone or with various organic diseases. The antianxiety agents are further grouped according to chemical similarity into (1) the benzodiazepines including clorazepate dipotassium, (2) the carbamates, and (3) hydroxyzine.

2. *Antidepressants*: These drugs counteract the symptoms characterizing psychotic depressive reactions or syndromes. The antidepressants are divided into the tricyclic antidepressants or dibenzazepine derivatives and the monoamine oxidase inhibitors (MAO-inhibitors).

3. *Antipsychotic Agents*: The antipsychotic agents modify the symptoms characterizing psychotic states, aggressive and overactive behavior, and disorganized mental patterns. These drugs are divided into (1) phenothiazines and also molindone hydrochloride and haloperidol, (2) thioxanthenes, (3) dibenzazepine (loxapine), (4) reserpine and rauwolfia serpentina, (5) lithium salts.

4. *Psychostimulants*: These cerebrocortical stimulants have been used to improve athletic performance, to induce wakefulness, to improve mentation, and to overcome hangover. Their use in treating mild depression or drug-induced depression is not officially approved. The psychostimulants are divided into three groups: (1) amphetamines, (2) caffeine and (3) methylphenidate.

Antianxiety Agents

GENERAL CLINICAL USES

The antianxiety agents or minor tranquilizers relieve anxiety, tension, and related symptoms without altering critical mental faculties. The antianxiety agents have been used with success in the therapy of psychosomatic disturbances, emotional stresses, and emotional disorders accompanying various physical diseases. They are of limited, if any, value in disturbed psychotic patients. The combination of two drugs provides control of a spectrum of symptoms with one dosage form for administration.

Parenteral administration is useful in controlling acute or severe anxiety and tension, as may be seen preoperatively, and also in controlling withdrawal symptoms of acute alcoholism.

SPECIFIC PRODUCTS AND DOSAGES

The dosage of these drugs, as with many medications, should be adjusted to the needs of each patient. The lowest effective dose should always be used. When maximal clinical response is achieved, the dosage may be reduced gradually to a maintenance level.

	GENERIC NAME	TRADE NAME	ROUTE OF ADMIN.	SUGGESTED DAILY DOSAGE		
				ADULTS	GERIATRICS	CHILDREN
CIV	*Benzodiazepines:* chlordiazepoxide	(G)† LIBRITABS LIBRIUM	po	15–100 mg/day divided in 3–4 doses	10–40 mg/day in divided doses	**Over 6 yrs.:** 5 mg bid to qid; maximum 10 mg bid to qid
			im/iv	50–100 mg initially then 75–200 mg/day divided in 3–4 doses; maximal recommended dose 300 mg/day	75–150 mg/day in divided doses	**Over 12 yrs.:** 25–50 mg bid or tid; **Under 12 yrs.:** not recommended
CIV*	clorazepate dipotassium	TRANXENE	po	7.5–15 mg bid to qid	3.75 mg bid to qid	**Under 18 yrs.:** not recommended
CIV	clorazepate monopotassium	AZENE	po	13–52 mg/day in divided doses	6.5–13 mg in divided doses	**Under 18 yrs.:** not recommended
CIV	chlordiazepoxide +amitriptyline	LIMBITROL 10–25 LIMBITROL 5–12.5	po	3–5 tablets/day	Not established	Not established
CIV	diazepam	VALIUM	po	2–10 mg bid to qid	2–2.5 mg od or bid	**Over 6 months:** 1–2.5 mg tid or qid
			im/iv	2–20 mg; may repeat	2–5 mg; may repeat	**Over 12 yrs.:** 2–5 mg; may repeat

*Designates schedule listing under Federal Controlled Substances Act.
†(G) Designates availability as a generic product.

(continued overleaf)

	GENERIC NAME	TRADE NAME	ROUTE OF ADMIN.	SUGGESTED DAILY DOSAGE		
				ADULTS	GERIATRICS	CHILDREN
CIV	lorazepam	ATIVAN	po	2–4 mg/day in single or divided doses	1–2 mg/day in divided doses	Not established
CIV	oxazepam	SERAX	po	10–30 mg od to qid	0.0–15 mg tid to qid	Not established
CIV	prazepam	VERSTRAN	po	20–60 mg/day in divided doses	10–15 mg/day in divided doses	**Under 6 yrs.:** not established
	Carbamates; Chlormezanone: chlormezanone	TRANCOPAL	po	100–200 mg tid or qid	Not established	**5–12 yrs.:** 50–100 mg tid or qid
CIV	meprobamate	(G) MILTOWN EQUANIL KESSOBAMATE SK-BAMATE	po	400 mg tid or qid; maximal recommended dose 2400 mg daily See Chapter 13, *Skeletal Muscle Relaxants,* page 494.	reduce dosage	**6–12 yrs.:** 100–200 mg bid or tid
	tybamate	SOLACEN	po	250–500 mg tid or qid	reduce dosage	**6–12 yrs.:** 20–35 mg/kg/day in 3–4 equally divided doses
	Hydroxyzine: hydroxyzine HCl or pamoate	ATARAX VISTARIL	po	25–100 mg tid or qid	25–100 mg tid or qid	**Over 6 yrs.:** 25 mg bid to qid **Under 6 yrs.:** 25 mg bid
	hydroxyzine HCl	VISTARIL	im	50–100 mg; repeat 4–6 hours prn	Not established	Not established

Benzodiazepines and Clorazepate

Clorazepate Dipotassium
Clorazepate Monopotassium
Chlordiazepoxide
Diazepam
Lorazepam
Oxazepam
Prazepam

PHARMACOLOGY

Following oral administration the benzodiazepines are absorbed rapidly from the gastrointestinal tract. Clinical effects are noted within 1 hour and last from 4 to 6 hours. The benzodiazepines are metabolized in the liver and excreted primarily in the urine.

Chlordiazepoxide and diazepam may be administered intramuscularly or intravenously; a rapid effect is obtained with intravenous administration.

The benzodiazepines are central nervous system depressants. The exact mechanism of action is unknown. Extensive animal studies indicate an effect on the limbic system of the brain which may be involved in emotional responses.

Diazepam is also useful as adjunctive therapy for relief of skeletal muscle spasms. See page 494, *Central-Acting Skeletal Muscle Relaxants*, for drug and dosage information.

SPECIAL PRECAUTIONS
- Use cautiously in patients with compromised liver or kidney function.
- Abrupt withdrawal may result in withdrawal symptoms.
- Physical or psychological dependence may occur in susceptible persons.
- Do not administer diazepam or clorazepate dipotassium to patients with acute narrow—angle glaucoma.
- Do not use in patients known or suspected to be hypersensitive to that drug or related drugs.
- Excessive and prolonged use of these drugs in susceptible persons (such as alcoholics, former addicts) may result in dependence or habituation.
- Administer to pregnant patients when, in the judgment of the physician, the potential benefits outweigh the possible risks.

ADVERSE EFFECTS
CNS EFFECTS: abrupt withdrawal may result in epileptiform seizures; drowsiness, ataxia, confusion, syncope, fatigue, headache, dizziness, minor EEG changes, euphoria
RESPIRATORY EFFECTS: diazepam—apnea may follow intramuscular or intravenous administration

CARDIOVASCULAR EFFECTS: hypotension, bradycardia, cardiovascular collapse, tachycardia
URINARY TRACT EFFECTS: urinary retention, incontinence
GASTROINTESTINAL EFFECTS: nausea, vomiting, diarrhea, anorexia, dry mouth, constipation
METABOLIC AND ENDOCRINE EFFECTS: minor menstrual irregularities, increased or decreased libido
HEPATIC EFFECTS: jaundice, hepatic dysfunction
HEMATOLOGIC EFFECTS: agranulocytosis, neutropenia
ALLERGIC EFFECTS: itchy urticarial rash
DERMATOLOGIC EFFECTS: rash
OPHTHALMIC EFFECTS: blurred vision, diplopia, nystagmus
LOCAL EFFECTS: with intravenous administration—thrombosis, phlebitis; with intramuscular administration—pain

CLINICAL GUIDELINES
ADMINISTRATION:
- Patients receiving chlordiazepoxide or diazepam parenterally should be kept under close observation, preferably in bed, for a period of up to 3 hours.
- Intramuscular administration should be well within the body of a relatively large muscle.
- Do not administer to patients in shock or comatose states.
- Intravenous administration should be slow to avoid respiratory arrest.
EFFECTS:
- With long–term therapy, periodic blood counts and liver function tests are advised.
- Adverse effects occur more commonly in elderly and debilitated patients than in young, healthy patients; therefore, supervise closely, particularly during ambulation.

- Withdrawal symptoms consisting of tremors, abdominal and muscle cramps, anorexia, vomiting, agitation, insomnia may occur with discontinuance, particularly if treatment had been for a prolonged time.

DRUG INTERACTIONS:
- Hypotension has occurred when these drugs were administered concurrently with spinal anesthesia.
- Phenothiazines, narcotics, barbiturates. MAO–inhibitors, and ethyl alcohol may potentiate the action of the benzodiazepines.
- Do not mix diazepam injectable with other drugs or solutions.
- Potentiation can occur with simultaneous ingestion of alcoholic beverages and other CNS depressant drugs including other antianxiety drugs.

OVERDOSAGE/ANTIDOTE:
- Overdosage is manifested by somnolence, ataxia, confusion, coma and diminished reflexes.
- There is no specific antidote. Empty stomach. General supportive measures should be used. Caffeine and sodium benzoate may be given to combat the CNS depressive effects. Dialysis is of limited value.

Carbamates and Chlormezanone

Meprobamate
Tybamate
Chlormezanone

PHARMACOLOGY
Animal studies have indicated that the carbamates and chlormezanone have an effect on multiple sites in the central nervous system, including the thalamus and limbic system. The mechanism of action in man has not been resolved.

Carbamates and chlormezanone are absorbed rapidly from the gastrointestinal tract. Clinical effects are noted within 1 hour and last 4 to 6 hours. These drugs are metabolized primarily in the liver and excreted in the urine.

SPECIAL PRECAUTIONS
- Administer cautiously to patients with compromised liver and kidney function.
- Abrupt discontinuation of the drug may result in withdrawal symptoms including tremor and convulsions.
- Physical or psychological dependence may occur in susceptible patients.
- Do not administer to patients with intermittent porphyria.
- Do not administer to patients known to be hypersensitive to these or related drugs.
- Administer to pregnant patients only when, in the judgment of the physician, the potential benefits outweigh the possible risks.

ADVERSE EFFECTS
CNS EFFECTS: with meprobamate, tybamate—drowsiness, ataxia, confusion, syncope, fatigue, headache, dizziness, minor EEG changes, euphoria; abrupt withdrawal may result in epileptiform seizures, paradoxical excitement; with chlormezanone—dizziness, flushing, drowsiness, depression, weakness
CARDIOVASCULAR EFFECTS: with meprobamate, tybamate—hypotension, palpitations, tachycardia, arrhythmias
URINARY TRACT EFFECTS: with chlormezanone—inability to void
GASTROINTESTINAL EFFECTS: with meprobamate, tybamate—nausea, vomiting, diarrhea; with chlormezanone—nausea

METABOLIC AND ENDOCRINE EFFECTS: with meprobamate, tybamate—minor menstrual irregularities, increased or decreased libido

HEPATIC EFFECTS: with chlormezanone—jaundice rarely

HEMATOLOGIC EFFECTS: with meprobamate—agranulocytosis, aplastic anemia, thrombocytopenic purpura, leukopenia

ALLERGIC EFFECTS: with meprobamate, tybamate—itchy, urticarial, or erythematous maculopapular rash, petechiae, ecchymoses, peripheral edema, adenopathy, eosinophilia, fever, fixed drug eruption, severe hypersensitivity reactions including anaphylaxis, bronchospasm, oliguria, anuria, angioneurotic edema, erythema multiforme, exfoliative dermatitis, stomatitis, proctitis

DERMATOLOGIC EFFECTS: with chlormezanone—drug rash

OPHTHALMIC EFFECTS: with meprobamate, tybamate—diplopia, blurred vision

CLINICAL GUIDELINES

ADMINISTRATION:
• Supervise administration of meprobamate in patients with a history of excessive self-medication.
• Prevent withdrawal reactions with the carbamates by gradually tapering off the dose over 1 to 2 weeks.

EFFECTS:
• Advise ambulatory patients to avoid activities involving the operation of a motor vehicle or other machinery because of occurrence of drowsiness.
• With long-term therapy, periodic blood counts and liver function tests are advisable.
• Meprobamate may occasionally precipitate seizures in epileptic patients.
• Allergic reactions to meprobamate, characterized by an itchy, urticarial or maculopapular rash, usually occur within the period of the first to fourth doses in patients having had no previous contact with the drug.
• Adverse effects such as drowsiness occur more commonly in elderly and debilitated patients; therefore, supervise ambulation.
• Withdrawal symptoms consisting of tremors, abdominal and muscle cramps, anorexia, vomiting, agitation, and insomnia may occur with discontinuance of meprobamate, particularly if treatment has been prolonged.

DRUG INTERACTIONS:
• Hypotension has occurred when meprobamate was administered concurrently with spinal anesthesia.
• The effect of ethyl alcohol may be dangerously potentiated by the administration of meprobamate, tybamate, or chlormezanone; the effects of meperidine (DEMEROL) and the barbiturates may also be potentiated.
• Hazardous potentiation of general central nervous system depression can occur with concurrent ingestion of alcoholic beverages, chloral hydrate, barbiturates, analgesics, and other antianxiety agents.

OVERDOSAGE/ANTIDOTE:
• Overdosage is manifested by somnolence, ataxia, confusion, coma, and diminished reflexes.
• There is no specific antidote for the drugs in this group. Death has occurred with ingestion of as little as 12 gm and survival with as much as 40 gm. Empty stomach; treat supportively. Diuresis, osmotic (mannitol) diuresis, peritoneal dialysis and hemodialysis have been used successfully.

Hydroxyzine

PHARMACOLOGY

Following oral administration hydroxyzine is rapidly absorbed from the gastrointestinal tract. Clinical effects are usually noted within 15 to 30 minutes after oral administration.
• Hydroxyzine is not a cortical depressant but its action may be due to a suppression of activity in certain key regions of the subcortical areas of the central nervous system (CNS).

SPECIAL PRECAUTIONS

• Since drowsiness may occur, patients must be cautioned against driving a car or operating machinery.
• Involuntary motor activity including rare instances of tremor and convulsions have been reported, usually with doses above those recommended.
• Do not use in patients known to be hypersensitive to the drug or related drugs.
• Drugs should be administered to pregnant patients only when, in the judgment of the physician, the potential benefits outweigh the possible risks.

ADVERSE EFFECTS

CNS EFFECTS: drowsiness, involuntary motor activity, rarely tremors and convulsions
AUTONOMIC EFFECTS: dry mouth with high doses

CLINICAL GUIDELINES

ADMINISTRATION:
• Patients receiving hydroxyzine intramuscularly should be kept under close observation, preferably in bed, for a period of up to 3 hours.
• Intramuscular injections should be well within the body of a relatively large muscle; do not administer intravenously or subcutaneously.
• Do not administer to patients in shock or comatose states.
• The patient should be warned of drowsiness and the possibility of impaired coordination which may hazardously affect driving or operating other machinery.
EFFECTS:
• With long-term therapy, periodic blood counts and liver function tests are advisable.
DRUG INTERACTIONS:
• Hydroxyzine may potentiate the effects of CNS depressants such as meperidine (DEMEROL), barbiturates, ethyl alcohol, and coumarin derivatives; these drugs should be administered in reduced dosages when administered concurrently with hydroxyzine.
OVERDOSAGE/ANTIDOTE:
• Overdosage is characterized by an exaggeration of the pharmacological effects.
• There is no known antidote to hydroxyzine.

Antidepressants

GENERAL CLINICAL USES

The antidepressant agents have a pronounced effect on depressive syndromes or depressive reactions characterized by profound sadness, lack of communication, and withdrawal from society.

SPECIFIC PRODUCTS AND DOSAGES

Adjust dosage to the needs of the patient. The lowest effective dose should always be used. When maximal clinical response is achieved, the dosage may be reduced gradually to a maintenance level.

| GENERIC NAME | TRADE NAME | ROUTE OF ADMIN. | SUGGESTED DAILY DOSAGE | | | ADOLESCENTS AND GERIATRICS |
| | | | ADULTS | | | |
			HOSPITALIZED	OUTPATIENTS	MRDD*	
Tricyclic Antidepressants (dibenzazepine derivatives):						
amitriptyline hydrochloride	(G)‡ ELAVIL ENDEP	po	100–200 mg/ day in divided doses	75–150 mg/ day in divided doses	300 mg	50 mg/day in divided doses
	(G) ELAVIL	im	80–120 mg/ day in divided doses	80–120 mg/ day in divided doses	120 mg	Not established
desipramine hydrochloride	NORPRAMIN PERTOFRANE	po	75–300 mg/ day in divided doses	75–200 mg/ day in divided doses	200 mg 150 mg†	25–100 mg/ day in divided doses
doxepin hydrochloride	ADAPIN SINEQUAN	po	75–150 mg/ day in divided doses	75–150 mg/ day in divided doses	300 mg	Not established
imipramine hydrochloride	(G) JANIMINE PRESAMINE TOFRANIL	po	100 mg–300 mg/day in divided doses	75–150 mg/ day in divided doses	300 mg** 200 mg 100 mg†	30–40 mg/ day in divided doses
	TOFRANIL	im	up to 100 mg/ day in divided doses	up to 100 mg/ day in divided doses	100 mg**	Not established
nortriptyline hydrochloride	AVENTYL	po	75–100 mg/ day in divided doses	reduce dosage	100 mg	30–50 mg/ day in divided doses
protriptyline hydrochloride	VIVACTIL	po	15–60 mg/ day in divided doses	15–60 mg/ day in divided doses	60 mg 20 mg†	15 mg/day in divided doses

*Maximal recommended daily dose.
**Hospitalized patients.
†Adolescents and elderly patients.
‡(G) Designates availability as a generic product.

(continued overleaf)

		ROUTE OF ADMIN.	SUGGESTED DAILY DOSAGE			
GENERIC NAME	TRADE NAME		ADULTS		MRDD*	ADOLESCENTS AND GERIATRICS
			HOSPITALIZED	OUTPATIENTS		
MAO-inhibitors: isocarboxazid	MARPLAN	po	10–30 mg/day in divided doses	10–30 mg/day in divided doses	30 mg	Not recommended
phenelzine sulfate	NARDIL	po	15–60 mg/day in divided doses	15–60 mg/day in divided doses	75	Not recommended
tranylcypromine	PARNATE	po	20 mg/day in divided doses	20 mg/day in divided doses	30	Not recommended

*Maximal recommended daily dose.

Tricyclic Antidepressants (Dibenzazepine Derivatives)

Amitriptyline HCl
Desipramine HCl
Doxepin HCl
Imipramine HCl
Nortriptyline
Protriptyline HCl

PHARMACOLOGY

When administered orally, the tricyclic antidepressants are readily absorbed from the gastrointestinal tract. Parenteral administration should be used only for initiating therapy in patients unable or unwilling to use oral medication. The oral forms should supplant the injectable form as soon as possible.

The mechanism of action of the tricyclic antidepressants in man is unknown. These drugs are neither MAO-inhibitors nor psychostimulants. They inhibit the membrane pump mechanism responsible for re-uptake of norepinephrine into adrenergic neurons. This action may potentiate the central and peripheral action of adrenergic agents.

SPECIAL PRECAUTIONS

• Do not administer to patients with congestive heart failure, angina pectoris, and/or paroxysmal tachycardia.
• Convulsive threshold may be lowered.
• Use cautiously in patients with glaucoma or urinary retention or those receiving anticholinergic agents.
• Psychosis may be exacerbated.
• Do not use in patients known or suspected to be hypersensitive to the drug or related drugs.
• Drugs should be given to pregnant patients only when, in the judgment of the physician, the potential benefits outweigh the possible risks.

ADVERSE EFFECTS

CNS EFFECTS: confusional states, disorientation, hallucinations, excitement, anxiety, insomnia, nightmares, paresthesias, tremors, peripheral neuropathy, extrapyramidal symptoms, alterations in EEG patterns, numbness, tingling, convulsions

CARDIOVASCULAR EFFECTS: hypertension, orthostatic hypotension, tachycardia, palpitations, myocardial infarction, arrhythmias, heart block, stroke, prolonged cardiac conduction time

URINARY TRACT EFFECTS: dilatation of urinary tract, urinary retention

AUTONOMIC EFFECTS: dry mouth

GASTROINTESTINAL EFFECTS: nausea, epigastric distress, vomiting, constipation, anorexia, stomatitis, diarrhea, parotid swelling, black tongue, paralytic ileus

METABOLIC AND ENDOCRINE EFFECTS: testicular swelling and gynecomastia in the male; breast enlargement and galactorrhea in the female; increased or decreased libido; hyperglycemia or hypoglycemia

HEPATIC EFFECTS: jaundice

HEMATOLOGIC EFFECTS: agranulocytosis, leukopenia, eosinophilia, purpura, thrombocytopenia

ALLERGIC EFFECTS: rash, urticaria, photosensitization, edema of face and tongue, petechiae

OPHTHALMIC EFFECTS: blurred vision, disturbances of accommodation

OTIC EFFECTS: tinnitus

CLINICAL GUIDELINES

EFFECTS:
• Monitor the effect of the tricyclic antidepressants on the blood pressure, especially in patients with hypertension or low normal pressure.
• Note that risk of suicide is greatest toward the end of a depressive cycle; watch patients carefully when they begin to respond to therapy.

DRUG INTERACTIONS:
• Be aware that the tricyclic antidepressants may block the antihypertensive effects of guanethidine and similar agents.
• Do not administer tricyclic antidepressants and MAO-inhibitors concurrently or within 2 weeks of each other.
• Potentiation may occur when tricyclic antidepressants and anticholinergic agents, barbiturates, adrenergic agents, amphetamines, and thyroid preparations are administered concurrently.
• May potentiate the response to alcoholic beverages and other CNS depressants.

OVERDOSAGE/ANTIDOTE:
• Overdosage is characterized by respiratory depression, cardiac arrhythmias, stupor, ataxia, coma, athetoid and choreiform movements.
• Although there is no specific antidote, overdosage has been treated with physostigmine salicylate, 1 to 3 mg administered slowly intravenously. Because physostigmine salicylate is rapidly metabolized, the dosage may be repeated if required, particularly if life-threatening signs (such as arrhythmias, convulsions, and deep coma) occur or persist. Dialysis is not of value because of the high drug-protein binding of this group of drugs.

MAO-Inhibitors

Isocarboxazid
Phenelzine Sulfate
Tranylcypromine Sulfate

PHARMACOLOGY

The MAO-inhibitors with antidepressive activity are absorbed readily following oral administration. A clinical effect is usually observed within 48 hours to 3 weeks. When the MAO-inhibitors are withdrawn, the drugs are excreted in 24 hours but monoamine oxidase activity is recovered in 3 to 5 days.

The MAO-inhibitors, potent inhibitors of amine oxidase, increase the concentration of epinephrine, norepinephrine, and serotonin in storage sites throughout the nervous system. In theory, this increased concentration of monoamines in the brain stem is responsible for the antidepressant activity.

SPECIAL PRECAUTIONS

• Warn patient against self-medication with proprietary cold, hay fever, or reducing preparations containing sympathomimetic agents.
• Hypertensive reactions may occur if patients consume food containing tryptophan (broad beans) or tyramine (aged cheese, beers, wines, pickled herring, chicken livers, yeast extract), and excessive caffeine.
• Do not administer meperidine (DEMEROL) concurrently; circulatory collapse may occur.
• Do not administer to any patient over 60 years of age or with a confirmed or suspected cardiovascular defect, hypertension, history of headaches or liver disease, or with abnormal liver function.
• Do not administer to patients with pheochromocytoma since such tumors secrete pressor substances.
• Do not use in patients known or suspected to be hypersensitive to that drug or related drugs or to any of the components.
• Drugs should be given to pregnant patients only when, in the judgment of the physician, the potential benefits outweigh the possible risks.
• Do not administer to patients with congestive heart failure, angina pectoris, or/ and paroxysmal tachycardia.
• Use cautiously in patients with glaucoma, urinary retention, or those receiving medication with anticholinergic effects; in particular, watch elderly patients.

ADVERSE EFFECTS

CNS EFFECTS: overstimulation, weakness, drowsiness, dizziness, chills, headache, parkinsonian effects
CARDIOVASCULAR EFFECTS: tachycardia, palpitations, orthostatic hypotension, abnormal cardiac rate and rhythm
URINARY TRACT EFFECTS: urinary retention
AUTONOMIC EFFECTS: dry mouth
GASTROINTESTINAL EFFECTS: nausea, diarrhea, abdominal pain, constipation, significant anorexia
METABOLIC AND ENDOCRINE EFFECTS: impotence
HEPATIC EFFECTS: hepatitis
HEMATOLOGIC EFFECTS: leukopenia
ALLERGIC EFFECTS: edema, skin rash
OPHTHALMIC EFFECTS: blurred vision

CLINICAL GUIDELINES

ADMINISTRATION:
• Monitor blood pressure in patients receiving MAO-inhibitors because of possible hypertensive effects.
• Warn patients of the possible occurrence of drowsiness; driving a car or operating machinery may be dangerous.
EFFECTS:
• An antianxiety effect may be noted in patients prior to noting the antidepressant effect.
• Note that the most important reaction associated with MAO-inhibitors is hypertensive crises.
• MAO-inhibitors should be discontinued 7 days before surgery.
• In patients being transferred from one MAO-inhibitor to another or from diaza-

zepine derivatives, allow a medication-free interval of at least 1 week; institute new therapy at a low dose.

DRUG INTERACTIONS:

• MAO-inhibitors should not be administered in combination with other MAO-inhibitors, dibenzazepine derivatives, sympathomimetics (including antihistamines), some CNS depressants including alcoholic beverages and narcotics, antihypertensives, diuretics, sedatives or anesthetic drugs, meperidine (DEMEROL).

• Potentiation may occur if MAO-inhibitors and barbiturates, insulin, procaine, adrenergic agents, methyldopa, thiazide diuretics, amphetamines, furazolidone, anti-parkinson agents, and phenethiazines are administered concomitantly.

• Since some MAO-inhibitors have contributed to hypoglycemic episodes in diabetic patients receiving insulin or hypoglycemic agents, watch the diabetic patient carefully.

OVERDOSAGE/ANTIDOTE:

• Overdosage with the MAO-inhibitors is characterized by prominence and frequency of adverse effects including possible hypertensive crises. These adverse effects may be delayed or prolonged; the patient should be observed closely for 1 week.

• There is no known antidote to the MAO-inhibitors.

Antipsychotic Agents

GENERAL CLINICAL USES

The antipsychotic agents, frequently called the major tranquilizers, modify the symptoms of psychotic states by decreasing aggressive, overactive behavior and ameliorating disorganized behavioral and mental patterns. The treated patients may become sleepy or drowsy initially, but can be aroused readily by ordinary stimuli. Increasing the dose of drug will not readily induce loss of consciousness or general anesthesia as may occur with the sedative and hypnotic agents such as chloral hydrate and the barbiturates.

The combination of an antipsychotic agent and an antidepressant provides control symptoms of both psychoses and depression.

SPECIFIC PRODUCTS AND DOSAGES

The dosages of these drugs, as with most medications, should be adjusted to the needs of the patient. The lowest effective dose should always be used. When maximal clinical response is achieved, the dosage may be reduced gradually to a maintenance level.

GENERIC NAME	TRADE NAME	ROUTE OF ADMIN.	OUTPATIENTS ADULTS USUAL	MRDD*
Phenothiazines, Thioxanthenes, Molindone dihydrochloride, Haloperidol, Loxapine:				
acetophenazine	TINDAL	po	20 mg tid	80 mg
butaperazine maleate	REPOISE	po	5–10 mg tid	100 mg
chlorpromazine	(G)† THORAZINE	po	10–50 mg bid to qid	800 mg
	(G) THORAZINE	im	25–50 mg; may repeat in 1 hr.	———
	THORAZINE	pr	100 mg q 6–8 hr.	
fluphenazine decanoate	PROLIXIN DECANOATE	im/sc	12.5–25 mg single dose	100 mg
fluphenazine enanthate	PROLIXIN ENANTHATE	im/sc	25 mg every 2 wk.	100 mg
fluphenazine hydrochloride	PROLIXIN	im	2.5–10 mg/day in divided doses	10 mg
	PERMITIL PROLIXIN	po	0.5–10 mg/day in divided doses 6–8 hr.	20 mg
mesoridazine besylate	SERENTIL	po	25–50 mg tid	400 mg
		im	25 mg; repeat in 30–60 min. if necessary	200 mg
perphenazine	TRILAFON	po	2–8 mg tid	24 mg
		im	5 mg repeat q 6 hr.	15 mg
perphenazine-amitriptyline	ETRAFON 2–10 TRIAVIL 2–10 ETRAFON 2–25 TRIAVIL 2–25 ETRAFON-A (4–10) TRIAVIL 4–10 ETRAFON FORTE (4–25) TRIAVIL 4–25	po	perphenazine 2–8 mg with amitriptyline 25–50 mg tid or qid	———

SUGGESTED DAILY DOSAGE					
GERIATRICS	CHILDREN	ADULTS		HOSPITALIZED PATIENTS	
				GERIATRICS	CHILDREN
		USUAL	MRDD*		
1/4–1/2 usual dose	**Under 12 yrs.:** 0.8–1.1 mg/kg/day divided in 3 doses	80–120 mg/day in divided doses	600 mg	Reduce dosage	**Under 12 yrs.:** Not established
1/4–1/2 usual dose	**Under 12 yrs.:** not recommended	———	———	———	———
Reduce dosage	0.25 mg/lb q 4–6 hr. prn	25–50 mg. tid to qid	1000 mg	Reduce dosage	**Up to 5 yrs.:** not over 40 mg/day; **5–12 yrs.:** not over 75 mg/day
1/4–1/2 usual dose	0.25 mg/lb q 8 hr. prn	25–400 mg q 4–6 hr.	1000 mg	Reduce dosage	same as oral
———	0.5 mg/lb q 6–8 hr. prn	———	———	———	———
———	Not established	———	———	———	———
———	Not established	———	———	———	———
1.0–2.5 mg/day in divided doses	0.25–3.5 mg/day in divided doses	———	———	———	———
1.0–2.5 mg day in divided doses	Not established	———	———	———	———
1/4–1/2 usual dose	**Under 12 yrs.:** not established	———	———	———	———
Reduce dosage	**Under 12 yrs.:** not established	———	———	———	———
1/4–1/2 usual dose	**1–6 yrs.:** 4–6 mg/day in divided doses; **6–12 yrs.:** 6 mg/day in divided doses	16–64 mg/day in divided doses	64 mg	Reduce dosage	Reduce dosage
Reduce dosage	Not established	5–10 mg repeat q 6 hr.	30 mg	Reduce dosage	Reduce dosage
1 tab tid or qid	**Adolescents:** 1 tab tid or qid	———	———	———	———

*Maximal recommended daily dose.
†(G) Designates availability as a generic product.

(continued overleaf)

GENERIC NAME	TRADE NAME	ROUTE OF ADMIN.	OUTPATIENTS ADULTS	
			USUAL	MRDD*
piperacetazine	QUIDE	po	20–40 mg/day in divided doses	160 mg
prochlorperazine	COMPAZINE	pr	50 mg/day in divided doses	———
prochlorperazine edisylate	COMPAZINE	im	5–20 mg; repeat q 3–4 hr.	40 mg
prochlorperazine maleate	COMPAZINE	po	5–10 mg tid or qid	150 mg
thioridazine hydrochloride	MELLARIL	po	50–100 mg tid or qid	800 mg
trifluoperazine hydrochloride	STELAZINE	po	1–2 mg bid	4 mg
	STELAZINE	im	1–2 mg q 4–6 hr. prn	10 mg.
triflupromazine hydrochloride	VESPRIN	po	30–150 mg/day in divided doses	150 mg
	VESPRIN	im	———	———
Butyrophenones: haloperidol	HALDOL	po	0.5–5 mg bid or tid	100 mg
	HALDOL	im	2–5 mg; repeat in 4–8 hr.	15 mg
loxapine succinate	DAXOLIN LOXITANE	po	60–100 mg/day in divided doses	250 mg
Thioxanthenes: chlorprothixene	TARACTAN	po	25–50 mg tid or qid	600 mg
	TARACTAN	im	25–50 mg tid or qid	———

*Maximal recommended daily dose.

SUGGESTED DAILY DOSAGE

GERIATRICS	CHILDREN	HOSPITALIZED PATIENTS			
		ADULTS		GERIATRICS	CHILDREN
		USUAL	MRDD*		
1/4–1/2 usual dose	**Under 12 yrs.:** not established	——	——	——	——
1/4–1/2 usual dose	**2–12 yrs.:** 5–7.5 mg/ day in divided doses **2–5 yrs.:** do not exceed 20 mg/day **6–12 yrs.:** do not exceed 25 mg/day	——	——	——	——
1/4–1/2 usual dose	**Under 12 yrs.:** 0.06 mg/lb	——	——	——	——
1/4–1/2 usual dose	**2–12 yrs.:** 2.5 mg bid or tid **2–5 yrs.:** do not exceed 20 mg/day **6–12 yrs.:** do not exceed 25 mg/day	30–40 mg/day in divided doses	**Adults:** 150 mg **Children:** 10 mg	——	5–7.5 mg/day in divided doses
1/4–1/2 usual dose	**2–12 yrs.:** 0.5–3 mg/kg/day	——	——	——	0.5–3 mg/kg/day
1/4–1/2 usual dose	**6–12 yrs.:** 1–2 mg od or bid	2–5 mg bid	**Adults:** 40 mg; **Children:** 15 mg	1/4–1/2 usual dose	**6–12 yrs.:** 1 mg od or bid
1/4–1/2 usual dose	**6–12 yrs.:** 1 mg od or bid	1–2 mg q 4–6 hr. prn	——	1/4–1/2 usual dose	**6–12 yrs:** 1 mg od or bid
20–30 mg daily in divided doses	2 mg/kg/day in divided doses	100–150 mg/day in divided doses	150 mg	——	——
——	0.2–0.25 mg/kg/day in divided doses	100–150 mg/day	150 mg in divided doses	——	——
0.5–2 mg bid or tid 2–5 mg; repeat in 4–8 hr.	**Under 12 yrs.:** not established **Under 12 yrs.:** not established	—— ——	—— ——	—— ——	—— ——
——	——	**Initial:** 50 mg/day	250 mg	——	——
10–25 mg tid or qid 10–25 mg tid or qid	**Over 6 yrs.:** 10–25 mg tid or qid **Over 12 yrs.:** 25–50 tid or qid	—— ——	—— ——	—— ——	—— ——

*Maximal recommended daily dose.

(continued overleaf)

GENERIC NAME	TRADE NAME	ROUTE OF ADMIN.	OUTPATIENTS ADULTS	
			USUAL	MRDD*
thiothixene	NAVANE	po	2–5 mg bid or tid	60 mg
	NAVANE	im	4 mg bid to qid	30 mg
molindone hydrochloride	MOBAN	po	5–25 mg tid or qid	225 mg
Reserpine/Rauwolfia serpentina: rauwolfia serpentina	RAUDIXIN	po	100–200 mg bid	——
reserpine	(G) RAU-SED SERPASIL	po	0.1–1.0 mg daily	——
	(G) SERPASIL	im	2.5–5.0 mg single dose	——
Lithium Salts: lithium carbonate	(G) ESKALITH LITHANE LITHONATE LITHOTABS	po	300–600 mg tid	——
lithium citrate	LITHONATE–S**	po	15–30 ml/day divided in 3–4 doses (8mEq lithium/5 ml equivalent to 300 mg lithium carbonate)	——

*Maximal recommended daily dose.
**Designates sugar-free product.

Phenothiazines
Thioxanthenes
Molindone Hydrochloride
Haloperidol
Loxapine Succinate

PHARMACOLOGY

After oral administration of the phenothiazines, thioxanthenes, molindone, or haloperidol, the psychotherapeutic effects do not develop for several hours. To determine the maximal therapeutic effect therapy may have to be continued for 2 to 3 weeks. After intramuscular administration of a single dose, the therapeutic effect is noted usually in 10 minutes and is maximal in 1 to 2 hours. The average duration of effect is 6 hours but may last for 12 to 24 hours. The phenothiazines, thioxanthenes, molindone, haloperidol, and loxapine are rapidly absorbed from the gastrointestinal tract, metabolized in the liver, and excreted primarily in the urine.

Two phenothiazines, fluphenazine decanoate and fluphenazine enanthate, both products for parenteral administra-

		SUGGESTED DAILY DOSAGE				
			HOSPITALIZED PATIENTS			
GERIATRICS	CHILDREN	ADULTS		GERIATRICS	CHILDREN
		USUAL	MRDD*		
Reduce dosage 4 mg bid to qid	**Over 12 yrs.:** same as adult 4 mg bid to qid	—— ——	—— ——	—— ——	—— ——
Reduce dosage	**Under 12 yrs.:** not established	——	——	——	——
Reduce dosage	Reduce dosage	——	——	——	——
Reduce dosage	Reduce dosage	——	——	——	——
Reduce dosage	Reduce dosage	——	——	——	——
Reduce dosage	**Under 12 yrs.:** not established				
Reduce dosage	Not established	——	——	——	——

*Maximal recommended daily dose.

tion, are long-acting antipsychotic agents. Therapeutic effects are usually obvious between 48 and 98 hours, and the clinical effects may persist from 2 to 4 weeks.

The phenothiazines, thioxanthenes, molindone, haloperidol, and loxapine have actions at all levels of the central nervous system, particularly the hypothalamus. However, the site and exact mechanism of action in man are unknown.

The phenothiazines also have antiemetic activity which is manifested at lower doses than required for antipsychotic effects. For detailed information, see Chapter 8, Drugs Affecting the Gastrointestinal Tract.

SPECIAL PRECAUTIONS

• Use extreme caution in patients with a history of mental depression because of possible suicide attempts.
• Use cautiously in patients with compromised liver or kidney function and also with a history of cardiovascular disorders, convulsive disorders, and blood dyscrasias.
• Phenothiazines and haloperidol are contraindicated in patients with suspected or established subcortical brain damage or

CNS depression.
- The antiemetic activity of the phenothiazines may obscure nausea and vomiting associated with various organic disorders.
- Do not use in patients known or suspected to be hypersensitive to that drug or related drugs.
- In general elderly and/or debilitated patients require less drug than other patients.
- Caution patients that a sedative effect may occur initially and patients should avoid activities requiring alertness such as driving a car or operating machinery.
- Use in pregnant patients only when, in the judgment of the physician, the potential benefits outweigh the possible risks.

ADVERSE EFFECTS

CNS EFFECTS: dystonia, tight feeling in throat, slurred speech, dysphagia, oculogyric crisis, trismus, torticollis, retrocollis, muscle weakness, aching and numbness of limbs, akathisia, motor restlessness, dyskinesia, parkinsonism, hyper-reflexia, ataxia, tardive dyskinesia, headaches, mild insomnia, EEG abnormalities, reactivation of psychosis, paradoxical excitement, paranoid reaction, catatonia, hypnotic effects

RESPIRATORY EFFECTS: asthma, asphyxia due to failure of the cough reflex; haloperidol—laryngospasm, bronchospasm, increased depth of respiration

CARDIOVASCULAR EFFECTS: postural hypotension, simple tachycardia, syncope, peripheral edema; haloperidol—tachycardia, hypotension

AUTONOMIC EFFECTS: blurred vision, dry mouth or salivation, nasal congestion, adynamic ileus, urinary retention or frequency, constipation, impotence; haloperidol—dry mouth, blurred vision, urinary retention, diaphoresis

GASTROINTESTINAL EFFECTS: anorexia, diarrhea, hypersalivation, dyspepsia anorexia, nausea, vomiting, constipation; haloperidol—anorexia, constipation, diarrhea, hypersalivation, dyspepsia, nausea, vomiting

METABOLIC AND ENDOCRINE EFFECTS: lactation, gynecomastia, galactorrhea, disturbances in the menstrual cycle, hyperglycemia, false positive pregnancy tests, breast enlargement, amenorrhea, glycosuria, hyperglycemia

HEPATIC EFFECTS: impaired liver function and/or jaundice

HEMATOLOGIC EFFECTS: phenothiazines—agranulocytosis, eosinophilia, hemolytic anemia, thrombocytopenia, pancytopenia; thioxanthenes—leukopenia, leukocytosis; haloperidol—leukopenia, leukocytosis, minimal decrease in erythrocyte count, anemia, agranulocytosis, tendency toward lymphomonocytosis

ALLERGIC EFFECTS: phenothiazines—erythema, pruritus, urticaria, eczema, anaphylactoid reactions, local and generalized edema, photosensitization, asthma, exfoliative dermatitis; thioxanthenes—rash, pruritus, urticaria, photosensitivity, rarely anaphylaxis; molindone—rash

DERMATOLOGIC EFFECTS: phenothiazines—contact dermatitis in nursing personnel, skin pigmentation with long-term use; haloperidol—maculopapular and acneiform skin reactions, isolated cases of photosensitivity and loss of hair

OPHTHALMIC EFFECTS: phenothiazines—blurred vision, deposition of fine particulate matter in lens and cornea; star-shaped opacities; lesions may regress after withdrawal of drug.

CLINICAL GUIDELINES

ADMINISTRATION:
- It is usually necessary to adjust the dosage for each patient and for the severity of his condition. Consequently, it is important to report changes in symptoms and symptom severity so that the physician can adjust the dosage accordingly.
- When administering phenothiazines intramuscularly, inject slowly, deep into the upper outer quadrant of the buttock.

• After administering phenothiazines intramuscularly, keep the patient lying down for at least 30 minutes because of the possible hypotensive effects.

• Avoid getting phenothiazine solution on the hands or clothing since contact dermatitis has been reported.

• Protect phenothiazine solutions from light since discoloration may occur; slight yellowing will not alter potency.

EFFECTS:

• Since drowsiness may occur with initial and high doses of the antipsychotic agents, outpatients should be warned about driving a car or operating mechanical equipment. Hospitalized patients should be guided in ambulation.

• Orthostatic hypotension may occur with certain phenothiazines and thioxanthenes, particularly when they are administered parenterally.

• Increase dosage gradually in elderly or emaciated patients because of the greater likelihood of side effects.

• Remember that maximal improvement may not be seen for weeks or even months.

• Phenothiazines can suppress the cough reflex; therefore, aspiration of vomitus may occur.

• Because of the possibility of suicide attempts, use with caution in patients with psychic depression.

• A significant rise in body temperature may indicate an idiosyncratic reaction; discontinue treatment with the particular agent being administered.

DRUG INTERACTIONS:

• Phenothiazines may counteract the antihypertensive effect of guanethidine and related compounds.

• Avoid concomitant use of alcoholic beverages, barbiturates, antihistamines, narcotics, and other CNS depressants; additive effects and hypotension may occur.

• If hypotension develops, do not administer ephinephrine because its action is blocked and partly reversed by the phenothiazines and haloperidol.

• If the patient has been exposed to the effects of atropine, heat, or phosphorus insecticides, use phenothiazines cautiously.

• Haloperidol may lower the convulsive threshold; anticonvulsant therapy may be necessary.

OVERDOSAGE/ANTIDOTE:

• Signs of overdosage are an exaggeration of the pharmacological effects and involve primarily the extrapyramidal mechanisms.

• Although a specific antidote has not been established, the parkinson like symptoms may be controlled with drugs such as benztropine mesylate (COGENTIN) or TREMIN (trihexyphenidyl hydrochloride).

Reserpine
Rauwolfia Serpentina

PHARMACOLOGY

Reserpine and rauwolfia serpentina have both antipsychotic and antihypertensive activities. Following oral administration, the onset of antipsychotic action is relatively slow but the effects are sustained. Both the antipsychotic and antihypertensive effects may persist following withdrawal of the drug. The antipsychotic activity is attributed to depletion of norepinephrine, epinephrine, and 5-hydroxytryptamine from the brain.

For psychiatric emergencies, intramuscular administration results in a more rapid effect than that obtained following oral administration.

For use as an antihypertensive agent, see Chapter 5, page 228.

SPECIAL PRECAUTIONS

• Use with extreme caution in patients with a history of mental depression because of possible suicide attempts.

• Use cautiously in patients with compromised liver or kidney function, and also with a history of cardiovascular disorders, convulsive disorders, and blood dyscrasis.

• Use cautiously in patients with a history of peptic ulcer, ulcerative colitis, and biliary colic because of increased gastrointestinal motility and secretion.

• Do not use in patients with known or suspected hypersensitivity to that drug or related drugs.

• Use in pregnant patients only when, in the judgment of the physician, the potential benefits outweigh the possible risks.

ADVERSE EFFECTS

CNS EFFECTS: drowsiness, depression, dizziness, syncope, insomnia, nervousness, paradoxical anxiety, nightmares, rarely parkinsonian syndrome, other extrapyramidal tract symptoms, dull sensorium

RESPIRATORY EFFECTS: dyspnea, increased respiratory secretions

CARDIOVASCULAR EFFECTS: angina-like symptoms, arrhythmias (particularly when used concurrently with digitalis or quinidine), bradycardia, water retention with edema in patients with hypertensive vascular disease

URINARY TRACT EFFECTS: dysuria

AUTONOMIC EFFECTS: nasal congestion, dry mouth

GASTROINTESTINAL EFFECTS: hypersecretion, nausea, vomiting, anorexia, diarrhea

METABOLIC AND ENDOCRINE EFFECTS: impotence or decreased libido, weight gain, breast engorgement, pseudolactation, gynecomastia

HEMATOLOGIC EFFECTS: epistaxis, purpura

ALLERGIC EFFECTS: rash, pruritus

OPHTHALMIC EFFECTS: glaucoma, uveitis, optic atrophy, conjunctival injection

MUSCULOSKELETAL EFFECTS: muscular aches

CLINICAL GUIDELINES

ADMINISTRATION:

• Administer after meals to reduce gastric discomfort.

• A past history of bronchial asthma or al-lergy may increase the possibility of drug reactions.

EFFECTS:

• Biliary colic may be precipitated.

• Watch for signs of mental depression; discontinue therapy if depression occurs.

DRUG INTERACTIONS:

• Avoid concurrent use of MAO-inhibitors.

• In patients receiving digitalis or quinidine watch for cardiac arrhythmias since they have occurred in patients receiving rauwolfia preparations.

• The anesthesiologist should be aware of the patient's use of rauwolfia preparations because of possible hypotensive effects.

• Concomitant use with ganglionic blocking agents, guanethidine, veratrum, hydralazine, methyldopa, chlorthalidone, or thiazides necessitates titration of dosage with each agent.

OVERDOSAGE/ANTIDOTE:

• Overdosage is characterized by impairment of consciousness, flushing of skin, hypothermia, central respiratory depression, possible bradycardia, and diarrhea.

• There is no specific antidote known. Anticholinergic and/or adrenergic drugs, e.g., metaraminol and norepinephrine, have been used to treat the adverse vagocirculatory effects.

Lithium Carbonate
Lithium Citrate

PHARMACOLOGY

Lithium carbonate and lithium citrate administered orally are absorbed rapidly from the gastrointestinal tract and are excreted primarily in the urine with insignificant amounts excreted in the feces. Renal excretion of lithium is proportional to its plasma concentration. The desirable serum lithium level ranges between 1.0 and 1.5 mEq/liter.

Lithium decreases sodium reabsorption by the renal tubules, which can lead to sodium depletion. Lithium toxicity is closely related to serum lithium levels.

The specific biochemical mechanism of action of lithium in psychosis is unknown.

SPECIAL PRECAUTIONS

• Use extreme caution in patients with a history of mental depression because of possible suicide attempts.

• Do not administer to patients with severe debilitation or dehydration, sodium depletion, or to patients receiving diuretics or a low salt diet.

• Lithium is contraindicated in patients with cardiovascular or renal disease, and brain damage.

• Do not use in patients known or suspected to be hypersensitive to this drug.

• Drugs should be given to pregnant patients only when, in the judgment of the physician, the potential benefits outweigh the possible risks.

ADVERSE EFFECTS

CNS EFFECTS: drowsiness, blackout spells, epileptiform seizures, slurred speech, dizziness, vertigo, incontinence of urine and feces, somnolence, psychomotor retardation, restlessness, confusion, stupor, coma, transient EEG changes, lack of coordination, worsening of organic brain syndrome, fine hand tremor, muscle hyperirritability (fasciculations, twitching, clonic movements of whole limbs), ataxia, choreoathetotic movements, hyperactive deep tendon reflexes

CARDIOVASCULAR EFFECTS: arrhythmia, hypotension, peripheral circulatory collapse, EEG changes, edema of ankles and wrists

URINARY TRACT EFFECTS: albuminuria, oliguria, polyuria, glycosuria

AUTONOMIC EFFECTS: blurred vision, dry mouth

GASTROINTESTINAL EFFECTS: anorexia, nausea, vomiting, diarrhea

METABOLIC AND ENDOCRINE EFFECTS: euthyroid goiter and/or hypothyroidism (including myxedema), weight loss, dehydration, thirst or polyuria sometimes resembling diabetes insipidus

HEMATOLOGIC EFFECTS: leukocytosis

DERMATOLOGIC EFFECTS: drying and thinning of hair, anesthesia of skin, chronic folliculitis, generalized pruritus with or without rash, cutaneous ulcers

OPHTHALMIC EFFECTS: transient scotomata, blurred vision

CLINICAL GUIDELINES

ADMINISTRATION:

• Patient must maintain a normal diet including salt and fluid intake since lithium decreases sodium reabsorption which can lead to sodium depletion.

• Blood samples for serum lithium determinations should be drawn 8 to 12 hours after the previous dose when lithium concentrations are relatively stable. Total reliance must not be placed on serum concentrations alone. Accurate patient evaluation does require both clinical and laboratory analyses.

EFFECTS:

• Caution patients that lithium may impair mental and/or physical abilities.

• Protracted sweating or diarrhea or concomitant infection with elevated temperatures may decrease tolerance; reduce dose if necessary.

• Fine hand tremor, polyuria, mild thirst, transient and mild nausea, and general discomfort may occur during initial therapy; these effects usually subside with continued treatment or a temporary reduction of dosage or termination of medication.

• The earliest signs of toxicity include diarrhea, vomiting, drowsiness, muscular weakness, and lack of coordination; they can occur at lithium serum levels below 2.0 mEq/l. At higher levels, ataxia, giddiness, tinnitus, blurred vision, and a large output of dilute urine may be seen. Serum lithium levels should not be permitted to exceed 2.0 mEq/l during the acute treatment phase.

• Elderly patients may exhibit signs of toxicity at serum levels ordinarily tolerated by other patients.

OVERDOSAGE/ANTIDOTE:

• Overdosage with lithium salts is characterized by an exaggeration of the adverse effects.

• There is no specific antidote for lithium poisoning.

• Gastric lavage, correction of fluid and electrolyte imbalance, and regulation of kidney function are essential. Use of urea, mannitol, and aminophylline will increase lithium excretion.

Psychostimulants

GENERAL CLINICAL USES

The psychostimulants, caffeine, the amphetamines, and methylphenidate, exert an action upon consciousness by decreasing the sense of fatigue, increasing alertness, offsetting drowsiness, and by causing an elevation of mood. These effects are attributed to selective stimulation of the cerebral cortex. Although widely prescribed heretofore for mild depressive states, these drugs have been replaced by the antidepressant drugs.

The psychostimulants may be helpful in improving psychomotor mentation, in treating children's behavioral disorders, and in the management of narcolepsy.

SPECIFIC PRODUCTS AND DOSAGES

GENERIC NAME	TRADE NAME	ROUTE OF ADMIN.	ADULTS	MRD*	CHILDREN
Amphetamines: CII** amphetamine	(G)† BIPHETAMINE DELCOBESE		10–20 mg bid to qid	100 mg	**6–12 yrs.:** 5–10 mg tid; maximal daily dose 30 mg

*Maximal recommended dose.
**Designates schedule listing under Federal Controlled Substances Act.
†(G) Designates availability as a generic product.

(continued facing page)

	GENERIC NAME	TRADE NAME	ROUTE OF ADMIN.	ADULTS	MRD*	CHILDREN
CII	amphetamine sulfate	(G) BENZEDRINE	po	10–20 mg bid to qid	100 mg	**6–12 yrs.:** 5–10 mg tid; maximal daily dose 40 mg
CIII	benzphetamine hydrochloride	DIDREX	po	25–50 mg od to tid		
CII	dextroamphetamine hydrochloride	DARO	po	5–10 mg bid to qid	60 mg	**Over 5 yrs.:** 5–10 mg bid; maximal daily dose 20 mg
CII	dextroamphetamine phosphate	DEXTRO-PROFETHAMINE	po	5–10 mg bid to qid	60 mg	**Over 5 yrs.:** 5–10 mg bid; maximal daily dose 20 mg
CII	dextroamphetamine sulfate	(G) DEXEDRINE	po	5–10 mg bid to qid	60 mg	**Over 5 yrs.:** 5–10 mg bid; maximal daily dose 20 mg
CII	methamphetamine hydochloride	DESOXYN	po	2.5–5 mg tid	———	2.5–5 mg od to bid; maximum: 20–25 mg/day for behavioral syndrome
	Caffeine Preparations: caffeine citrate, NF caffeine and sodium benzoate, USP	(G) (G)	po im/iv	100 mg tid 500 mg as necessary	1000 mg 1000 mg	Not established 8 mg/kg; maximal daily dose 500 mg
CII	*Miscellaneous:* methylphenidate hydrochloride	RITALIN	po	5–20 mg bid to tid	60 mg	**Over 6 yrs.:** 5–20 mg bid to tid

*Maximal recommended dose.

Amphetamines

Amphetamine
Amphetamine Sulfate
Benzphetamine HCl
Dextroamphetamine HCl
Dextroamphetamine Phosphate
Dextroamphetamine Sulfate
Methamphetamine HCl

PHARMACOLOGY

The amphetamines distinctly modify the electroencephalogram by causing a shift to high frequencies and a reduction in the large delta waves such as are observed in narcolepsy. The desynchronization of the EEG in the adult is characteristic of behavioral arousal.

In the hyperkinetic syndrome in children, the paradoxical effect of amphetamines results in a beneficial effect on behavioral patterns. The amphetamines do not necessarily convert the EEG pattern, despite the improvement in clinical or behavioral criteria.

The amphetamines when administered orally have a rapid onset of action and a relatively short duration of action; tolerance develops rapidly. In high doses the amphetamines become medullary excitants with marked stimulating actions on respiration, the electrocardiogram, and peripheral circulation.

SPECIAL PRECAUTIONS

• These agents are classified as Schedule II drugs under the Controlled Substances Act.

• Do not administer to patients prone to or with a history of drug abuse.

• Avoid concomitant use with MAO-inhibitors and use in hyperthyroid patients or agitated patients; hypertensive crises have resulted from concomitant use or within 14 days following use of MAO-inhibitors.

• Do not administer to patients with coronary artery disease, or other cardiovascular disorders such as hypertension.

• Do not administer during pregnancy.

• May impair the ability to engage in potentially hazardous activities such as operating machinery or vehicles.

• Do not administer to patients with a known hypersensitivity or idiosyncrasy to sympathomimetic amines.

ADVERSE EFFECTS

CNS EFFECTS: restlessness, dizziness, tremors, hyperactive reflexes, anxiety, insomnia, irritability, confusion, headache, chills, hallucinations, convulsions, euphoria, tremor, dysphoria, rarely psychotic episodes

RESPIRATORY EFFECTS: increased rate and depth

CARDIOVASCULAR EFFECTS: hypertension, palpitations, arrhythmias, tachycardia

URINARY TRACT EFFECTS: dysuria

AUTONOMIC EFFECTS: excessive perspiration, dry mouth and nose

GASTROINTESTINAL EFFECTS: nausea, vomiting, diarrhea, constipation, anorexia

METABOLIC AND ENDOCRINE EFFECTS: weight loss, changes in libido, impotence

ALLERGIC EFFECTS: urticaria

DERMATOLOGIC EFFECTS: pallor, flushing

OPHTHALMIC EFFECTS: pupillary dilation

CLINICAL GUIDELINES

ADMINISTRATION:

• Avoid administering the drug in late afternoon to prevent drug-induced insomnia.

• Since amphetamines may be prescribed for weight loss, the patient should be queried to avoid overdosage.

• These drugs are subject to the Drug Abuse Control Amendments; they are classified as Schedule II Drugs.

EFFECTS:

• Amphetamines do not obviate the need for rest; they defer it by masking fatigue. When the drug effects disappear, severe fatigue and mental depression may follow.

• Tolerance develops rapidly; with increased dosages and frequency of administration, physical and psychological dependence can occur.

• After prolonged use, the amphetamines should be withdrawn gradually to prevent withdrawal symptoms.

DRUG INTERACTIONS:

• Overdosage is manifested by tremors, chills, pupillary dilation, convulsions, confusion, hallucinations, and possibly coma. Respiration and pulse are accelerated and blood pressure is elevated. Chronic intoxication is manifested by severe dermatoses, marked insomnia, irritability, hyperactivity, and personality changes. Psychosis often is indistinguishable from schizophrenia.

• There is no known antidote for amphetamine overdosage. However, antianxiety agents (minor tranquilizers) or short-acting barbiturates may be helpful.

Caffeine Preparations

PHARMACOLOGY
Caffeine is readily absorbed from the gastrointestinal tract or from the site of injection. The clinical response is usually seen within 1 hour and persists for 2 to 4 hours. The improvement in sensory awareness is attributed to stimulation of regions of the cerebral cortex.

Larger than threshold doses of caffeine stimulate the medullary centers associated with respiration, vascular balance, and integration. Increased respiratory rate and an increase in blood pressure are frequently measured. An influence upon the spinal cord also is evidenced by the intensified patellar response.

SPECIAL PRECAUTIONS
• Caffeine citrate should not be injected for cortical psychostimulating effects; administer only by mouth. Only caffeine and sodium benzoate, USP, is suitable for intramuscular administration.
• Do not use in patients known or suspected to be hypersensitive to that drug or related drugs.
• Do not administer to patients with gastric or duodenal ulcer.
• Administer to pregnant patients only when, in the judgment of the physician, the potential benefits outweigh the possible risks.

ADVERSE EFFECTS
CNS EFFECTS: insomnia, restlessness, excitement, tremor, irritability, delirium, clonic convulsions, headache, hyperesthesia

RESPIRATORY EFFECTS: hyperpnea followed by apnea
CARDIOVASCULAR EFFECTS: hypertension, palpitation, tachycardia, bradycardia, extrasystoles
URINARY TRACT EFFECTS: polyuria
AUTONOMIC EFFECTS: increased vagal tone
GASTROINTESTINAL EFFECTS: nausea, vomiting
METABOLIC AND ENDOCRINE EFFECTS: increased basal metabolic rate
OPHTHALMIC EFFECTS: scintillating scotomata
MUSCULOSKELETAL EFFECTS: muscular tremor
OTIC EFFECTS: tinnitus

CLINICAL GUIDELINES
ADMINISTRATION:
• Patients receiving caffeine and sodium benzoate, USP, intramuscularly should be closely observed, preferably in bed, for a period of up to 3 hours.
• Intramuscular injection should be given well within the body of a relatively large muscle.
EFFECTS:
• Beverages high in caffeine should be omitted from the diet of patients with peptic ulcer or gastrointestinal complaints because of the increased vagal time produced by caffeine.
• The tremor may impede eye-hand coordinating tasks.
• The insomnia may interfere with or exacerbate an underlying anxiety state.
DRUG INTERACTIONS:
• Caffeine may interact with amphetamines or antidepressants in an idiosyncratic manner
OVERDOSAGE/ANTIDOTE:
• Overdosage is manifested by insomnolence, hyperexcitability, confusion, exaggerated reflexes.

• There is no specific antidote to caffeine. An antianxiety agent (minor tranquilizer) or short-acting barbiturate may be administered to control anxiety.

Methylphenidate Hydrochloride

PHARMACOLOGY

Methylphenidate hydrochloride, a mild central nervous system stimulant, is similar to the amphetamines; it is more potent than caffeine. Maximal effect develops in several days.

SPECIAL PRECAUTIONS

• Do not administer to patients with marked anxiety, tension, and agitation since the drug may aggravate these symptoms.
• Do not administer to patients hypersensitive to the drug or to patients with glaucoma.
• May lower the convulsive threshold in patients with prior history of seizures, and no prior EEG evidence of seizures.
• Note that safe concomitant use of anticonvulsants and methylphenidate has not been established.
• Discontinue the drug in the presence of seizures.
• Use with caution in patients with hypertension; monitor blood pressure at appropriate intervals.
• Drugs should not be prescribed for pregnant women unless, in the judgment of the physician, the potential benefits outweigh the possible risks.

ADVERSE EFFECTS

CNS EFFECTS: nervousness, insomnia, dizziness, headache, dyskinesia, drowsiness, toxic psychosis
CARDIOVASCULAR EFFECTS: palpitations, increased and decreased blood pressure and pulse, tachycardia, angina, arrhythmias
GASTROINTESTINAL EFFECTS: nausea, loss of weight during prolonged therapy, abdominal pain
HEMATOLOGIC EFFECTS: leukopenia; also anemia
ALLERGIC EFFECTS: rash, urticaria, fever, arthralgia, exfoliative dermatitis, erythema multiforme, thrombocytopenic purpura
DERMATOLOGIC EFFECTS: hair loss

CLINICAL GUIDELINES

ADMINISTRATION:
• Monitor the patient's blood pressure frequently.
EFFECTS:
• Periodic CBC, leukocyte differential, and platelet counts are advised during prolonged therapy.
DRUG INTERACTIONS:
• May decrease the hypotensive effect of guanethidine.
• Use cautiously with pressor agents and MAO-inhibitors.
• May inhibit metabolism of coumarin anticoagulants, phenobarbital, diphenylhydantoin, primidone, phenylbutazone, imipramine, and desipramine; dosage reduction may be required.
OVERDOSAGE/ANTIDOTE:
• Overdosage is characterized by overstimulation of the central nervous system and excessive sympathomimetic effects. Symptoms include vomiting, agitation, tremors, hyperreflexia, muscle twitching, convulsions, coma, euphoria, confusion, hallucinations, delirium, sweating, flushing, headache, hyperpyrexia, tachycardia, palpitations, mydriasis, and dryness of mucous membranes.
• There is no known antidote. Efficacy of peritoneal dialysis or extracorporeal hemodialysis has not been established.

Drugs affecting the brain and spinal cord

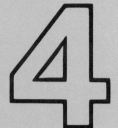

INTRODUCTION

The medicinal drugs affecting the brain and spinal cord may be classified as depressants, stimulants, or those associated with metabolic changes or which produce vascular alterations within the central nervous system. Drugs which act upon the central nervous system but have their primary effect elsewhere in the body such as the muscle relaxants are discussed in the appropriate chapter but are cross referenced in this chapter.

SPECIFIC THERAPEUTIC CLASSIFICATION

The central nervous system depressants encompass the following major groups of drugs:

1. Analgesics: They are grouped as antipyretic analgesics, opiate-type analgesics, and others.
2. Anesthetic agents, general: The general anesthetic agents are divided into injectable and inhalation anes-

thetics.
3. Anesthetic agents, regional
4. Anticerebral edema agents
5. Anticonvulsants: The anticonvulsants are grouped as the barbiturates, long acting; diphenylhydantoin and derivatives; trimethadione and related compounds; succinimides; and miscellaneous drugs. The classification of seizure, drug choice, and dosage is extremely complex since many patients are affected with more than one type of seizure.
6. Anti-infective agents
7. Antimigraine preparations: These preparations are grouped as the standard analgesic agents and the ergot alkaloids.
8. Antiparkinsonian agents: Drugs used to treat parkinsonism are divided into 3 groups: (1) atropinelike anticholinergic agents; (2) dopaminergic agents, and (3) miscellaneous agents including amantadine hydrochloride.
9. Antivertigo agents: Please refer to the discussion of antinauseants, antiemetics, and antivertigo agents, in Chapter 8, page 379, for detailed information.
10. Central nervous system stimulants: Please refer to Chapter 3, page 122.
11. Cerebrovasodilators: Please see Chapter 5, page 283, for detailed information.
12. Muscle relaxants: Please refer to Chapter 13, page 493, for detailed information.
13. Sedative-hypnotic drugs: These drugs are grouped as follows: nonbarbiturate sedative-hypnotic agents, other agents employed as sedative-hypnotic agents, and barbiturates.

Analgesic Agents

Antipyretic Analgesic Agents

SPECIFIC PRODUCTS AND DOSAGES

			SUGGESTED DAILY DOSAGE		
GENERIC NAME	TRADE NAME	ROUTE OF ADMIN.	ADULT SINGLE DOSE (mg)	MRDD* (mg)	CHILDREN SINGLE DOSE
acetaminophen (APAP)	(G)‡ DATRIL TYLENOL	po	325–650 q 4–6 hr	3900	Under 1 yr.: 60 mg q 4–6 hrs. **1–3 yrs.:** 60–120

*MRDD = maximal recommended daily dose.
‡(G) Designates availability as a generic product.

(continued facing page)

| | | ROUTE OF ADMIN. | SUGGESTED DAILY DOSAGE | | |
GENERIC NAME	TRADE NAME		ADULT SINGLE DOSE (mg)	MRDD* (mg)	CHILDREN SINGLE DOSE
acetaminophen (APAP) (continued)					mg q 4–6 hrs. **4–5 yrs.:** 120 mg q 4–6 hrs. **6–12 yrs.:** 150–300 mg q 4–6 hrs.
acetophenetidin (phenacetin)	(G)‡	po	300–600 q 3 hr	2400	———
acetylsalicylic acid (aspirin)	(G)‡ ASCRIPTIN† BUFFERIN†	po	300–1000 q 4 hr	5000	65 mg/kg/day divided in 4–6 doses
choline salicylate	ARTHROPAN TRILISATE†	po	1000–1500 bid	3400	Not established
fenoprofen calcium	NALFON	po	See Chapter 13 for detailed information, page 472		
ibuprofen	MOTRIN	po	See Chapter 13 for detailed information, page 472		
indomethacin	INDOCIN	po	See Chapter 13 for detailed information, page 472		
magnesium salicylate	MOBIDIN HYALEX† PABALATE†	po	See Chapter 13 for detailed information, page 492		
mefenamic acid	PONSTEL	po	250–500 qid	2000	Not established
naproxen	NAPROSYN	po	See Chapter 13 for detailed information, page 472		
oxyphenbutazone	OXALID TANDEARIL	po	See Chapter 13 for detailed information, page 472		
phenylbutazone	AZOLID BUTAZOLIDIN	po	See Chapter 13 for detailed information, page 472		
tolmetin sodium	TOLECTIN	po	See Chapter 13 for detailed information, page 472		

* MRDD = maximal recommended daily dose.
† Contains more than one active ingredient.
‡ (G) Designates availability as a generic product.

Acetaminophen Acetophenetidin (Phenacetin)

GENERAL CLINICAL USES

Acetaminophen and acetophenetidin may be used in place of salicylates as analgesic and antipyretic agents for mild to moderate pain such as with headache. They differ from salicylates by the absence of anti-inflammatory effects and, therefore, are not recommended for the treatment of rheumatic diseases.

PHARMACOLOGY

Acetophenetidin is absorbed readily after oral administration; it is metabolized to active acetaminophen. The antipyretic action may be central as well as peripheral. The analgesic effect, comparable to that of acetylsalicylic acid, reflects an elevation in threshold to pain, but the pharmacologic basis for the relief of the pain remains undetermined. A single recommended dose remains effective for 3 to 4 hours. Elimination is through the kidneys following metabolism and conjugation by the liver.

SPECIAL PRECAUTIONS
• Do not administer to patients with a history of hypersensitivity or with cardiac or pulmonary disease.
• Mild chronic hemolytic anemia has been associated with prolonged use.

ADVERSE EFFECTS
CNS EFFECTS: drowsiness, euphoria, relaxation
URINARY TRACT EFFECTS: renal papillary necrosis (infrequent)
HEPATIC EFFECTS: jaundice (rare)
HEMATOLOGIC EFFECTS: hemolytic anemia, agranulocytosis (rare)
ALLERGIC EFFECTS: mouth lesions
DERMATOLOGIC EFFECTS: rash

CLINICAL GUIDELINES
ADMINISTRATION:
• Caution patients against driving a car or operating machinery.
DRUG INTERACTIONS:
• Acetaminophen has been reported to potentiate the effects of oral anticoagulants.
OVERDOSAGE/ANTIDOTE:
• Overdosage is characterized by methemoglobinemia, cyanosis, dizziness, toxic psychosis, convulsions, fever, respiratory depression, and apnea.

• No specific antidote is known. Gastric lavage should be performed if the drug was ingested recently. Management is symptomatic. Vital respiratory, circulatory, and renal functions must be adequately supported and maintained. Blood transfusions may be required to offset hemolytic anemia and shock in cases of severe intoxication.

Acetylsalicylic Acid (Aspirin)
Choline Salicylate
Magnesium Salicylate

GENERAL CLINICAL USES
Aspirin is the drug of choice when mild to moderate analgesia and antipyresis are desired. Since it exerts both analgesic and anti-inflammatory effects, the drug is recommended in various rheumatic and musculoskeletal diseases. For additional information on its use as an anti-inflammatory agent, please refer to Chapter 13, *Drugs Affecting the Musculoskeletal System.* See page 492.

PHARMACOLOGY
The antipyretic analgesics relieve certain types of pain, usually of low to moderate intensity (such as headache, myalgia, arthralgia), arising from musculoskeletal structures rather than from the viscera. Orally administered salicylates are rapidly and completely absorbed from the gastrointestinal tract. Much of the absorbed aspirin is hydrolyzed to salicylate in tissues and blood. The analgesic effect exerted by salicylates is not understood despite evidence to support increased pain threshold. In contrast to opiate-type analgesics, salicylates fail to induce sedation, drowsiness, or euphoria in recommended analgesic doses. The salicylates also lower the tem-

perature in fever by a dilatation of superficial skin blood vessels, an action accompanied by profuse sweating, associated evaporation of perspiration, and further cooling.

Salicylates do not depress respiration, but may cause serious hyperventilation with overdosage. Ordinary doses have no effect on the cardiovascular system. Large doses do not appear to alter hepatic or cardiovascular function. However, renal function may be modified to the extent that uric acid is more readily eliminated in the urine. The uricosuric action of salicylates has been used in treating acute and chronic gout. Autonomic and gastrointestinal functions are not affected pharmacologically.

The usual salicylate dose for analgesia remains effective for 3 to 4 hours. These compounds are metabolized in the liver and excreted in the urine.

Salicylates may induce hypoprothrombinemia and modify blood platelet aggregation, therefore interfering with normal blood clotting processes.

Salicylates inhibit synthesis of prostaglandins, which may be responsible for the analgesic and antipyretic effects, and also anti-inflammatory or antirheumatic effects.

SPECIAL PRECAUTIONS

- Do not use in patients with a history of salicylate hypersensitivity.
- Do not use in patients with asthma, hay fever, or nasal polyps; these patients have a higher incidence of hypersensitivity to salicylates than other patients.
- Caution should be observed in patients with gastric ulcers, bleeding tendencies, hypothrombinemia, or those receiving anticoagulant therapy.
- Avoid excessive or prolonged medication in patients with impaired renal or hepatic function.

ADVERSE EFFECTS

CNS EFFECTS: stimulation, confusion, dizziness, drowsiness, hyperthermia, stupor, coma; toxic psychosis rarely

RESPIRATORY EFFECTS: hyperventilation

URINARY TRACT EFFECTS: uricosuria

AUTONOMIC EFFECTS: sweating

GASTROINTESTINAL EFFECTS: nausea, vomiting, heartburn, irritation and bleeding, melena

HEMATOLOGIC   EFFECTS: hypoprothrombinemia, hemolytic anemia (rare)

ALLERGIC EFFECTS: coryza

DERMATOLOGIC EFFECTS: urticaria, angioneurotic edema

OPHTHALMIC EFFECTS: dimness of vision

OTIC EFFECTS: tinnitus, impaired hearing

CLINICAL GUIDELINES

ADMINISTRATION:

- Since salicylates may cause irritation of the gastric lining, administer with food, ample water, milk, or other nonalcoholic beverages.
- Carefully observe patient for signs of nasal, subcutaneous, or gastric bleeding (melena).
- Exposed to humid air, aspirin tablets decompose to salicylic acid and acetic acid. Since the free salicylic acid is highly irritating to the gastrointestinal tract, the tablets should be discarded.

DRUG INTERACTIONS:

- The salicylates enhance the analgesic actions of codeine, propoxyphene, pentazocine, and related opiate-type analgesics.
- Salicylates may potentiate anticoagulants and thereby increase coagulation time excessively.
- The hypoglycemic response to salicylates does not alter actions of insulin or oral antidiabetic agents.

OVERDOSAGE/ANTIDOTE:

- Symptoms of overdosage include high-pitched tinnitus, dizziness, deafness, impaired vision, alkalosis, tachycardia, renal irritation, hypoglycemia, and elevated body temperature; restlessness, agitation, confusion, and convulsions are followed by stupor or coma. Acidosis may occur in young children. Initial respiratory stimulation converts to respiratory depression and metabolic acidosis.

• No specific antidote is known. Initial treatment consists of gastric lavage. Hyperthermia should be combated with alcohol sponges or ice packs. Urine volume should be maintained by oral or parenteral fluids to keep acid-base values on the alkaline side with intravenously administered sodium bicarbonate and thereby increase renal excretion of the salicylate.

Mefenamic Acid

GENERAL CLINICAL USES

Mefenamic acid is used for relief of mild to moderate pain when therapy will not exceed 1 week.

PHARMACOLOGY

Mefenamic acid has analgesic, antipyretic, and anti-inflammatory actions. It is absorbed rapidly, and excreted in urine and feces as unchanged drug and metabolites.

SPECIAL PRECAUTIONS

• Do not use in patients with ulceration or chronic inflammation of either the upper or lower gastrointestinal tract.
• Do not use in patients with a history of hypersensitivity to mefenamic acid.
• Safe use in pregnancy and in children less than 14 years old has not been established.
• If diarrhea occurs, discontinue drug; patient usually will be unable to tolerate the drug thereafter.

• Use with caution in patients with a history of kidney or liver disease.
• Use with caution in asthmatic patients; an acute exacerbation may occur.

ADVERSE EFFECTS

CNS EFFECTS: drowsiness, dizziness, nervousness, headache, insomnia
CARDIOVASCULAR EFFECTS: palpitations, rarely
URINARY TRACT EFFECTS: dysuria, hematuria
HEPATIC EFFECTS: mild toxicity
HEMATOLOGIC EFFECTS: hemolytic anemia, leukopenia, eosinophilia, thrombocytopenic purpura, agranulocytosis, pancytopenia, bone marrow hypoplasia
AUTONOMIC EFFECTS: perspiration
GASTROINTESTINAL EFFECTS: nausea, discomfort, vomiting, gas; diarrhea, possibly associated with inflammation or hemorrhage of the bowel
DERMATOLOGIC EFFECTS: rash, and facial edema
ALLERGIC EFFECTS: urticaria
OPHTHALMIC EFFECTS: blurred vision, irritation, reversible loss of color vision

CLINICAL GUIDELINES

ADMINISTRATION:
• Give with food to minimize gastric irritation.
• Do not administer for longer than 1 week.
DRUG INTERACTIONS:
• Insulin requirements may be increased in the diabetic patient.
• The effects of oral anticoagulant agents are enhanced by prolonged prothrombin time; should monitor prothrombin time frequently.
• A false positive reaction for urinary bile (diazo tablet test) may result; perform other diagnostic procedures such as the Harrison test.

Opiate-Type Analgesic Agents

SPECIFIC PRODUCTS AND DOSAGES

	GENERIC NAME	TRADE NAME	ROUTE OF ADMIN.	SUGGESTED DAILY DOSAGE		
				ADULT SINGLE DOSE	MRDD†	CHILDREN SINGLE DOSE
*CII	alphaprodine HCl	NISENTIL	sc	0.4–1.2 mg/kg	240 mg	Not recommended
			iv	0.4–0.6 mg/kg	———	Not recommended
			im	Not recommended	———	Not recommended
CII	anileridine HCl	LERITINE	po	25–50 mg q 4–6 hr.	200 mg	Not recommended
CII	anileridine phosphate	LERITINE	sc/im	25–50 mg q 4–6 hr.	200 mg	Not recommended
			iv	5–10 mg, 0.6 mg/ min.	———	Not recommended
CII	codeine phosphate	(G)‡	po	15–60 mg q 4 hr. mg	300 mg	3 mg/kg/day divided in 6 doses
CII	codeine sulfate	(G)	sc/im	15–60 mg q 4 hr.	300 mg	3 mg/kg/day divided in 6 doses
			iv	Not recommended	———	Not recommended
CII	fentanyl citrate	SUBLIMAZE	iv/im	0.05–0.1 mg, repeat at 2 to 3 min, intervals **In elderly patients:** 0.025–0.05 mg	———	**From 2–12 yrs:** 0.02–0.03 mg/ 20–25 lbs single dose
CII	hydromorphone HCl or sulfate	(G) DILAUDID	po sc/im iv pr	2 mg q 4–6 hr. 2–4 mg q 4–6 hr. 2–4 mg q 4–6 hr. 3 mg q 4–6 hr.	16 mg 16 mg 16 mg 16 mg	Not recommended Not recommended Not recommended Not recommended
CII	levorphanol tartrate	LEVO-DROMORAN	po sc/im	2–3 mg q 4–6 hr. 2–3 mg q 4–6 hr.	12 mg 12 mg	Not recommended Not recommended
*CII	meperidine HCl	(G)‡ DEMEROL	po	50–150 mg q 4 hr.	600 mg	0.5–0.8 mg/lb q 3–4 hr.

*C denotes schedule listing under Controlled Substances Act.
†MRDD = maximal recommended daily dose.
‡(G) Designates availability as a generic product.

(continued overleaf)

		ROUTE OF ADMIN.	SUGGESTED DAILY DOSAGE		
GENERIC NAME	**TRADE NAME**		**ADULT SINGLE DOSE**	**MRDD†**	**CHILDREN SINGLE DOSE**
meperidine HCl (continued)		im/sc	50–150 mg q 4 hr.	600 mg	0.5–0.8 mg/lb q 3–4 hr.
		iv	50–150 mg q 4 hr. (10 mg/ml)	600 mg	Not recommended
*CII methadone hydrochloride	(G)‡ DOLOPHINE WESTADONE	po sc/im	2.5–10 mg q 3–4 hr. 2.5–10 mg q 3–4 hr.	40 mg 40 mg	Not recommended Not recommended
methotrimeprazine	LEVOPROME	im	5–40 mg q 1–2 hr. **In elderly:** 5–10 mg	———	Not recommended
Opiate-type Narcotic Analgesics:					
CII morphine sulfate	(G)	po sc	5–15 mg q 4 hr. 2–20 mg q 4 hr.	——— 60 mg	Not recommended 0.1–0.2 mg/kg every 4 hr.
		iv	2.5–15 mg	48 mg	Not recommended
CII oxymorphone HCl	(G) NUMORPHAN	iv pr sc/im	0.5 mg 5 mg q 4–6 hr. 1–1.5 mg q 4–6 hr.	40 mg 40 mg 40 mg	Not recommended Not recommended Not recommended
CIV pentazocine lactate	TALWIN	im/sc iv	30 mg q 3–4 hr. 15–30 mg single dose	360 mg ———	Not recommended Not recommended
CIV pentazocine HCl	TALWIN	po	50–100 mg q 3–4 hr.	600 mg	Not recommended
CIV propoxyphene HCl	(G) DARVON	po	65 mg q 4 hr.	1200 mg	Not recommended
CIV propoxyphene nasylate	DARVON–N	po	100 mg every 4 hr.	800 mg	Not recommended
Other: butorphanol tartrate	STADOL	im iv	1–4 mg q 3–4 hr. 0.5–2 mg q 3–4 hr.	——— ———	Not recommended Not recommended

*C denotes schedule listing under the Controlled Substances Act.
†MRDD = maximal recommended daily dose.
‡(G) Designates availability as a generic product.

Alphaprodine Hydrochloride
Anileridine Phosphate
Anileridine Hydrochloride

GENERAL CLINICAL USES

Alphaprodine and anileridine are indicated for relief of moderate to severe pain. These agents are related chemically and pharmacologically to meperidine.

PHARMACOLOGY

Alphaprodine hydrochloride and anileridine phosphate are for parenteral administration whereas anileridine is for oral administration. Generally, the pharmacologic properties of these compounds are the same as for merperidine. However, about one-half the dosage by injection is required for analgesia as compared to meperidine. Parenteral administration results in prompt onset and short duration of action. Oral administration results in a slower effect.

SPECIAL PRECAUTIONS, ADVERSE
REACTIONS, GUIDELINES
See *Meperidine,* page 139.

Codeine Phosphate
Codeine Sulfate

GENERAL CLINICAL USES
Codeine is indicated for the relief of moderate to moderately severe pain. It is frequently prescribed in combination with an antipyretic analgesic such as aspirin. It also has been widely used for its oral antitussive action (about one-sixth the analgesic oral dose). Because the abuse liability of codeine is considerably less than for morphine, patients maintained on injected morphine may be shifted successfully to codeine in order to diminish morphine addiction potential.

PHARMACOLOGY
Codeine is well absorbed after subcutaneous or oral administration. It is much less potent than morphine on a weight basis. Codeine produces less sedation and much less respiratory depression than morphine. It has considerably fewer pharmacologic effects in the gastrointestinal and urinary tracts. Although very large doses of codeine can produce tolerance and physi-

cal dependence, the severity and incidence generally are much smaller than with morphine. Codeine has little, if any, effect upon the vasomotor center, and consequently changes in blood pressure occur only with severe overdosage. Unlike morphine, codeine does not readily induce nausea and vomiting. Similarly, the pinpoint pupil characteristic of morphine use does not readily appear following codeine administration.

The usual dose remains effective for 3 to 6 hours. Codeine, like morphine, is metabolized by the liver, and the metabolic products are excreted primarily in the urine.

SPECIAL PRECAUTIONS
• Ambulatory patients should be cautioned that codeine may impair physical abilities required for potentially hazardous tasks such as driving a car or operating machinery.
• May fatally potentiate other CNS depressant drugs such as ethyl alcohol, tranquilizers, sedative-hypnotic agents, and other analgesics.
• Prolonged use can result in habituation and physical dependence.

ADVERSE EFFECTS
CNS EFFECTS: drowsiness, restlessness, dizziness
RESPIRATORY TRACT EFFECTS: suppression of cough
GASTROINTESTINAL EFFECTS: nausea, vomiting, constipation infrequently
ALLERGIC EFFECTS: urticaria, rarely
OPHTHALMIC EFFECTS: constricted pupils, rarely

CLINICAL GUIDELINES
ADMINISTRATION:
• Ambulatory patients must be cautioned against driving a car or operating machin-

ery while taking codeine.
• Record patient's response as indicated by relief of pain.
• Record patient's coughing frequency, particularly noting his breathing efficiency and discharge of sputum.

DRUG INTERACTIONS:
• Potentiation of central nervous system depression reflecting synergistic action with barbiturates, other opiate-type analgesics, muscle relaxants, ethyl alcohol, sedative-hypnotic agents, tranquilizers, and general anesthetics can result in fatal respiratory depression.

OVERDOSAGE/ANTIDOTE:
• Symptoms of overdosage include disorientation, respiratory depression (slow, shallow, irregular); skin may be pale or cyanotic, pulse rate and blood pressure may be lowered.
• The specific antidotes are levallorphan, and naloxone. They must be given cautiously to avoid precipitation of a withdrawal crisis. Treat symptomatically and supportively. For additional information about these antidotes please refer to Chapter 20, page 696.

Fentanyl Citrate

GENERAL CLINICAL USE
Fentanyl, a narcotic analgesic with actions qualitatively similar to those of morphine and meperidine, is used for analgesic action of short duration during the anesthetic periods (premedication, induction, and maintenance) and in the immediate postoperative period (recovery room).

PHARMACOLOGY
Following intravenous injection, onset of analgesia is almost immediate with maximal action occurring after several minutes; duration is 30 to 60 minutes. When given intramuscularly, onset occurs within 10 minutes and is maintained for 1 to 2 hours. Respiration is depressed; this depression may persist longer than the analgesic effect. Fentanyl apparently is metabolized in the liver and excreted by the kidneys.

SPECIAL PRECAUTIONS, ADVERSE EFFECTS, CLINICAL GUIDELINES
See *Morphine* and *Meperidine*, pages 137 and 139, respectively.

Hydromorphone Hydrochloride
Hydromorphone Sulfate
Oxymorphone Hydrochloride

GENERAL CLINICAL USES
Hydromorphone and oxymorphone, potent semisynthetic derivatives of morphine, are indicated for relief of moderate to severe pain. They are employed in a manner similar to morphine.

PHARMACOLOGY
Parenteral, rectal, and oral administration result in uniform absorption. The onset of action after injection is more rapid than for morphine and the duration of action is somewhat shorter. Respiratory depression may be as marked as with morphine; nausea, vomiting, and constipation appear to be less frequent. Hydromorphone depresses the cough reflex, whereas oxymorphone shows little if any effect. They may be somewhat less sedative and less euphoriant than morphine, but the potential for addiction remains as great.

SPECIAL PRECAUTIONS
• Use in pregnancy only when expected benefits outweigh risks.

• Do not use in patients with status asthmaticus.

• Prolonged use can result in habituation and physical dependence.

ADVERSE EFFECTS

CNS EFFECTS: dizziness

RESPIRATORY EFFECTS: depression

CARDIOVASCULAR EFFECTS: hypotension, bradycardia

URINARY TRACT EFFECTS: urinary retention minimal

GASTROINTESTINAL EFFECTS: nausea, vomiting, anorexia, constipation minimal

ALLERGIC EFFECTS: urticaria

OPHTHALMIC EFFECTS: constricted pupils

LOCAL EFFECTS: irritation, induration

CLINICAL GUIDELINES

ADMINISTRATION:

• Elderly and debilitated patients, and also patients receiving tranquilizers or sedative-hypnotic agents, usually require a lower dosage.

• Record patient's response as indicated by relief of pain.

• Be alert for local irritation and induration after repeated subcutaneous injection in the same area.

• Ambulatory patients should be cautioned that physical abilities required for potentially hazardous tasks such as driving a car or operating machinery may be impaired.

EFFECTS:

• After repeated daily use, withdrawal symptoms, characteristic of addiction, may appear within 16 hours if drug administration is terminated suddenly. Withdrawal symptoms include sweating, restlessness, nausea, vomiting, diarrhea, abdominal cramps; increased temperature, heart rate, blood pressure, and respiratory rate.

DRUG INTERACTIONS:

• The action of most CNS depressants is potentiated by hydromorphone or oxymorphone. The synergistic action with barbiturates, other opiate-type analgesics, muscle relaxants, ethyl alcohol, sedative-hypnotic agents, tranquilizers, and general anesthetics can cause fatal respiratory failure.

OVERDOSAGE/ANTIDOTE:

• Overdosage is characterized by disorientation, respiratory depression (rate and tidal volume), extreme somnolence progressing to stupor or coma, bradycardia, and hypotension. The skin is pale initially and then cyanotic.

• The specific antidotes are levallorphan and naloxone. They must be given cautiously to avoid precipitation of a withdrawal crisis. Treat symptomatically and supportively.

Morphine Sulfate
Levorphanol Tartrate

GENERAL CLINICAL USES

Morphine sulfate and levorphanol tartrate are used for relief of pain of diverse origin, obstetric analgesia, preanesthetic medication, sedation, and hypnosis. They are also used for sedation and hypnosis when pain is present; as a preanesthetic medication; in dyspneic seizures of acute ventricular failure, and pulmonary edema.

PHARMACOLOGY

Morphine is well absorbed following parenteral administration. However, after oral administration absorption is erratic. Morphine exerts a combination of depression and stimulation in the central nervous system. In addition to analgesia and sedation, euphoria appears. In the usual analgesic dose, drowsiness and sleep also follow. In moderate to large doses the vasomotor center is depressed resulting in vasodilatation and hypotension. Respiratory depression occurs at analgesic dosages, and features decreased sensitivity of the respiratory center to carbon dioxide.

Levorphanol tartrate, a synthetic analgesic related chemically and pharmacologically to morphine, is more potent than morphine and longer acting. It is less likely to produce nausea, vomiting, and constipation.

In contrast morphine stimulates the vomiting center of the medulla and causes nausea and vomiting; it increases the tone of most smooth muscles and consequently may be harmful in patients with asthma by causing constriction of the bronchioles. By contracting the smooth muscle of the gastrointestinal tract it causes constipation. Similarly, contraction of smooth muscle of the urinary bladder and ureters may lead to urinary retention. Contraction of biliary tract smooth muscle may result in reduced bile flow. A marked contraction of the iris (eye) follows the administration of morphine and results in a pinpoint pupil.

The usual dose is effective for about 4 hours. Morphine is metabolized by the liver and excreted primarily in the urine.

SPECIAL PRECAUTIONS
• Use caution in debilitated patients, patients in traumatic shock, or those with impaired function of respiratory, hepatic or renal systems.
• Do not use in patients with increased intracranial pressure from head injury or in patients with convulsive disorders, acute alcoholism, Addison's disease, hypothyroidism, or asthma.

• Prolonged use can result in habituation and physical dependence.
• Safe use in pregnancy has not been established.
• Pre-existing convulsive disorders may be aggravated.
• May fatally potentiate other CNS depressants such as tranquilizers, sedative-hypnotic agents, other analgesics, and general anesthetics.

ADVERSE EFFECTS
CNS EFFECTS: drowsiness, dizziness, confusion, decreased temperature, increased intracranial pressure, euphoria, dysphoria, delirium, paradoxical excitement, deep sleep, coma, weakness, headache, insomnia
RESPIRATORY EFFECTS: depression of rate and amplitude (less than 12 per minute), cyanosis, Cheyne-Stokes breathing, apnea
CARDIOVASCULAR EFFECTS: tachycardia, palpitation, peripheral circulatory collapse, cardiac arrest, slowed pulse, hypotension
URINARY TRACT EFFECTS: retention or hesitancy
GASTROINTESTINAL EFFECTS: nausea, vomiting, constipation, abdominal distention and cramps, dry mouth
METABOLIC AND ENDOCRINE EFFECTS: antidiuretic effect, reduced libido and/or potency, hyperglycemia
HEPATIC EFFECTS: biliary tract spasm
DERMATOLOGIC EFFECTS: urticaria, itching about nose, rarely contact dermatitis
OPHTHALMIC EFFECTS: constricted pupils
LOCAL EFFECTS: following subcutaneous administration, pain, tissue irritation and induration

CLINICAL GUIDELINES
ADMINISTRATION:
• When administering intravenously inject slowly, preferably in form of a diluted

solution; rapid injection increases the incidence of adverse reactions.

• Verify the narcotic order; morphine is subject to federal and state narcotic laws.

• Record patient's response as indicated by relief of pain.

• Patient should lie down prior to injection to minimize nausea and vomiting.

• Caution ambulatory patients that mental and/or physical abilities may be impaired.

EFFECTS:

• Prolonged use may result in severe dependence. After repeated daily use, withdrawal symptoms, characteristic of addiction, may appear within 16 hours if drug injection is stopped suddenly. Withdrawal symptoms include sweating, restlessness, nausea, vomiting, diarrhea, abdominal cramps; increased temperature, heart rate, blood pressure, and respiratory rate.

DRUG INTERACTIONS:

• Elderly and debilitated patients, also patients receiving tranquilizers or sedative-hypnotic agents, usually require lower morphine dosage.

• The action of most central nervous system depressants is potentiated by these drugs. The synergistic action can cause fatal respiratory failure.

OVERDOSAGE/ANTIDOTE:

• Symptoms of overdosage are disorientation, respiratory depression (slow, shallow, irregular), extreme somnolence progressing to stupor or coma, and skeletal muscle flaccidity. A history of addiction will be suggested by needle-marked arms or other regions of the body. Pinpoint pupils are seen initially, but in terminal narcosis pupils become dilated. The skin is initially pale and then cyanotic. Pulse is slow and blood pressure lowered.

• The specific antidotes are levallorphan or naloxone. (See Chapter 20, page 696, for detailed information on use of these anti-

dotes). Use cautiously to avoid precipitation of a withdrawal crisis. Treat supportively and symptomatically.

Meperidine Hydrochloride

GENERAL CLINICAL USES

Meperidine, a synthetic analgesic with multiple actions characteristic of morphine, has been employed widely in treating moderate to severe pain of visceral, cardiovascular, and neuromuscular origin; also in obstetric delivery and as preanesthetic analgesia.

PHARMACOLOGY

Meperidine has an analgesic effect intermediate between codeine and morphine. Absorption occurs readily from the gastrointestinal tract as well as from subcutaneous or intramuscular sites. It is less effective after oral than parenteral administration. Maximal analgesia occurs 30 to 60 minutes after injection. Meperidine facilitates relaxation and dilatation of the cervix but may decrease uterine contractions. Respiratory depression reflects a reduction in depth of breathing rather than the rapid decline in respiratory rate characteristic of morphine. Only minimal depression of the cough reflex occurs, and actions on the gastrointestinal tract are less than with morphine. Meperidine is primarily metabolized in the liver, then excreted in the urine. Like morphine it crosses the placental barrier and may induce respiratory depression and other opiate-type actions in the newborn.

SPECIAL PRECAUTIONS

• Ambulatory patients must be cautioned against driving a motor vehicle or operat-

ing machinery since mental or physical abilities may be impaired.
• Administer intravenously only if necessary; injection must be very slow; a narcotic antagonist agent, as well as facilities for assisted respiration, must be available immediately.
• Extreme caution should be used in patients with inadequate respiratory reserve (asthma, chronic obstructive pulmonary disease, cor pulmonale, pre-existing hypoxia, or hypercapnia).
• Do not use in pregnant women prior to the labor period since safe use relative to possible adverse effects on fetal development has not been established.
• Caution should be exercised in debilitated patients, patients in traumatic shock, or those with impaired function of hepatic or renal systems.
• Contraindicated in the presence of increased intracranial pressure from head injury, in convulsive disorders, acute alcoholism, Addison's disease, hypothyroidism, and asthma.
• Prolonged use can result in habituation and physical dependence.

ADVERSE EFFECTS
CNS EFFECTS: light-headedness, euphoria, hallucinations, dizziness, sedation, delirium, excitement, syncope
RESPIRATORY EFFECTS: depression, apnea
CARDIOVASCULAR EFFECTS: altered pulse, cardiac arrest, circulatory hypotension
URINARY TRACT EFFECTS: retention infrequently
AUTONOMIC EFFECTS: sweating, dry mouth
GASTROINTESTINAL EFFECTS: dry mouth, nausea, vomiting; constipation infrequently; biliary colic infrequently
ALLERGIC EFFECTS: urticaria

DERMATOLOGIC EFFECTS: pruritus
OPHTHALMIC EFFECTS: mydriasis
LOCAL EFFECTS: pain, induration after subcutaneous injection

CLINICAL GUIDELINES
ADMINISTRATION:
• Elderly and debilitated patients, also those receiving tranquilizers, sedative-hypnotic agents, or other central nervous system depressants, usually require lowered dosages.
• Patients should lie down prior to administration of meperidine parenterally to minimize dizziness and syncope. Instruct patient not to ambulate without supervision.
• Intramuscular route is preferred for parenteral administration; subcutaneous administration is painful. Intravenous administration is hazardous and should be avoided.
• Record patient's response as indicated by relief of pain or appearance of side effects.
EFFECTS:
• If patient develops diminished rate or depth of breathing prior to administering the drug, respiration may be severely impaired following administration of meperidine. Monitor patient closely and inform physician.
• Prolonged use may result in severe dependence. After repeated daily use, withdrawal symptoms characteristic of addiction may appear if drug administration is stopped suddenly. Withdrawal symptoms include profuse sweating, restlessness, insomnia, tremors, nausea, vomiting, diarrhea; increased temperature, pulse, and blood pressure.
• Laboratory tests may show elevated transaminase, amylase, and BSP values.

DRUG INTERACTIONS:
- The action of most CNS depressants is potentiated by meperidine. The synergistic action with barbiturates, other opiate-type analgesics, muscle relaxants, ethyl alcohol, sedative-hypnotic agents, tranquilizers, tricyclic antidepressants, and general anesthetics can cause fatal respiratory arrest.
- Meperidine may enhance the anticholinergic action of atropine and related drugs.
- Do not administer concomitantly with monoamine oxidase inhibitors (MAOI); also in patients who received MAO-inhibitors within 14 days; rare fatal reactions have occurred.

OVERDOSAGE/ANTIDOTE:
- Overdosage is characterized by decreased respiratory rate and shallow irregular breathing and cyanosis; somnolence progressing to stupor or coma, cold and clammy skin, skeletal muscle flaccidity, and sometimes slowed pulse and reduced blood pressure can occur. In severe overdosage, fatal apnea, circulatory collapse, and cardiac arrest may occur.
- Specific antidotes are levallorphan or naloxone. (See Chapter 20, page 696, for detailed information on use of antidotes). They should preferably be administered intravenously, simultaneously with efforts at respiratory resuscitation. Oxygen, intravenous fluids, vasopressors, and other supportive measures should be employed as indicated.

Methadone Hydrochloride

GENERAL CLINICAL USES
Methadone is indicated for relief of severe pain and for detoxification or temporary maintenance in patients addicted to narcotics. It is used to control severe pain in malignant and metastatic cancer; also visceral pain including renal colic.

Methadone is not recommended for obstetric analgesia because its long duration of action increases the probability of infant respiratory depression.

PHARMACOLOGY
Methadone, a synthetic narcotic analgesic, is well absorbed after injection or ingestion. It has multiple actions quantitatively similar to morphine. However, considerably less euphoria occurs.

Methadone, like morphine, increases smooth muscle tone. Consequently, harmful constriction of bronchioles may follow in patients with asthma; urinary retention, biliary tract spasm, and constipation may occur. The pinpoint pupil caused by contraction of the eye iris, characteristic of morphine, becomes evident.

Appreciable amounts of methadone appear in plasma within 10 minutes after injection; the onset of action may be somewhat more rapid than for morphine. The usual analgesic dose remains effective for 4 to 6 hours. Peak brain levels can be found 1 to 2 hours after administration. The longer duration of action as compared to morphine reflects slower metabolism by the liver and associated reduced rate of excretion in the urine and feces.

SPECIAL PRECAUTIONS
- Extreme caution should be used in patients with inadequate respiratory reserve (asthma, chronic obstructive pulmonary disease, cor pulmonale, pre-existing hypoxia or hypercapnia).
- Caution should be exercised in debilitated patients, patients in traumatic shock, or those with impaired function of hepatic or renal systems.

• Do not use in presence of increased intracranial pressure from head injury, or in patients with convulsive disorders, acute alcoholism, Addison's disease, hypothyroidism, or asthma.

• Severe hypotension may occur in individuals whose ability to maintain blood pressure has already been compromised by a depleted blood volume or concurrent administration of drugs such as phenothiazine or certain anesthetics.

• Prolonged use can result in habituation and physical dependence.

• Methadone is not recommended for use as an analgesic in children.

• Do not use in pregnant women or for obstetric analgesia because of its long duration of action which increases probability of respiratory depression in the newborn.

• Do not use in patients with a history of hypersensitivity to methadone.

ADVERSE EFFECTS

CNS EFFECTS: light-headedness, sedation, dysphoria, drowsiness, dizziness, confusion, euphoria, delirium, agitation, headache, insomnia, syncope

RESPIRATORY EFFECTS: depression of rate and amplitude, cyanosis, apnea

CARDIOVASCULAR EFFECTS: bradycardia, palpitation, hypotension

URINARY TRACT EFFECTS: retention or hesitancy

AUTONOMIC EFFECTS: dry mouth, sweating, flushing of face

GASTROINTESTINAL EFFECTS: nausea, vomiting, anorexia, constipation, abdominal distention and cramps

METABOLIC AND ENDOCRINE EFFECTS: loss of weight, reduced libido and/or potency, antidiuretic effect

HEPATIC EFFECTS: biliary tract spasm

ALLERGIC EFFECTS: pruritus, rash, edema, urticaria; hemorrhagic urticaria rarely

OPHTHALMIC EFFECTS: constricted pupils, visual disturbances

CLINICAL GUIDELINES

ADMINISTRATION:

• Ambulatory patients should be cautioned against driving a car or operating machinery since mental or physical abilities may be impaired.

• Administer intravenously only if necessary. Injection must be very slow. A narcotic antagonist as well as facilities for assisted respiration must be immediately available.

EFFECTS:

• Methadone elevates cerebrospinal fluid pressure which may be markedly exaggerated in the presence of increased intraocular pressure.

DRUG INTERACTIONS:

• Do not use concurrently with monoamine oxidase inhibitors; also patients who received MAO-inhibitors within 14 days. Rare fatal reactions have occurred.

OVERDOSAGE/ANTIDOTE:

• Overdosage is characterized by respiratory depression (a decrease in rate and/or tidal volume), Cheyne-Stokes respiration, cyanosis, extreme somnolence progressing to stupor or coma; maximally constricted pupils, skeletal muscle flaccidity, cold and clammy skin, and sometimes bradycardia and hypotension.

• In serious overdosage, particularly following intravenous administration, apnea, circulatory collapse, cardiac arrest, and death may occur.

• Re-establish adequate respiratory exchange through provision of a patent airway and institution of assisted or controlled respiration. Narcotic antagonists (naloxone, levallorphan) may be useful, particularly in children, to overcome potentially lethal respiratory depression. Remember, methadone is a long-acting depressant (36 to 48 hours), whereas the antagonists act for much shorter periods (1 to 3 hours). See

Chapter 20, page 696, for detailed information on use of narcotic antagonists.

Methotrimeprazine

GENERAL CLINICAL USES

Methotrimeprazine is indicated for relief of moderate to severe pain in non-ambulatory patients; for obstetrical analgesia; and sedation where respiratory depression is to be avoided; as a pre-anesthetic for producing sedation, somnolence, and the relief of apprehension and anxiety.

PHARMACOLOGY

Methotrimeprazine, a phenothiazine derivative, is a CNS depressant. It raises the pain threshold and produces amnesia. It also has antihistaminic, anticholinergic, and antiadrenaline effects. It is metabolized, conjugated, and excreted primarily in the urine. The analgesic effect is comparable to morphine and meperidine.

After intramuscular administration the maximal analgesic effect usually occurs within 20 to 40 minutes and is maintained for about 4 hours.

SPECIAL PRECAUTIONS

• Do not use in patients with a history of phenothiazine hypersensitivity, or in presence of overdosage of CNS depressants, or comatose state.
• Do not use in patients with severe myocardial, renal, or hepatic disease.
• It is not recommended for patients less than 12 years old.
• Use with caution in women who are of childbearing potential and during early pregnancy.
• Elderly and debilitated patients with heart disease are sensitive to phenothiazine effects; a low initial dose is recommended.

ADVERSE EFFECTS

CNS EFFECTS: syncope, weakness, fainting, disorientation, dizziness, excessive sedation, slurring of speech,
CARDIOVASCULAR EFFECTS: orthostatic hypotension
GASTROINTESTINAL EFFECTS: abdominal discomfort, nausea, vomiting
AUTONOMIC EFFECTS: dry mouth, nasal congestion, chills
URINARY TRACT EFFECTS: difficulties in urination
METABOLIC AND ENDOCRINE EFFECTS: uterine inertia, rarely
HEMATOLOGIC EFFECTS: agranulocytosis
HEPATIC EFFECTS: jaundice
LOCAL EFFECTS: pain, inflammation, and swelling

CLINICAL GUIDELINES

ADMINISTRATION:
• Patients should remain in bed or be closely supervised for about 6 hours after each of the first several injections; orthostatic hypotension, fainting, or dizziness may occur.
DRUG INTERACTIONS:
• Concurrent use of epinephrine may result in a paradoxical decrease in blood pressure.
• Additive effects may occur with CNS depressant drugs such as narcotics, barbiturates, general anesthetics, acetylsalicylic acid, meprobamate, and reserpine; dosage reduction may be necessary.
• Do not use concurrently with antihypertensive drugs including MAO-inhibitors.
• Concurrent use with atropine, scopolamine, and succinylcholine may result in tachycardia, decrease in blood pressure, stimulation, delirium, and extrapyramidal symptoms.
OVERDOSAGE/ANTIDOTE:
• Overdosage is characterized by hypotension, fainting, and disorientation.

• Treat supportively as indicated by condition of patient.

Pentazocine Hydrochloride
Pentazocine Lactate

GENERAL CLINICAL USE

Pentazocine is indicated for the relief of moderate to severe pain. The drug may be administered parenterally for preoperative or preanesthetic medication and as a supplement to surgical anesthesia.

PHARMACOLOGY

Pentazocine is a potent analgesic. With oral administration an effect occurs in 15 to 30 minutes and persists for 3 hours or more. With parenteral administration an effect is noted within 20 minutes (subcutaneous) or 3 minutes (intravenous). The effect lasts 3 to 4 hours. In addition, it produces incomplete reversal of cardiovascular, respiratory, and behavioral depression induced by morphine or meperidine. Pentazocine is metabolized by the liver and excreted primarily in the urine.

SPECIAL PRECAUTIONS

• Do not use in patients with a history of hypersensitivity to pentazocine.
• Administer subcutaneously only if necessary because of possible severe tissue damage at injection sites; pentazocine should be administered intramuscularly when frequent injections are needed.
• Prolonged use can result in habituation and physical dependence.
• Patients previously given narcotic analgesics, including methadone, have experienced withdrawal symptoms after receiving pentazocine.

• Do not use in patients with increased intracranial pressure from head injury.
• Ambulatory patients must be cautioned against driving a car or operating machinery since mental or physical abilities may be impaired.
• Patients receiving therapeutic doses have rarely experienced hallucinations, disorientation, and confusion.
• Extreme caution should be used in patients with inadequate respiratory reserve (asthma, chronic obstructive pulmonary disease, cor pulmonale, pre-existing hypoxia, or hypercapnia).
• Caution should be exercised in debilitated patients, patients in traumatic shock, or those with impaired function of hepatic or renal systems.
• Do not use in pregnant women prior to the labor period since safe use relative to possible adverse effects on fetal development has not been established.
• Do not use in patients with convulsive disorders, acute alcoholism, Addison's disease, hypothyroidism, or asthma.
• Pentazocine should be used with caution in patients with myocardial infarction or those about to undergo surgery of the biliary tract.
• Safe use in children under 12 years of age has not been established.

ADVERSE EFFECTS

CNS EFFECTS: light-headedness, euphoria, disorientation, confusion, hallucinations, disturbed dreams, weakness, dizziness, insomnia, sedation, alterations in mood, tremors, excitement, coma, paresthesias.
RESPIRATORY EFFECTS: depression; apnea, transient
CARDIOVASCULAR EFFECTS: decrease in blood pressure, tachycardia, circulatory depression, shock, hypertension
URINARY TRACT EFFECTS: retention

AUTONOMIC EFFECTS: sweating, chills, flushing

GASTROINTESTINAL EFFECTS: nausea, vomiting, constipation, dry mouth; diarrhea, rarely; cramps, taste alteration

METABOLIC AND ENDOCRINE EFFECTS: alterations in rate and strength of uterine contractions during labor

HEMATOLOGIC EFFECTS: depression (reversible) of leukocyte count; transient eosinophilia

ALLERGIC EFFECTS: rash, urticaria, edema of face (rare)

DERMATOLOGIC EFFECTS: diaphoresis, flushing, dermatitis

OPHTHALMIC EFFECTS: blurred vision, focusing difficulties, nystagmus, diplopia, miosis

OTIC EFFECTS: tinnitus

LOCAL EFFECTS: sting on injection, induration, ulceration, nodules, severe sclerosis of the skin and protuberances, epidermal necrosis

CLINICAL GUIDELINES

ADMINISTRATION:
• Confirm whether patient recently has received other narcotic analgesics since withdrawal syndrome may be elicited after administration of pentazocine.
• Intramuscular administration is preferred for repeated parenteral injections.

EFFECTS:
• If patient experiences diminished rate or depth of breathing prior to administering this drug, respiration may be severely impaired. Monitor patient closely and consult the physician.
• Prolonged use may result in severe dependence. After repeated daily use, withdrawal symptoms characteristic of addiction may appear if drug administration is suddenly stopped. Withdrawal symptoms include profuse sweating, restlessness, insomnia, tremors, nausea, vomiting, diarrhea; increased temperature, pulse and blood pressure.

DRUG INTERACTIONS:
• The action of most CNS depressants is potentiated by pentazocine. The synergistic action with barbiturates, muscle relaxants, ethyl alcohol, sedative-hypnotic agents, tranquilizers, tricyclic antidepressants, and general anesthetics may cause fatal respiratory arrest.
• Do not mix pentazocine in same syringe with barbiturates; precipitation will occur.

OVERDOSAGE/ANTIDOTE:
• Although signs of overdosage are insufficiently defined because of limited clinical experience, serious overdosage may decrease respiratory rate, result in shallow irregular breathing, and cyanosis; somnolence progressing to stupor or coma may occur. The skin will be cold and clammy, skeletal muscles flaccid, and pulse slowed and blood pressure reduced. In severe overdosage, fatal apnea, circulatory collapse and cardiac arrest may occur.
• The only specific and effective antidote for pentazocine is naloxone and should preferably be administered intravenously simultaneously with efforts at respiratory resuscitation (see Chapter 20, page 696, for detailed information concerning use). Nalorphine or levallorphan are *not* effective antidotes. Use supportive measures as indicated.

Propoxyphene Hydrochloride
Propoxyphene Napsylate

GENERAL CLINICAL USE

Propoxyphene, like codeine, is used for the treatment of mild to moderate pain, particularly to pain unresponsive to aspirin or phenacetin. When combined with aspirin, the drug approximates the combination of codeine and aspirin in effectiveness.

PHARMACOLOGY

Although as an analgesic, propoxyphene is similar to codeine in effectiveness, actions upon the gastrointestinal tract are less. Actions on the respiratory or cardiovascular systems are usually encountered only infrequently at recommended dosages. An oral dose is absorbed efficiently and remains effective for 4 to 6 hours. The drug is metabolized by the liver and excreted in the urine.

Unlike codeine, no relief of cough is obtained with propoxyphene. Also, it retains only minimal drug dependence liability. It is a controlled drug.

SPECIAL PRECAUTIONS

• Do not use in patients with a history of hypersensitivity to propoxyphene.
• Ambulatory patients should be cautioned that propoxyphene may impair physical abilities required for potentially hazardous tasks such as driving a car or operating machinery.
• Prolonged use can result in habituation and physical dependence.
• Safe use in pregnancy has not been established.
• Usage in children is not recommended because insufficient documented clinical experience exists to establish safety and dosage in the pediatric age group.

ADVERSE EFFECTS

CNS EFFECTS: dizziness, sedation, restlessness, light-headedness, euphoria, paradoxical excitement
RESPIRATORY EFFECTS: respiratory depression, minimal
GASTROINTESTINAL EFFECTS: nausea, vomiting; constipation, rarely; abdominal pain

DERMATOLOGIC EFFECTS: rash, rarely
OPHTHALMIC EFFECTS: visual disturbances, rarely

CLINICAL GUIDELINES

ADMINISTRATION:
• Ambulatory patients must be cautioned against driving a car or operating any machinery.
• Prolonged use may result in dependence.
DRUG INTERACTIONS:
• Potentiation of CNS depression may result from concomitant use of barbiturates, other opiate-type analgesics, muscle relaxants, ethyl alcohol, sedative-hypnotic agents, tranquilizers, and general anesthetics; fatal respiratory depression can result.
OVERDOSAGE/ANTIDOTE:
• Overdosage is characterized by disorientation, slow and irregular respiration; occasionally pulmonary edema. Skin may be pale or cyanotic; pulse rate and blood pressure may be irregular. In addition, local and generalized convulsions occur in most cases of severe propoxyphene poisoning.
• The specific antidotes are levallorphan or naloxone. (See Chapter 20, page 696, for detailed information concerning use of narcotic antagonists.) They must be given cautiously to avoid precipitation of a withdrawal crisis or exacerbation of convulsions. The principal supportive measures are directed at maintaining adequate lung ventilation and control of cardiac arrhythmias. Patient may require careful titration with an anticonvulsant to control the seizures.

Butorphanol Tartrate

GENERAL CLINICAL USES

Butorphanol tartrate is recommended for the relief of moderate to severe pain.

PHARMACOLOGY

Butorphanol tartrate is a potent analgesic with a duration of action of 3 to 4 hours. The analgesic activity is equivalent to that of morphine. After intramuscular administration, analgesia appears within 30 minutes, and in less time after intravenous administration. Peak analgesia is obtained at 1 hour after intramuscular administration and at 30 minutes after intravenous administration.

The mechanism of action of butorphanol tartrate is unknown. It has narcotic antagonist activity which is approximately equivalent to that of nalorphine, 30 times that of pentazocine, and 1/40 that of naloxone.

SPECIAL PRECAUTIONS

• Administer with caution and in low dosage to patients with respiratory depression (e.g., from other medication, uremia, or severe infection), severely limited respiratory reserve, bronchial asthma, obstructive respiratory conditions, or cyanosis; butorphanol tartrate causes some respiratory depression.
• Use with caution in patients with impaired renal or hepatic function.
• Use in pregnant patients only when the physician deems it essential to the welfare of the patient.

ADVERSE EFFECTS

CNS EFFECTS: sedation, headache, vertigo, floating feeling, dizziness, lethargy, confusion, light-headedness, nervousness, unusual dreams, agitation, euphoria, hallucinations
RESPIRATORY EFFECTS: slowing of respiration, shallow breathing
CARDIOVASCULAR EFFECTS: palpitation, increase or decrease in blood pressure

GASTROINTESTINAL EFFECTS: nausea, vomiting
AUTONOMIC EFFECTS: flushing and warmth, dry mouth, sensitivity to cold
DERMATOLOGIC EFFECTS: rash, hives
OPHTHALMIC EFFECTS: diplopia, blurred vision

CLINICAL GUIDELINES

ADMINISTRATION:
• Be aware that respiratory depression occurs.
• In patients physically dependent on narcotics, it is advisable to detoxify patient prior to use of butorphanol tartrate because of its antagonist properties.
• Use special care when administering to emotionally unstable patients and to those with a history of drug misuse.
EFFECTS:
• Since butorphanol tartrate, like other potent analgesics, elevates cerebrospinal fluid pressure, use in cases of head injury can produce effects (e.g., miosis) which may obscure the clinical course of patient with head injuries.
• Butorphanol tartrate increases the work of the heart, especially the pulmonary circuit. Therefore, use in patients with acute myocardial infarction, ventricular dysfunction, or coronary insufficiency should be limited to those who are hypersensitive to morphine sulfate or meperidine.
OVERDOSAGE/ANTIDOTE:
• Overdosage could produce some degree of respiratory depression and variable cardiovascular and central nervous system effects.
• Overdosage is treated with naloxone administered intravenously. Evaluate cardiac and respiratory status constantly. Use supportive measures such as oxygen, intravenous fluids, vasopressors, and assisted or controlled respiration.

General Anesthetics

General Anesthetics, Injectable

SPECIFIC PRODUCTS AND DOSAGES

	GENERIC NAME	TRADE NAME	ROUTE OF ADMIN.	SUGGESTED DOSAGES (For detailed information consult current labeling.)
CII*	fentanyl citrate and droperidol	INNOVAR	im iv	**Adults:** 0.5–2 ml; **Children:** 0.25–25 ml/20 lbs. **Adults:** 1 ml/20–25 lbs; **Children:** 0.5 ml/20 lbs.
	ketamine HCl	KETALAR KETAJECT	iv im	1–4.5 mg/kg; inject over a period of 60 sec. **Adults:** 6.5–13 mg/kg; 6.5–13 mg; titrate subsequent doses to response of patient; **Children:** 9–13 mg/kg (4–6 mg/lb) produces anesthesia in 3–4 min.; duration of anesthesia 12–25 min.
CIV	methohexital sodium	BREVITAL Sodium	iv	5–12 ml of 1.0% solution (50–120 mg) at rate of 1.0 ml/5 sec. with supplemental small increases
CIII	thiamylal sodium	SURITAL	iv	Initially 3–6 ml of 2.5% solution at rate of 1.0 ml/5 sec. with supplemental small increases.
CIII	thiopental sodium	PENTOTHAL	iv pr	210–280 (3–4 mg/kg) or 2–3 ml of a 3.5% solution at intervals of 20–40 sec.; repeat until anesthesia is achieved. Adult or robust child: up to 1 gm/50–75 lb (22.5 kg) or 20 mg/lb; inactive or debilitated patients: use lower dosage

*C designates schedule classification under the Controlled Substances Act.

Fentanyl Citrate and Droperidol

GENERAL CLINICAL USES

Fentanyl citrate and droperidol are combined to provide tranquilization and analgesia required for surgical and diagnostic procedures. Also, this combination is useful as a preanesthetic medication.

PHARMACOLOGY

Fentanyl citrate, a narcotic analgesic, in combination with droperidol, a major tranquilizer, produces anesthesia in 3 to 5 minutes. The onset of anesthesia is slow but the analgesia frequently persists into the postoperative period. Complete loss of consciousness does not occur from use of this drug combination alone.

SPECIAL PRECAUTIONS
• Mild to moderate hypotension and bradycardia may occur.
• Do not administer to patients with parkinsonism.
• Use with caution in patients with head injuries who may be particularly susceptible to respiratory depression, such as comatose patients.
• Safe use in children less than 2 years old and in pregnant women has not been established.
• Use with caution in patients with chronic obstructive pulmonary disease, patients with decreased respiratory reserve, and others with potentially compromised ventilation.
• Administer with caution to patients with liver and kidney dysfunction since these organs are important in the metabolism and excretion of these drugs.

ADVERSE EFFECTS
CNS EFFECTS: extrapyramidal symptoms (dystonia, akathisia, oculogyric crisis), restlessness, hyperactivity, anxiety, dizziness, chills and/or shivering, twitching, emergence delirium, postoperative hallucinatory episodes, drowsiness
RESPIRATORY EFFECTS: depression, apnea, respiratory arrest, laryngospasm, bronchospasm, slowing of respiratory rate
CARDIOVASCULAR EFFECTS: hypotension, circulatory depression, elevated blood pressure with and without pre-existing hypertension, bradycardia, tachycardia
GASTROINTESTINAL EFFECTS: nausea and emesis
AUTONOMIC EFFECTS: diaphoresis
OPHTHALMIC EFFECTS: blurred vision

MUSCULOSKELETAL EFFECTS: muscular rigidity

CLINICAL GUIDELINES
ADMINISTRATION:
• Appropriate rescucitative equipment should be readily available during drug administration.
• The initial dose should be appropriately reduced in elderly, debilitated, or other poor-risk patients.
• Patient's vital signs should be monitored routinely.
EFFECTS:
• When the EEG is used for postoperative monitoring, it may be noted that the EEG pattern returns to normal slowly.
• Diminished sensitivity to CO_2 stimulation may persist longer than depression respiratory rate.
DRUG INTERACTIONS:
• Effects may be potentiated by other CNS depressant drugs (barbiturates, tranquilizers, narcotics, and general anesthetics). Dosage reduction may be required.
OVERDOSAGE/ANTIDOTE:
• Overdosage is characterized by an exaggeration of the pharmacologic effects. Large doses may produce apnea, hypotension, hypovolemia, and decreased pulmonary arterial pressure.
• There is no specific antidote but the narcotic antagonists can reverse the respiratory depression caused by narcotic analgesics. See Chapter 20, page 695, for detailed information on the narcotic antagonists, levallorphan, and naloxone. Extrapyramidal symptoms may be controlled with the antiparkinsonian agents. Oxygen should be administered; a patent airway must be maintained. The duration of respiratory depression following overdose may be longer than the duration of the narcotic antagonist action.

Ketamine Hydrochloride

GENERAL CLINICAL USES

Ketamine hydrochloride, a nonbarbiturate ultra-short-acting agent (15 minutes or less), produces general anesthesia with analgesia following intravenous or intramuscular administration. It is recommended for diagnostic or surgical procedures that require muscle relaxation. It also may be used for the induction of anesthesia prior to the administration of other general anesthetic agents.

PHARMACOLOGY

Ketamine hydrochloride appears to interrupt selectively pathways of the brain before eliciting somesthetic sensory blockage. It does not impede pharyngeal-laryngeal reflexes or induce any skeletal muscle relaxation. It causes cardiovascular stimulation including an increase in blood pressure. On occasion a transient respiratory depression can be seen. The elevation of blood pressure begins shortly after injection, reaches a maximum in a few minutes, and usually returns to preanesthetic values within 15 minutes after injection. The mean peak rise has ranged from 20 to 25 percent of preanesthetic values. Ketamine hydrochloride and its metabolites are excreted primarily in the urine.

SPECIAL PRECAUTIONS

- Do not use in patients in whom a significant elevation of blood pressure would constitute a serious hazard.
- Do not use in patients with a history of hypersensitivity to ketamine.
- Should be used only by or under the direction of physicians experienced in administering general anesthetics, in maintenance of an airway, and in control of respiration.
- Resuscitative equipment should be available and ready for use.
- Do not use alone in surgery or diagnostic procedures of the pharynx, larynx, or bronchial tree; mechanical stimulation of the pharynx should be avoided.
- In surgical procedures involving visceral pain tracts, supplemental agents which relieve such pain are required.
- Use with caution in the chronic alcoholic or any acutely alcohol-intoxicated patient.
- Use with extreme caution in patients with preanesthetic elevated spinal fluid pressure.
- Safe use in pregnancy including obstetrics has not been established; such use is not recommended.

ADVERSE EFFECTS

CNS EFFECTS: emergence reactions, disorientation, excitement, hallucinations, increased cerebrospinal fluid pressure

RESPIRATORY EFFECTS: depression of respiration, apnea, laryngospasm other forms of airway obstruction

CARDIOVASCULAR EFFECTS: hypertension, an increased pulse rate, hypotension, tachycardia

GASTROINTESTINAL EFFECTS: anorexia, nausea, vomiting

ALLERGIC EFFECTS: erythema, morbilliform rash

OPHTHALMIC EFFECTS: diplopia, nystagmus, elevated intraocular pressure

MUSCULOSKELETAL EFFECTS: tonic-clonic movements sometimes resembling seizures

LOCAL EFFECTS: pain, exanthema, transient erythema

CLINICAL GUIDELINES

ADMINISTRATION:

- The increased incidence of emergence reactions may be reduced if verbal and tactile stimulation of the patient is minimized during the recovery period. This does not preclude continuous monitoring of vital signs.

• The intravenous dose should be injected over a period of 60 seconds. More rapid injection may result in respiratory depression, apnea, and enhanced rise in blood pressure.

• Resuscitative equipment should be available and ready for use.

• During administration the possibility of vomiting and aspiration must be considered. It should be used in patients whose stomach is *not* empty *only* when the benefits outweigh the risks.

• During injection be on the alert for sudden respiratory arrest.

• Atropine, scopolamine or other anticholinergic agents should be given at appropriate prior intervals.

• Because of the rapid induction, the patient should be in an appropriate supported position during the injection.

• Increments of one-half to the full induction dose may be repeated for maintenance of anesthesia.

• Purposeless and tonic-clonic movements may occur during the course of the anesthesia and are indicative of need for additional anesthetic.

EFFECTS:

• Postoperative confusional states may occur during the recovery period.

• Emergence reactions have occurred in approximately 12 percent of patients. The psychological manifestations vary in severity between dreamlike states, hallucinations, and emergence delirium. In some cases, confusion, excitement, and irrational behavior (without amnesia) have occurred. The incidence appears lower in preadolescent and elderly patients.

• A small dose of a very short-acting barbiturate may be required to terminate a serious emergence reaction.

• If used on an outpatient basis, the patient should not be released until recovery from anesthesia is complete, and then should be accompanied by an adult.

DRUG INTERACTIONS:

• When adequate respiratory exchange is maintained, ketamine is compatible with commonly used general local anesthetic agents, skeletal muscle relaxants, atropine, scopolamine, and also analgesics including morphine.

• Prolonged recovery time may occur if barbiturates, tranquilizers, or opiates are used concomitantly.

• Barbiturates and ketamine are chemically incompatible; a precipitate forms; do not inject these materials from the same syringe.

OVERDOSAGE/ANTIDOTE:

• Ketamine has a relatively wide margin of safety. Instances of unintentional injection of overdoses (up to ten times usually required) have been followed by prolonged but successful recovery. Overdosage may result in respiratory arrest.

• There is no specific antidote. Supportive ventilation should be employed. Mechanical support of respiration is preferred to administration of analeptic agents.

Methohexital Sodium
Thiamylal Sodium
Thiopental Sodium

GENERAL CLINICAL USES

The injectable general anesthetics include the ultra-short-acting barbiturates, methohexital, thiamylal, and thiopental. They are indicated (1) as the sole agent for brief (15 minutes or less) procedures; (2) for induction of anesthesia prior to administration of other longer-acting anesthetic agents; (3) to supplement regional anesthetics or (4) in combination with other agents for analgesia or skeletal muscle relaxation.

PHARMACOLOGY

Methohexital, thiamylal, and thiopental are ultra-short-acting barbiturates which when administered intravenously cause hypnosis, rapid loss of consciousness, and anesthesia. Recovery after small anesthetic doses is rapid with a period of drowsiness and retrograde amnesia. Repeated intravenous doses may lead to a prolonged anesthesia because fatty or other tissues act as a reservoir and then release the drug slowly. The analgesia produced is not profound. The short-acting barbiturates are metabolized in the liver and excreted in the urine.

Methohexital sodium, a potent rapid-acting barbiturate, is similar in action to thiopental sodium, but more potent. The duration of anesthesia is 5 to 8 minutes.

Thiamylal sodium, also a short-acting barbiturate, is essentially the equivalent of pentothal sodium in its pharmacology.

Thiopental sodium can induce general anesthesia within 30 to 60 seconds after intravenous administration. It is a potent respiratory depressant; rate and depth of respiration are reduced.

SPECIAL PRECAUTIONS

- Drug should be administered only by personnel qualified in the use of intravenous anesthetics.
- Keep resuscitative and endotracheal intubation equipment and oxygen readily available; maintain patency of airway at all times.
- Contraindicated in hypersensitivity to barbiturates, status asthmaticus, or latent or manifest porphyria.
- Respiratory depression, apnea, or hypotension may occur.
- Use caution in debilitated patients and in those with impaired function of respiratory, circulatory, hepatic, renal, or endocrine systems.
- If used in above conditions, reduce dosage and administer slowly.
- Repeated use could potentially be habit-forming.
- Safe use in pregnancy with respect to possible adverse effects on human fetal development has not been established. If to be given to pregnant women, benefits to the mother should be weighed against risks to the fetus.

ADVERSE EFFECTS

CNS EFFECTS: emergence delirium, headache, severe generalized depression, prolonged somnolence and recovery, shivering, restlessness, anxiety

RESPIRATORY EFFECTS: apnea, depression, sneezing, coughing, bronchospasm, laryngospasm, dyspnea, rhinitis

CARDIOVASCULAR EFFECTS: arrhythmias, myocardial depression, hypotension

AUTONOMIC EFFECTS: hiccups

GASTROINTESTINAL EFFECTS: hypersalivation, nausea, vomiting

ALLERGIC EFFECTS: pruritus, urticaria, rash, erythema

LOCAL EFFECTS: with intravenous administration, thrombophlebitis, pain, swelling, ulceration, necrosis

CLINICAL GUIDELINES

ADMINISTRATION:

- Observe aseptic precautions at all times in preparation and handling of all intravenous solutions.
- Since no bacteriostatic agent is present, unused drug should be discarded.

EFFECTS:

- Since prolonged drowsiness and muscular incoordination may occur during the recovery from the general anesthetic, institutionalized patients should be assisted in any ambulatory activity; outpatients should be warned about driving a motor vehicle or operating any mechanical device.

• During recovery from anesthesia, vomiting may occur and may be complicated by aspiration since the cough reflex may have been paralyzed.

• In patients with impaired liver function prolonged somnolence with a delay in recovery from the anesthetic will occur.

• Adjust dosage for each patient; consider age, sex, body weight, clinical signs, and stages of induction. It is advisable to administer a test dose to assess tolerance or unusual sensitivity to the general anesthetic, pausing for 60 seconds before resuming the injection.

• Be prepared with pretested auxiliary equipment including oxygen, and alert for prompt remedial procedures should respiratory arrest occur during the induction of anesthesia and during recovery.

• The patient must be monitored continuously for vital signs (particularly for any respiratory difficulties) during anesthesia and immediately thereafter until there is full recovery from the anesthesia.

• Respiratory depression, apnea, or hypotension may occur.

DRUG INTERACTIONS:

• Separate premedication with atropine or scopolamine to suppress vagal reflexes, and to minimize salivation is compatible pharmacologically.

• Separate premedication with a tranquilizer, barbiturate, or opiate is also compatible provided a precautionary reduction in dosage is made since an unpredictable degree of potentiation of CNS depression may occur.

• Potentiation may also occur with ethyl alcohol, chloral hydrate, or other CNS depressants.

• Inhalation anesthesia with nitrous oxide, ethyl ether, and other similar anesthetics is compatible provided precautionary measures have been taken to assure an adequate airway passage, especially to overcome laryngospasm. The use of a skeletal muscle relaxant or positive pressure oxygen will usually relieve the laryngospasm.

• Curarelike skeletal muscle relaxants (d-tubocurarine, succinylcholine) may further depress respiration or cause respiratory arrest.

• Solutions of any muscle relaxant or anticholinergic agent should not be administered in the same solution or syringe with these barbiturates since a dangerous precipitate will form.

• Solutions of methohexital are incompatible with silicone and should not be allowed to come in contact with equipment treated with silicone.

OVERDOSAGE/ANTIDOTE:

• Overdosage is characterized by an exaggeration of the pharmacologic effects. Respiration and myocardial depression may occur.

• There is no specific antidote. In the event of suspected or apparent overdosage, injection of drug should be discontinued, a patent airway promptly established or maintained, and oxygen administered with artificial or supported respiration as necessary.

General Anesthetics, Inhalation

The inhalation anesthetics are used when general anesthesia must be maintained 30 minutes or longer; when extensive or radical surgical procedures are undertaken. The inhalation anesthetics, whether gas or volatile liquids, are absorbed via the lungs and circulated throughout the body tissues by the bloodstream. Most of these anesthetics are not metabolized within the body; they are returned unchanged to the lungs for discharge in expired

SPECIFIC PRODUCTS AND DOSAGES

GENERIC NAME	TRADE NAME	FLAMMABLE AND EXPLOSIVE	INHALATION ANESTHESIA APPARATUS	ANALGESIA
cyclopropane	(G)†	yes	closed	3–5% with oxygen
ether	(G)	yes	open, closed or semiclosed	not recommended
halothane	(G) FLUOTHANE	no	calibrated flow, closed or semiclosed	not recommended
methoxyflurane	PENTHRANE	no	closed or semiclosed	0.3–0.8% with oxygen
nitrous oxide	(G)	no	closed or semiclosed	20% with oxygen 80%

†(G) Designates availability as a generic product.

Cyclopropane

GENERAL CLINICAL USES

Cyclopropane induces deep anesthesia suitable for most surgical procedures. It is often the drug of choice for patients in shock or classified as poor surgical risks.

PHARMACOLOGY

Cyclopropane is the most potent of the inhalation general anesthetic agents. Induction of anesthesia is extremely rapid (2 to 3 minutes) and recovery is more rapid than for ether anesthesia. Analgesia is readily obtained along with adequate muscle relaxation.

Cyclopropane is both absorbed and eliminated primarily through the lungs. It depresses the rate and depth of respiration in relation to depth of anesthesia, but does not cause increased bronchial secretions. Occasionally, laryngospasm or bronchial constriction may occur, but it does not cause hepatic injury and has little or no effect on gastrointestinal motility.

The cardiovascular system usually is not impaired during anesthesia with cyclopropane. Myocardial contractility and cardiac output are maintained; the heart rate may be slightly increased and arterial blood pressure is maintained. Peripheral resistance is increased. Cyclopropane sensitizes the heart to epinephrine so that ventricular arrhythmias may occur.

SPECIAL PRECAUTIONS
• Use with caution, if at all, in patients with bronchial asthma.
• A marked decrease in blood pressure may occur postoperatively without tachycardia, pallor, or other signs of shock.

air. In contrast, the intravenous general anesthetics are dependent upon the liver and kidneys for their metabolism and excretion from the body.

ANESTHESIA	MAINTENANCE OF ANESTHESIA	DURATION OF INDUCTION (MINUTES)	RECOVERY
15–30% with oxygen	10–20% with oxygen	3–5	5–10
10–15% with oxygen	5% with oxygen	10–20	10–20
2.0–2.5% with oxygen	0.5–1.5% with oxygen	3–5	5–15
1.5–3.0% oxygen 50%	0.1–0.5% with oxygen	5–20	5–20
80% with oxygen 20%	70% with oxygen 34%	3–10	3–10

ADVERSE EFFECTS

CNS EFFECTS: postoperative delirium, headache

RESPIRATORY EFFECTS: depression of rate and depth of respiration, occasional laryngospasm or bronchial constriction

CARDIOVASCULAR EFFECTS: cardiac arrhythmias following myocardial sensitization to epinephrine; rarely severe postanesthetic hypotension

URINARY TRACT EFFECTS: reduced urine output

AUTONOMIC EFFECTS: increased mucous secretions, rarely

GASTROINTESTINAL EFFECTS: nausea, vomiting, retching

METABOLIC AND ENDOCRINE EFFECTS: elevation of blood glucose

HEPATIC EFFECTS: abnormal liver function tests for several days after anesthesia

HEMATOLOGIC EFFECTS: increased capillary bleeding with no disturbances of the blood-clotting mechanism

CLINICAL GUIDELINES

ADMINISTRATION:
• Cyclopropane is highly flammable and explosive; a completely closed (total rebreathing) anesthesia apparatus with carbon dioxide absorption system is required.
• Monitor all electrical services to be absolutely certain that no spark, direct or indirect, may be discharged to cause a fire or explosion. No open flame should be allowed in the same room.
• Monitor all clothing fabrics, plastics, surgical instruments, and metallic surfaces to be certain that no static charges can accumulate and cause sparking.
• Monitor patient continuously during induction to assure maintenance of a patent airway.

EFFECTS:
• The delirium during induction or recov-

ery may be associated with exaggerated psychomotor limb and trunk movement.

• The nausea, retching, and vomiting during the relatively long recovery demands continuous alertness to the danger of aspiration of vomitus and the postoperative risk of suture rupture.

• Cyclopropane anesthesia usually leaves an unpleasant aftertaste in the mouth which frequently persists for 24 hours or longer, the patient should be forewarned or informed immediately after recovery from anesthesia.

• Anticipate a postoperative reduction in urinary output and a tendency to constipation as a result of cyclopropane anesthesia, particularly when anesthesia has been prolonged.

DRUG INTERACTIONS:
• Cyclopropane potentiates the central nervous system depression caused by ethyl alcohol, sedatives, hypnotics, tranquilizers, or analgesics.

• Cyclopropane potentiates the neuromuscular blocking action of the curarelike skeletal muscle relaxants (e.g., succinylcholine).

OVERDOSAGE/ANTIDOTE:
• Overdosage is characterized by respiratory depression, dyspnea, progressive signs of cyanosis or respiratory arrest followed immediately by signs of cardiovascular inadequacy.

• No specific antidote is available. Supportive measures must be initiated at once and maintained until adequate spontaneous respiratory function returns.

Ether

GENERAL CLINICAL USES
Ether, a volatile liquid inhalation general anesthetic, induces profound general analgesia and anesthesia.

PHARMACOLOGY
Induction of anesthesia with ether is relatively slow (10 to 20 minutes) and the recovery is prolonged. The electroencephalogram shows characteristic changes in cortical potentials as anesthesia deepens. Ether stimulates bronchial and salivary secretions which can be controlled by preanesthetic administration of anticholinergic drugs such as atropine. Respiration is not depressed during moderate anesthesia but is during deep anesthesia; respiratory depression with paralysis of thoracic muscles may occur. Ether also causes curarelike neuromuscular blockage and thereby significant skeletal muscle relaxation. Although ether does not sensitize the heart to epinephrine, cardiac arrhythmias have developed during deep anesthesia. Ether is eliminated from the body via the lungs in the expired air; its elimination is not dependent upon metabolic conversion by the liver or kidneys. Nevertheless, slight transient impairment of liver function has been reported. Ether passes the placental barrier and the concentration in the fetal circulation is similar to that in maternal blood.

SPECIAL PRECAUTIONS
• Ether is highly volatile and flammable and its vapor, when mixed with air and ignited, may explode violently.

• Ether causes excessive salivation, stimulation of bronchial secretions, and irritation of respiratory passages which may compromise airway maintenance.

• Postoperative nausea and vomiting occur frequently; and consequently, aspiration of vomitus is a continuing hazard during recovery.

• Use with caution in patients with liver disease or abnormal liver function tests since these impairments may be prolonged after ether anesthesia.

ADVERSE EFFECTS

CNS EFFECTS: delirium during induction and recovery

RESPIRATORY EFFECTS: irritation of bronchial tree, with excessive bronchial secretion, postoperative atelectasis pneumonia, and respiratory depression during deep anesthesia

CARDIOVASCULAR EFFECTS: increased heart rate

URINARY TRACT EFFECTS: reduced urine output

GASTROINTESTINAL EFFECTS: nausea, vomiting during recovery; increased salivation, depression of gastric tone and motility

METABOLIC AND ENDOCRINE EFFECTS: transient hyperglycemia, metabolic acidosis in children

CLINICAL GUIDELINES

ADMINISTRATION:

• Monitor all electrical services to be absolutely certain that no spark, direct or indirect, may be discharged to cause a fire or explosion. No open flame can be allowed in the same room as ether.

• Monitor all clothing fabrics, plastics, surgical instruments, and metallic surfaces to be certain that no static charges can accumulate and cause sparking.

• Use ether from freshly opened container. Never utilize any ether that has been removed from the approved USP container for 24 hours or longer.

• The patient must be continuously monitored during induction to ensure maintenance of a patent airway.

EFFECTS:

• The delirium during induction or recovery may be associated with exaggerated psychomotor limb and trunk movement.

• The nausea, retching, and vomiting during the relatively long recovery demands continuous alertness to avoid the danger of aspiration of vomitus and the postoperative risk of rupture of sutures.

• Ether anesthesia usually leaves an unpleasant aftertaste in the mouth which frequently persists for 24 hours or longer; the patient should be forewarned or informed immediately after recovery from the effects of anesthesia.

• Anticipate a postoperative reduction in urinary output and a tendency to constipation as a result of ether anesthesia, particularly when anesthesia has been prolonged.

• Liver function tests may be altered transiently.

• Ether can produce profound muscular relaxation.

DRUG INTERACTIONS:

• Ether potentiates the central nervous system depression caused by ethyl alcohol, sedatives, hypnotics, tranquilizers, or analgesics.

• Ether potentiates the neuromuscular blocking action of the curarelike skeletal muscle relaxants; dosage of these agents should be reduced.

• The ether-stimulated mucous secretion in the bronchial tree and of the salivary glands is readily counteracted by anticholinergic drugs.

OVERDOSAGE/ANTIDOTE:

• Overdosage is characterized by respiratory depression, dyspnea, progressive signs of cyanosis of respiratory arrest followed immediately by signs of cardiovascular inadequacy.

• Supportive respiratory measures must be initiated at once and maintained until adequate spontaneous respiratory function returns. No specific antidote is available.

Halothane

GENERAL CLINICAL USES

Halothane is the preferred inhalation general anesthetic when deep and prolonged anesthia is required. It is the anesthetic of choice for asthmatics. Halothane is not recommended for light plane anesthesia or minor surgical procedures such as obstetric delivery. If it becomes necessary to induce anesthesia in a patient who has recently received halothane, a different inhalation anesthetic should be used.

PHARMACOLOGY

Anesthesia is induced rapidly with little or no excitement. Halothane does not irritate the respiratory tissues. It dilates bronchioles; salivation, coughing, laryngospasm, and bronchospasm are uncommon. As surgical anesthesia deepens, it causes progressive respiratory depression while respiratory tidal volume increases. Hypoxia, acidosis, or apnea may develop. Because halothane does not produce adequate skeletal muscle relaxation, curarelike agents are required. Halothane is a potent uterine muscle relaxant. Induction and recovery are rapid and depth of anesthesia can be rapidly altered. Recovery is relatively smooth and rapid after short procedures and delayed 10 to 15 minutes after long procedures.

The cardiovascular system is markedly affected by halothane anesthesia. The contractility of heart muscle and vascular smooth muscle is diminished resulting in reduced blood pressure.

SPECIAL PRECAUTIONS

• Do not use for obstetric anesthesia except when uterine relaxation is required.
• Do not use in patients with known or suspected liver disease, or in a patient recently anesthetized with halothane.
• Do not use in pregnancy, unless in the judgment of the physician, the potential benefit outweighs the unknown hazards to the fetus.

ADVERSE EFFECTS

CNS EFFECTS: hyperpyrexia, increased spinal fluid pressure, shivering
RESPIRATORY EFFECTS: progressive depression, slowed rate and reduced tidal volume, hypoxia, apnea with deep anesthesia, respiratory arrest
CARDIOVASCULAR EFFECTS: hypotension, bradycardia, decreased pulse rate, dilation of the blood vessels of the skin and skeletal muscles, cardiac arrhythmias, cardiac arrest
URINARY TRACT EFFECTS: oliguria (reversible)
AUTONOMIC EFFECTS: relaxation of uterine muscle
GASTROINTESTINAL EFFECTS: nausea, vomiting
METABOLIC AND ENDOCRINE EFFECTS: acidosis after prolonged deep anesthesia
HEPATIC EFFECTS: necrosis, hepatitis

CLINICAL GUIDELINES
ADMINISTRATION:
• Monitor patient continuously for signs of overdosage; blood pressure, pulse rate, respiration changes; or arrhythmias.
• A calibrated flow and temperature-compensated flow meter must be used.
• Halothane should be kept only in vaporizer bottles that are calibrated for its use. They should be placed out of circuit, in closed circuit rebreathing system; otherwise, overdosage is difficult to avoid. These vaporizers should be emptied at the end of each operating day.
• Thymol serves as a stabilizer for the halothane, but does not volatilize. Its accumulation, evidenced by yellow discoloration, serves as an indicator that the vaporizer should be drained, cleaned, and the discolored halothane discarded.
• Halothane interacts with rubber, some plastics, and similar materials, but not polyethylene.
• Halothane is not explosive.

• Be prepared with pretested auxiliary equipment including oxygen and be alert for prompt remedial procedures should respiratory arrest occur during induction of anesthesia or during recovery.

• The patient should be monitored closely for signs of depression of blood pressure, pulse rate, and ventilation. Drugs to counteract cardiac depression and hypotension should be available.

EFFECTS:

• The incidence of postanesthetic nausea and vomiting is lower than after either ether or cyclopropane.

DRUG INTERACTIONS:

• The uterine response to ergot derivatives or oxytocic posterior pituitary extract may be blocked by halothane.

• Epinephrine, levarterenol, or norepinephrine should not be employed during halothane anesthesia since ventricular tachycardia or fibrillation may be induced.

• Halothane augments the action of curarelike muscle relaxants (e.g., succinylcholine) and ganglion blocking agents (e.g., pancuronium, gallamine); dosage of these agents should be reduced.

OVERDOSAGE/ANTIDOTE:

• Overdosage is characterized by reduction of blood pressure, circulatory collapse, and decreased ventilation.

• No specific antidote is available. Standard resuscitative procedures must be instituted to support respiration and to restore cardiovascular function.

Methoxyflurane

GENERAL CLINICAL USES

Methoxyflurane is useful in inducing anesthesia necessary for performing minor surgical procedures and obstetric delivery. It is not recommended for deep anesthesia.

PHARMACOLOGY

Methoxyflurane, a volatile liquid anesthetic, induces anesthesia slowly; recovery is prolonged. Methoxyflurane has good analgesic and muscle-relaxing properties. Respiration is readily depressed and, therefore, must be assisted. Cardiovascular effects are comparable to fluroxene, and ordinarily methoxyflurane does not induce laryngospasm or bronchial constriction.

Blood pressure may decrease and be accompanied by bradycardia and reduced cardiac output. In light planes of anesthesia, it has little effect on uterine contractions.

Methoxyflurane is metabolized to several metabolites which may cause significant renal damage which results in renal failure.

SPECIAL PRECAUTIONS

• Induce only a light plane of anesthesia since severe renal damage which appears to be dose-related may occur; limit duration of anesthesia to surgical procedures not exceeding 1 hour.

• Use cautiously in obese patients because of storage potential.

• Use of methoxyflurane is extremely hazardous in aged or obese patients or in surgical procedures of long duration.

• Do not employ in patients with preexisting renal disease, toxemia of pregnancy, or patients undergoing vascular surgery.

• Minimize possible cumulative renal toxic effects by not repeating use.

• Use with extreme caution in patients receiving tetracyclines or antibiotics with nephrotoxic potential.

ADVERSE EFFECTS

CNS EFFECTS: occasional excitement during induction and recovery from anesthesia; malignant hyperpyrexia, emergence somnolence

RESPIRATORY EFFECTS: reduction in rate and volume

CARDIOVASCULAR EFFECTS: sinus bradycardia, readily reversible ventricular arrhythmias (rare), cardiac arrest (rare)

URINARY TRACT EFFECTS: increased urine volume with low specific gravity, increase in blood urea nitrogen

AUTONOMIC EFFECTS: laryngospasm, bronchospasm

GASTROINTESTINAL EFFECTS: nausea, vomiting

METABOLIC AND ENDOCRINE EFFECTS: increased excretion of oxalic acid, slight metabolic acidosis

HEPATIC EFFECTS: increased BSP retention, jaundice, fatal hepatic necrosis

CLINICAL GUIDELINES

ADMINISTRATION:
• Administer with calibrated temperature-compensated, out-of-circle vaporizers or other methods which provide accurately delivered vapor concentration.
• Methoxyflurane is nonflammable.
• Monitor patients for urine output and laboratory signs of renal function at appropriate intervals; oxylate crystals and acute tubular necrosis have often been noted at autopsy.
• An antioxidant is added to insure stability on standing; it slowly turns yellow, then brown, and may accumulate in vaporizer wick. Clean with diethyl ether but be careful to dry the wick afterward to avoid introduction of any diethyl ether into the apparatus.
• Methoxyflurane dissolves rubber and other plastics; disposable conductive plastic circuits should be discarded after a single use to avoid crosscontamination with other agents.

• Asthmatic patients tolerate this drug well.

EFFECTS:
• Limit depth of anesthesia to light planes when given alone.
• An odor of methoxyflurane may persist in the breath for days.
• Postoperative polyuric failure is characterized by early development of weight loss and changes in urinalysis: low specific gravity, decreased osmolality; elevated serum or blood sodium chloride, uric acid, BUN and creatinine.

DRUG INTERACTIONS:
• Concomitant use with antibiotics of known nephrotoxic potential may enhance nephrotoxicity.
• The neuromuscular blocking effects of the nondepolarizing muscle relaxants (tubocurarine, gallamine, pancuronium) are augmented; therefore dosage reduction of these agents is required.
• Compatible with oxytocic agents.

OVERDOSAGE/ANTIDOTE:
• The earliest signs of overdosage include an abrupt drop in blood pressure and respiratory depression; acute renal failure may follow shortly thereafter.
• Since no specific antidote is available, standard resuscitative procedures must be promptly instituted to restore respiratory adequacy and cardiovascular function. In addition, measures to remedy any renal inadequacy must be instituted.

Nitrous Oxide

GENERAL CLINICAL USES
The only significant usage for nitrous oxide by itself is intermittent analgesia during brief procedures such as delivery, although it was formerly used for dental extractions. However, nitrous oxide is often utilized to facilitate induction as a compo-

nent of "balanced" general anesthesia (for example, with ether or halothane).

PHARMACOLOGY

Nitrous oxide (laughing gas) is not an unpleasant-smelling gas, but has a low anesthetic potency (about 1/7 of ether). Alone, it cannot induce stage 3 anesthesia in a patient at the usual safe concentration (85 percent nitrous oxide, 15 percent oxygen) for 2 or 3 minutes. It acts rapidly (2 to 4 minutes) and recovery is equally so (2 to 10 minutes). By itself it will ordinarily produce analgesia. A few breaths of 100 percent nitrous oxide, or prolonged breathing of 85 percent nitrous oxide and 15 percent oxygen, can carry the patient to stage 2 with euphoria or altered perception.

Nitrous oxide does not stimulate salivation nor afford adequate muscle relaxation. It does not appear to have any toxic effect on any organ systems. It is excreted unaltered by the lungs.

SPECIAL PRECAUTIONS

• Dangerous hypoxia may develop after discontinuing prolonged nitrous oxide anesthesia because of its very high solubility in blood (35 times that of nitrogen); to minimize this hazard, additional oxygen should be inhaled during emergence from anesthesia.
• Do not use in presence of pneumothorax, adynamic ileus, and pneumoencephalopathy.

ADVERSE EFFECTS

CNS EFFECTS: euphoria, dreaming, altered perception
RESPIRATORY EFFECTS: postanesthetic hypoxia with embolism after high concentrations or prolonged anesthesia

CARDIOVASCULAR EFFECTS: depression of blood pressure, heart rate, and muscle tone
GASTROINTESTINAL EFFECTS: nausea, vomiting
HEMATOLOGIC EFFECTS: bone marrow depression with prolonged exposure (24 hours)

CLINICAL GUIDELINES

ADMINISTRATION:
• Atropinelike drug premedication is *not* required to be administered concomitantly since respiratory and salivary secretions are not stimulated by nitrous oxide.
• Administer by semiclosed or nonrebreathing methods; it is not explosive or flammable (except when mixed with ether or cyclopropane).
• The amount of anesthetic must be adjusted for each patient as governed by age, sex, body weight, clinical signs and stages of induction.
• Monitor patient continuously for signs of hypoxia or asphyxia when anesthesia is prolonged or high concentrations (greater than 85 percent nitrous oxide, less than 15 percent oxygen) are used.
EFFECTS:
• Postanesthetic hypoxia or asphyxia should be offset by administering 100 percent oxygen on an intermittent basis until full recovery from the asphyxia has been established.
• The euphoria and distorted perception during induction or the recovery from anesthesia rarely produces psychomotor aberrations.
• When nitrous oxide is used in combination with another general anesthetic (for example, ether, halothane, or an intravenous barbiturate), the patient response will reflect those of these potent agents rather than those for nitrous oxide.
DRUG INTERACTIONS:
• Nitrous oxide has been clinically com-

patible with a wide variety of drugs including anticholinergics, curarelike agents, tranquilizers, strong analgesics, mild analgesics, local anesthetics; also intravenous and inhalation anesthetics.

OVERDOSAGE/ANTIDOTE:
• Overdosage for a short period of time does not depress or impair respiratory function. When nitrous oxide, 85 percent, is given for a prolonged time, or 100 percent for a few minutes, hypoxia and embolism can occur.
• Discontinue nitrous oxide and administer oxygen 100 percent, intermittently until blood oxygenation has been reestablished.

Regional Anesthetics

Regional anesthetics are those which can be administered by infiltration, specific nerve block, spinally, saddle block; into the perineum, lower limbs, lower or upper abdomen.

In contrast, the topical surface, or local anesthetics are applied to the surface of the skin or mucous membranes. For detailed information concerning these agents please refer to the following chapters: Chapter 7, *Drugs Affecting the Urinary Tract*, Chapter 9, *Drugs Affecting the Skin*, Chapter 10, *Drugs Affecting the Mouth and Teeth*, Chapter 11, *Drugs Affecting the Eye*, Chapter 12, *Drugs Affecting the Ear*.

SPECIFIC PRODUCTS AND DOSAGES
Children, elderly patients, or debilitated patients should be given doses commensurate with their age and physical status. In all patients, dosage depends on the area to be anesthetized, vascularity, neuronal segments to be blocked, and technique of administration. Use lowest dosage required for effective anesthesia.

| | | | | SUGGESTED DOSAGE | |
| | | ROUTE OF | | MAXIMAL SINGLE | DURATION |
GENERIC NAME	TRADE NAME	ADMIN.	USUAL ADULT DOSAGE	DOSE (mg)	(min.)
bupivacaine HCl	(G)† MARCAINE	Infiltration Nerve block	0.25% solution 0.25–0.75% solution	500	240–300

† (G) Designates availability as a generic product.

(continued facing page)

GENERIC NAME	TRADE NAME	ROUTE OF ADMIN.	USUAL ADULT DOSAGE	SUGGESTED DOSAGE MAXIMAL SINGLE DOSE (mg)	DURATION (min.)
chloroprocaine HCl	NESACAINE	Infiltration	Up to 80 ml of 1% soln.	1000	30–60
		Nerve block	Up to 40 ml of 1–2% soln.	800	40–60
		Epidural block	2–3%; 1.5–2.5 ml/segment	800	40–60
		Caudal block	2–3%; 15–25 ml	800	40–60
dibucaine HCl	NUPERCAINE	Spinal block	1:200 solution, 0.5–1.5 ml	10	60–360
			1:1500 solution, 6–18 ml (4–12 mg)	12	60–360
			Heavy solution, 1–2 ml		
etidocaine HCl	DURANEST	Caudal block	1.0% solution, 10–30 ml	300	————
		Nerve block	0.5–1.5% solution, 5–30 ml	400	8–10 hr.
		Infiltration	0.5% solution, 1–80 ml	400	————
lidocaine HCl	(G)	Dental	2% solution; 1–5 ml		
	XYLOCAINE	Infiltration	0.5% solution, 1–60 ml	300	60–90
	L-CAINE	Epidural block	1–2% solution, 10–30 ml	300	100
	ULTRACAINE	Caudal block	1–2% solution, 15–30 ml	300	75–135
		Peripheral nerve block	1–2% solution, 1–20 ml	50–300	————
		Sympathetic nerve block	1% solution, 5–10 ml	100	————
mepivacaine HCl, mepivacaine	CARBOCAINE	Infiltration	0.5–1% solution, 1–40 ml	5–7 mg/kg	30–120+
		Nerve block	1–2% solution, 5–20 ml	400 mg	30–90
		Epidural block	1–2% solution, 10–30 ml	400	115–150
		Caudal block	1–2% solution, 10–30 ml	400	100–170
		Dental	3% solution, 0.7–1.8 ml		
piperocaine HCl	METYCAINE	Infiltration	0.5–1% solution, up to 100 ml	800	30–90
		Nerve block	0.5–2% solution, up to 35 ml		————
		Caudal block	1.5% solution, up to 50 ml		————
prilocaine HCl	CITANEST	Infiltration	1–2% solution, 20–30 ml	600	30–120 +
		Peripheral nerve block	1–3% solution, 3–30 ml	600	120–180
		Epidural block	1–3% solution, 15–30 ml	600–3%	120–180
		Caudal block	1–3% solution, 15–30 ml	600–3%	120–180
procaine HCl	(G)	Infiltration	0.25–0.5% solution	25–50	30–90
	NOVOCAIN	Nerve block	1–2% solution, up to 25 ml	300–600	————
		Epidural block	1–2% solution, 15–30 ml	300–600	————
		Caudal block	1–2% solution, 15–30 ml	300–600	————
		Spinal block	10% solution, 0.5–2 ml	50–200	————
tetracaine HCl	(G) PONTOCAINE	Spinal block	0.5–2% solution, 1–3 ml	15	120–180

Bupivacaine HCl
Chloroprocaine HCl
Dibucaine HCl
Etidocaine HCl
Lidocaine HCl
Mepivacaine HCl
Piperocaine HCl
Prilocaine HCl
Procaine HCl
Tetraczine HCl

GENERAL CLINICAL USES

The regional anesthetic agents are administered by injection to produce anesthesia in a specific or relatively specific area of the body. They may be used in patients unable to tolerate general anesthesia and are employed in minor or major surgical procedures.

The most common methods for inducing regional anesthesia by injection are infiltration, nerve block, spinal (subarachoid or intrathecal) block, epidural or caudal block; certain products are used for dental anesthesia.

The region to be anesthetized depends upon the application site, total volume of drug injected, and the penetrating capacity of the drug. The degree and duration of action depends on concentration, duration of exposure, size of nerve fibers, and type of nerves (medullated or nonmedullated).

Of the regional anesthetic agents, lidocaine is also used as an antiarrhythmic agent. For detailed information concerning this use, please refer to Chapter 5, page 213.

PHARMACOLOGY

Knowledge about the absorption, fate, and distribution of these drugs is limited. After parenteral administration, they enter the circulation, reversibly block the conduction of sensory impulses, and prevent their transmission from a localized area without causing the patient to lose consciousness. Generally these drugs are broken down by cholinesterases in the blood or liver with portions excreted unchanged in the urine.

Since regional anesthetic agents paralyze vasoconstrictor nerves, vasodilatation usually occurs. Consequently, a vasoconstrictor agent such as epinephrine hydrochloride is generally added to anesthetic solutions.

SPECIAL PRECAUTIONS
• Avoid administration, if possible, to patients with known history of allergic reaction or intolerance to the drug.
• Since most regional anesthetic solutions contain epinephrine, avoid use in elderly patients or those with hypertension, cardiovascular disease, diabetes, or thyrotoxicosis; avoid use with inhalation anesthetics known to sensitize the heart to epinephrine.
• Avoid solutions containing epinephrine for nerve block in patients in labor; it may produce a decreased placental circulation and prolonged labor.
• Patients allergic to penicillin may be allergic to the procaine in penicillin and not penicillin itself. Therefore patients "allergic to penicillin" should be closely questioned before using procaine as a local anesthetic agent.
• Prilocaine should not be used in patients with methemoglobinemia; a dose exceeding 400 mg may produce significant methemoglobin blood levels.
• Large doses of regional anesthetics should not be used in patients with heart block.
• Preparations containing preservatives should not be used for spinal or epidural anesthesia.

• Use these (amide-type) anesthetic agents with caution in patients with severe liver disease.

• Safe use in pregnancy with respect to adverse fetal development has not been established.

• Fetal bradycardia frequently follows paracervical block and may be associated with fetal acidosis; added risk appears to be present in prematurity, toxemia of pregnancy, and fetal distress.

ADVERSE EFFECTS

CNS EFFECTS: postanesthetic headache, euphoria, nervousness, restlessness, dizziness, anxiety, excitement, disorientation, coma, drowsiness, tremors, paresthesia

RESPIRATORY EFFECTS: dyspnea, bronchoconstriction, respiratory arrest, status asthmaticus

CARDIOVASCULAR EFFECTS: palpitations, hypotension, bradycardia, thready pulse, shock, cardiac arrest

URINARY TRACT EFFECTS: with high or total spinal block, urinary retention

GASTROINTESTINAL EFFECTS: nausea, vomiting, swelling and persistant paresthesia of the lips and oral tissues, fecal incontinence

METABOLIC AND ENDOCRINE EFFECTS: loss of perineal sensation and sexual functions.

HEMATOLOGIC EFFECTS: with prilocaine, methemoglobinemia

ALLERGIC EFFECTS: cutaneous lesions, urticaria, edema, anaphylactoid reactions

DERMATOLOGIC EFFECTS: angioneurotic edema, eczematoid dermatitis, skin discoloration, sloughing, neuritis, vesiculation, pruritus

OPHTHALMIC EFFECTS: blurred vision

MUSCULOSKELETAL EFFECTS: muscle twitching, tremors, convulsions, backache

CLINICAL GUIDELINES

ADMINISTRATION:

• Aseptic technique is mandatory in preparing the various solutions for administration.

• To prevent accidental intravascular injection, frequent syringe aspirations to check for blood vessel puncture should be made.

• Assure that proper concentration and proper diluent for the specific application or specific formulation for indication is utilized.

• Special hypobasic, isobasic, or hyperbasic solutions (usually containing dextrose) are employed for spinal anesthesia.

• Single-dose vials should be used for caudal, epidural, and spinal blocks since the chemical preservatives used in multiple-dose vials are contraindicated in these applications.

• Large doses of local anesthetics should not be made into or through infected or inflamed tissues.

• Resuscitative equipment and drugs should be immediately available when any regional anesthetic is used.

EFFECTS:

• Cardiovascular effects are a result of myocardial depression and peripheral vasodilation followed by hypotension, thready pulse, and shock.

• Systemic reactions of allergic or idiosyncratic origin may occur, and these are manifested by urticaria, dermatitis, angioneurotic edema, bronchoconstriction, syncope, and respiratory failure.

• If preparations containing epinephrine or similar vasoconstrictors are used in patients during or following the administration of chloroform, halothane, cyclopropane, trichloroethylene, or related drugs, serious dose-related cardiac arrhythmias may occur.

DRUG INTERACTIONS:

• Regional anesthetics may react with certain metals and cause the release of their respective ions which, if injected, may cause severe local irritation.

• Since certain regional anesthetics (chloroprocaine, procaine, piperocaine, tetracaine) may be metabolized to or derivatives of aminobenzoic acid, they may inhibit the action of sulfonamides if administered concomitantly.

• Anesthetics containing a vasoconstrictor should be used with extreme caution in patients receiving drugs known to produce blood pressure alterations such as MAO-inhibitors, tricyclic antidepressants, and phenothiazines; severe and sustained hypotension or hypertension may occur.

• Serious dose-related cardiac arrhythmias may occur if preparations containing epinephrine are used concurrently with chloroform, halothane, cyclopropane, trichloroethylene, or other related drugs.

• Concurrent administration of oxytocic drugs in postpartum patients receiving anesthetics containing epinephrine may cause severe persistent hypertension or even rupture of a cerebral blood vessel.

OVERDOSAGE/ANTIDOTE:

• Overdosage is characterized by nausea, cardiovascular and respiratory inefficiency.

• There are no specific antidotes. Supportive measures must be initiated at once and maintained until spontaneous and adequate function returns. Vasopressors such as ephedrine or metaraminol and intravenous fluids may be necessary. If convulsions occur or persist, small increments of an ultra-short-acting barbiturate (thiopental or thiamylal) may be administered intravenously.

Anticerebral Edema Agents

SPECIFIC PRODUCTS AND DOSAGES

GENERIC NAME	TRADE NAME	ROUTE OF ADMIN.	SUGGESTED DAILY DOSAGE		
			ADULT	MRDD*	CHILDREN
dexamethasone sodium phosphate	(G)† DECADRON	im/iv	10 mg, then 4 mg every 6 hr. for 24 hr.; then reduce dosage	40 mg	Individualize by age and weight
mannitol	(G) OSMITROL	iv	1.5–2 gm/kg as 15–25% solution over 30–60 min.	200 mg	Individualize by age and weight

*MRDD = maximal recommended daily dose.
†(G) Designates availability as a generic product.

Dexamethasone Sodium Phosphate

GENERAL CLINICAL USE

Dexamethasone, a synthetic glucocorticoid used primarily for its potent anti-inflammatory activity, is particularly useful in the treatment of patients with cerebral edema of diverse origin. Administered orally or parenterally, it may be used in the preoperative preparation of patients with increased intracranial pressure secondary to brain tumors; for palliative management of patients with inoperable or recurrent brain tumors; and also in the management of cerebral edema associated with surgery or head injury. However, the use of dexamethasone is not a substitute for neurosurgical evaluation, neurosurgery, or other specialized therapy.

PHARMACOLOGY, SPECIAL PRECAUTIONS, ADVERSE EFFECTS, CLINICAL GUIDELINES

For detailed information, see Chapter 15, page 532, *Endocrine and Other Drugs Affecting Metabolism.*

Mannitol

GENERAL CLINICAL USES

Mannitol, an obligatory osmotic diuretic when administered parenterally, causes a reduction of intracranial pressure and brain mass.

PHARMACOLOGY, SPECIAL PRECAUTIONS, ADVERSE EFFECTS, CLINICAL GUIDELINES

For detailed information, see the discussion of diuretic agents in Chapter 5, page 245.

Anticonvulsant Agents

SPECIFIC PRODUCTS AND DOSAGES

	GENERIC NAME	TRADE NAME	ROUTE OF ADMIN.	SUGGESTED DAILY DOSAGE		
				ADULTS		CHILDREN SINGLE DOSE
				SINGLE DOSE	MRDD[†]	
	Barbiturates, Long acting, and Primidone:					
CII*	amobarbital sodium (G)[‡]	AMYTAL Sodium	po	65 mg bid to qid	260 mg	Not established

*C denotes schedule listing under the Controlled Substances Act.
[†]MRDD = maximal recommended daily dose.
[‡](G) Designates availability as a generic product.

(continued overleaf)

	GENERIC NAME	TRADE NAME	ROUTE OF ADMIN.	SUGGESTED DAILY DOSAGE		
				ADULTS		CHILDREN SINGLE DOSE
				SINGLE DOSE	MRDD†	
CIV*	mephobarbital	(G)‡ MEBARAL	po	100–200 mg tid	600 mg	**Under 5 yrs.:** 16–32 mg tid or qid **Over 5 yrs.:** 32–64 mg tid or qid
CIII	metharbital	GEMONIL	po	100 mg od to tid	800 mg	50–100 mg od to tid; 5–15 mg/kg/day in divided doses
CII	pentobarbital	(G) NEMBUTAL	im	150–200 mg	500 mg	25–80 mg
CIV	phenobarbital	(G) LUMINAL	po	50–100 mg bid to tid	350 mg	15–50 mg bid or tid
CIV	phenobarbital sodium	(G)	sc/im/ iv	200–300 mg; repeat in 6 hrs.	600 mg	3–5 mg/kg single dose
CII	secobarbital sodium	(G) SECONAL Sodium	im/iv	2.5 mg/lb every 3–4 hr.	————	Not established
CIII	thiopental sodium	PENTOTHAL	iv	No fixed dosage; 75–125 mg initially	————	Not established
	primidone	(G) MYSOLINE RO-PRIMIDONE	po	0.75–1.5 gm/day in divided doses	2 gm	**Under 8 yrs.:** 500– 750 mg/day in divided doses
	Diphenylhydantoin and Derivatives: diphenylhydantoin (phenytoin)	(G) DIPHENYLAN DILANTIN	po	100 mg tid	600 mg	4–8 mg/kg/day in single or 2–3 equally divided doses
	diphenylhydantoin sodium	DILANTIN	im/iv	150–250 mg; 100–150 mg after 30 min.	500 mg	3–8 mg/kg/24 hr single dose or divided in 2 doses
	ethotoin	PEGANONE	po	2–3 gm divided in 4–6 equal doses/ 24 hr.	3000 mg	up to 80 mg/kg/24 hr divided in 3 or 4 equal doses
	mephenytoin	MESANTOIN	po	200–600 mg/day in single or divided doses	800 mg	100–400 mg/day in single or divided doses
	Trimethadione and Related Agents: paramethadione	PARADIONE	po	300–600 mg tid or qid	2400 mg	40 mg/kg/day divided in 3–4 doses
	trimethadione	TRIDIONE	po	300–600 mg tid or qid	2400 mg	300–900 mg/day divided in 3–4 doses or 40 mg/kg/day divided in 3–4 doses

*C denotes schedule listing under the Controlled Substances Act.
†MRDD = maximal recommended daily dose.
‡(G) Designates availability as a generic product.

(continued facing page)

	GENERIC NAME	TRADE NAME	ROUTE OF ADMIN.	SUGGESTED DAILY DOSAGE		CHILDREN SINGLE DOSE
				ADULTS		
				SINGLE DOSE	MRDD*	
	Succinimides:					
	ethosuximide	ZARONTIN	po	250 mg bid to qid	1500 mg	**Under 6 yrs.:** 250 mg/24 hr. **Over 6 yrs.:** 500 mg/24 hr. divided in 2 doses
	methsuximide	CELONTIN	po	300 mg hs to qid	1200 mg	300–1200 mg/day in divided doses
	phensuximide	MILONTIN	po	500–1000 mg bid to tid	3000 mg	600–1000 mg bid or tid
	Miscellaneous Drugs:					
	acetazolamide	(G)† DIAMOX	po	375–1000 mg/day in divided doses	1000 mg	8–30 mg/kg in divided doses
	carbamazepine	TEGRETOL	po	200–400 mg bid to qid	1600 mg 1000 mg in children	**12–15 yrs.;** 1000 mg/day in divided doses **Under 12 yrs.:** not established
	clonazepan	CLONOPIN	po	0.5 mq tid, then increase by 0.5–1 mg every 3rd day	20 mg	**Infants up to 10 yrs.:** 0.01–0.03 mg/kg/day; do not exceed 0.05 mg/kg/24 hr.; give in divided doses
CIV	diazepam	VALIUM	im/iv	5–10 mg See Chapter 3, page 101, for detailed information	30 mg	**Over 30 days and children under 5 yrs.:** 0.2–0.5 mg **5 yrs. and older:** 1–10 mg
	magnesium sulfate	(G)	im/iv	1–2 gm	———	———
CIV	paraldehyde	(G) PARAL	im iv	5 ml 3–5 ml See *Nonbarbiturate sedative-hypnotic agents.*	——— ———	——— ———
	phenacemide	PHENURONE	po	500 mg tid, then increase to 2000–3000 mg/day	5000 mg	**Children 5–10 yrs.:** one half the adult dose
	valproic acid	DEPAKENE	po	15–30 mg/kg/day; if total daily dose exceeds 250 mg, give in a divided regimen	1500 mg	15–30 mg/kg/day in divided doses

*MRDD = maximal recommended daily dose.
†(G) Designates availability as a generic product.

Barbiturates, Long-Acting

Amobarbital Sodium
Mephobarbital
Metharbital
Pentobarbital
Phenobarbital Sodium
Secobarbital Sodium
Thiopental Sodium

GENERAL CLINICAL USES

The long-acting barbiturates are standard anticonvulsant agents used primarily in grand mal epilepsy. For detailed information, please refer to the section *Sedative-Hypnotic Agents* at the end of this chapter.

Primidone

GENERAL CLINICAL USES

Primidone, either alone or in combination with other anticonvulsants, is indicated in grand mal epilepsy, particularly in cases refractory to other anticonvulsant therapy. It is also prescribed in psychomotor and focal epileptic seizures.

PHARMACOLOGY

Primidone, although not actually a barbiturate, is closely related chemically and pharmacologically. It acts on the central nervous system to raise seizure threshold or to alter seizure pattern. The drug is metabolized to phenobarbital and phenylethylmalonamide in the liver and excreted in the urine. A single oral dose remains effective for 5 to 9 hours.

SPECIAL PRECAUTIONS

• Do not use in patients with porphyria or those hypersensitive to phenobarbital.

• Abrupt withdrawal of medication may precipitate status epilepticus.
• Safe use in pregnancy has not been established.
• Do not use in nursing mothers; a substantial quantity appears in milk.

ADVERSE EFFECTS

CNS EFFECTS: drowsiness, sedation, ataxia, vertigo, headache, hyperirritability
HEMATOLOGIC EFFECTS: megaloblastic anemia, rare
DERMATOLOGIC EFFECTS: morbilliform rash, pitting edema
OPHTHALMIC EFFECTS: diplopia, and nystagmus

CLINICAL GUIDELINES

ADMINISTRATION:
• Therapeutic efficacy of a dosage regimen takes several days for assessment.
EFFECTS:
• Although sedation may be severe at the beginning of therapy, it tends to disappear with continued use.
OVERDOSAGE/ANTIDOTE:
• Overdosage is characterized by CNS depression, namely, respiratory depression, depression of superficial and deep reflexes, constriction of pupils, decreased urine formation, lowered body temperature; later fever, gradual appearance of circulatory collapse and pulmonary edema, coma.
• No specific antidote is known; the use of analeptic agents is controversial.
• If the patient is seen within a few hours of overdosage, empty stomach by lavage. A patent airway must be maintained. Mechanical ventilation and oxygen may be required. Endotracheal intubation may be necessary. Adequate cardiovascular function must be maintained. If renal failure occurs, drug removal by hemodialysis is effective.

Diphenylhydantoin and Derivatives

Diphenylhydantoin (Phenytoin)
Diphenylhydantoin Sodium
Ethotoin
Mephenytoin

GENERAL CLINICAL USES

Diphenylhydantoin is indicated for grand mal epilepsy and psychomotor seizures; it remains the drug of choice of the hydantoins.

Mephenytoin and ethotoin are employed in patients unresponsive or intolerant to diphenylhydantoin.

PHARMACOLOGY

Diphenylhydantoin and ethotoin have little or no sedative effects in recommended dosages. Mephenytoin exerts a sedative action and serious reactions are more common than with diphenylhydantoin and ethotoin. None of these drugs in recommended dosages exert any significant pharmacologic action on respiratory cardiovascular, or renal function. After oral administration of diphenylhydantoin, maximal blood levels are attached in about 8 hours. The drug is metabolized by the liver and excreted as a conjugate in the urine. However, metabolism is slow with a plasma half-life of 22 hours; a stable level is not reached until 7 to 10 days after initiation of a fixed dosage.

SPECIAL PRECAUTIONS

- Toxicity may occur early in elderly patients or in those with impaired liver function.
- Abrupt withdrawal of medication may precipitate status epilepticus.
- Safe use in pregnancy has not been established.

ADVERSE EFFECTS

CNS EFFECTS: slurred speech, drowsiness, ataxia, mental confusion, dizziness, insomnia, headache, nervousness, tremors, toxic psychoses, stupor, coma

URINARY TRACT EFFECTS: nephrosis rarely

AUTONOMIC EFFECTS: fever

GASTROINTESTINAL EFFECTS: nausea, vomiting, constipation, gingival hyperplasia

METABOLIC AND ENDOCRINE EFFECTS: periarteritis nodosa, hyperglycemia

HEPATIC EFFECTS: jaundice, liver damage, toxic hepatitis

HEMATOLOGIC EFFECTS: thrombocytopenia, leukopenia, agranulocytosis, megaloblastic anemia, lymphadenopathy

DERMATOLOGIC EFFECTS: hirsutism, alopecia, morbilliform rash; bullous, exfoliative or purpuric dermatitis, lupus, erythematosus, Stevens-Johnson syndrome

OPHTHALMIC EFFECTS: nystagmus, diplopia, photophobia

MUSCULOSKELETAL EFFECTS: polyarthropathy

CLINICAL GUIDELINES

ADMINISTRATION:

- Oral preparations should be given after meals or with ample water to minimize gastric irritation.
- Parenteral solutions should be discarded if not used within a few hours of preparation.
- Therapeutic efficacy of a dosage regimen takes a week or more for assessment. Subsequent adjustment in dosage may diminish side effects.
- Blood counts and urinalyses should be performed on a regular fixed schedule.
- In multiple seizure crises protect patient from injury by placing in padded bed with side rails; emergency apparatus to maintain patent airway must be at bedside;

do not unduly restrain patient during an attack.
• Record frequency and nature of limb, head, and trunk contractions in order to facilitate characterization of seizures.

EFFECTS:
• Hyperglycemia may occur in patients with previously normal blood sugar levels and diabetics may show further elevations of sugar levels in blood.
• Patients should be advised of possible side effects and instructed to report them promptly. Since hydantoins may cause a pink or red urine, the patient should be informed of this possibility.
• Advise patient that because of possible gum hypertrophy it is particularly important to diligently massage the gums and care for the mouth and teeth.

DRUG INTERACTIONS:
• Concomitant use of tricyclic antidepressants may precipitate seizures.
• Hyperglycemia in diabetics induced by hydantoins may require adjustment in dosage of insulin or oral antidiabetic agents.
• Metabolism of hydantoins may be significantly altered by concomitant use of other drugs. Coumarin anticoagulants, phenylbutazone, and isoniazid may inhibit metabolism resulting in elevated serum levels and increasing the incidence of adverse effects.

Trimethadione and Related Agents

Paramethadione
Trimethadione

GENERAL CLINICAL USES

Paramethadione and trimethadione are relatively specific for the control of petit mal seizures; they are recommended for petit mal seizures refractory to other drugs. They may be used concomitantly with phenobarbital in patients with grand mal seizures.

PHARMACOLOGY

In contrast to the long-acting barbiturates and hydantoins, paramethadione and trimethadione fail to modify maximal seizures in humans receiving electroshock therapy. The two drugs have a slight to moderate sedative effect which progresses to ataxia with overdosage.

Paramethadione and trimethadione are readily absorbed from the gastrointestinal tract, degraded by the liver, and excreted slowly by the kidneys.

SPECIAL PRECAUTIONS

• Withdraw promptly if skin rash appears to minimize grave possiblity of exfoliative dermatitis or erythema multiforme. Rash must clear completely before cautiously resuming administration of medication.
• Use with caution in patients with diseases of the retina or optic nerve.
• Discontinue therapy if scotomata are encountered.
• Do not use in patients with confirmed liver or kidney disease or with blood dyscrasias.
• Safe use in pregnancy has not been established.

ADVERSE EFFECTS

CNS EFFECTS: fever, headache, drowsiness, dizziness, ataxia, personality changes, precipitation of grand mal seizures, a myasthenia-gravislike syndrome (with trimethadione)
RESPIRATORY EFFECTS: depression
CARDIOVASCULAR EFFECTS: alterations in blood pressure
URINARY TRACT EFFECTS: albuminuria, nephrosis
GASTROINTESTINAL EFFECTS: nausea, vomiting, abdominal pain, gastric distress, an-

orexia, hiccups, bleeding gums
METABOLIC AND ENDOCRINE EFFECTS: vaginal bleeding
HEPATIC EFFECTS: hepatitis
HEMATOLOGIC EFFECTS: neutropenia, aplastic anemia (rare), leukopenia, lymphadenopathy, agranulocytosis, and thrombocytopenia
DERMATOLOGIC EFFECTS: alopecia, lupus erythematosus, petechial hemorrhages
OPHTHALMIC EFFECTS: photophobia, blurred vision, scotomata, diplopia, and retinal petechiae

CLINICAL GUIDELINES
ADMINISTRATION:
• Blood counts, blood chemistries, and urinalyses should be completed before initiating medication. These tests should be repeated weekly or monthly on a fixed schedule once medication begins.
• Caution patient to avoid driving a motor vehicle or operating machinery while taking these medications; drowsiness may be offset by judicious prescribing of amphetamine.
EFFECTS:
• Patients should be advised of possible side effects and instructed to report them promptly.
• If jaundice or dark frothy urine is noted, medication should be withheld; notify attending physician promptly.
• Sudden onset of heavy scalp hair loss should also be promptly reported after discontinuing therapy.
• Inform patient that a regular daily body skin check for rash will minimize risk of exfoliative dermatitis.
DRUG INTERACTIONS:
• Amphetamine can be given to offset drowsiness without impairing anticonvulsant activity.
OVERDOSAGE/ANTIDOTE:
• Overdosage is characterized by stupor,

coma, and possibly grand mal seizures.
• No antidote is known. Treat symptomatically and supportively. Protect patient against injury during seizures.

Succinimides

Ethosuximide
Methsuximide
Phensuximide

GENERAL CLINICAL USES
Ethosuximide is the current drug of choice in the control of petit mal epilepsy. Methsuximide and phensuximide are less effective and fail to demonstrate reduced side effects. They may be useful when other drugs fail.

PHARMACOLOGY
In the electroencephalogram, ethosuximide and related agents suppress the paroxysmal spike and wave pattern which is common in petit mal seizures. The incidence of epileptiform attacks is apparently reduced by depression of the motor cortex and elevation of the CNS threshold to convulsive stimuli. The succinimides are absorbed from the gastrointestinal tract completely with peak plasma concentrations occurring in 1 to 7 hours. Ten to 20 percent of the drug is excreted in the urine; the remainder is metabolized in the liver.

SPECIAL PRECAUTIONS
• Do not use in patients with a history of hypersensitivity to any of these drugs.
• When used in mixed types of epilepsy, succinimides may increase the frequency of grand mal seizures in some patients.
• Patients should be cautioned against engaging in activities requiring mental alertness and physical dexterity such as driving

a car or operating machinery.
• Proceed slowly with dosage increases or decreases to minimize side effects and to minimize the danger of precipitating petit mal status.
• Succinimides should be withdrawn promptly if skin rash appears to minimize possibility of exfoliative dermatitis or erythema multiforme.
• Do not use in patients with confirmed liver and kidney disease or with blood dyscrasias.

ADVERSE EFFECTS

CNS EFFECTS: Drowsiness, headache, dizziness, euphoria, irritability, lethargy, ataxia, night terrors, inability to concentrate, toxic psychosis; depression with overt suicidal intentions (rare)
URINARY TRACT EFFECTS: nephrosis, hematuria
GASTROINTESTINAL EFFECTS: anorexia, gastric upset, cramps, nausea, vomiting, epigastric pain, diarrhea, hiccups, swelling of tongue, gum hypertrophy
METABOLIC AND ENDOCRINE EFFECTS: vaginal bleeding
HEPATIC EFFECTS: hepatitis
HEMATOLOGIC EFFECTS: leukopenia, agranulocytosis, pancytopenia, aplastic anemia and eosinopenia
DERMATOLOGIC EFFECTS: lupus erythematous, Stevens-Johnson syndrome, pruritic erythematous rashes, hirsutism, alopecia
OPHTHALMIC EFFECTS: myopia

CLINICAL GUIDELINES

ADMINISTRATION:
• Blood counts, blood chemistries, and urinalyses should be performed on a regular fixed schedule to minimize the risk of irreversible liver, kidney, and erythrocyte and leukocyte toxicity.
EFFECTS:
• Patient should be advised of possible side effects and instructed to report them promptly.
• If jaundice or dark frothy urine is noted, medication should be withheld; notify attending physician promptly.
• Sudden onset of heavy scalp hair loss should also be promptly reported after discontinuing treatment.
• Inform patient that a regular daily body skin check for rash will minimize risk of exfoliative dermatitis.
DRUG INTERACTIONS:
• To date none confirmed.
OVERDOSAGE/ANTIDOTE:
• Overdosage is characterized by stupor and/or coma, and grand mal seizures may occur.
• No antidote is known. Treat symptomatically and supportively. Protect patient against injury during seizures.

Miscellaneous Drugs

Acetazolamide

GENERAL CLINICAL USES
Acetazolamide is indicated for adjunctive treatment of centrocephalic epilepsies (petit mal, unlocalized seizures). It is used also for adjunctive treatment of edema due to congestive heart failure, chronic simple (open-angle) glaucoma, secondary glaucoma, and preoperatively in acute angle closure glaucoma.

PHARMACOLOGY, SPECIAL PRECAUTIONS, ADVERSE EFFECTS, CLINICAL GUIDELINES
See Chapter 11, page 454.

Carbamazepine

GENERAL CLINICAL USES

Carbamazepine is used for treatment of patients with epilepsy who have not responded satisfactorily to treatment with other drugs such as the hydantoins, phenobarbital, or primidone. Petit mal does not appear to be controlled. Carbamazepine is also useful in treating the pain associated with trigeminal neuralgia or glossopharyngeal neuralgia.

PHARMACOLOGY

Carbamazepine is chemically and pharmacologically related to the tricyclic antidepressants. It is absorbed rapidly after oral administration and is metabolized in the liver. The half-life is somewhere between 14 and 29 days. Carbamazepine has mild anticholinergic activity.

SPECIAL PRECAUTIONS

• Do not use in patients with a history of bone marrow depression and/or hypersensitivity to the drug.
• Do not use in patients with a known sensitivity to any of the tricyclic compounds such as amitriptyline, desipramine, or imipramine.
• If evidence of significant bone marrow depression occurs, discontinue drug.
• Patients with a history of adverse hematologic reactions may be particularly at risk.
• Safe use in pregnancy and nursing infants has not been established.
• Use with caution and frequent monitoring in patients with increased intraocular pressure.
• Use with caution in patients with a history of cardiovascular, hepatic, or renal impairment.

ADVERSE EFFECTS

CNS EFFECTS: dizziness, drowsiness, unsteadiness, speech disturbances, abnormal voluntary movements, peripheral neuritis, paresthesias, depression with agitation, talkativeness

CARDIOVASCULAR EFFECTS: congestive heart failure, aggravation of hypertension, hypotension, syncope and collapse, primary thrombophlebitis, recurrence of thrombophlebitis, aggravation of coronary artery disease

URINARY TRACT EFFECTS: frequency, retention, oliguria with elevated blood pressure, increase in deposits in urine

AUTONOMIC EFFECTS: diaphoresis, dry mouth and pharynx

GASTROINTESTINAL EFFECTS: nausea, vomiting, pain, diarrhea, constipation, anorexia, glossitis, stomatitis

METABOLIC AND ENDOCRINE EFFECTS: impotence, albuminuria, glycosuria, elevated BUN, adenopathy, lymphadenopathy, fever, chills, edema

ALLERGIC EFFECTS: urticaria

HEMATOLOGIC EFFECTS: aplastic anemia, leukopenia, agranulocytosis, eosinophilia, leukocytosis, thrombocytopenia, purpura

DERMATOLOGIC EFFECTS: rash, Stevens–Johnson syndrome, photosensitivity, alterations in pigmentation, exfoliative dermatitis, alopecia, erythema multiforme and nodosum, aggravation of disseminated lupus erythematosus

OPHTHALMIC EFFECTS: blurred vision, also visual hallucinations, transient diplopia, oculomotor disturbances, nystagmus; punctate, cortical lens opacities, conjunctivitis

OTIC EFFECTS: tinnitus, hyperacusis

MUSCULOSKELETAL EFFECTS: aching joints and muscles, leg cramps

CLINICAL GUIDELINES

ADMINISTRATION:

- Warn patients that dizziness and drowsiness may occur; use caution in operating machinery, motor vehicles, or in other potentially dangerous tasks.
- Complete pretreatment blood counts (including platelet and reticulocytes) and serum iron should be obtained; significant abnormalities rule out use of this drug.
- Monitor hematologic, renal, and ophthalmic parameters frequently.

EFFECTS:

- Be aware of the possible activation of a latent psychosis and, in elderly patients, of confusion and agitation. This is because of the relationship of carbamazepine to other tricyclic compounds.

DRUG INTERACTIONS:

- Do not use in patients receiving MAO-inhibitors; the MAO-inhibitors should be discontinued for at least 14 days before administration of carbamazepine.

OVERDOSAGE/ANTIDOTE:

- Overdosage is characterized by dizziness, ataxia, drowsiness, stupor, nausea, and vomiting. The patient frequently is restless, agitated, disoriented, and exhibits tremors, involuntary movements, and opisthotonus. Reflexes may be abnormal and mydriasis, nystagmus, flushing, and cyanosis may be present. Urinary retention may occur. Hypotension or hypertension may develop. Coma ensues.
- There is no specific antidote. Empty stomach by inducing emesis or gastric lavage. Treat supportively. Parenteral barbiturates may be used if hyperirritability is present; do not use if MAO-inhibitors have been taken during the last 7 days. Paraldehyde may be used in children to counteract muscular hypertonus. Monitor ECG to detect arrhythmias or conduction defects.

Clonazepam

GENERAL CLINICAL USES

Clonazepam may be useful for patients with petit mal epilepsy who have failed to respond to succinimides.

PHARMACOLOGY

Clonazepam is chemically related to the benzodiazepines; abrupt discontinuance may induce withdrawal symptoms similar to those noted with barbiturates or ethyl alcohol. A single oral dose results in maximal blood levels within 2 hours; significant blood levels persist for 20 to 40 hours. Biotransformation occurs in the liver and excretion with metabolites by way of the kidneys.

SPECIAL PRECAUTIONS

- In mixed types of epilepsy an increase in grand mal seizures may occur.
- Patients must be cautioned against driving a motor vehicle, operating machinery, or other hazardous operations requiring alertness.
- Do not use in patients with significant liver or kidney disease, acute narrow-angle glaucoma.
- Safe use during pregnancy or lactation and in pediatric patients has not been established.
- Use cautiously in patients with chronic respiratory disease since clonazepam may produce respiratory depression and an increase in salivation.

ADVERSE EFFECTS

CNS EFFECTS: depression, drowsiness, ataxia, behavior problems, aphonia, choreiform movements, coma, headache, slurred speech, vertigo, fever, hemiparesis, confusion, hallucinations, hysteria, insomnia, psychosis, suicide attempt

RESPIRATORY EFFECTS: depression, chest congestion, shortness of breath, rhinorrhea,

hypersecretion in upper respiratory tract
CARDIOVASCULAR EFFECTS: palpitations
URINARY TRACT EFFECTS: dysuria, enuresis, nocturia, urinary retention
GASTROINTESTINAL EFFECTS: anorexia, constipation, diarrhea, dry mouth, gastritis, nausea, sore gums
METABOLIC AND ENDOCRINE EFFECTS: dehydration
HEPATIC EFFECTS: transient elevations of serum transaminase and alkaline phosphatase; hepatomegaly
HEMATOLOGIC EFFECTS: anemia, leukopenia, thrombocytopenia, eosinophilia, lymphadenopathy
DERMATOLOGIC EFFECTS: alopecia, hirsutism, rash, ankle and facial edema
OPHTHALMIC EFFECTS: abnormal eye movements, "glassy eye," nystagmus
MUSCULOSKELETAL EFFECTS: dysarthria, muscle pain and weakness

CLINICAL GUIDELINES

ADMINISTRATION:
• Monitor hepatic, renal, and hematologic parameters prior to and frequently during therapy.
DRUG INTERACTIONS:
• CNS depressant action may be potentiated by ethyl alcohol, barbiturates, sedative-hypnotic agents, tranquilizers, antipsychotic agents, MAO-inhibitors, or tricyclic antidepressants.
OVERDOSAGE/ANTIDOTE:
• Overdosage is characterized by exaggeration of the CNS adverse effects.
• There is no specific antidote; treat supportively as necessary.

Magnesium Sulfate

GENERAL CLINICAL USES
Magnesium sulfate may be used for seizures associated with toxemia of pregnancy and in low levels of plasma magnesium.

PHARMACOLOGY
Magnesium sulfate solution replaces depleted magnesium in the plasma when administered intravenously or intramuscularly. Following intramuscular administration, the action is slower than after intravenous administration. The duration of action after intramuscular administration is several hours, whereas after intravenous administration the effect lasts only about 30 minutes.

SPECIAL PRECAUTIONS
• Do not administer to patients with heart block or myocardial damage.
• Use with extreme caution in patients with serious impairment of renal function.

ADVERSE EFFECTS
CNS EFFECTS: depressed CNS function
RESPIRATORY EFFECTS: depression
CARDIOVASCULAR EFFECTS: hypotension, circulatory collapse, depression of cardiac function
DERMATOLOGIC EFFECTS: flushing, and sweating

CLINICAL GUIDELINES
ADMINISTRATION:
• Watch patient carefully for signs of overdosage.
• Have on hand for intravenous administration solutions of calcium gluconate or gluceptate.
EFFECTS:
• Do not exceed administration rate of 1.5 ml (10% solution)/min intravenously.
DRUG INTERACTIONS:
• Dosage of concurrently administered barbiturates, narcotics, or other hypnotics (or systemic anesthetics) may require adjustment because of additive CNS depressant effects.

• Administer to patients receiving digitalis preparations with great care since serious alterations of cardiac conduction or heart block may occur.

OVERDOSAGE/ANTIDOTE:

• Overdosage is characterized by flushing, sweating, hypotension, circulatory collapse, and depression of cardiac and CNS function. Respiratory depression is the most immediate danger to life.

• Calcium gluconate and gluceptate are the antidotes.

Paraldehyde See p. 201.

Phenacemide

GENERAL CLINICAL USES

Phenacemide is indicated for the control of severe epilepsy; it is used particularly in mixed forms of psychomotor seizures refractory to action of other drugs.

PHARMACOLOGY

Phenacemide is well absorbed from the intestines after oral administration. The duration of action is about 5 hours. Phenacemide is metabolized in the liver and excreted in the urine as inactive metabolites.

SPECIAL PRECAUTIONS

• Do not administer unless other available anticonvulsants have been found to be ineffective in controlling seizures.

• Safe use during pregnancy has not been established.

• Personality changes, including attempts at suicide and occurrence of psychoses requiring hospitalization have been reported during therapy.

• Extreme caution is essential if administering concurrently with any other anticonvulsant which is known to cause similar toxic effects.

• Use with caution in patients with a history of previous liver dysfunction; death attributable to liver damage during therapy has been reported.

• If jaundice or other signs of hepatitis appear, discontinue drug immediately.

• Administer with caution to patients with a history of allergy, particularly in association with the administration of other anticonvulsants.

• Discontinue at first sign of skin rash or other allergic manifestation.

ADVERSE EFFECTS

CNS EFFECTS: drowsiness, dizziness, insomnia, paresthesias, psychic changes, personality changes (severe)

URINARY TRACT EFFECTS: nephritis

GASTROINTESTINAL EFFECTS: anorexia, weight loss, gastrointestinal disturbances

HEPATIC EFFECTS: jaundice

HEMATOLOGIC EFFECTS: blood dyscrasias including leukopenia, aplastic anemia

DERMATOLOGIC EFFECTS: rash

CLINICAL GUIDELINES

ADMINISTRATION:

• Monitor hematologic, hepatic, and renal parameters before and during therapy; blood counts should be performed at monthly intervals.

EFFECTS:

• Depression (marked) of the blood count is an indication for withdrawal of the drug.

• Abnormal urinary findings are an indication for discontinuance of therapy.

• Discontinue drug if jaundice or signs of hepatitis occur.

• Watch for suicidal ideation or severe personality changes. Chart and report to physician.

DRUG INTERACTIONS:

• Concurrent administration with other

anticonvulsant medication may result in enhanced toxic effects.

OVERDOSAGE/ANTIDOTE:

• Overdosage is characterized by excitement or mania. Drowsiness, ataxia, and coma follow.

• Treatment consists of inducing emesis or gastric lavage to empty stomach. General supportive measures will be necessary.

Valproic Acid

GENERAL CLINICAL USES

Valproic acid is indicated for sole and adjunctive therapy of simple and complex absence seizures, including petit mal, and in patients with multiple seizure types which include absence seizures.

PHARMACOLOGY

Valproic acid is an anticonvulsant agent. The mechanism of action has not been established.

Valproic acid is rapidly absorbed after oral administration with peak serum levels occurring at 1 to 4 hours. It is excreted primarily in the urine as the glucuronide conjugate.

SPECIAL PRECAUTIONS

• Do not use in patients with known hypersensitivity to valproic acid.

• Use caution when administering to patients with pre-existing hepatic disease. Liver dysfunction, including hepatic failure resulting in fatalities, has occurred in a few patients receiving valproic acid and concomitant anticonvulsant drugs.

• The effects of valproic acid in human pregnancy are unknown. Animal studies have demonstrated teratogenicity.

• Caution is recommended when valproic acid is administered with drugs affecting coagulation, such as aspirin and warfarin.

ADVERSE EFFECTS

CNS EFFECTS: drowsiness, ataxia, headache, tremor, dizziness, dysarthria, incoordination, coma rarely when used in patients receiving phenobarbital; emotional upset, depression, psychosis, aggression, hyperactivity, behavioral deterioration, asterixis

GASTROINTESTINAL EFFECTS: nausea, vomiting, indigestion, diarrhea, abdominal cramps, constipation, anorexia

HEPATIC EFFECTS: increases in serum alkaline phosphatase and serum glutamic oxaloacetic transaminase (SGOT), severe hepatotoxicity (isolated cases)

MUSCULOSKELETAL EFFECTS: weakness

HEMATOLOGIC EFFECTS: inhibition of secondary phase of platelet aggregation, lymphocytosis, mild thrombocytopenia, leukopenia

DERMATOLOGIC EFFECTS: hair loss, rash, petechiae

OPHTHALMIC EFFECTS: nystagmus, diplopia, "spots before eyes"

CLINICAL GUIDELINES

ADMINISTRATION:

• Conduct liver function tests, platelet counts, and bleeding time tests prior to drug administration and at periodic intervals thereafter.

EFFECTS:

• Since valproic acid may interact with concurrently administered anticonvulsant drugs, it is advisable to monitor serum levels of these drugs during the early course of therapy.

• Valproic acid is excreted in breast milk. It is not known what effect this would have on a nursing infant. Nursing should not be undertaken while a patient is receiving valproic acid.

DRUG INTERACTIONS:

• A ketone-containing metabolite of valproic acid may lead to a false interpretation of the urine ketone test.

• Concomitant administration of another CNS depressant (ethyl alcohol, tranquilizers, barbiturates) may interfere with driving a car, operating dangerous machinery, or other hazardous activities.

• Concomitant use of valproic acid and clonazepam may produce absence status.

• Phenytoin dosage may require adjustment.

OVERDOSAGE/ANTIDOTE:

• One patient who ingested valproic acid, 36 grams, in combination with phenobarbital and phenytoin, went into a deep coma. An electroencephalogram recorded diffuse slowing, compatible with the state of unconsciousness. The patient made an uneventful recovery.

• There is no specific antidote. Gastric lavage may be of limited value since valproic acid is absorbed very rapidly. General supportive measures should be applied. In particular, be sure to maintain an adequate urinary output.

Anti-Infective Agents

GENERAL CLINICAL USE

Few anti-infective agents cross the blood-brain barrier unless inflammation is present. However, certain drugs are known to cross the blood-brain barrier in the presence of meningitis: amikacin sulfate, ampicillin, chloramphenicol (crosses the blood-brain barrier in absence of infection), flucytosine, gentamicin sulfate, tobramycin sulfate. Although polymyxin B sulfate does not pass the blood-brain barrier, it may be administered intrathecally to treat CNS infections caused by susceptible organisms.

PHARMACOLOGY, SPECIAL
PRECAUTIONS, ADVERSE EFFECTS,
CLINICAL GUIDELINES

For detailed information for each specific drug, see the appropriate section in Chapter 2, *Anti-Infective Agents,* page 10.

Antimigraine Agents

INTRODUCTION

The so-called antimigraine agents are used to treat and prevent vascular headaches. The antimigraine agents are divided into two groups: (1) the standard analgesic groups which have been discussed in previous sections and (2) the ergot alkaloids which affect the cerebral vasculature.

SPECIFIC PRODUCTS AND DOSAGES: ERGOT ALKALOIDS

GENERIC NAME	TRADE NAME	ROUTE OF ADMIN.	SUGGESTED DAILY DOSAGE		
			ADULT	MRDD*	CHILDREN
dihydroergotamine mesylate	D.H.E. 45	im	1 mg initially, repeat at 1-hr. intervals to a total of 3 mg	3 mg	Not recommended
		iv	2 mg	2 mg	Not recommended
ergotamine tartrate	(G)† GYNERGEN	im	0.25–0.5 mg	1.0 mg/wk	Not recommended
		po	2–6 mg/attack	10.0 mg/wk	Not recommended
methysergide maleate	SANSERT	po	1–2 mg bid or qid	8 mg	Not recommended

*MRDD = maximal recommended dosage.
†(G) Designates availability as a generic product.

Dihydroergotamine Mesylate

GENERAL CLINICAL USES

Dihydroergotamine mesylate is indicated as therapy to abort or prevent vascular headache, e.g., migraine, migraine variants, or so-called histaminic cephalalgia, when rapid control is desired or when other routes of administration are not feasible.

PHARMACOLOGY

Dihydroergotamine mesylate, an alpha adrenergic blocking agent, has a direct stimulating effect on the smooth muscle of peripheral and cranial blood vessels. It produces depression of central vasomotor centers and antagonizes serotonin. In comparison with ergotamine, the adrenergic blocking actions are more pronounced, the vasoconstrictive actions somewhat less pronounced, and there is reduced incidence and degree of nausea and vomiting.

An effect is noted 15 to 30 minutes after intramuscular administration; the effect persists for 3 to 4 hours. Repeated dosage at 1-hour intervals up to 3 hours may be required to obtain maximal effect.

SPECIAL PRECAUTIONS

• Do not use in patients with peripheral vascular disease, coronary heart disease, hypertension, impaired hepatic or renal function; sepsis; hypersensitivity.
• It is contraindicated in pregnancy.

ADVERSE EFFECTS

CARDIOVASCULAR EFFECTS: precordial distress and pain, transient tachycardia or bradycardia
METABOLIC AND ENDOCRINE EFFECTS: localized edema and itching
GASTROINTESTINAL EFFECTS: nausea, vomiting
MUSCULOSKELETAL EFFECTS: numbness

and tingling of fingers and toes, muscle pains in the extremities, weakness in the legs

CLINICAL GUIDELINES

ADMINISTRATION:
- Administer at the first warning sign of headache; repeat at 1-hour intervals for 3 hours.
- Optimal results are obtained by adjusting the dose for several headaches to find the minimal effective dose for each patient.

EFFECTS:
- For rapid effect, administer intravenously.

OVERDOSAGE/ANTIDOTE:
- Overdosage is characterized by onset of peripheral toxic signs and symptoms of ergotism.
- Treatment includes discontinuance of the drug, warmth, vasodilators (such as nitroprusside), and good nursing care to prevent tissue damage.

Ergotamine Tartrate

GENERAL CLINICAL USES

Ergotamine tartrate, the drug of choice in the treatment of various types of acute migraine headaches, is most effective when administered intramuscularly. This is important since many patients cannot ingest oral medication because of migraine-related nausea and vomiting. It is not recommended as a prophylactic agent in patients with migraine.

PHARMACOLOGY

Ergotamine is a vasoconstrictor agent which prevents the distention of cerebral arterioles and arteries. Absorption after oral administration may be erratic. However, after a single intramuscular injection, the onset of action appears in 20 minutes and may persist for 24 hours. Detoxification occurs in the liver.

SPECIAL PRECAUTIONS
- Do not use in patients with peripheral vascular disease, coronary heart disease, hypertension, impaired hepatic or renal function, active infection, known or suspected hypersensitivity.
- Because of its oxytocic properties, avoid use during pregnancy.
- Severe vasoconstriction and endarteritis may occur with long-term uninterrupted use and can result in gangrene.

ADVERSE EFFECTS

CNS EFFECTS: ergotism rarely, headaches, dizziness, weakness
CARDIOVASCULAR EFFECTS: numbness and tingling of fingers and toes, cold extremities, transient alterations in heart rate, precordial distress and pain
GASTROINTESTINAL EFFECTS: nausea, vomiting, abdominal cramps
DERMATOLOGIC EFFECTS: edema, itching
MUSCULOSKELETAL EFFECTS: muscle pain in extremities

CLINICAL GUIDELINES

ADMINISTRATION:
- A test dose of ergotamine should be injected prior to administering the recommended dose.
- Ergotamine should be given at the onset of the migraine, but not as a preventive.
- The response will be enhanced if the patient is lying down in a darkened quiet room.

EFFECTS:
- Patient may experience transient numbness or chilling of fingers and toes.

DRUG INTERACTIONS:
- Ergotamine will lower blood pressure,

block, and actually reverse the rise in blood pressure that usually follows the administration of epinephrine.

OVERDOSAGE/ANTIDOTE:
- Overdosage results in spastic arteriolar disease, coldness of extremities, and arterial occlusion (especially the legs). Gangrene may ensue.
- No specific antidote is known. Treatment includes discontinuance of drug, administration of vasodilators, warmth, and miminization of tissue damage.

Methysergide Maleate

GENERAL CLINICAL USES

Methysergide maleate is recommended for oral medication in patients with vascular headache (migraine, histaminic cephalalgia), primarily for the prevention or reduction of the intensity and frequency of attacks. It is not useful in the management of an acute migraine attack.

SPECIAL PRECAUTIONS

- With long-term uninterrupted use, retroperitoneal fibrosis, pleuropulmonary fibrosis, and cardiovascular disorders with murmurs or vascular bruits have been reported.
- Patients must be warned to report promptly the following symptoms: cold, numb or painful hands and feet; leg cramps on walking; any type of pelvic, flank, or chest pain. If any of these symptoms appear, drug should be stopped.
- Continuous dosage should not be used for more than 6 months without providing for a 4- to 8-week drug-free interval. Dosage should be reduced gradually after the first 5 months to avoid "headache rebound."
- Not recommended for use in children.
- Do not use in patients with peripheral

vascular disease, valvular heart disease, severe hypertension, coronary artery disease, thrombophlebitis, pulmonary disorders, peptic ulcer, renal or liver disease, rheumatoid arthritis, and other collagen disorders.

ADVERSE EFFECTS

CNS EFFECTS: ataxia, dizziness, vertigo, behavioral changes (depersonalization, confusion, drowsiness, restlessness, insomnia), paresthesias of extremities

RESPIRATORY EFFECTS: pleural-pulmonary fibrosis

CARDIOVASCULAR EFFECTS: tachycardia, postural hypotension, peripheral arterial insufficiency (rare)

URINARY TRACT EFFECTS: retroperitoneal fibrosis with obstruction of the urinary tract

GASTROINTESTINAL EFFECTS: nausea, epigastric pain, vomiting, diarrhea, constipation, increased gastric hydrochloric acid in peptic ulcer

METABOLIC AND ENDOCRINE EFFECTS: peripheral edema

HEMATOLOGIC EFFECTS: neutropenia, eosinophilia

DERMATOLOGIC EFFECTS: alopecia, facial flush, nonspecific rash (rare)

MUSCULOSKELETAL EFFECTS: arthralgia, myalgia, leg cramps

CLINICAL GUIDELINES

ADMINISTRATION:
- Recommended only for the prevention or reduction of the intensity and frequency of migraine; not for the treatment of acute attacks.
- Patients should be seen frequently during therapy and must be instructed to report symptoms such as chest pain, leg cramps, peripheral edema, or paresthesias in the extremities.

DRUG INTERACTIONS:
- When epinephrine is administered, the

adrenolytic action will lower blood pressure rather than cause an increase.

OVERDOSAGE/ANTIDOTE:

• Symptoms of overdosage include spastic arteriolar disease, coldness of extremities, and arterial occlusion, especially in the legs. Gangrene may ensue.

• No antidote is known. Discontinue drug. Administer vasodilators, warmth, and special nursing care to minimize or prevent tissue damage.

Antiparkinsonian Agents

SPECIFIC PRODUCTS AND DOSAGES

GENERIC NAME	TRADE NAME	ROUTE OF ADMIN.	USUAL DOSAGE	MRDD*
Atropinelike Anticholinergic Agents:				
benztropine mesylate	COGENTIN	po	0.5–6.0 mg daily	8 mg
		im/iv	0.5–6.0 mg daily	8 mg
biperiden HCl and lactate	AKINETON	po	2 mg tid to qid	8 mg
		im/iv	2 mg; may repeat every 30 min. until symptoms abate; maximum: 4 doses/24 hrs.	8 mg
chlorphenoxamine HCl	PHENOXENE	po	50–100 mg tid or qid	400 mg
cycrimine HCl	PAGITANE	po	1.25–5.0 mg bid to qid	20 mg
diphenhydramine HCl	BENADRYL	po	25–50 mg tid to qid	300 mg
		im/iv	10–50 mg	400 mg
ethopropazine HCl	PARSIDOL	po	10–100 mg tid to qid	600 mg
orphenadrine HCl	DISIPAL	po	50 mg tid to qid	250 mg
procyclidine HCl	KEMADRIN	po	2–5 mg tid to qid	20 mg
trihexyphenidyl HCl	(G)† ANTITREM ARTANE TREMIN	po	1–2 mg daily; increase up 12–15 mg in divided doses	15 mg

*MRDD = maximal recommended dosage.
†(G) Designates availability as a generic product.

(continued facing page)

GENERIC NAME	TRADE NAME	ROUTE OF ADMIN.	USUAL DOSAGE	MRDD*
Dopaminergic Agents: carbidopa and levodopa	SINEMET	po	1–2.5 tablets tid	8 tablets
levodopa	(G)† BENDOPA DOPAR LARODOPA	po	0.5–1.0 gm daily divided in 2 or more doses	8 gm
Miscellaneous Agent: amantadine HCl	SYMMETREL	po	100 mg bid or qid	400 mg

*MRDD = maximal recommended dosage.
†(G) Designates availability as a keneric product.

Anticholinergic Agents

Benztropine Mesylate
Biperiden HCl and Lactate
Chlorphenoxamine HCl
Cycrimine HCl
Diphenhydramine HCl
Ethopropazine HCl
Orphenadrine HCl
Procyclidine HCl
Trihexyphenidyl HCl

GENERAL CLINICAL USES

The atropinelike anticholinergic agents are used as adjunctive treatment in therapy of parkinsonism (postencephalitic, arteriosclerotic, and idiopathic) and also in the control of drug-induced extrapyramidal disorders such as those caused by phenothiazines. Procyclidine hydrochloride is especially advantageous in treating rigidity.

PHARMACOLOGY

The atropinelike anticholinergic agents act by blocking acetylcholine at certain cerebral synaptic sites. They are absorbed adequately following oral administration with no accumulation in the body during continued administration.

SPECIAL PRECAUTIONS

• Do not use in patients with a history of hypersensitivity to any of these agents.
• In patients with glaucoma, urinary retention benign prostatic hypertrophy, cardiac arrhythmias or other conditions which might be adversely affected by anticholinergic action, the benefits of therapy must be carefully weighed because of the possible adverse anticholinergic effects.
• May impair mental and/or physical abilities required for the performance of potentially harzardous tasks such as driving a vehicle or operating machinery.
• Use with caution in patients with cardiovascular, hepatic, or renal pathology.
• Tolerance may develop necessitating adjustment of dosage and/or use of combination therapy.
• Geriatric patients frequently develop increased responsiveness to the actions of anticholinergic agents and require strict dosage regulation.

ADVERSE EFFECTS

CNS EFFECTS: light-headedness, memory loss, disorientation, confusion, excitement, delirium, visual hallucinations, psycosis, headache

CARDIOVASCULAR EFFECTS: tachycardia
URINARY TRACT EFFECTS: retention
AUTONOMIC EFFECTS: dry mouth, with rare and isolated cases of suppurative parotitis; blurred vision, decreased sweating
GASTROINTESTINAL EFFECTS: constipation, dilatation of colon, paralytic ileus, vomiting
DERMATOLOGIC EFFECTS: rash
OPHTHALMIC EFFECTS: dilatation of pupil

CLINICAL GUIDELINES

ADMINISTRATION:
• Caution patients of possible effects on mental and/or physical abilities.
• Younger and postencephalitic patients require and tolerate somewhat larger doses than older patients and those with arteriosclerotic types of parkinsonism.
• If patient experiences increased pupillary dilatation, advise use of sunglasses.
• Monitor blood and biochemical parameters in patients with cardiovascular, hepatic, or renal pathology.
EFFECTS:
• Patients on long-term therapy must be supervised continuously.
DRUG INTERACTIONS:
• In patients taking anticholinergic-type antiparkinsonism drugs in combination with phenothiazines and/or tricyclic antidepressants, paralytic ileus (sometimes fatal) or other gastrointestinal complaints may develop.
OVERDOSAGE/ANTIDOTE:
• Overdosage is characterized by an exaggeration of the adverse effects, namely dryness of mucous membranes, hyperpyrexia, dilatation of pupils, hot, dry, and flushed skin, tachycardia, nausea, and vomiting. Circulatory collapse and respiratory depression may also occur.
• Treatment is symptomatic. Empty stomach by inducing vomiting or gastric lavage. Pilocarpine may be given to relieve peripheral effects. Artificial respiration and oxygen therapy may be required.

Dopaminergic Agents

Carbidopa/Levodopa
Levodopa

GENERAL CLINICAL USES
The dopaminergic agents administered orally are useful in alleviating the symptoms of parkinsonism. Improvement can be seen within 2 weeks after beginning treatment. The most significant finding is usually seen after 6 months or longer. These agents, in comparison to the atropinelike drugs, appear to exert a more desirable improvement in balance, posture, gait, and speech.

PHARMACOLOGY
Levodopa, the metabolic precursor of dopamine, crosses the blood brain barrier and is converted presumably into dopamine in the basal ganglia. Dopamine relieves the symptoms of Parkinson's disease in which a deficiency of striatal dopamine is recognized. With increased doses, systolic and diastolic blood pressures often decrease 20 to 30 mm Hg. Significant orthostatic hypotension may occur.

Carbidopa inhibits decarboxylation of peripheral levodopa. This action makes more levodopa available for transport to the brain. It does not cross the blood-brain barrier and also does not affect the metabolism of levodopa within the central nervous system.

SPECIAL PRECAUTIONS
• Do not use in patients with a history of hypersensitivity to levodopa or to carbidopa or with narrow-angle glaucoma.

- Do not use carbidopa in patients with suspicious, undiagnosed skin lesions or a history of melanoma; carbidopa may activate malignant melanoma.
- Use with caution in patients with cardiovascular or pulmonary disease, bronchial asthma, renal, hepatic, or endocrine disease.
- Use with caution in patients with a history of myocardial infarction who have residual atrial, nodal or ventricular arrhythmias; monitor patient in coronary care unit or intensive care unit.
- Be alert for possible upper gastrointestinal tract hemorrhage in patients with a history of active peptic ulcer disease.
- Use caution in treating psychotic patients; depression may develop with concomitant suicidal tendencies.
- Safe use in women who are or who may become pregnant, and in children less than 12 years old, has not been established.
- Use with caution in patients with chronic wide-angle glaucoma; monitor intraocular pressure for changes.

ADVERSE EFFECTS

CNS EFFECTS: adventitious movements (choreiform and/or dystonic movements), paranoid ideation, psychotic episodes, depression with or without suicidal tendencies, dementia, convulsions, ataxia, increased head tremor, headache, dizziness, numbness, weakness, faintness, bruxism, confusion, insomnia, nightmares, hallucinations, delusions, agitation, anxiety, malaise, fatigue, euphoria, sense of stimulation

RESPIRATORY EFFECTS: bizarre breathing patterns, hoarseness

CARDIOVASCULAR EFFECTS: irregularities, palpitations, orthostatic hypotension, bradykinetic episodes, hypertension, phlebitis

URINARY TRACT EFFECTS: retention, incontinence

AUTONOMIC EFFECTS: dry mouth, sialorrhea, increased sweating, hot flashes

GASTROINTESTINAL EFFECTS: bleeding rarely, duodenal ulcer, anorexia, nausea, vomiting, abdominal pain and distress, dysphagia, burning sensation of tongue, bitter taste, diarrhea, constipation, flatulence, hiccups

METABOLIC AND ENDOCRINE EFFECTS: weight gain or loss, dark sweat and/or urine, edema, priapism

HEMATOLOGIC EFFECTS: hemolytic anemia and agranulocytosis rarely; decreased hemoglobin and hematocrit; leukopenia; positive Coombs test

DERMATOLOGIC EFFECTS: alopecia, pallor, urticaria, edema, rash

OPHTHALMIC EFFECTS: diplopia, blurred vision, dilated pupils; oculogyric crisis rarely; activation of latent Horner's syndrome

CLINICAL GUIDELINES

ADMINISTRATION:
- Therapeutic efficacy of a regimen of gradually increasing dosage takes 2 weeks or more for assessment. Subsequent adjustment in dosage may diminish side effects.
- Observe patients carefully for development of depression with concomitant suicidal tendencies.
- Monitor hepatic, hematopoietic, cardiovascular, and renal functions periodically during extended therapy.
- Administer with food to minimize adverse gastrointestinal effects.
- Patients over 60 years of age generally require lower doses and appear to be more sensitive to the drug.

EFFECTS:
- The adverse reactions due to levodopa are not decreased by carbidopa when they are administered together.
- Occurrence of dyskinesia may require reduction in dosage of carbidopa.

DRUG INTERACTIONS:

- Use with caution in patients receiving antihypertensive drugs such as pargyline and MAO-inhibitors; dosage adjustment may be necessary.
- Discontinue monoamine oxidase inhibitors 2 weeks prior to initiating therapy with levodopa.
- Pyridoxine hydrochloride (vitamin B[6]), 10 to 25 mg administered orally, may reverse the toxic and therapeutic effects of levodopa.
- Since phenothiazines and butyrophenones may reduce the therapeutic effects of levodopa, they should be administered with caution if concomitant administration is necessary; observe patients carefully for loss of antiparkinsonian effect.
- Elevations of blood urea nitrogen (BUN), serum glutamic oxaloacetic transaminase (SGOT), serum glutamic pyruvic transaminase (SGPT), lactic dehydrogenase, bilirubin, alkaline phosphatase, protein bound iodine have been reported; positive Coombs test has been reported; decreases in BUN, creatinine, uric acid have been reported with levodopa.

OVERDOSAGE/ANTIDOTE:

- Overdosage is characterized by an exaggeration of the adverse effects, namely, dry mouth, mydriasis, dry flushed skin, hyperpyrexia, tachycardia, nausea, vomiting, confusion, coma, circulatory collapse, and respiratory depression.
- For treating acute overdosage, general supportive measures should be employed along with immediate gastric lavage. Use intravenously administered fluids judiciously; maintain an adequate airway; monitor the electrocardiogram. There has been no experience with dialysis. Although pyridoxine hydrochloride (vitamin B[6]) may reverse the antiparkinson effects of levodopa, its usefulness in the management of acute overdosage has not been established.

Amantadine Hydrochloride

GENERAL CLINICAL USES

Amantadine hydrochloride is indicated in the treatment of idiopathic Parkinson's disease (paralysis agitans), postencephalitic parkinsonism, in drug-induced extrapyramidal reactions, and symptomatic parkinsonism which may follow injury to the nervous system by carbon monoxide intoxication. It is indicated in elderly patients believed to develop parkinsonism in association with cerebral arteriosclerosis.

PHARMACOLOGY

Amantadine hydrochloride has been shown to cause an increase in dopamine release in the animal brain but its mechanism of action in the treatment of parkinsonism is not known. Amantadine is not an anticholinergic agent. It is not metabolized but excreted primarily in the urine. The onset of action is usually within 48 hours.

SPECIAL PRECAUTIONS

- Do not use in patients with a history of hypersensitivity to amantadine hydrochloride.
- Observe closely patients with a history of epilepsy or other "seizures" since seizure activity may possibly increase.
- Since patients receiving amantadine hydrochloride have developed congestive heart failure, use caution and observe closely the patients with a history of congestive heart failure or peripheral edema.
- Caution patients that they may experience blurring of vision or central nervous system effects which may interfere with driving a motor vehicle or operating machinery where alertness is required.
- Safe use in pregnancy or in women of childbearing potential has not been established.
- Do not use in nursing mothers since

amantadine is secreted in the milk.
- Do not discontinue amantadine abruptly since a few patients with Parkinson's disease experience a parkinsonian crisis, i.e., a sudden marked clinical deterioration, when this medication was stopped suddenly.
- Use with caution in patients with renal impairment, congestive heart failure, peripheral edema, or orthostatic hypotension; dosage adjustment may be necessary.
- If renal function is impaired, amantadine hydrochloride may accumulate since it is excreted primarily by the kidneys.
- Use caution in administering to patients with liver disease, a history of recurrent eczematoid rash, or to patients with psychosis or severe psychoneurosis not controlled by chemotherapeutic agents.

ADVERSE EFFECTS

CNS EFFECTS: depression, psychosis; convulsions, hallucinations, confusion, anxiety, irritability, ataxia, dizziness (lightheadedness), headache, fatigue, insomnia, weakness, slurred speech
RESPIRATORY EFFECTS: dyspnea
CARDIOVASCULAR EFFECTS: congestive heart failure, orthostatic hypotensive episodes
URINARY TRACT EFFECTS: retention
AUTONOMIC EFFECTS: dry mouth
GASTROINTESTINAL EFFECTS: anorexia, nausea, constipation, vomiting

METABOLIC AND ENDOCRINE EFFECTS: livedo reticularis, peripheral edema
HEMATOLOGIC EFFECTS: leukopenia, neutropenia
DERMATOLOGIC EFFECTS: rash, eczematoid dermatitis
OPHTHALMIC EFFECTS: visual disturbances, oculogyric episodes

CLINICAL GUIDELINES

ADMINISTRATION:
- If atropinelike symptoms appear when amantadine hydrochloride and anticholinergic agents are administered concurrently, dosage adjustment of both compounds may be necessary.
DRUG INTERACTIONS:
- May be used concomitantly with anticholinergic agents or levodora; dosage adjustment may be required.
- Careful observation is required when amantadine hydrochloride is administered concurrently with central nervous system stimulants.
OVERDOSAGE/ANTIDOTE:
- Overdosage is characterized by an exaggeration of the adverse effects.
- No antidote is known. Empty stomach by inducing vomiting or gastric lavage. Use supportive measures; force fluids; administer fluids intravenously if necessary. Since the excretion rate increases when the urine is acidic, administer urine acidifying products to increase elimination of amantadine.

Antivertigo Agents

For detailed information, see Chapter 8, page 379.

Central Nervous System Stimulants
For detailed information, see Chapter 3, page 122.

Cerebrovasodilators
For detailed information, see Chapter 5, page 283

Muscle Relaxants
For detailed information, see Chapter 13, page 493.

Sedative-Hypnotic Drugs

Nonbarbiturate Sedative-Hypnotic Agents

SPECIFIC PRODUCTS AND DOSAGES—Refer to table, pages 192 and 193.

Chloral Betaine
Chloral Hydrate
Triclofos Sodium

GENERAL CLINICAL USES

Chloral betaine, chloral hydrate, and triclofos sodium are indicated for sleep induction and preoperative sedation. Chloral hydrate is prescribed infrequently as a daytime sedative. Many clinicians prefer to use chloral hydrate to barbiturates for elderly patients. These products may be used as hypnotics in children and prior to EEG to induce the sleeping state for this examination. These drugs are usually administered orally but chloral hydrate may also be administered rectally.

PHARMACOLOGY

Chloral betamine, chloral hydrate, and triclofos sodium induce sedation 15 to 30 minutes after oral administration. After rectal administration, chloral hydrate induces sedation in 20 to 60 minutes; the duration is from 5 to 8 hours.

Chloral betaine 870 mg is equivalent to chloral hydrate 500 mg. Triclofos sodium, a phosphate ester of trichlorethanol, yields the same pharmacologically active metabolite as chloral hydrate. At hypnotic doses, little, if any, respiratory or cardiovascular depression occurs. With large doses or prolonged use, peripheral vasodilatation, hypotension, and some myocardial depression may be observed. Chloral hydrate has no significant analgesic action; it has no effect upon the contraction of the uterus during labor.

SPECIAL PRECAUTIONS

- Avoid administration to patients with gastric or duodenal ulcers or gastritis, or with a history of hypersensitivity to chloral hydrate.
- Do not administer to patients with renal, hepatic, or cardiac disease.
- Prolonged use of moderate to large amounts can result in habituation and physical dependence.
- Do not use in pregnant patients or nursing mothers; chloral hydrate passes the placental barrier and also appears in breast milk.

ADVERSE EFFECTS

CNS EFFECTS: confusion, delirium, impaired mental function, psychic or physical dependence, headache, hangover, drowsiness, excitement

RESPIRATORY EFFECTS: depression with large doses

CARDIOVASCULAR EFFECTS: myocardial depression with large doses; peripheral vasodilatation, hypotension

URINARY TRACT EFFECTS: ketonuria, albuminuria

GASTROINTESTINAL EFFECTS: gastric distress, nausea, vomiting, flatulence

HEPATIC EFFECTS: liver damage, icterus

HEMATOLOGIC EFFECTS: eosinophilia, decreased leukocytes

ALLERGIC EFFECTS: urticaria

DERMATOLOGIC EFFECTS: erythema, exfoliative dermatitis, eruptions of face, neck, and trunk

OPHTHALMIC EFFECTS: constricted pupils

MUSCULOSKELETAL EFFECTS: ataxia, staggering gait

CLINICAL GUIDELINES

ADMINISTRATION:

- Give orally with ample water, juice, or other suitable beverage to minimize esophageal and stomach irritation and to offset unpleasant taste.

	GENERIC NAME	TRADE NAME	ROUTE OF ADMIN.	ADULTS HYPNOTIC DOSE (single) mg
CIV‡	chloral betaine	BETA-CHLOR	po	870–1740
CIV	chloral hydrate	(G)‡‡ NOTEC Felsules	po	500–1000
		(G)	pr	500–1000
CIV	ethchlorvynol	PLACIDYL	po	500–1000
CIV	ethinamate	VALMID	po	500–1000
	ethyl alcohol (brandy, whiskey, sherry wine, beer)	(G)	po	5–15 ml
CIV	flurazepam HCl	DALMANE	po	15–30
CII	glutethimide	(G) DORIDEN	po	250–1000
CIII	methaqualone	QUAALUDE SOPOR	po	150–300
CII	methaqualone HCl	PAREST	po	200–400
CIII	methyprylon	NOLUDAR	po	200–400
CIV	paraldehyde	(G) PARAL	po im iv pr	5–30 ml 10 ml 10 ml 5–30 ml
	triclofos sodium	TRICLOS	po	1500

‡C denotes schedule listing under the Controlled Substances Act.
‡‡(G) Designates availability as a generic product.

• If rectal suppositories are not available, administer by olive oil retention enema.

EFFECTS:
• Large doses may give false positive results for sugar in urine (copper sulfate test).
• Large doses may elevate blood BUN.

• Sudden withdrawal after prolonged use may result in delirium tremens.

DRUG INTERACTIONS:
• Dangerous potentiation of depressant action may occur when taken with ethyl alcohol; the combination is known as

| DAYTIME SEDATIVE (bid or qid) mg | MRDD* mg | CHILDREN | |
		HYPNOTIC DOSE (single) mg	DAYTIME SEDATIVE (bid or qid) mg
870–1740†	——	0.1 ml/lb††	——
250	2000	50 mg/kg	25 mg/kg
250	1000 for children	50 mg/kg	25 mg/kg
100–200	1000	NR**	NR
NR	2000	NR	NR
——	50 ml	NR	NR
NR	30	NR	NR
250	1000	NR	NR
75	300	NR	NR
NR	400	NR	NR
NR	400	NR	NR
5–10 ml	30 ml	NR	NR
5 ml	30 ml	0.3 ml/kg	0.15 ml/kg
5 ml	5 ml	NR	NR
NR	30 ml	NR	NR

* Maximal recommended daily dose.
** Not recommended.
† Preoperative sedation.
†† Sleep induction in EEG.

"Mickey Finn" or "knockout drops."
• Synergistic depressant action on the CNS with other sedative-hypnotic agents, analgesics, tranquilizers, or general anesthetics may be severe and can cause brain damage or fatal respiratory failure

• In patients receiving furosemide intravenously, prior oral administration of chloral hydrate may result in a hemodynamic reaction consisting of vasodilatation, diaphoresis, flushing, hypertension, and tachycardia.

OVERDOSAGE/ANTIDOTE:
• Patient overdosage is characterized by respiratory depression, dyspnea, signs of progressive cyanosis, and shallow respiration. Cardiovascular inadequacy may follow, particularly in those with heart disease.
• No specific antidote is available. Supportive measures should be initiated immediately and sustained until respiratory function returns.

Ethchlorvynol

GENERAL CLINICAL USES
Ethchlorvynol is indicated for short-term hypnotic therapy in patients with uncomplicated insomina.

PHARMACOLOGY
Ethchlorvynol, a tertiary acetylenic alcohol, induces sleep within 15 to 60 minutes and is effective for approximately 5 hours. Sleep is less profound than that obtained with barbiturates. It has no significant analgesic action. The drug is metabolized primarily by the liver.

SPECIAL PRECAUTIONS
• Do not use in patients in the first or second trimester of pregnancy, during lactation with known hypersensitivity to the drug, or with porphyria.
• Use with caution in patients with impaired function of the renal or hespatic system.
• Tolerance and physical dependence may occur.

ADVERSE EFFECTS
CNS EFFECTS: Dizziness, ataxia, confusion, facial numbness, disorientation; rarely hallucinations

RESPIRATORY EFFECTS: depression
CARDIOVASCULAR EFFECTS: hypotension
GASTROINTESTINAL EFFECTS: nausea, vomiting, gastric upset, unpleasant aftertaste
HEPATIC EFFECTS: cholestatic jaundice rarely
HEMATOLOGIC EFFECTS: thrombocytopenia rarely
ALLERGIC EFFECTS: skin rash, urticaria
OPHTHALMIC EFFECTS: blurred vision, reversible toxic amblyopia after prolonged use
MUSCULOSKELETAL EFFECTS: profound muscular weakness

CLINICAL GUIDELINES
ADMINISTRATION:
• Administration with food may control the transient giddiness and taxia which have occurred.
• Patients must be cautioned against driving a motor vehicle, operating machinery or other hazardous operations requiring alertness.
• Inform patient of hazardous potentiation with concomitant ingestion of central depressants such as ethyl alcohol.
EFFECTS:
• Sudden withdrawal of drug after prolonged use may result in tremors, mental confusion, hallucinations and convulsions; drug should be withdrawn gradually.
• No relief of pain is to be expected.
DRUG INTERACTIONS:
• Dangerous potentiation of CNS depressant action, in particular severe respiratory inadequacy, may occur when taken with ethyl alcohol, other sedative-hypnotic agents, analgesics, tranquilizers or general anesthetics.
• Caution should be exercised in giving the drug to patients receiving antidepres-

sants such as MAO-inhibitors or amitripty-line; transient delirium has been reported.
• It may be necessary to re-adjust dosage of oral anticoagulants since ethchlorvynol may decrease prothrombin time.

OVERDOSAGE/ANTIDOTE:
• Overdosage is characterized by stupor, coma, respiratory depression, hypotension, bradycardia, and hypothermia; pancyto-penia has also been noted.
• Peritoneal dialysis and hemodialysis have been reported to be of value in the management of overdosage. There is no specific antidote. Treat supportively until effects of drug have dissipated.

Ethinamate

GENERAL CLINICAL USES

Ethinamate is indicated in patients with uncomplicated insomnia caused by excessive fatigue, apprehension, or excitement.

PHARMACOLOGY

Ethinamate, a carbamate, is a non-selective CNS depressant. The onset of central depressant effects after oral administration is rapid, 15 to 30 minutes; the duration of action is about 4 hours. In hypnotic doses, no analgesic or antipyretic effects are seen. Little, if any, changes occur in the pulse, blood pressure, or respiration. Ethinamate is inactivated by the liver. The rapid metabolism may be responsible for the low incidence of aftereffects.

SPECIAL PRECAUTIONS
• Safe use during pregnancy, lactation, or in pediatric patients has not been established.

• Patients must be cautioned against driving a motor vehicle, operating machinery, or other hazardous operations requiring alertness.
• Physical and psychic dependence may occur.

ADVERSE EFFECTS

CNS EFFECTS: stupor, coma, rare idiosyncrasy with fever, paradoxical excitement
RESPIRATORY EFFECTS: depression
GASTROINTESTINAL EFFECTS: mild gastrointestinal disturbances
HEMATOLOGIC EFFECTS: thrombocytopenia rarely
DERMATOLOGIC EFFECTS: rash

CLINICAL GUIDELINES

ADMINISTRATION:
• Therapy in debilitated or elderly patients should be initiated with low doses.
• Inform patient of hazardous potentiation if ethyl alcohol is taken concomitantly.
EFFECTS:
• Sudden withdrawal after prolonged use may result in hallucinations and convulsions; gradual withdrawal should be made.
• No relief of pain is to be expected.
DRUG INTERACTIONS:
• Dangerous potentiation of CNS depressant action, namely, respiratory inadequacy, may occur when taken concomitantly with ethyl alcohol, other sedative-hypnotic agents, analgesics, tranquilizers, or general anesthetics.
OVERDOSAGE/ANTIDOTE:
• Overdosage is characterized by severe respiratory depression, stupor, and/or coma. Death has occurred from ingestion of 15 gm; recovery has occurred after ingestion of 28 gm.
• There is no specific antidote. Treat

supportively and assist respiration until the effects of the drug have dissipated.

Ethyl Alcohol (Ethanol)

Brandy, Whiskey,
Sherry wine, etc.

GENERAL CLINICAL USES

Ethyl alcohol is indicated for use in patients requiring sedation and/or sleep. The sedative-hypnotic effect is basically a function of the amount ingested and not that of the particular type of alcoholic beverage.

PHARMACOLOGY

Ethyl alcohol is a central nervous system depressant. The initial site of action seems to be the reticular activating system. In small amounts the sedative and hypnotic characteristics are prominent. In moderate to large amounts, disinhibition frequently occurs with a lessening of self-restraint, mood changes, ataxia, faulty judgment, aggressive behavior, and impaired mental and physical performance. With ingestion of very large amounts, advanced intoxication, loss of consciousness, and general anesthesia can occur.

Vasodilatation follows the ingestion of ethyl alcohol and reflects a direct action on central vasomotor centers. Unusually large amounts of alcohol will cause bradycardia and a reduction in blood pressure. The vasodilatation accounts for substantial body heat loss and antipyretic response after ethyl alcohol ingestion.

Ethyl alcohol is absorbed effectively from the stomach and small intestine, and is distributed rapidly to all tissues. It is metabolized primarily by the liver at a uniform rate of 10 to 20 ml per hour.

SPECIAL PRECAUTIONS

• Caution should be exercised in debilitated patients or in those with impaired function of the respiratory, hepatic, or renal systems.

• Since visual acuity, diminished skeletal muscular tone and coordination, and drowsiness frequently occur, patients must be cautioned against driving a car or operating machinery.

• Ethyl alcohol may potentiate fatally other central nervous system depressants such as tranquilizers, other sedative-hypnotics, analgesics, and general anesthetics. Consequently, it should be avoided or given in very small amounts to patients receiving such medications.

• Prolonged use of moderate to large amounts can result in habituation and physical dependence (chronic alcoholism).

ADVERSE EFFECTS

CNS EFFECTS: disorientation, impulsive behavior, impaired judgment, slowed reaction time, euphoria, slurred speech, psychic and physical dependence hallucinations, convulsions upon abrupt withdrawal from ethyl alcohol, delirium tremens.

RESPIRATORY EFFECTS: reduction in respiratory efficiency; respiratory failure with asphyxia after overdosage

CARDIOVASCULAR EFFECTS: vasodilatation

URINARY TRACT EFFECTS: increased output

GASTROINTESTINAL EFFECTS: vomiting, motility and secretion inhibition; irritation to gastric mucosa; delayed gastric emptying

HEPATIC EFFECTS: impaired liver function

OPHTHALMIC EFFECTS: blurred vision, nystagmus

MUSCULOSKELETAL EFFECTS: muscular incoordination, slowed reaction time

CLINICAL GUIDELINES

ADMINISTRATION:
- Do not give to patients with gastric or peptic ulcer.
- Caution patients against driving a motor vehicle or operating machinery.
- Prolonged use may result in severe dependence (alcoholism); the higher the dose the greater the potential for habituation and dependence.
- Caution patients against excessive self-medication.

EFFECTS:
- Severe withdrawal reactions consisting of insomnia, anorexia, delirium tremens, hallucinations, tremors, psychotic behavior, convulsions, and/or coma may accompany abrupt withdrawal after prolonged ingestion
- Psychic disinhibition, aggressive behavior, ataxia, and incoordination may occur.

DRUG INTERACTIONS:
- The action of most central nervous system depressants is potentiated by ethyl alcohol.
- The synergistic action with barbiturates, opiate-type analgesics, muscle relaxants, other sedative-hypnotics, tranquilizers, and general anesthetics may be severe and can cause fatal respiratory depression.

OVERDOSAGE/ANTIDOTE:
- Severe overdosage is characterized by respiratory depression, dyspnea, signs of progressive cyanosis, and shallow respiration. Respiratory arrest usually is followed by cardiovascular inadequacy.
- No specific antidote is available. Supportive respiratory measures including oxygen must be initated at once and sustained until respiratory function returns.

Flurazepam Hydrochloride

GENERAL CLINICAL USES
Flurazepam is indicated for relief of all types of insomnia and in acute or chronic medical conditions requiring sleep induction.

PHARMACOLOGY
Flurazepam hydrochloride, a benzodiazepine compound, acts within the central nervous system at unknown sites. Sleep is induced in 15 to 45 minutes after oral administration and persists for 6 to 8 hours. At recommended hypnotic doses, no significant effects on the cardiovascular or renal systems have been reported. Large doses induce generalized central nervous system depression and hypotension. Flurazepam presumably is metabolized primarily in the liver and excreted in the urine.

SPECIAL PRECAUTIONS
- Do not use in patients with a history of hypersensitivity to flurazepam.
- Do not use in patients with a history of drug abuse.
- Weigh risks to benefits carefully before use during pregnancy or lactation.
- Usual precautions are indicated for severely depressed patients or those with latent depression or suicidal tendencies.
- Patients must be warned not to operate machinery, drive motor vehicles, or engage in activities requiring alertness.
- Safe use in children less than 15 years has not been established.
- Use with caution in patients with impaired renal or hepatic function.

ADVERSE EFFECTS
CNS EFFECTS: headache, dizziness, lightheadedness, drowsiness, slurred speech, euphoria, ataxia (particularly in the elderly or

debilitated patient), nervousness, talkativeness, apprehension, irritability, weakness, excitement and hyperactivity rarely
RESPIRATORY EFFECTS: shortness of
breath, respiratory depression
CARDIOVASCULAR EFFECTS: palpitations,
hypotension, chest pains
URINARY TRACT EFFECTS: genitourinary
discomfort
AUTONOMIC EFFECTS: sweating, flushing,
excessive salivation
GASTROINTESTINAL EFFECTS: upset stomach, dry mouth, bitter taste, diarrhea,
heartburn, constipation
HEPATIC EFFECTS: elevated SGOT, SGPT,
total and direct bilirubin, and alkaline
phosphatase
HEMATOLOGIC EFFECTS: leukopenia and
granulocytopenia rarely
DERMATOLOGIC EFFECTS: rash, pruritus
OPHTHALMIC EFFECTS: difficulty in focusing, blurred vision, burning sensation
MUSCULOSKELETAL EFFECTS: body and
joint pain

CLINICAL GUIDELINES
ADMINISTRATION:
• In elderly and debilitated patients, the
initial dosage should be limited to 15 mg.
• With repeated use, periodic blood
counts, liver and kidney function tests,
should be performed.
• Inform patient of dangerous potentia-
tion of ethyl alcohol if taken concomitantly.
• Caution patient not to participate in ac-
tivities that require alertness.
EFFECTS:
• No relief of pain is to be expected.
• Sudden withdrawal after prolonged use
may result in an abstinence syndrome characterized by hallucinations, tremors, convulsions, etc.
DRUG INTERACTIONS:
• Dangerous potentiation of CNS depressant action, characterized by severe respi-

ratory inadequacy, may occur when taken
with ethyl alcohol, other sedative-hypnotic
agents, analgesics, tranquilizers, or general
anesthetics.
OVERDOSAGE/ANTIDOTE:
• Overdosage is characterized by somnolence, confusion and coma. Severe sedation, lethargy, disorientation are also probably indicative of overdosage or of drug
intolerance.
• No specific antidote is known. Empty
stomach by gastric lavage with due caution
to prevent aspiration of gastric contents.
Treat symptomatically. Adequate respiratory exchange and cardiovascular function
must be maintained; urinary output must
be monitored.

Glutethimide

GENERAL CLINICAL USES
Glutethimide is useful in treating
most types of insomnia, and also for daytime or preoperative sedation. It is suitable
for use in the elderly and in patients with
chronic illnesses. Impaired respiratory or
renal function is not a contraindication.

PHARMACOLOGY
The sedative-hypnotic action is comparable to that observed for pentobarbital.
The usual hypnotic dose does not produce
analgesic, anticonvulsant, or antipyretic action. Generally, recommended doses of glutethimide have no important effects on organ systems other than the CNS. Sleep is
usually induced within 30 minutes after ingestion and persists for 4 to 8 hours. Glutethimide is detoxified by metabolic processes in the liver, and the by-products are
excreted in the bile and urine.

SPECIAL PRECAUTIONS
• Do not use in patients with a history of
drug abuse; both physical and psychological

dependence has occurred.
• Weigh the risk to benefits carefully before using during pregnancy and lactation.
• Do not use in children less than 12 years old.
• Do not use in patients with a history of hypersensitivity to glutethimide.

ADVERSE EFFECTS
CNS EFFECTS: psychosis, hangover, ataxia, tremors, paradoxical excitation
RESPIRATORY EFFECTS: cyanosis, pulmonary edema
CARDIOVASCULAR EFFECTS: tachycardia
AUTONOMIC EFFECTS: dry mouth
GASTROINTESTINAL EFFECTS: nausea
HEMATOLOGIC EFFECTS: rarely thrombocytopenic purpura, leukopenia, aplastic anemia
DERMATOLOGIC EFFECTS: urticarial rash, exfoliative dermatitis
OPHTHALMIC EFFECTS: mydriasis, blurred vision

CLINICAL GUIDELINES
ADMINISTRATION:
• Caution patient not to participate in activities that require alertness.
EFFECTS:
• No relief of pain is to be expected.
• Sudden withdrawal after prolonged use may result in an abstinence syndrome consisting of hallucinations, tremors, convulsions, etc.
DRUG INTERACTIONS:
• Dangerous potentiation of CNS depressant action, namely, severe respiratory inadequacy, may occur when administered concomitantly with ethyl alcohol, other sedative-hypnotic agents, analgesics, tranquilizers, or general anesthetics.
• Dosage of coumarin anticoagulants may require adjustment during and upon cessation of glutethimide.
• The action of anticholinergic agents will be enhanced by moderate doses of glutethimide.

OVERDOSAGE/ANTIDOTE:
• Overdosage is characterized by coma, hypothermia, convulsions, cerebral edema, sudden apnea, hypotension, and/or atony of the urinary bladder. Fever without apparent infection may also occur. Reflexes are depressed. With gastric lavage or endotracheal intubation, apnea may occur.
• There is no specific antidote. Empty stomach by lavage with due caution to prevent aspiration of gastric contents. Treat symptomatically and supportively.

Methaqualone
Methaqualone Hydrochloride

GENERAL CLINICAL USES
Methaqualone is useful to produce sleep and daytime sedation.

PHARMACOLOGY
The mode of sedative-hypnotic action is not known. Large doses exert a selective depressant effect on polysynaptic spinal reflexes. Action of methaqualone is apparent within 20 minutes; it lasts for 6 to 8 hours. Methaqualone is metabolized by the liver and excreted in the urine and in the feces.

SPECIAL PRECAUTIONS
• Do not use in patients with a history of hypersensitivity to methaqualone.
• Hypnotic doses should be taken only at bedtime, since methaqualone may produce drowsiness in 10 to 20 minutes.
• Do not use in women who may become or who are pregnant. When administered in high doses to the pregnant animal, skeletal abnormalities have been observed in the offspring.

- Do not use continuously for periods exceeding 3 months or in patients with a history of ethyl alcohol or drug abuse.
- Warn patients against operating a motor vehicle or machinery while receiving the drug.
- Use in reduced dosages in patients with impaired hepatic function.

ADVERSE EFFECTS

CNS EFFECTS: headache, hangover, fatigue, dizziness, stupor, transient paresthesias of the extremities, restlessness, and anxiety

GASTROINTESTINAL EFFECTS: anorexia, nausea, dry mouth, emesis, epigastric discomfort, diarrhea

HEMATOLOGIC EFFECTS: aplastic anemia rarely; prothrombin deficiencies, hemorrhage

ALLERGIC EFFECTS: urticaria

DERMATOLOGIC EFFECTS: diaphoresis, bromhidrosis, exanthema

CLINICAL GUIDELINES

ADMINISTRATION:

- Inform patient of hazardous potentiation of ethyl alcohol if taken concurrently.
- Caution patients not to participate in activities requiring alertness.

EFFECTS:

- No relief of pain is to be expected.
- Sudden withdrawal after prolonged use may result in an abstinence syndrome characterized by hallucinations, tremors, convulsions, etc.

DRUG INTERACTIONS:

- Dangerous potentiation of CNS depressant action characterized by severe respiratory inadequacy may occur when taken with ethyl alcohol, other sedative-hypnotic drugs, analgesics, tranquilizers, or general anesthetics.

OVERDOSAGE/ANTIDOTE:

- Overdosage is characterized by delirium and coma; restlessness and hypertonia may progress to convulsions. Spontaneous vomiting and secretions are common. Cutaneous edema, pulmonary edema, hepatic damage, renal insufficiency, and bleeding may occur with large overdoses. Cardiac and respiratory depression occur less frequently than with barbiturates. Coma has occurred with acute overdosages of 2.4 gm; death has occurred with 8 gm. Most fatalities have occurred with concomitant ingestion of alcohol.
- There is no specific antidote. Gastric lavage should be done in all cases; use caution to prevent aspiration of gastric contents. Treat symptomatically. Adequate respiratory exchange and cardiovascular function must be monitored; urinary output must be monitored. Dialysis may be helpful.

Methyprylon

GENERAL CLINICAL USES

Methyprylon is indicated for relief of insomnia of varied etiology in adults and children. It has been prescribed in patients who cannot tolerate barbiturates.

PHARMACOLOGY

Methyprylon administered orally usually induces sleep within 45 minutes; sleep persists for 5 to 8 hours. It apparently increases the threshold of the arousal centers of the brain stem. Large doses induce depression of the respiratory center but no prominent effects have been seen on the cardiovascular system. The autonomic nervous system and gastrointestinal tract remain unaltered. Methyprylon is dehydrogenated by the liver and excreted in the urine and feces.

SPECIAL PRECAUTIONS
- Do not use in patients with a history of drug abuse or with porphyria.
- Weigh risk to benefits carefully before use in pregnancy and lactation.
- Concomitant use with ethyl alcohol or other CNS depressants may cause abrupt respiratory failure.
- Warn patients not to operate motor vehicles, machinery, or engage in activities requiring alertness.
- Do not use in children less than 3 months old.

ADVERSE EFFECTS

CNS EFFECTS: morning drowsiness, rarely; dizziness, headache, parodoxical excitement, hangover

GASTROINTESTINAL EFFECTS: vomiting, diarrhea, esophagitis

HEMATOLOGIC   EFFECTS: neutropenia, thrombocytopenia rarely

DERMATOLOGIC EFFECTS: rash

CLINICAL GUIDELINES

ADMINISTRATION:
- Inform patient of hazardous potentiation which may occur with concomitant ingestion of ethyl alcohol.
- Caution patient not to participate in activities requiring alertness.

EFFECTS:
- No relief of pain is to be expected.
- Sudden withdrawal after prolonged use may result in an abstinence syndrome characterized by hallucinations, tremors, convulsions, etc.

DRUG INTERACTIONS:
- Dangerous potentiation of CNS depressant action, namely, severe respiratory inadequacy, may occur when concomitantly administered with ethyl alcohol, other sedative-hypnotic agents, analgesics, tranquilizers, or general anesthetics.

OVERDOSAGE/ANTIDOTE:
- Overdosage is characterized by somnolence, coma, confusion, constricted pupils, respiratory depression, and hypotension.
- No specific antidote is known. Gastric lavage should be done in all cases with due caution to prevent aspiration of gastric contents. Treat symptomatically. Hypotension may be treated with levarterenol, metaraminol, or other hypotensive agents. Adequate respiratory exchange and cardiovascular function must be maintained. Urinary output must be monitored. Hemodialysis may be of value.

Paraldehyde

GENERAL CLINICAL USES

Paraldehyde, a potent hypnotic with a wide margin of safety, is restricted in use because of a pungent odor imparted to the patient's breath. Consequently, it is used primarily in institutional patients or outpatients with limited social contact. Frequently paraldehyde is prescribed for patients with delirium tremens and other acute behavioral abnormalities characterized by hyperexcitability.

It may be given intravenously for the emergency management of tetanus, epileptic seizures, eclampsia, or seizures induced by toxic substances.

PHARMACOLOGY

Paraldehyde produces a hypnotic effect within 30 minutes after oral, rectal, or intravenous administration. It produces moderately prolonged sleep, 6 to 12 hours.

The sedative-hypnotic actions are similar to those obtained with ethyl alcohol or chloral hydrate. Minimal actions upon motor or medullary functions occur with hypnotic doses. A reduction in perception of pain accompanies its use; this is apparently accomplished by inducing amnesia rather than an insensibility to pain characteristic of analgesia.

Paraldehyde is metabolized extensively in the liver and is excreted by the lungs and kidneys. It crosses the placental barrier and appears in the fetal circulation.

SPECIAL PRECAUTIONS

- Avoid administration to patients with gastritis and gastric or duodenal ulcers.
- Do not use in patients with known pulmonory or hepatic disease.
- May be habit-forming.

ADVERSE EFFECTS

CNS EFFECTS: generalized depression with large doses, coma, psychic and physical dependence

RESPIRATORY EFFECTS: pulmonary edema with large doses, respiratory depression

CARDIOVASCULAR   EFFECTS: right   side heart failure with large doses, rapid pulse

GASTROINTESTINAL EFFECTS: irritation of throat, esophagus, stomach; nausea, vomiting

METABOLIC   AND   ENDOCRINE   EFFECTS: metabolic acidosis with prolonged use

CLINICAL GUIDELINES

ADMINISTRATION:

- Administer orally with ample water, juice or other suitable beverage to minimize esophageal and gastric irritation and to offset unpleasant taste.
- For rectal administration, administer in olive oil retention enema.
- Parenteral injections are dangerous and should be used only in emergency situations.

EFFECTS:

- Amnesia is induced in obstretric and preoperative preparation of patients; no relief of pain is obtained.

DRUG INTERACTIONS:

- Dangerous potentiation of CNS depressant action featuring severe respiratory inadequacy may occur when taken concomitantly with ethyl alcohol, other sedative-hypnotics, analgesics, tranquilizers, or general anesthetics.
- Do not administer concomitantly with disulfiram.

OVERDOSAGE/ANTIDOTE:

- Overdosage is characterized by severe respiratory depression.
- There is no specific antidote. Treat supportively.

Other Agents Employed as Sedative-Hypnotics

Tranquilizers are employed as sedative-hypnotics for patients with complaints of mild insomnia. The action of the tranquilizers in these circumstances is predominantly that of removing the anxiety which contributes to the inability of the patient to sleep. However, some tranquilizers possess hypnotic properties as secondary pharmacologic actions. Therefore by increasing the dose, the hypnotic action of the drug may predominate. For detailed information about the tranquilizers, see Chapter 3, page 100.

The opium alkaloids (morphine, codeine, etc.) and related synthetic narcotic analgesics also can facilitate sleep. Obviously their ability to alleviate organic pain will facilitate sleep. Beyond their analgesic properties, these drugs allay anxiety; they are also capable of exerting a soporific action. For detailed information, refer to the discussion of opiate-type analgesics in this chapter.

In addition, certain antihistamines cause a high incidence of somnolence. This side effect has been utilized as a sleep-inducing action. Included are diphenhydramine, methapyrilene, and promethazine. Diphenhydramine, as an elixir, is widely prescribed in pediatrics. For detailed information, see Chapter 6, page 302.

Barbiturates

SPECIFIC PRODUCTS AND DOSAGES
Appropriate dosages for anticonvulsant use are presented in the section *Anticonvulsant Agents*. Refer to table, pages 167 and 168.

Long-Acting Barbiturates

Mephobarbital
Phenobarbital

GENERAL CLINICAL USES
Mephobarbital and phenobarbital, long-acting sedative-hypnotic agents, have been prescribed extensively in a variety of conditions characterized by anxiety and tension and for preoperative and postoperative apprehension.

Phenobarbital is also useful in the management of epilepsy. (For information concerning drugs used in treating convulsive discorders, see the discussion of anticonvulsant agent in this chapter).

PHARMACOLOGY
Mephobarbital and phenobarbital administered orally are slow in onset of hypnotic action in comparison with secobarbital or pentobarbital. The posthypnotic drowsiness or "hangover" lethargy may persist for many hours after the patient awakens. The prolonged actions reflect very slow metabolism. The half-life of phenobarbital is 2 to 5 days. As much as 35 percent of the phenobarbital is found in unchanged form in the urine.

At sedative-hypnotic doses, no significant actions are seen upon respiratory, cardiovascular, renal, or autonomic function. The barbiturates produce depression of the CNS, cross the blood-brain barrier, and have a selective anticonvulsant effect, but no analgesic action.

SPECIAL PRECAUTIONS
• Do not administer to patients with known sensitivity to barbiturates or with porphyria.
• Cautious and careful downward adjustment of dosage is required when prescribed for patients with impaired liver, kidney, cardiac or respiratory function.
• Lower doses are required in elderly or debilitated patients to preclude excessive accumulation and oversedation.
• Safe use in pregnancy has not been established.
• The patient should be warned against performance of tasks requiring mental alertness.
• Tolerance, psychological and physical dependence may occur.
• Rarely rickets and osteomalacia have been reported following prolonged use; thus vitamin D requirements may increase.
• Avoid use in patients with mental

GENERIC NAME.	TRADE NAME	ROUTE OF ADMIN.	ADULTS HYPNOTIC DOSE (single)
Long-Acting Barbiturates:			
CIV* mephobarbital	(G)‡‡ MEBARAL	po	NR‡
CIV phenobarbital	(G) ESKABARB SOLFOTON LUMINAL	po	50–200 mg
CIV phenobarbital sodium	(G) LUMINAL Sodium	sc/im/iv	50–200 mg
Intermediate-Acting Barbiturates:			
CII amobarbital	(G) AMYTAL	po	65–200 mg
CII amobarbital sodium	(G) AMYTAL Sodium	im	65–500 mg
		iv	65–500 mg
CIII aprobarbital	ALURATE ALURATE VERDUM	po	80–160 mg
CIII butabarbital sodium	(G) BUTISOL BUTAZEM	po	50–100 mg
CIII talbutal	LOTUSATE	po	120 mg
Short-Acting Barbiturates:			
CIV pentobarbital	(G) NEMBUTAL	po	100–200 mg
		iv	100–200 mg
		im	150–200 mg
		pr	120–200 mg
CII secobarbital	(G) SECONAL	po	100–200 mg
		iv	75–250 mg
		im	100–200 mg
		pr	120–200 mg
Ultra-Short-Acting Barbiturates:			
CIII hexobarbital	SOMBULEX	po	250–500 mg

*C denotes schedule listing under the Controlled Substances Act.
‡Not recommended.
‡‡(G) Designates availability as a generic product.

DAYTIME SEDATIVE DOSE (bid or qid) (single)	MRDD†	CHILDREN	
		HYPNOTIC DOSE (single)	DAYTIME SEDATIVE DOSE (bid or qid) (single)
32–100 mg	600 mg	NR‡	16–32 mg
16–32 mg	600 mg	NR	2 mg/kg/day in divided doses
16–32 mg	600 mg	3–6 mg/kg	2 mg/kg/day in divided doses
15–120 mg	1000 mg	NR	6 mg/kg/day in divided doses
———	500 mg	3–5 mg/kg	NR
———	500–1000 mg	3–5 mg/kg	NR
40 mg	160 mg	NR	NR
15–30 mg	240 mg	7.5–30 mg by age and weight	NR
NR	120 mg	NR	NR
20–40 mg.	500 mg	By age and weight	6 mg/kg/24 hrs in 3 divided doses
20–50 mg	500 mg	30 mg	6 mg/kg/24 hrs in 3 divided doses
20–50 mg	500 mg	3–5 mg/kg	3–6 mg/kg/24 hrs in 3 divided doses
———	———	30–60 mg	6 mg/kg/24 hrs in 3 divided doses. See labeling
30–50 mg	300 mg	50–100 mg	6 mg/kg/24 hrs in divided doses
NR	250 mg	NR	Same as po
0.5–0.75 mg/lb	250 mg	2–3 mg/kg	Same as po
30 mg	———	60–120 mg	15–60 mg
NR	500 mg	NR	NR

‡ Not recommended.
† MRDD = maximal recommended daily dose.

depression, suicidal tendency or known history of drug alcohol abuse.

ADVERSE EFFECTS

CNS EFFECTS: drowsiness, dizziness, mental sluggishness, delirium, memory disturbances, euphoria, paradoxical excitement, ataxia.

RESPIRATORY EFFECTS: depression; coughing, hiccups, laryngospasm, and chest wall spasm following intravenous administration; bronchospasm

CARDIOVASCULAR EFFECTS: hypotension with intravenous administration

GASTROINTESTINAL EFFECTS: nausea, vomiting, epigastric pain

METABOLIC AND ENDOCRINE EFFECTS: vitamin D deficiency

HEPATIC EFFECTS: altered liver metabolism

HEMATOLOGIC EFFECTS: megaloblastic anemia rarely; agranulocytosis, and thrombocytopenia

ALLERGIC EFFECTS: facial edema, allergic degenerative changes in the liver, urticaria

DERMATOLOGIC EFFECTS: eruptions, angioneurotic edema, morbilliform rash, bullous erythema multiforme, exfoliative dermatitis

LOCAL EFFECTS: with intravenous administration, thrombophlebitis

CLINICAL GUIDELINES

ADMINISTRATION:
- Warn patient about concomitant use of ethyl alcohol, tranquilizers, and other sedative-hypnotic agents.
- Patients must be instructed not to keep any barbiturate in the bedroom; poor memory induced by the drug may result in repetitive swallowing of the drug with possible fatal poisoning.
- Caution patients not to participate in activities that require alertness.

EFFECTS:
- No relief of pain is obtained.
- Cumulative action may result in drowsiness, lethargy, and impaired memory for several days or weeks after discontinuation of medication.
- Sudden withdrawal after prolonged use of moderate or high doses may result in an abstinence syndrome characterized by hallucinations, tremors, and convulsions.

DRUG INTERACTIONS:
- Dangerous potentiation of CNS depressant action (characterized by respiratory inadequacy) may occur when the drug is taken concomitantly with ethyl alcohol, other sedative-hypnotic agents, analgesics, tranquilizers, or general anesthetics.
- Certain drug-metabolizing hepatic functions may be increased, thus decreasing blood levels and clinical efficacy of drugs (antihistamines, steroids, anticonvulsants) given concurrently.
- Phenobarbital may lower blood levels of coumarin anticoagulants and thus shorten prothrombin time.

OVERDOSAGE/ANTIDOTE:
- Overdosage is characterized by CNS depression, namely, respiratory depression, depression of superficial and deep reflexes; constriction of pupils, decreased urine formation, lowered body temperature, later fever, gradual appearance of circulatory collapse and pulmonary edema; coma.
- No specific antidote is known; the use of analeptic agents is controversial.
- If the patient is seen within a few hours of overdosage, empty stomach by lavage. A patent airway must be maintained. Mechanical ventilation and oxygen may be required. Endotracheal intubation may be necessary. Adequate cardiovascular function must be maintained. If renal failure occurs, drug removal by hemodialysis is effective.

Intermediate-Acting Barbiturates

Amobarbital
Amobarbital Sodium
Aprobarbital
Butabarbital Sodium
Talbutal

Short-Acting Barbiturates

Pentobarbital
Secobarbital

Ultra-Short-Acting Barbiturate

Hexobarbital

GENERAL CLINICAL USES

The intermediate-acting barbiturates are indicated for conditions requiring sedation for relief of anxiety and tension and also for hypnotic effects, prior to anesthesia administration, or for treating insomnia.

The short-acting barbiturates are used to treat insomnia, for preoperative sedation, and in dental procedures.

The ultra-short-acting barbiturate, hexobarbital, is used similarly to the short-acting barbiturates.

The sodium salts of these agents are used for parenteral administration.

PHARMACOLOGY

The intermediate-acting barbiturates are more dependable, more rapid and distinctly shorter acting than the long-acting barbiturates. Sleep is induced in 15 to 30 minutes after oral or rectal administration. Sleep can be maintained for 4 to 8 hours following a single dose. These barbiturates are metabolized more rapidly and extensively by the liver than the long-acting

compounds. Consequently, only small amounts of the intermediate-acting compounds are excreted unchanged in the urine.

Following administration of sedative-hypnotic dosages, no significant actions are ordinarily observed upon respiration, cardiovascular, renal, or autonomic functions.

The short-acting and ultra-short-acting barbiturates are similar in all respects to the intermediate-acting compounds with the exception that they exert an effect in a shorter time and for a shorter duration of time.

SPECIAL PRECAUTIONS

• Do not administer to patients with known sensitivity to barbiturates or with porphyria.
• In patients with impaired liver, kidney, cardiac, or respiratory function, cautious downward adjustment of dosage is required.
• Safe use in pregnancy has not been established.
• The patient should be warned against performance of tasks requiring mental alertness such as driving a car or operating machinery.
• Tolerance or psychological and physical dependence may occur with barbiturates.
• Avoid use in patients with mental depression, suicidal tendency, or known history of drug or alcohol abuse.

ADVERSE EFFECTS

CNS EFFECTS: drowsiness, dizziness, mental sluggishness, delirium, memory disturbances, euphoria, paradoxical excitement, ataxia
RESPIRATORY EFFECTS: depression, pulmonary edema, insensitivity of carbon dioxide receptors

URINARY TRACT EFFECTS: reduced output

GASTROINTESTINAL EFFECTS: nausea, vomiting, epigastric pain

HEPATIC EFFECTS: altered liver metabolism

HEMATOLOGIC EFFECTS: megaloblastic anemia rarely, agranulocytosis, thrombocytopenia

ALLERGIC EFFECTS: facial edema, allergic degenerative changes in the liver

DERMATOLOGIC EFFECTS: rash, eruptions, urticaria, angioneurotic edema, morbilliform rash, bullous erythema multiforme, exfoliative dermatitis

LOCAL EFFECTS: with extravasation or accidental intra-arterial injection, severe local pain

CLINICAL GUIDELINES

ADMINISTRATION:

• Lower doses are required in elderly and debilitated patients to preclude excessive accumulation and oversedation.

• The outpatient should be warned against concomitant use of ethyl alcohol, tranquilizers, other psychotherapeutic agents, other sedative-hypnotic agents, and analgesics.

• Patient must be instructed not to keep barbiturates in the bedroom; poor memory induced by the drug may result in repetitive swallowing of the drug with possible fatal poisoning.

• Caution patients not to participate in activities requiring alertness.

• For parenterally administered barbiturates, avoid extravasation or accidental intra-arterial injection; severe local necrosis may result.

EFFECTS:

• No relief of pain is obtained; infrequent pain sensation may intensify.

• Cumulative action may result in drowsiness, lethargy, and impaired memory for several days or weeks after discontinuation of medication.

• Sudden withdrawal after prolonged use of moderate or high doses may result in an abstinence syndrome characterized by hallucinations, tremors, and convulsions.

DRUG INTERACTIONS:

• Dangerous potentiation of CNS depressant action (characterized by respiratory inadequacy) may occur when the drug is taken concomitantly with ethyl alcohol, other sedative-hypnotics, analgesics, tranquilizers or other psychotherapeutic agents, and general anesthetics.

• Certain drug-metabolizing hepatic functions may be increased, thus decreasing blood levels and clinical efficacy of drugs (antihistamines, adrenal steroids, anticonvulsants) administered concurrently.

• Barbiturates may lower blood levels of coumarin anticoagulants and thus shorten prothrombin time and necessitate dosage adjustment.

OVERDOSAGE/ANTIDOTE:

• Overdosage is characterized by severe respiratory insufficiency, amnesia, nystagmus, ataxia, delirium, or shock. Coma and exacerbation of pre-existing pain, hypotension, anuria or oliguria, impaired liver function, or jaundice may occur.

• No specific antidote is known; the use of analeptic agents is controversial.

• If the patient is seen within a few hours of overdosage, gastric lavage may be performed. Treat symptomatically and supportively. If renal failure occurs, drug removal by hemodialysis is effective.

Drugs affecting the heart, circulation, blood vessels, and blood

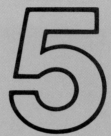

INTRODUCTION

The drugs affecting the heart, circulation, blood vessels, and blood include those products acting on cardiac contraction, cardiac and peripheral circulation, hemostasis, coagulation, and blood volume. All products will be grouped according to therapeutic use.

SPECIFIC THERAPEUTIC CLASSIFICATION

The drugs affecting the heart, circulation, blood vessels, and blood are grouped as follows:

1. Antiarrhythmic agents
2. Anticoagulants
3. Antihypertensive agents/Diuretics
4. Congestive heart failure agents
5. Electrolyte solutions
6. Hemostatic agents
7. Plasma substitutes/Blood extenders

8. Sclerosing agents
9. Thrombolytic agents
10. Vasodilating agents/Antianginal agents
11. Vasopressor agents

The antilipemic/hypocholesterolemic agents are included in Chapter 15, *Endocrine and Other Drugs Affecting Metabolism—Cholesterol and Lipid-Reducing Agents*, page 547.

Antiarrhythmic Agents

Since use of each antiarrhythmic agent is relatively specific, the general clinical uses are presented with the information for each drug.

SPECIFIC PRODUCTS AND DOSAGES

GENERIC NAME	TRADE NAME	ROUTE OF ADMIN.	USUAL DOSE	
			ADULTS	CHILDREN
bretylium tosylate	BRETYLOL	im	5–10 mg/kg	Not established
		iv	5–30 mg/kg	
disopyramide phosphate	NORPACE	po	400–800 mg/day divided in 4 doses	Not established
lidocaine HCl	XYLOCAINE	im	300 mg (4.3 mg/kg)	Not established
		iv	50–100 mg; 25–50 mg/min; maximum: 200–300 mg/hr.	Not established
procainamide HCl	(G)* PRONESTYL	po im/iv	0.2–1 gm; 6 mg/kg every 3 hrs. 0.2–1.0 gm; repeat as required	Not established
propranolol HCl	INDERAL	po iv	10–30 mg tid or qid 1–3 mg; may repeat in 2 min, then every 4 hrs.	Not established Not established
quinidine gluconate	(G) QUINAGLUTE	iv im po	330–750 as needed 400–600 mg as needed 324 mg bid or qid	Not established Not established
quinidine polygalacturonate	CARDIOQUIN	po	275–825 mg; adjust as needed	Not established
quinidine sulfate	(G) QUINIDEX QUINORA CIN–QUIN	po	0.2–0.4 gm tid or qid as needed	Not established

*(G) designates availability as a generic product.

Bretylium Tosylate

GENERAL CLINICAL USES

Bretylium tosylate is indicated for treating life-threatening ventricular arrhythmias, principally ventricular fibrillation and ventricular tachycardia that have failed to respond to first-line antiarrhythmic agents such as lidocaine or procainamide.

PHARMACOLOGY

Bretylium tosylate suppresses ventricular fibrillation and ventricular arrhythmias. The mechanism of action is not established. Bretylium tosylate inhibits norepinephrine release by depressing adrenergic nerve terminal excitability.

Peak hypotensive effects are measured within 1 hour after intramuscular administration. Suppression of premature ventricular beats is not maximal until 6 to 9 hours after dosing.

Following intravenous administration, ventricular fibrillation is suppressed rapidly, usually within minutes. Ventricular tachycardia and other ventricular arrhythmias are suppressed, usually within 20 minutes to 2 hours following parenteral administration.

Bretylium tosylate is eliminated unchanged by the kidneys. No metabolites have been identified.

SPECIAL PRECAUTIONS

• Bretylium tosylate regularly results in postural hypotension, subjectively recognized by dizziness, light-headedness, vertigo, or fainting.

• Transient hypertension or increased frequency of premature ventricular contractions and other arrhythmias may occur in some patients.

• Exert caution when used with digitalis glycosides. Be sure the etiology of the arrhythmia is not digitalis toxicity.

• Avoid use in patients with severe aortic stenosis or severe pulmonary hypertension.

• Safe use in pregnancy and in children has not been established.

• Dosage should be reduced in patients with impaired renal function.

ADVERSE EFFECTS

CNS EFFECTS: vertigo, dizziness, light-headedness, syncope, confusion, paranoid psychosis, emotional lability, lethargy, and anxiety

RESPIRATORY EFFECTS: hiccups, shortness of breath, nasal stuffiness

CARDIOVASCULAR EFFECTS: transitory hypotension, postural hypotension, bradycardia, increased frequency of premature ventricular contractions, initial increase in arrhythmias, precipitation of anginal attacks, sensation of substernal pressure

URINARY TRACT EFFECTS: dysfunction of the kidneys

GASTROINTESTINAL EFFECTS: nausea, vomiting, diarrhea, abdominal pain

METABOLIC AND ENDOCRINE EFFECTS: hyperthermia, diaphoresis

DERMATOLOGIC EFFECTS: erythematous macular rash, flushing, generalized tenderness

OPHTHALMIC EFFECTS: conjunctivitis

LOCAL EFFECTS: with intramuscular administration, atrophy and necrosis of muscle tissue, fibrosis, vascular degeneration, and inflammatory changes

CLINICAL GUIDELINES

ADMINISTRATION:

• Patients should be kept supine until tolerance to the hypotensive effect of bretylium tosylate develops (usually several days).

• Caution patients that postural hypoten-

sion will probably occur. It is recognized by dizziness, light-headedness, vertigo, or fainting.
• Dilute bretylium tosylate for intravenous use. Consult package directions.
• When administering intramuscularly, vary sites of administration to avoid tissue damage.

EFFECTS:
• There is a delay in onset of the antiarrhythmic action; do not consider it a replacement for rapidly acting antiarrhythmic agents currently in use.
• Rapid intravenous administration may cause severe nausea and vomiting.

DRUG INTERACTIONS:
• The pressor effects of the catecholamines are enhanced by bretylium tosylate.
• Bretylium tosylate may aggravate digitalis toxicity.

OVERDOSAGE/ANTIDOTE:
• To date there has been little experience with dosages greater than 30 mg/kg/day.
• Treat supportively.

Disopyramide Phosphate

GENERAL CLINICAL USES
Disopyramide phosphate is indicated for suppression or prevention of recurrence of the following cardiac arrhythmias: unifocal premature (ectopic) ventricular contractions; premature (ectopic) ventricular contractions of multifocal origin; paired premature ventricular contractions (couplets).

Disopyramide is effective in treating the above arrhythmias in both digitalized and nondigitalized patients; in treating primary cardiac arrhythmias and those occurring in association with coronary artery disease.

PHARMACOLOGY
Disopyramide phosphate decreases the rate of diastolic depolarization and the uptake velocity, and increases the action potential of normal cardiac cells. At therapeutic blood levels, disopyramide shortens the sinus node recovery time, lengthens the effective refractory period of the atrium, and has a minimal effect on the effective refractory period of the A-V node.

Following oral administration significant alterations in blood pressure are rarely produced. Intravenous administration produces a transient and moderate increase in heart rate and total peripheral resistance. Therepeutic effects are obvious 30 minutes to 3 hours after administration. Disopyramide has anticholinergic properties.

Disopyramide is absorbed rapidly and completely after oral administration. The plasma half-life in healthy subjects ranges from 4 to 10 hours; in patients with impaired renal function it ranges from 8 to 18 hours. Disopyramide is excreted primarily in the urine and also in the feces; the majority is excreted as unchanged drug.

SPECIAL PRECAUTIONS
• Do not administer to patients in cardiogenic shock, pre-existing second or third degree A-V block (if no pacemaker is present) or with known hypersensitivity to the drug.
• Severe hypotension may occur, particularly in patients with primary cardiomyopathy or inadequately compensated congestive heart failure.
• Do not use in presence of poorly compensated or uncompensated congestive heart failure unless exacerbated or caused by an arrhythmia and proper treatment has been accomplished.
• In patients with marginally compensated heart failure, administration may cause cardiac decompensation.
• If first degree heart block develops, reduce dosage.
• Do not use in patients with glaucoma or

urinary retention unless adequate measures are taken to compensate for anticholinergic activity.

• Use in pregnant women only when clearly indicated and the benefit to risk ratio has been carefully evaluated.

• Effects on labor, delivery, and the fetus are unknown.

• It is not known if it is excreted in human milk.

• Safety and effectiveness in children has not been established.

• Digitalize patients with atrial flutter or fibrillation before administration.

• In patients with impaired renal function, dosage reduction may be required; monitor ECG.

• Impaired hepatic function causes an increase in plasma half-life; dosage reduction may be required.

• Antiarrhythmic drugs may be ineffective in patients with hypokalemia; correct potassium defect before instituting therapy.

ADVERSE EFFECTS

CNS EFFECTS: dizziness, general fatigue, headache, malaise, nervousness, depression, insomnia, acute psychosis (1 case)

RESPIRATORY EFFECTS: dry nose, throat; shortness of breath, syncope, chest pain

CARDIOVASCULAR EFFECTS: hypotension

URINARY TRACT EFFECTS: hesitancy, urinary frequency and urgency, retention, dysuria

AUTONOMIC EFFECTS: dry mouth

GASTROINTESTINAL EFFECTS: constipation, nausea, pain, bloating, gas, anorexia, diarrhea, vomiting

METABOLIC AND ENDOCRINE EFFECTS: impotence

DERMATOLOGIC EFFECTS: rash, various dermatoses

OPHTHALMIC EFFECTS: blurred vision, dry eyes

MUSCULOSKELETAL EFFECTS: muscle weakness

CLINICAL GUIDELINES

ADMINISTRATION:

• Patients of small stature or those with moderate renal insufficiency or hepatic insufficiency, cardiomyopathy, or possible cardiac decompensation may require lower doses than other patients.

• Patients should be hospitalized for evaluation and continuous monitoring.

• Monitor ECG frequently.

DRUG INTERACTIONS:

• Other antiarrhythmic drugs (e.g., quinidine, procainamide, lidocaine, propranolol) have been used concomitantly.

• Administer with caution to patients receiving other antiarrhythmic drugs. Excessive widening of QRS complex may occur.

OVERDOSAGE

• Overdosage is characterized by prolongation of PR interval, QRS widening; also worsening of congestive heart failure, hypotension, varying kinds and degrees of conduction disturbance, bradycardia, and asystole. Anticholinergic effects may also be observed.

• No specific antidote is known. Treat supportively. Supportive therapy with vasopressors, cardiac glycosides, and diuretics may be used as required. Disopyramide is dialyzable (*in vitro*).

Lidocaine Hydrochloride

GENERAL CLINICAL USES

Lidocaine hydrochloride is indicated in the management of cardiac arrhythmias paticularly those of ventricular origin such as occurs with acute myocardial infarction. Information concerning analgesic use may be found in the discussion of regional anesthetics in Chapter 4, *Drugs Affecting the Brain and Spinal Cord,* page 162.

PHARMACOLOGY

Lidocaine hydrochloride increases the electrical stimulation threshold of the ventricle during diastole, and thereby exerts an antiarrhythmic effect. Effective antiarrhythmic blood levels may be attained in 5 to 15 minutes and usually persist for 60 to 90 minutes. Lidocaine is metabolized in the liver and excreted in the urine.

SPECIAL PRECAUTIONS

• Do not use in patients with a history of hypersensitivity to local anesthetics of the amide type and in patients with severe degrees of sinoatrial, atrioventricular or intraventricular block.
• Intramuscular injections should be made with frequent aspirations to avoid possible inadvertent intravascular administration.
• Not recommended for pediatric use.
• Prolonged use in patients with renal or hepatic disease may result in possible accumulation.
• Use with caution in patients with hypovolemia and shock, and all forms of heart block.
• Lidocaine solutions containing epinephrine should not be used to treat arrhythmias or administered intravenously.

ADVERSE EFFECTS

CNS EFFECTS: light-headedness, drowsiness, dizziness, apprehension, euphoria, sensations of cold or numbness, twitching, tremors, convulsions, unconsciousness
RESPIRATORY EFFECTS: depression, respiratory arrest
CARDIOVASCULAR EFFECTS: hypotension, cardiovascular collapse, bradycardia, cardiac arrest
GASTROINTESTINAL EFFECTS: vomiting, nausea
OPHTHALMIC EFFECTS: blurred or double vision
OTIC EFFECTS: tinnitus
LOCAL EFFECTS: soreness at injection site

CLINICAL GUIDELINES

ADMINISTRATION:
• Monitor effects with ECG.
• Monitor flow rate when administered by intravenous infusion.
• Administer intramuscularly in deltoid; aspirate frequently.
• Reduce dosage in presence of congestive heart failure or liver damage.
EFFECTS:
• Increased creatine phosphokinase levels may occur.
DRUG INTERACTIONS:
• There have been no reports of cross sensitivity between lidocaine hydrochloride and procainamide or between lidocaine hydrochloride and quinidine.
• The preferred diluent for intravenous administration is 5% dextrose in water.
• Do not add to blood transfusion assemblies.
OVERDOSAGE/ANTIDOTE:
• Overdosage is characterized by an exaggeration of the adverse effects. Severe convulsions may occur.
• Institute emergency resuscitative procedures including maintenance of patent airway and assisted respiration if necessary. For severe convulsions, parenteral administration of a rapidly acting anticonvulsant may be used, and small doses of an ultrashort-acting barbiturate or a short-acting muscle relaxant are suggested.

Procainamide Hydrochloride

GENERAL CLINICAL USES

Procainamide hydrochloride is indicated in the treatment of premature ventricular contractions and ventricular tachycardia, atrial fibrillation and paroxysmal atrial tachycardia.

PHARMACOLOGY

Procainamide hydrochloride depresses the excitability of the cardiac muscle to electrical stimulation and slows conduction in the atrium, the bundle of His, and the ventricle. The refractory period of the atrium is considerably more prolonged than that of the ventricle. Large doses can induce atrioventricular block and ventricular extrasystoles which may proceed to ventricular fibrillation.

The action of procainamide begins almost immediately after intramuscular or intravenous administration. Peak plasma levels are reached in 15 to 60 minutes; after oral administration comparable plasma levels are obtained with maximal effect in 1 hour. Therapeutic levels are usually attained in half that time. The drug is excreted in the urine.

SPECIAL PRECAUTIONS

• Do not use in patients with myasthenia gravis or a history of hypersensitivity to this drug; cross sensitivity to procaine and related drugs must be borne in mind.
• Do not administer to patients with complete atrioventricular block, or in cases of second and third degree A-V block unless an electrical pacemaker is operative.
• Reduce dosage in patients with decreased creatinine clearance.
• In atrial fibrillation or flutter, the ventricular rate may increase suddenly as the atrial rate is slowed; adequate digitalization reduces but does not abolish this danger.
• If myocardial damage exists, ventricular

tachysystole is particularly hazardous; other untoward responses may occur.
• Correction of atrial fibrillation, with resultant forceful contractions of the atrium, may cause a dislodgement of mural thrombi and produce an embolic episode; in a patient already discharging emboli, procainamide hydrochloride is more likely to stop than aggravate the process.
• Attempts to adjust the heart rate in a patient who has developed ventricular tachycardia during an occlusive coronary episode should be carried out with extreme caution.
• Caution is also required in marked disturbances of A-V conduction time such as second and third degree A-V block, bundle branch block, or severe digitalis intoxication, where use of procainamide may result in additional depression of conduction and ventricular asystole or fibrillation.
• If the ventricular rate is significantly slowed by procainamide without attaining regular atrioventricular conduction, the drug should be stopped and the patient reevaluated, as asystole may result under these circumstances.
• In patients with liver and kidney disease who are receiving normal dosage, symptoms of overdosage (principally ventricular tachycardia and severe hypotension) may result.

ADVERSE EFFECTS

CNS EFFECTS: weakness, mental depression, giddiness, psychosis with hallucinations
CARDIOVASCULAR EFFECTS: hypotension, ventricular asystole, fibrillation
GASTROINTESTINAL EFFECTS: anorexia, nausea, bitter taste, diarrhea
HEMATOLOGIC EFFECTS: thrombocytopenia, Coombs-positive hemolytic anemia,

lupuslike reaction (fever, chills, nausea, vomiting, abdominal pain, acute hepatomegaly; also an increase in SGOT), agranulocytosis

ALLERGIC EFFECTS: urticaria, pruritus, angioneurotic edema

DERMATOLOGIC EFFECTS: maculopapular rash

CLINICAL GUIDELINES

ADMINISTRATION:
- Watch closely for evidence of untoward myocardial responses.
- Routine blood counts are advisable during maintenance therapy because of hematologic effects.
- Dilute parenteral form for intravenous use; do not administer over 25–50 mg/min.
- Keep patients supine and monitor blood pressure continuously during intravenous infusion.
- Limit intravenous use to extreme emergencies.
- If injectable solution develops a slightly yellow color, it may be used. However, if color is darker than light amber or any other color, discard.
- Store injection at temperature between 50 and 90°F.

EFFECTS:
- Prolonged administration often leads to development of a positive antinuclear antibody (ANA) test with or without symptoms of lupus-erythematouslike syndrome, polyarthralgia, arthritis, pleuritic pain, fever, skin lesions, myalgia, pleural effusion, and pericarditis. If a positive ANA antibody titer develops, the benefit to risk ratio related to continued procainamide therapy should be assessed.

OVERDOSAGE/ANTIDOTE:
- Overdosage is characterized by ventricular tachycardia and severe hypotension.

- Solutions of phenylephrine hydrochloride injection, USP, or levarterenol bitartrate injection, USP, should be available to counteract severe hypotensive responses.

Propranolol Hydrochloride

GENERAL CLINICAL USES

Propranolol hydrochloride is indicated for treatment of cardiac arrhythmias, namely, supraventricular arrhythmias (paroxysmal atrial tachycardias), persistent sinus tachycardia, tachycardias and arrhythmias due to thyrotoxicosis, persistent atrial extrasystoles, atrial flutter and fibrillation, ventricular arrhythmias, tachyarrhythmias of digitalis intoxication, resistant tachyarrhythmias due to excessive catecholamine action during anesthesia.

Additionally, propranolol hydrochloride is used in treating hypertension, angina pectoris due to coronary atherosclerosis, pheochromocytoma, and hypertrophic subaortic stenosis.

PHARMACOLOGY

Propranolol, a beta adrenergic blocking drug, exerts its antiarrhythmic activity through this action. It also decreases heart rate, cardiac output and blood pressure; the mechanism of action is unclear.

Propranolol is absorbed from the gastrointestinal act; peak effect occurs in 1 to 1½ hours. The biologic half-life is approximately 2 to 3 hours. There is no direct correlation between dose or plasma level.

SPECIAL PRECAUTIONS

- Do not use in patients with bronchial asthma, allergic rhinitis during the pollen season, sinus bradycardia and greater than first degree block, cardiogenic shock.

- Do not use in patients with right ventricular failure secondary to pulmonary hypertension, congestive heart failure, patients receiving adrenergic-augmenting psychotherapeutic agents or MAO-inhibitors, and during 2-week withdrawal from such drugs.
- Use with caution in patients with cardiac failure; digitalis and propranolol are additive in depressing A-V conduction.
- In certain patients, depression of the myocardium can occur which may lead to cardiac failure.
- Angina pectoris may be exacerbated during and following abrupt discontinuation of propranolol therapy.
- In patients with thyrothxicosis, abrupt withdrawal may result in exacerbation of hyperthyroidism.
- In patients undergoing major surgery, beta blockade impairs the ability of the heart to respond to reflex stimuli; withdraw propranolol 48 hours prior to surgery.
- In patients with nonallergic bronchospasm, bronchodilation may be blocked.
- Safe use in pregnancy has not been established; physician should weigh the benefits versus the risks.
- May produce hypotension and/or marked bradycardia.

ADVERSE EFFECTS

CNS EFFECTS: light-headedness, insomnia, weakness, fatigue, lassitude, depression, hallucinations, disorientation, memory loss, emotional lability, clouded sensorium, paresthesias
CARDIOVASCULAR EFFECTS: bradycardia, congestive heart failure, A-V block, hypotension, atrial insufficiency
RESPIRATORY EFFECTS: bronchospasm
GASTROINTESTINAL EFFECTS: nausea, vomiting, abdominal cramps, epigastric distress, diarrhea, constipation

DERMATOLOGIC EFFECTS: thrombocytopenic purpura, agranulocytosis, nonthrombocytopenic purpura
ALLERGIC EFFECTS: pharyngitis, erythematous rash, fever, aching, sore throat, laryngospasm, respiratory distress

CLINICAL GUIDELINES

ADMINISTRATION:
- Monitor patient continuously.
- If treatment is discontinued, reduce dosage over a period of several weeks.
- If initially administered intravenously, transfer to oral route as soon as possible.

EFFECTS:
- In diabetic patients and patients prone to hypoglycemia, the usual premonitory signs and symptoms of acute hypoglycemia may be prevented. Particularly caution patients with labile diabetes. A precipitous elevation of blood pressure may accompany the hypoglycemia.

DRUG INTERACTIONS:
- In patients receiving MAO-inhibitors and adrenergic-augmenting psychotherapeutic drugs, the inotropic effect of diagitalis may be reduced, whereas an additive depression of A-V conduction may occur.
- With anesthetics requiring catecholamine release for maintenance of cardiac function, beta blockade will impair the desired inotropic effect.
- Isoproterenol or levarterenol may reverse the effect of propranolol; patients receiving these drugs may experience protracted severe hypotension.
- Catecholamine-depleting drugs such as reserpine may produce excessive reduction of sympathetic tone.

OVERDOSAGE/ANTIDOTE:
- Overdosage is characterized by bradycardia, cardiac failure, hypotension, and bronchospasm.

• There is no specific antidote for propranolol; but for bradycardia, atropine, isoproterenol, or levarterenol may be administered; for cardiac failure, digitalis and diuretics; for hypotension, levarterenol or epinephrine; for bronchospasm, isoproterenol or aminophylline.

Quinidine Salts

Quinidine Gluconate
Quinidine Polygalacturonate
Quinidine Sulfate

GENERAL CLINICAL USES

The quinidine salts are indicated in the treatment of certain cardiac arrhythmias: premature atrial and ventricular contractions, paroxysmal atrial tachycardia, paroxysmal A-V junctional rhythm, atrial flutter, paroxysmal atrial flutter, established atrial fibrillation, paroxysmal ventricular tachycardia when not associated with complete heart block, maintenance therapy after electrical conversion of atrial fibrillation and/or flutter.

PHARMACOLOGY

Quinidine depresses myocardial excitability, conduction velocity, and contractility. It also exerts some indirect activity on the heart through an anticholinergic action. Large oral doses may reduce the atrial pressure by means of peripheral vasodilation.

Following oral administration of quinidine salts, the maximal effect usually occurs in 1 to 3 hours and activity lasts for 6 to 8 hours or more.

Quinidine polygalacturonate, also administered orally, has a slower incidence of local gastrointestinal irritation than does quinidine sulfate.

Quinidine gluconate may be administered orally, intramuscularly, or intravenously.

SPECIAL PRECAUTIONS

• In the treatment of atrial flutter, reversion to sinus rhythms may be preceded by a progressive reduction in the degree of A-V block to a 1:1 ratio and resulting extremely rapid ventricular rate.

• Usage in pregnancy should be reserved only for those cases in which the benefits outweigh the possible hazards to the patient and fetus.

• Do not use in patients known to be hypersensitive to or have idiosyncratic reactions to these drugs; with a history of thrombocytopenic purpura associated with previous quinidine administration; digitalis intoxication manifested by A-V or A-V nodal or idioventricular pacemaker; and ectopic impulses and rhythms due to escape mechanisms.

• Use with extreme caution where there is A-V block, since complete block and asystole may result.

• These drugs may cause unpredictable abnormalities of rhythm in digitalized patients; use with special caution in the presence of digitalis intoxication.

• The depressant effects on cardiac contractility and arterial blood pressure limit its use in congestive heart failure and in hypotensive states unless these conditions are due to or aggravated by the arrhythmia.

• The dangers of the parenteral use of quinidine are increased in the presence of atrioventricular heart block or in the absence of atrial activity.

• The administration of quinidine is more hazardous in patients with extensive myocardial damage than it is in persons with a normal heart muscle who have a cardiac arrhythmia.

• Patients sensitive to quinine (for malaria) may be sensitive to quinidine.

• Occasionally a cardiac arrhythmia may have been produced by digitalis intoxication, and the use of quinidine in this situation is extremely dangerous because the cardiac glycoside may already have caused serious impairment of the intracardiac conduction system.

• Use with extreme caution when given with any drug that can depress conduction at the myoneuronal junction (e.g., polymyxin B, neomycin, kanamycin).

ADVERSE EFFECTS

CNS EFFECTS: headache, fever, vertigo, apprehension, excitement, confusion, delirium, syncope, cold sweat

CARDIOVASCULAR EFFECTS: widening of QRS complex, cardiac asystole, ventricular ectopic beats, and idioventricular rhythms (including ventricular tachycardia and fibrillation), paradoxical tachycardia, atrial embolism, hypotension with parenteral administration

GASTROINTESTINAL EFFECTS: nausea, vomiting, abdominal pain, diarrhea

ALLERGIC EFFECTS: angioedema, acute asthmatic episode, vascular collapse, respiratory arrest

DERMATOLOGIC EFFECTS: cutaneous flushing with intense pruritus

OPHTHALMIC EFFECTS: visual disturbances, mydriasis, blurred vision, disturbed color perception, photophobia, diplopia, nightblindness, scotomata, optic neuritis

OTIC EFFECTS: tinnitus, decreased auditory acuity

CLINICAL GUIDELINES

ADMINISTRATION:

• When administering orally, give with food to minimize gastrointestinal effects.

• Discontinue drug if any one of the following occurs: side effects of more than trivial nature; restoration of sinus rhythm; prolongation of QRS complex in excess of 25 percent beyond that observed prior to the injection; disappearance of the P wave; decrease in heart rate to 120 beats per minute.

• Administer intravenously slowly; inject at rate of 1 ml/min; too rapid injection may cause a fall in arterial pressure of 25 to 50 mm Hg.

• Frequent or continuous ECG monitoring is necessary, especially during intravenous administration to detect any change in rate or rhythm.

EFFECTS:

• Large doses may have a deleterious effect on the heart and result in heart block or standstill diastole.

DRUG INTERACTIONS:

• Dilute in 5% glucose.

• Do not administer with neuromuscular blocking agents.

OVERDOSAGE/ANTIDOTE:

• Overdosage is characterized by the symptoms of cinchonism, namely, vertigo, tinnitus, headache, fever, and visual disturbances.

• Discontinue drug. Treat symptomatically and supportively. Cardiotoxic effects may be reversed in part by molar sodium lactate, the hypotension by vasoconstrictors and cateholamines (since the vasodilation is partly due to adrenergic blockage).

Anticoagulants

SPECIFIC PRODUCTS AND DOSAGES

GENERIC NAME	TRADE NAME	ROUTE OF ADMIN.	USUAL DOSAGE
heparin sodium	(G)* LIQUAEMIN HEPATHROM	iv infusion	**Individualize; 20,000–40,000 units**
		sc	8,000–20,000 units bid or tid; individualize
Coumarin Derivatives: acenocoumarol	SINTROM	po	**Initial:** 16–28 mg; **Maintenance:** 2–10 mg
bishydroxycoumarin	(G) DICUMAROL	po	**Initial:** 200–300 mg **Maintenance:** 25–200 mg
phenprocoumon	LIQUAMAR	po	**Initial:** 9–24 mg **Maintenance:** 0.75–6 mg
warfarin potassium	ATHROMBIN-K	po	**Initial:** 40–60 mg; **Maintenance:** 2.5–10 mg
warfarin sodium	COUMADIN PANWARFIN	po	**Initial:** 40–60 mg; **In elderly and/or debilitated:** 20–30 mg **Maintenance:** 2–10 mg
Indandione Derivatives: anisindione	MIRADON	po	**Initial:** 300 mg **Maintenance:** 25–250 mg
phenindione	HEDULIN DANILONE	po	**Initial:** 200–300 mg **Maintenance:** 100–200 mg

*(G) designates availability as a generic product.

Heparin Sodium

GENERAL CLINICAL USES

Heparin sodium is indicated for anticoagulant therapy in prophylaxis of thrombosis and as treatment to prevent its extension. It is also used to prevent clotting in arterial and heart surgery, in blood transfusions, extracorporeal circulation, dialysis procedures, and in blood samples for laboratory tests.

PHARMACOLOGY

Heparin sodium, administered parenterally, inhibits the clotting of blood and the formation of fibrin clots both *in vitro* and *in vivo*. It inactivates thrombin, preventing the conversion of fibrinogen to fibrin and the formation of a stable fibrin clot. Although clotting time is prolonged by therapeutic doses, bleeding time is usually unaffected. The drug does not have fibrinolytic activity and will not lyse clots. Heparin is metabolized in the liver and excreted in the urine. Heparin does not cross the placental barrier.

SPECIAL PRECAUTIONS

- Do not use in patients known to be sensitive to the drug.
- Do not use if facilities are not available for performance of suitable blood coagulation tests (Lee-White whole blood clotting time, activated partial thromboplastin time).
- Do not use during any uncontrolled active bleeding state.
- Safe use in pregnancy has not been established.
- Use with extreme caution in disease states in which there is increased danger of hemorrhage.
- Use with caution in patients with allergies, since heparin sodium is derived from animal tissue.
- Use with caution during the last trimester of pregnancy and during the immediate postpartum period; also in the presence of mild hepatic or renal disease, in hypertension, during menstruation, or in patients with indwelling catheters.

ADVERSE EFFECTS

URINARY TRACT EFFECTS: suppression of renal function after long-term administration of high doses.
METABOLIC AND ENDOCRINE EFFECTS: osteoporosis, aldosterone suppression, priapism, rebound hyperlipidemia
HEMATOLOGIC EFFECTS: hemorrhage, reversible thrombocytopenia

ALLERGIC EFFECTS: hypersensitivity reactions manifested as chills, fever, urticaria asthma, rhinitis, lacrimation, anaphylactoid reactions
DERMATOLOGIC EFFECTS: delayed transient alopecia
LOCAL EFFECTS: with intramuscular administration, irritation, mild pain, hematoma; histaminelike reaction

CLINICAL GUIDELINES

ADMINISTRATION:
- Monitor prothrombin time frequently.
- Advise patients to report signs of bleeding and bruising; they indicate drug overdosage.

EFFECTS:
- It may be necessary to increase dosage in febrile states.
- An increased resistance to the drug is frequently encountered in thrombosis, thrombophlebitis, infection with thrombosing tendencies, myocardial infarction, cancer, and postsurgical patients.
- A higher incidence of bleeding may be seen in women over 60 years of age than in younger women.

DRUG INTERACTIONS:
- Heparin sodium may prolong the one-step prothrombin time.
- When heparin sodium is given with dicumarol or sodium warfarin, a period of 4 to 5 hours after the last intravenous dose or 12 to 24 hours after the last subcutaneous dose should elapse before blood is drawn if a valid prothrombin time is to be obtained.
- Drugs such as aspirin that interfere with platelet aggregation reactions (the main hemostatic defense of heparinized patients) may induce bleeding and should be used with caution in patients receiving heparin.
- Heparin may antagonize the action of ACTH, insulin, or corticoids.
- The anticoagulant action may be par-

tially counteracted by digitalis, tetracyclines, nicotine, or antihistamines.

OVERDOSAGE/ANTIDOTE:
- Overdosage is characterized by hemorrhage and bruising.
- Protamine sulfate 1% solution, administered by slow infusion, will neutralize heparin sodium. No more than 50 mg should be administered very slowly in any 10-minute period. Each mg neutralizes approximately 100 USP heparin units. Plasma or whole blood transfusions may be necessary. See Chapter 20, page 694.

Coumarin Derivatives

Acenocoumarol
Bishydroxycoumarin
Phenprocoumon
Warfarin Potassium
Warfarin Sodium

GENERAL CLINICAL USES
The coumarin derivatives are indicated for the prophylaxis and treatment of venous thrombosis and its extension, the treatment of atrial fibrillation with embolization, the prophylaxis and treatment of pulmonary embolism, and as an adjunct in the treatment of coronary occlusion.

PHARMACOLOGY
The coumarin derivatives, administered orally, reduce the concentration of prothrombin in the blood by inhibiting the formation of prothrombin in the liver and thus, increasing the prothrombin time. These drugs also interfere with the production of factors VII, IX, and X, so that the concentration in the blood is lowered during therapy. The coumarin derivatives pass the placental barrier and also appear in human milk.

Acenocoumarol is an intermediate-acting coumarin derivative. The peak effect is reached in 2 to 8 hours; the maximal effect is reached in 36 to 48 hours. Restoration of normal prothrombin activity occurs 2 to 7 days after the last dose is given.

Bishydroxycoumarin is absorbed effectively after oral administration. It is a long-acting anticoagulant. Peak action develops in 3 to 5 days and the hypoprothrombinemia persists for 2 to 10 days following discontinuance of therapy.

Phenprocoumon is also a long-acting coumarin derivative. The onset of peak action is 48 to 72 hours after initial administration; recovery may take up to 7 days after the last dose.

After oral administration of warfarin sodium and potassium, the maximal plasma concentration is reached in 2 to 8 hours and the maximal effect on prothrombin time is achieved in 36 to 72 hours. Following a single therapeutic dose, the effect on prothrombin time persists for 4 to 5 days.

SPECIAL PRECAUTIONS
- Do not use in patients who are bleeding or who have hemorrhagic tendencies, blood dyscrasias, purpura, open ulcerations, traumatic or surgical wounds, ulceration of the gastrointestinal tract, visceral carcinoma, diverticulitis, colitis, or subacute bacterial endocarditis.
- Do not use in the presence of threatened abortion, recent operations on the eye, brain, or spinal cord, regional and lumbar block anesthesia, vitamin K deficiency, severe hypertension, severe hepatic or renal disease, and continuous tube drainage of the stomach or small intestine.
- Use in pregnancy ONLY when the potential benefits of its use outweigh the possible hazards; congenital malformations have occurred in children born to mothers receiving oral anticoagulants.

• The effects of warfarin tend to be cumulative and prolonged; at earliest sign of bleeding withdraw drug.

• If administered to nursing mothers, observe infant for evidence of unexpected bleeding.

• Use with caution in patients with active tuberculosis, moderate hypertension, mild liver or kidney disease, and in those with severe diabetes.

• Use with caution in patients with indwelling catheters, during menstruation and the postpartum period, or in patients with a past history of ulcerative disease of the gastrointestinal tract or any occupation which carries a hazard of significant physical injury.

• Patients with congestive heart failure frequently become more sensitive to the drug and an appropriate reduction in dosage may be necessary.

ADVERSE EFFECTS

CNS EFFECTS: fever

URINARY TRACT EFFECTS: hematuria

GASTROINTESTINAL EFFECTS: paralytic ileus, intestinal obstruction, nausea, vomiting abdominal cramps, diarrhea

METABOLIC AND ENDOCRINE EFFECTS: excessive uterine bleeding, hemorrhagic necrosis of the female breast, priapism, elevated SGOT

HEMATOLOGIC EFFECTS: bleeding from mucous membranes, wounds, or ulcerative lesions, petechiae, purpuric hemorrhage, leukopenia

ALLERGIC EFFECTS: urticaria rarely

DERMATOLOGIC EFFECTS: dermatitis, loss of hair.

CLINICAL GUIDELINES

ADMINISTRATION:

• Frequent monitoring of prothrombin time is essential, particularly if other drugs have been added to the patient's treatment regimen.

• Dosage can be controlled only by periodic determinations of prothrombin time; determinations of clotting and bleeding times are not effective measures for control of therapy.

• Advise patient of signs of overdosage, namely, bleeding and bruising.

EFFECTS:

• The effects of coumarin derivatives tend to be cumulative and prolonged; at earliest signs of bleeding, withdraw drug.

• Bleeding is an inherent risk of treatment with any anticoagulant; its frequency and severity can be minimized by careful management.

DRUG INTERACTIONS:

• Use of vitamin K complicates subsequent anticoagulant therapy.

• A change in intake of dietary fat may influence anticoagulant response.

• Renal insufficiency, fever, alcoholism, and scurvy enhance or prolong the anticoagulant response.

• Heparin prolongs the one-stage prothrombin time; therefore, when heparin is given with coumarin derivatives, a period of from 4 to 5 hours after the last intravenous dose and 12 to 24 hours after the last subcutaneous dose of heparin sodium should elapse before blood is drawn if a valid prothrombin time is to be obtained.

• Drugs which may stimulate metabolic degradation of coumarin derivatives include phenobarbital as well as some other barbiturates, glutethimide, meprobamate, ethchlorvynol, and griseofulvin.

• Oral contraceptives may reduce the response to coumarin anticoagulants. Patients may require larger doses of anticoagulant than are usually needed.

• There have been conflicting reports of both potentiation and inhibition of the anticoagulant response by ACTH and the adrenocorticosteroids.

• Drugs which depress prothrombin formation in the liver and thus increase patient's sensitivity to warfarin sodium and cause hemorrhage include quinine and quinidine as well as salicylates in large doses.

• Drugs which potentiate the danger of hemorrhage in patients receiving oral anticoagulants include aspirin, phenylbutazone, phenytoin, chlorpromazine, guaifenesin, chloral hydrate, oxyphenbutazone, diazoxide; mefenamic, ethacrynic and nalidixic acids, antimetabolites, alkalyating agents, salicylates, indomethacin, and streptokinase-streptodornase.

• Broad-spectrum antibiotics which suppress the organisms comprising the normal bacterial flora of the intestines and reduce production of vitamin K_1 may increase anticoagulant activity.

• Drugs which may cause an exaggerated response and a prolonged prothrombin time include methylthiouracil, propylthiouracil, methyldopa, phenyramidol, disulfiram, dextrothyroxine, clofibrate, and various anabolic steroids, as well as some radioactive compounds.

• Diphenylhydantoin may increase the anticoagulant effect by displacing coumarin derivatives from plasma binding sites; however, coumarin derivatives elevate the serum hydantoin concentration, thus possibly leading to drug intoxication due to diphenylhydantoin.

• Tolbutamide will accumulate in the body if administered concurrently with dicumarol.

• Coumarin anticoagulants potentiate the hypoglycemic effects of tolbutamide by inhibiting its degradation in the liver.

OVERDOSAGE/ANTIDOTE:

• Overdosage is characterized by bruising and/or bleeding.

• Phytonadione (vitamin K) or fresh whole blood will counteract the effects of these agents.

Indandione Derivatives

Anisindione
Phenindione

GENERAL CLINICAL USES

The indandione derivatives are indicated for the prophylaxis and treatment of venous thrombosis and its extensions, the treatment of atrial fibrillation with embolization, the prophylaxis and treatment of pulmonary embolism, and as an adjunct in the treatment of coronary occlusion.

PHARMACOLOGY

The indandione derivatives, synthetic anticoagulants for oral administration, inhibit synthesis or prothrombin in the liver. They are metabolized in the liver and excreted in the urine.

Anisindione is a long-acting, orally effective anticoagulant. The peak effect is reached in 48 to 72 hours and lasts 1 to 3 days. Phenindione is a prompt acting compound; the onset of action is noted in 2 to 8 hours and a therapeutic effect is reached in 18 to 24 hours and persists for 4 to 5 days.

These indandione derivatives are secreted in mother's milk and can cause hemorrhage in the nursing infant. These drugs cross the placental barrier.

SPECIAL PRECAUTIONS

• Do not use in patients who are bleeding or who have hemorrhagic tendencies, blood dyscrasias, purpura, open ulcerations, traumatic or surgical wounds, ulceration of the gastrointestinal tract, visceral carcinoma, deverticulitis, colitis, or subacute bacterial endocarditis.

• Do not use in the presence of threatened abortion, recent opera tions on the eye, brain, or spinal cord; regional and lumbar block anesthesia, vitamin K deficiency, severe hypertension, severe hepatic or renal disease, and continuous tube drainage of the stomach or small intestine.

• Use in pregnancy ONLY when the potential benefits of its use outweigh the possible hazards; congenital malformations have occurred in children born to mothers receiving oral anticoagulants.

• If administered to nursing mothers, observe infant for evidence of unexpected bleeding.

• Use with caution in patients with active tuberculosis, moderate hypertension, mild liver or kidney disease, and severe diabetes.

• Use with caution in patients with indwelling catheters, during menstruation, and the postpartum period, or in patients with a past history of ulcerative disease of the gastrointestinal tract, or any occupation which carries a hazard of significant physical injury.

• Patients with congestive heart failure frequently become more sensitive to the drug and an appropriate reduction in dosage may be necessary.

• Discontinue if fever or skin rash occurs; these reactions may signal the development of severe complications.

ADVERSE EFFECTS

CNS EFFECTS: neuropathy, fever
URINARY TRACT EFFECTS: albuminuria
GASTROINTESTINAL EFFECTS: diarrhea
METABOLIC AND ENDOCRINE EFFECTS: edema

HEPATIC EFFECTS: jaundice, hepatitis
HEMATOLOGIC EFFECTS: agranulocytosis, leukopenia, leukocytosis
ALLERGIC EFFECTS: urticaria
DERMATOLOGIC EFFECTS: exfoliative dermatitis

CLINICAL GUIDELINES

ADMINISTRATION:
• Monitor prothrombin time frequently.
• Advise patients to report signs of bleeding and bruising immediately; these effects indicate overdosage.
• Discontinue promptly if fever or rash appears; these symptoms may signal the onset of a more severe complication.

EFFECTS:
• In patients with alkaline urine, the urine color may change to orange.
• Any acute illness that causes fever, vomiting, diarrhea may alter the response to these drugs.

DRUG INTERACTIONS:
• Alcohol may increase or decrease the effect of these drugs.
• A large intake of vitamin K or vitamin K containing foods may reduce the effectiveness of these drugs. Vitamin K containing foods include cabbage, cauliflower, fish, liver, kale, spinach.
• May increase the effects of insulin, phenylhydantoin, and sulfonylureas.
• Anticoagulant effect is decreased by antacids, barbiturates, carbamazepine, chlorpromazine, digitalis preparations, estrogens, ethchlorvynol, furosemide, glutehimide, griseofulvin, haloperidol, meprobamate, oral contraceptives, phenylbutazone, and phenylpropanolamine.

OVERDOSAGE/ANTIDOTE:
• Overdosage is characterized by bruising and hemorrhage.
• Discontinue drug. Fresh whole blood transfusions may be necessary.

Antihypertensive Agents

The antihypertensive agents are indicated for reduction of blood pressure in patients with blood pressure elevated to varying degrees of severity, with hypertensive crises, in controlled hypotension during anesthesia, and in the hypertension associated with pheochromocytoma. Since each antihypertensive agent has relatively specific uses, the clinical indications for each will be summarized below and also repeated with the information for each product.

Other products used in treating hypertension, either alone or in combination with the agents listed below, are the diuretic agents, namely, the thiazides, ethacrynate sodium, triamterene, and furosemide. For detailed information refer to the discussion of diuretic agents in this chapter.

HYPERTENSIVE CRISES:

cryptenamine acetates, iv/im
diazoxide, iv
hydralazine HCl, iv
methyldopa, parenteral

nitroprusside sodium
reserpine, im
trimethaphan camsylate

SEVERE HYPERTENSION:

guanethidine sulfate
hydralazine HCl
mecamylamine hydrochloride

methyldopa
pargyline HCl
propranolol HCl

MODERATE HYPERTENSION:

clonidine HCl
cryptenamine tannate
guanethidine sulfate
mecamylamine hydrochloride
methyldopa/methyldopate HCl

metoprolol tartrate
pargyline HCl
prazosin HCl
propranolol HCl

MILD HYPERTENSION:

alseroxylon
clonidine HCl
deserpidine
metoprolol tartrate
prazosin HCl

rauwolfia, whole root
rauwolfia serpentina alkaloids
rescinnamine
reserpine

CONTROLLED HYPERTENSION:

trimethaphan camsylate

HYPERTENSION OF PHEOCHROMOCYTOMA:

phenoxybenzamine hydrochloride
phentolamine

SPECIFIC PRODUCTS AND DOSAGES

GENERIC NAME	TRADE NAME	ROUTE OF ADMIN.	USUAL ADULT DOSAGE
alseroxylon	RAUTENSIN RAUWILOID	po	**Initial:** 2–4 mg/day in divided doses **Maintenance:** 2 mg/day
clonidine HCl	CATAPRES	po	**Initial:** 0.1 mg bid **Maintenance:** 0.2–0.8 mg/day in divided doses
cryptenamine acetates	UNITENSEN	iv im	**Initial:** 0.5 ml **Initial:** 0.5 ml; increase by 0.1 ml increments
cryptenamine tannate	UNITENSEN	po	**Initial:** 4 mg/day **Mainenance:** 4–12 mg/day in divided doses
deserpidine	HARMONYL	po	**Initial:** 0.75–1 mg/day **Maintenance:** 0.25–0.75 mg/day
diazoxide	HYPERSTAT I.V.	iv	300 mg administered in 30 sec. as a bolus; if no response, repeat in 30 min, then every 4–24 hrs as needed
guanethidine sulfate	ISMELIN	po	**Initial:** 10–50 mg/day **Maintenance:** adjust according to response
hydralazine HCl	(G)* APRESOLINE	po iv/im	10–25 mg qid; adjust as necessary 20–40 mg; repeat as necessary
mecamylamine HCl	INVERSINE	po	**Initial:** 2.5 mg bid; increase by 2.5 mg increments every 2 days
methyldopa/methyldopate hydrochloride	ALDOMET	po iv	**Initial:** 250 mg bid or tid **Maintenance:** 0.5–2.0 gm in divided doses; usual 250–500 mg qid; maximum: 1 gm every 6 hrs.
metoprolol tartrate	LOPRESSOR	po	**Initial:** 50 mg bid **Maintenance:** 100–450 mg/day
nitroprusside sodium	(G)* NIPRIDE	iv infusion	0.5–10 mcg/kg/min.
pargyline HCL	EUTONYL	po	**Initial:** 25 mg od; increase by 10 mg increments once a wk.; max 200 mg/day
phenoxybenzamine HCl	DIBENZYLINE	po	**Initial:** 10 mg/day **Maintenance:** 20–60 mg/day
phentolamine	REGITINE	po im/iv	50 mg 4–6 times/day **Adults:** 5 mg 1–2 hr. before surgery **Children:** 1 mg 1–2 hr. before surgery

*(G) designates availability as a generic product.

(continued overleaf)

GENERIC NAME	TRADE NAME	ROUTE OF ADMIN.	USUAL ADULT DOSAGE
prazosin HCl	MINIPRESS	po	**Initial:** 1 mg tid; **Maintenance:** 6–15 mg/day
propranolol HCl	INDERAL	po iv	**Initial:** 20–80 mg/day **Maintenance:** 160–480 mg/day 1–3 mg; may repeat after 2 min.
Rauwolfia serpentina alkaloids	(G)* HYPERLOID	po	2–6 mg/day
rescinnamine	CINNASIL MODERIL	po	**Initial:** 0.5 mg bid **Maintenance:** 0.25–0.5 mg/day
reserpine	(G) RAU-SED SERPASIL	po im	**Initial:** 0.5 mg/day for 1–2 wks. **Maintenance:** 0.1–0.25 mg/day 0.5–1.0 mg, then 2–4 mg every 3 hr.
trimethaphan camsylate	ARFONAD	iv infusion	0.1% (1 mg/ml) in 5% Dextrose Injection; adjust rate individually
rauwolfia, whole root	(G) RAUDIXIN SERFOLIA	po	200–400 mg/day in divided doses

*(G) designates availability as a generic product.

Rauwolfia Alkaloids

Alseroxlon
Deserpidine
Rauwolfia Serpentina Alkaloids
Rauwolfia, Whole Root
Rescinninamine
Reserpine

GENERAL CLINICAL USES

These drugs administered orally are indicated in the treatment of mild hypertension. However, reserpine administered intramuscularly may be useful in hypertensive crises.

PHARMACOLOGY

These drugs deplete the tissue stores of catecholamines (epinephrine and norepinephrine) from peripheral sites, lowering the blood pressure. They have sedative and tranquilizing properties which may be related to the depletion of 5-hydroxytryptamine from the brain.

After oral administration the onset of action is slow but the effect sustained. Following withdrawal both the cardiovascular and central nervous system effects may persist. These drugs are excreted in mother's milk.

SPECIAL PRECAUTIONS

• Do not use in patients with known hypersensitivity, mental depression (especially suicidal tendencies), active peptic ulcer, and ulcerative colitis.

• Do not use in patients receiving electroconvulsive therapy.

• Discontinue drug at first signs of despondency, early morning insomnia, loss of appetite, impotence, or mild depression.

• Safe use in pregnancy or lactation has not been established.

• Use with caution in patients with a history of peptic ulcer, ulcerative colitis, or gallstones; biliary colic may be precipitated.

• Use with caution in treating hypertensive patients with renal insufficiency since they adjust poorly to lowered blood pressure levels.

• Preoperative withdrawal of this drug does not assure that circulatory instability will not occur.

ADVERSE EFFECTS

CNS EFFECTS: drowsiness, depression, nervousness, paradoxical anxiety, nightmares, rare parkinsonian syndrome, dull sensorium, dizziness, headache, extrapyramidal tract symptoms

RESPIRATORY EFFECTS: nasal congestion, dyspnea

CARDIOVASCULAR EFFECTS: anginalike symptoms, arrhythmias, bradycardia

URINARY TRACT EFFECTS: dysuria

AUTONOMIC EFFECTS: dry mouth

GASTROINTESTINAL EFFECTS: hypersecretion, nausea, vomiting, anorexia, diarrhea, gastrointestinal bleeding

METABOLIC AND ENDOCRINE EFFECTS: impotence or decreased libido, weight gain, water retention with edema rarely

HEMATOLOGIC EFFECTS: purpura

DERMATOLOGIC EFFECTS: pruritus, rash

MUSCULOSKELETAL EFFECTS: muscular aches

OPHTHALMIC EFFECTS: glaucoma, uveitis, optic atrophy, conjunctival injection

OTIC EFFECTS: deafness

CLINICAL GUIDELINES

ADMINISTRATION:

• Caution patients that drowsiness usually occurs.

EFFECTS:

• Drug-induced depression may persist for several months after drug withdrawal and may be severe enough to result in suicide.

• Increased respiratory secretion, nasal congestion, cyanosis, and anorexia may occur in infants born to rescinnamine-treated mothers since the drug crosses the placental barrier and appears in cord blood and breast milk.

DRUG INTERACTIONS:

• When used in patients receiving digitalis and quinidine, cardiac arrhythmias have occurred.

• Concomitant administration with ganglionic blocking agents, guanethidine, veratrum, hydralazine, methyldopa, chlorthalidone, or thiazides necessitates careful titration of dosage of each agent.

OVERDOSAGE/ANTIDOTE:

• Overdosage is characterized by exaggerated sedative effects and/or hypotension.

• Discontinue drug and empty stomach. Hypotension may be treated by use of an adrenergic drug such as levarterenol administered intravenously.

Clonidine Hydrochloride

GENERAL CLINICAL USES

Clonidine hydrochloride is indicated in the treatment of mild to moderate hypertension.

PHARMACOLOGY

Clonidine hydrochloride appears to reduce blood pressure by central alpha adrenergic stimulation. In addition, it stimulates peripheral alpha adrenergic receptors producing transient vasoconstriction. Clonidine hydrochloride acts relatively rapidly following oral administration; blood pressure declines within 30 to 60 minutes with a maximal decrease occurring within 2 to 4 hours. The antihypertensive effect lasts 6 to 8 hours. Clonidine hydrochloride is excreted in the urine.

SPECIAL PRECAUTIONS

• Tolerance may develop, necessitating a re-evaluation of therapy.
• This drug is not recommended for use in women who are or may become pregnant unless the potential benefit outweighs the potential risk to the mother and infant.
• No clinical experience is available for use in children.
• When discontinuing clonidine hydrochloride therapy, reduce gradually over 2 to 4 days to avoid a possible rapid rise in blood pressure and associated symptoms.
• Use with caution in patients with severe coronary insufficiency, recent myocardial infarction, cerebrovascular disease, or chronic renal failure.

ADVERSE EFFECTS

CNS EFFECTS: drowsiness, sedation, dizziness, headache, fatigue, vivid dreams, nightmares, insomnia, other behavioral changes, nervousness, restlessness, anxiety, mental depression
RESPIRATORY EFFECTS: dry nasal mucosa
CARDIOVASCULAR EFFECTS: congestive heart failure, Raynaud's phenomena, ECG abnormalities manifested as Wenckebach period or ventricular trigeminy
URINARY TRACT EFFECTS: urinary retention

AUTONOMIC EFFECTS: dry mouth
GASTROINTESTINAL EFFECTS: constipation, anorexia, malaise, nausea, vomiting, parotid pain
METABOLIC AND ENDOCRINE EFFECTS: weight gain, transient elevation of blood glucose or serum creatinine phosphokinase, gynecomastia, impotence, increased sensitivity to alcohol
HEPATIC EFFECTS: mild transient abnormalities of liver function tests; hepatitis (1 case)
HEMATOLOGIC EFFECTS: weakly positive Coombs' test
ALLERGIC EFFECTS: urticaria
DERMATOLOGIC EFFECTS: rash, angioneurotic edema, thinning of hair, pruritus, dryness, pallor
OPHTHALMIC EFFECTS: burning of eyes

CLINICAL GUIDELINES

ADMINISTRATION:
• Caution patients not to discontinue drug without physicians' advice.
EFFECTS:
• Caution patients that the sedative effect may interfere with potentially hazardous activities such as operating machinery or driving a motor vehicle.
DRUG INTERACTIONS:
• Concurrent administration of diuretics may enhance effects of antihypertensive agents.
• May enhance central nervous system depressive effects of alcohol, barbiturates, and other sedatives.
• May be administered with hydralazine, guanethidine, methyldopa, reserpine, spironolactone, furosemide, chlorthalidone, and thiazide diuretics without drug to drug interactions.
OVERDOSAGE/ANTIDOTE:
• Overdosage is characterized by profound weakness, somnolence, diminished or absent reflexes or vomiting.

• Empty stomach by gastric lavage and administer an analeptic and a vasopressor. In children 19 months to 5 years, recovery was within 24 hours after overdosage. Tolazoline, 1 mg intravenously, at 3-minute intervals usually abolishes all effects.

Cryptenamine Acetate
Cryptenamine Tannate

GENERAL CLINICAL USES

Cryptenamine acetate administered intravenously or intramuscularly is indicated for short-term parenteral treatment of hypertensive crises, whereas cryptenamine tannate is indicated for treatment of mild to moderate hypertension.

PHARMACOLOGY

Cryptenamine acetate, an alkaloidal fraction of *Veratrum viride*, reduces blood pressure by widespread arteriolar dilatation mediated centrally without peripheral adrenergic or ganglionic blockage. It may be administered intramuscularly or intravenously. Cryptenamine tannate, for oral administration, acts similarly but more slowly than the acetate salt.

SPECIAL PRECAUTIONS

• Do not use in patients with known idiosyncrasy or hypersensitivity to *Veratrum viride*.
• Safe use in pregnancy, lactation, or in women of childbearing age has not been established.
• Use with care in hypertensive patients with angina pectoris or those with extensive cardiovascular disease.
• Use with caution in patients who have experienced a recent coronary or cerebral thrombosis.
• Special caution is warranted when treating patients with a history of bronchial asthma who may respond adversely to the cholinergic effects of cryptenamine.
• Use with caution when treating patients with renal insufficiency or pre-existing uremia; they may adjust poorly to lowered blood pressure levels.

ADVERSE EFFECTS

CNS EFFECTS: prostration, mental confusion
RESPIRATORY EFFECTS: bronchiolar constriction, respiratory depression
CARDIOVASCULAR EFFECTS: hypotension, cardial arrhythmias, bradycardia
AUTONOMIC EFFECTS: sweating, blurring of vision
GASTROINTESTINAL EFFECTS: anorexia, nausea, vomiting, epigastric and substernal burning, unpleasant taste, salivation, hiccups

CLINICAL GUIDELINES

ADMINISTRATION:
• Dilute for intravenous administration.
• Use undiluted for intramuscular injection.
EFFECTS:
• A narrow margin exists between the dose reducing the blood pressure and that producing side effects such as nausea and vomiting.
DRUG INTERACTIONS:
• Veratrum alkaloids may increase the high toned cardiac irritability produced by digitalis; concurrent use of cryptenamine with digitalis may lead to ectopic cardiac rhythms.
• The bradycardic effect of Veratrum alkaloids is additive to, but not synergistic with, that produced by morphine and related drugs.
• Concurrent administration with a saluretic agent can result in greater reduction in blood pressure than does therapy with either agent alone.

• An additive hypotensive effect occurs with preanesthetic and anesthetic agents.
OVERDOSAGE/ANTIDOTE:
• Overdosage is characterized by an exaggeration of the pharmacologic effects, namely, hypotension and severe bradycardia.
• Discontinue drug. Monitor ECG. Treat supportively. Atropine administration and positioning of patient to facilitate venous return may be adequate.

Diazoxide

GENERAL CLINICAL USES
Diazoxide, an intravenously administered agent, is indicated for emergency reduction of blood pressure in malignant hypertension in hospitalized patients, when prompt and urgent decrease of diastolic pressure is required. It is ineffective in hypertension caused by pheochromocytoma.

PHARMACOLOGY
Diazoxide, a nondiuretic thiazide, administered intravenously as a bolus reduces the blood pressure promptly by relaxing smooth muscle in peripheral arterioles. Cardiac output is increased as blood pressure is reduced; coronary and cerebral blood flow is maintained. Diazoxide crosses the placental barrier. The lowest level of blood pressure may be reached in 2 to 3 minutes.

Diazoxide has no known central nervous system effects. Renal blood flow is increased after an initial decrease.

SPECIAL PRECAUTIONS
• Do not use in the treatment of compensatory hypertension such as that associated with aortic coarctation or arteriovenous shunt.
• Do not use in patients with a history of hypersensitivity to diazoxide or other thiazides, unless the potential benefits outweigh the possible risks.
• Safe use in pregnancy or in children has not been established.
• Since diazoxide crosses the placental barrier, as with other thiazides, it may produce fetal or neonatal hyperbilirubinemia, thrombocytopenia, altered carbohydrate metabolism, and possibly adverse effects which have occurred in adults.
• Hypotension may occasionally occur; if therapy is required, it will respond to sympathomimetic agents such as norepinephrine.
• Since diazoxide causes sodium retention, repeated injections may precipitate edema.
• Use with caution in patients with impaired cerebral or cardiac circulation.
• Use with caution in diabetic patients because of hyperglycemic effect, and sodium and water retention.
• Since peritoneal dialysis and hemodialysis can reduce blood levels of diazoxide, patients undergoing dialysis may require more than one injection.

ADVERSE EFFECTS
CNS EFFECTS: shock, unconsciousness, convulsions, paralysis, confusion, numbness of hands with cerebral ischemia and thrombosis, headache, dizziness, light-headedness, sleepiness, euphoria, weakness, apprehension, anxiety, malaise.
RESPIRATORY   EFFECTS: "tightness"   in chest, dyspnea, cough, choking sensation
CARDIOVASCULAR   EFFECTS: hypotension to shock levels, myocardial ischemia, cerebral ischemia (usually transient), vasodilation phenomenons such as orthostatic hypotension, sweating, flushing, sensation of warmth, supra-ventricular tachycardia and palpitation, bradycardia
URINARY TRACT EFFECTS: nocturia
GASTROINTESTINAL EFFECTS: nausea, vom-

iting, abdominal discomfort, anorexia, alteration in taste, parotid swelling, salivation, dry mouth, constipation, diarrhea
METABOLIC AND ENDOCRINE EFFECTS: sodium and water retention, transient hyperglycemia, acute pancreatitis, rarely; transient retention of nitrogenous wastes
HEMATOLOGIC EFFECTS: leukopenia
ALLERGIC EFFECTS: rash, fever
MUSCULOSKELETAL EFFECTS: back pain
OPHTHALMIC EFFECTS: papilledema, lacrimation, blurred vision
OTIC EFFECTS: ringing in ears, momentary hearing loss
LOCAL EFFECTS: warmth along injected vein; cellulitis without sloughing and/or phlebitis at site of extravasation

CLINICAL GUIDELINES

ADMINISTRATION:
• Must be administered rapidly; slow injection may fail to reduce blood pressure.
• Blood pressure must be monitored closely and frequently during therapy.
• Administer only in peripheral vein; alkalinity of solution is irritating to tissue if leakage or extravasation occurs.
• Patient should remain recumbent for 30 minutes after injection.
EFFECTS:
• Since hyperglycemia occurs in the majority of patients, blood glucose should be monitored, particularly in patients with diabetes mellitus.
DRUG INTERACTIONS:
• Anticoagulant dosage may require reduction, particularly in patients who are hypoalbuminemic and receiving diazoxide intravenously and coumarin and its derivatives.
• Hyperglycemia caused by diazoxide may be treated with insulin.
OVERDOSAGE/ANTIDOTE:
• Overdosage effects have not been characterized.

• Peritoneal dialysis or hemodialysis can reduce levels of diazoxide in blood.

Guanethidine Sulfate

GENERAL CLINICAL USES
Guanethidine is indicated for treatment of moderate and severe hypertension either alone or as an adjunct and in treatment of renal hypertension including that secondary to pyelonephritis, renal amyloidosis, and renal artery stenosis. Do not use in patients with pheochromocytoma.

PHARMACOLOGY
Guanethidine may act by depleting norepinephrine stores. The maximal hypotensive effect does not occur until 2 to 3 days after initial administration and may persist for 7 to 10 days after withdrawal of the drug. Guanethidine causes sodium and water retention.

SPECIAL PRECAUTIONS
• Do not use in patients with hypersensitivity, with frank congestive heart failure not due to hypertension, or those using MAO-inhibitors.
• Orthostatic hypotension can occur frequently; instruct patients about this hazard.
• Postural hypotension may occur and is most marked in the morning and is accentuated by hot weather, alcohol, or exercise.
• If possible withdraw therapy 2 weeks prior to surgery to reduce the possibility of vascular collapse and cardiac arrest during anesthesia.
• If emergency surgery is required, preanesthetic and anesthetic agents should be administered cautiously and in reduced dosages.
• Use vasopressors only with extreme caution since guanethidine augments the re-

sponsiveness of exogenously administered norepinephrine and vasopressors with respect to blood pressure and their propensity for the production of cardiac arrhythmias.

• Use special care in patients with a history of bronchial asthma; asthmatics are more apt to be hypersensitive to catecholamine depletion and conditions may be aggravated.

• Safe use in pregnancy has not been established.

• Effects are cumulative over long periods; initial doses should be small and increased gradually in small increments.

• Use very cautiously in hypertensive patients with renal disease and nitrogen retention or rising BUN levels. Decreased blood pressure may further compromise renal function.

• Use very cautiously in patients with coronary disease with insufficiency or recent myocardial infarction, and cerebral vascular disease, especially with encephalopathy.

• Do not give to patients with severe cardiac failure except with extreme caution since guanethidine may interfere with the compensatory role of the adrenergic system in producing circulatory adjustment in congestive heart failure.

• Use cautiously in patients with a history of peptic ulcer or other chronic disorders which may be aggravated by a relative increase in parasympathetic tone.

ADVERSE EFFECTS

CNS EFFECTS: dizziness, weakness, lassitude, syncope, fatigue, depression, chest paresthesias

RESPIRATORY EFFECTS: dyspnea, nasal congestion, asthma in susceptible individuals

CARDIOVASCULAR EFFECTS: bradycardia, angina (chest pain)

URINARY TRACT EFFECTS: nocturia, incontinence

AUTONOMIC EFFECTS: dry mouth

GASTROINTESTINAL EFFECTS: increased bowel movements, diarrhea, nausea, vomiting, parotid tenderness

METABOLIC AND ENDOCRINE EFFECTS: inhibition of ejaculation, fluid retention and edema, increase in BUN, weight gain

HEMATOLOGIC EFFECTS: anemia, thrombocytopenia, leukopenia

DERMATOLOGIC EFFECTS: dermatitis, scalp hair loss

OPHTHALMIC EFFECTS: ptosis of lids, blurring of vision

MUSCULOSKELETAL EFFECTS: myalgia, muscle tremor

CLINICAL GUIDELINES

ADMINISTRATION:

• Caution patient about occurrence of postural and orthostatic hypotension.

• Dosage requirements may be reduced in presence of fever.

EFFECTS:

• Watch for weight gain or edema; may be averted with concomitant administration of a thiazide.

DRUG INTERACTIONS:

• When thiazides are added to regimen, guanethidine dosage may require reduction.

• Alcohol may accentuate postural hypotension.

• Concurrent use with rauwolfia derivatives may cause excessive postural hypotension, bradycardia, and mental depression.

• Both digitalis and guanethidine slow the heart rate.

• Amphetaminelike compounds, stimulants (such as ephedrine, methylphenidate), tricyclic antidepressants (amitriptyline, imipramine, desipramine) and other psychopharmaceutical agents (phenothiazines and related compounds), and oral contraceptives may reduce the hypotensive effect of guanethidine.

• MAO-inhibitors should be discontinued for at least 1 week before starting therapy with guanethidine.

OVERDOSAGE/ANTIDOTE:

• Overdosage is characterized by postural hypotension (with dizziness, blurring of vision, possibly progressing to syncope) and bradycardia; diarrhea, possibly severe, may also occur. Unconsciousness is unlikely if adequate blood pressure and cerebral perfusion can be maintained by appropriate positioning (supine).

• Treatment consists of restoring blood pressure and heart rate to normal by keeping patient supine. Normal hemostatic control usually returns gradually over a 72-hour period in normotensive patients. In previously hypertensive patients, particularly those with impaired cardiac reserve or other cardiovascular-renal disease, intensive treatment may be required. Supine position and vasopressors may be required. If diarrhea is severe or persists, treat symptomatically to reduce intestinal hypermotility; maintain hydration and electrolyte balance.

Hydralazine Hydrochloride

GENERAL CLINICAL USES

Hydralazine hydrochloride is indicated as sole or adjunctive therapy of essential hypertension. When administered intravenously it is useful in hypertensive crises.

PHARMACOLOGY

Hydralazine acts directly by relaxing arteriolar smooth muscle, thereby reducing blood pressure. It may be administered orally or intravenously.

SPECIAL PRECAUTIONS

• Do not use in patients with a history of hypersensitivity to hydralazine hydrochloride; with coronary artery disease; or with mitral valvular rheumatic heart disease.

• May produce a clinical picture simulating systemic lupus erythematosus; discontinue drug if this occurs.

• Use monoamine oxidase inhibitors with caution in patients receiving hydralazine.

• Use in pregnancy only when, in the judgment of the physician, it is essential to the welfare of the patient.

• May cause anginal attacks and ECG changes typical of myocardial ischemia; it has been implicated in myocardial infarction.

• Use with caution in all patients with suspected coronary artery disease or with cerebrovascular accidents.

ADVERSE EFFECTS

CNS EFFECTS: fever, malaise, headache, dizziness, tremors, psychotic reactions characterized by disorientaton and anxiety

RESPIRATORY EFFECTS: chest pain, dyspnea, nasal congestion

CARDIOVASCULAR EFFECTS: postural hypotension, palpitations, tachycardia, angina pectoris, paradoxical pressor response

URINARY TRACT EFFECTS: difficulty urinating

GASTROINTESTINAL EFFECTS: anorexia, nausea, vomiting, diarrhea, constipation, paralytic ileus

METABOLIC AND ENDOCRINE EFFECTS: edema, lymphadenopathy, splenomegaly

HEPATIC EFFECTS: hepatitis rarely

HEMATOLOGIC EFFECTS: reduction of hemoglobin and erythrocytes; leukopenia, agranulocytosis, eosinophilia

ALLERGIC EFFECTS: rash, urticaria, pruritus, fever, chills

DERMATOLOGIC EFFECTS: purpura and flushing

OPHTHALMIC EFFECTS: lacrimation

CLINICAL GUIDELINES
ADMINISTRATION:
- Conduct CBC, LE cell preparation, and antinuclear antibody titer determinations prior to and periodically during prolonged therapy.

EFFECTS:
- Incidence of toxic effects, particularly LE cell syndrome, is high in patients receiving large doses.

DRUG INTERACTIONS:
- Use MAO-inhibitors with caution; blood pressure may decrease.
- Effects are increased by tricyclic antidepressants (ELAVIL, TOFRANIL, SINEQUAN, etc.)

OVERDOSAGE/ANTIDOTE:
- Overdosage is characterized by hypotension, tachycardia, headache, and generalized skin flushing; myocardial ischemia and cardiac arrhythmias can develop and profound shock can occur with severe overdosage.
- Evacuate stomach; instill activated charcoal slurry if condition permits. Use supportive measures. Renal function must be monitored. No experience has been reported with either extracorporeal or peritoneal dialysis.

Mecamylamine Hydrochloride

GENERAL CLINICAL USES
Mecamylamine is indicated for treatment of moderatively severe to severe essential hypertension; also, malignant hypertension when uncomplicated.

PHARMACOLOGY
Mecamylamine, a ganglionic blocking agent, is absorbed almost completely from the gastrointestinal tract after oral administration. Blood pressure is reduced in both the normotensive and hypertensive patients. The onset of action is noted in 1/2 to 3 hours; the effects last from 6 to 12 hours.

SPECIAL PRECAUTIONS
- Do not use in patients with coronary insufficiency, glaucoma, pyloric stenosis, uremia, recent myocardial infarction, or mild or labile hypertension.
- Use with caution in patients with renal insufficiency, particularly if the blood urea nitrogen is elevated or rising.
- In patients with cerebral or renal insufficiency, central nervous systems effects may occur.
- When renal, cerebral, or coronary blood flow is impaired, any additional impairment should be avoided.
- Use with caution in patients with marked cerebral and coronary atherosclerosis or after a recent cerebral vascular accident.
- Do not restrict sodium; if necessary, adjust mecamylamine dosage.
- Use with caution in patients with prostatic hypertrophy, bladder neck obstruction, and urethral stricture; urinary retention may occur.

ADVERSE EFFECTS
CNS EFFECTS: weakness, fatigue, sedation, syncope, paresthesias, dizziness
RESPIRATORY EFFECTS: interstitial pulmonary edema, fibrosis
CARDIOVASCULAR EFFECTS: orthostatic and postural hypotension
URINARY TRACT EFFECTS: retention
GASTROINTESTINAL EFFECTS: anorexia, dry mouth glossitis, nausea, vomiting, constipation, ileus
METABOLIC AND ENDOCRINE EFFECTS: decreased libido

OPHTHALMIC EFFECTS: dilated pupils, blurred vision

CLINICAL GUIDELINES

ADMINISTRATION:
• Administer after meals for gradual absorption and smoother control of excessively high blood pressure.
• Drug administration in relation to meals should be consistent.
• Give larger drug doses at noontime and evening since blood pressure response is increased in the early morning.

EFFECTS:
• When discontinued suddenly, hypertensive levels return; this may be abrupt and cause fatal cerebral vascular accident or acute congestive heart failure.
• Withdraw therapy gradually; effects may last from hours to days after therapy is discontinued.

DRUG INTERACTIONS:
• May be potentiated by anesthesia, other antihypertensive drugs, and alcohol.
• Action may also be potentiated by excessive heat, infection, fever, hemorrhage, pregnancy, surgery, vigorous exercise, salt depletion (due to diarrhea, vomiting, sweating, diuretics).

OVERDOSAGE/ANTIDOTE:
• Overdosage is characterized by hypotension and an exaggeration of the adverse effects.
• Treat with small doses of pressor amines; use other supportive measures as indicated.

Methyldopa
Methyldopate Hydrochloride

GENERAL CLINICAL USES
Methyldopa and methyldopate hydrochloride, administered orally or parenterally repeatedly, are indicated for treatment of sustained moderate to severe hypertension.

Parenteral administration may be useful in hypertensive crises.

PHARMACOLOGY
Methyldopa is a dopa decarboxylase inhibitor. The antihypertensive action is probably due to its metabolism of alpha-methylnorepinephrine, which then lowers arterial pressure by stimulating central inhibitory alpha adrenergic receptors. Also, methyldopa has no direct effect on cardiac function and usually does not reduce glomerular filtration rate, renal blood flow, or filtration fraction. Cardiac output usually is maintained without cardiac acceleration; the heart rate may be slowed in some patients. Methyldopa is excreted by the kidney.

With parenteral administration (methyldopate hydrochloride), a decline in blood pressure may begin in 4 to 6 hours and last 10 to 16 hours after injection.

SPECIAL PRECAUTIONS
• Do not use in patients with active hepatic disease such as acute hepatitis and active cirrhosis; use with caution in patients with a history of previous liver disease or dysfunction.
• Do not use if previous methyldopa therapy was associated with liver disorders.
• Do not use in patients with a history of hypersensitivity to methyldopa or methyldopate hydrochloride.
• Use in women of childbearing age requires that the potential benefits be weighed against the possible hazards to the mother and fetus.
• If involuntary choreoathetotic movements occur, particularly in patients with severe bilateral cerebrovascular disease, discontinue therapy.
• Patients may require reduced doses of

anesthesia when on methyldopa; if hypotension occurs, it may be controlled with vasopressors.
• After dialysis, hypertension has occurred occasionally because the methyldopa is removed by this procedure.
• Use with caution in patients with impaired renal function.

ADVERSE EFFECTS

CNS EFFECTS: fever, involuntary choreothetotic movements rarely; sedation, headache, asthenia, weakness, dizziness lightheadedness, symptoms of cerebrovascular insufficiency, paresthesias, parkinsonism, Bell's palsy, nightmares, reversible mild psychosis or depression
RESPIRATORY EFFECTS: nasal stuffiness
CARDIOVASCULAR EFFECTS: bradycardia, aggravation of angina pectoris, orthostatic hypotension
GASTROINTESTINAL EFFECTS: nausea, vomiting, distention, constipation, flatus, diarrhea, mild dryness of mouth, sore or "black tongue," pancreatitis, sialadenitis
METABOLIC AND ENDOCRINE EFFECTS: increased BUN, breast enlargement, gynecomastia, lactation, impotence, decreased libido, edema
HEPATIC EFFECTS: jaundice with or without fever; hepatic necrosis, rarely fatal; abnormal liver function tests
HEMATOLOGIC EFFECTS: hemolytic anemia, eosinophilia, granulocytopenia, thrombocytopenia, positive Coombs' test, leukopenia
ALLERGIC EFFECTS: drug-related fever, myocarditis
DERMATOLOGIC EFFECTS: eczema, lichenoid eruptions
MUSCULOSKELETAL EFFECTS: myalgia, mild arthralgia

CLINICAL GUIDELINES

ADMINISTRATION:
• Perform CBC (hematocrit, hemoglobin, RBC in particular) prior to drug use; periodically repeat.
• Increased dosage at evening may minimize daytime drowsiness.
EFFECTS:
• Sedation usually occurs during the initial period of therapy or whenever the dose is increased.
• A positive Coombs' test, hemolytic anemia, and liver disorders may occur.
• A positive Coombs' test usually occurs between 6 and 12 months of therapy in 10 to 20 percent of patients.
• Syncope in older patients may be related to increased sensitivity and advanced arteriosclerosis; lower dosage.
• Occasionally tolerance occurs, usually between the second and third months of therapy.
• Urine may darken after voiding because of breakdown of methyldopa to its metabolites.
DRUG INTERACTIONS:
• Abnormalities of serum alkaline phosphatase, SGOT, SGPT, bilirubin, cephalin flocculation, prothrombin time, and BSP may occur.
• May interfere with measurement of uric acid by the phosphotungstate method; creatinine, by the alkaline picrate method; and SGOT by colorimetric methods; interference with spectrophotometric methods for SGOT analysis has not been reported.
• False high levels of urinary catecholamines may be reported since methyldopa causes fluorescence in urine samples at the same wavelengths as catecholamines.
OVERDOSAGE/ANTIDOTE:
• Overdosage is characterized by an exag-

geration of the pharmacologic effects, namely, hypotension.
• Treat supportively. Methyldopa can be removed by dialysis.

Metoprolol Tartrate

GENERAL CLINICAL USES

Metoprolol tartrate is indicated for the management of hypertension. It may be used alone or in combination with other antihypertensive agents.

PHARMACOLOGY

Metoprolol tartrate, a beta-adrenergic blocking agent, lowers blood pressure. The exact mechanism of action is unknown. Following oral administration, absorption is rapid and complete. Plasma levels are approximately 50 percent of those obtained after intravenous administration. The drug is metabolized in the liver.

Significant beta blocking effect occurs within 1 hour after oral administration.

SPECIAL PRECAUTIONS

• Do not use in patients with sinus bradycardia, heart block greater than first degree, cardiogenic shock, and overt cardiac failure.
• Administer cautiously to patients with hypertension who also have congestive heart failure controlled by digitalis and diuretics. Both digitalis and metoprolol slow A-V conduction.
• Continued depression of the myocardium as with metoprolol tartrate can lead to cardiac failure.
• Following abrupt cessation of therapy, exacerbations of angina pectoris and, in some cases, myocardial infarction have been reported.

• Do not administer any beta blocker (including metoprolol tartrate) to patients with bronchospastic diseases.
• Prior to surgery it may be desirable to withdraw any beta blocker since the ability of the heart to respond to reflex adrenergic stimuli may be impaired.
• May mask the symptoms of hypoglycemia in patients with diabetes mellitus; use with caution in diabetic patients.
• May mask the signs of hyperthyroidism. Avoid abrupt withdrawal since this may precipitate a thyroid storm.
• Use with caution in patients with impaired hepatic or renal function.
• Safe use in pregnancy has not been established; use only when clearly needed.
• Breast-feeding should not be undertaken by mothers receiving metoprolol tartrate.
• Safe use in children has not been established.

ADVERSE EFFECTS

CNS EFFECTS: tiredness, dizziness, depression, headache, nightmares, insomnia, mental depression progressing to catatonia, hallucinations, short-memory loss, emotional lability, clouded sensorium, drowsiness
CARDIOVASCULAR EFFECTS: shortness of breath, bradycardia, cold extremities, Raynaud's disease, palpitations, congestive heart failure, intensification of A-V block
RESPIRATORY EFFECTS: wheezing (bronchospasm), laryngospasm, respiratory distress
GASTROINTESTINAL EFFECTS: nausea, gastric pain, constipation, flatulence, heartburn
ENDOCRINE AND METABOLIC EFFECTS: elevated blood urea levels in patients with severe heart disease, elevated serum trans-

aminase, alkaline phosphatase, lactate dehydrogenase

DERMATOLOGIC EFFECTS: reversible alopecia

HEMATOLOGIC EFFECTS: agranulocytosis, nonthrombocytopenic purpura, thrombocytopenic purpura

ALLERGIC EFFECTS: pruritus, erythematous rash, fever

OPHTHALMIC EFFECTS: visual disturbances

CLINICAL GUIDELINES

ADMINISTRATION:

• Advise patients to notify physician if dizziness or diarrhea occurs.

• Caution patients not to discontinue medication except on the advice of a physician. Angina may be precipitated.

EFFECTS:

• The maximal effect of therapy will be apparent after 1 week of therapy.

• Note that beta 1 selectivity diminishes as dosage is increased.

DRUG INTERACTIONS:

• Catecholamine-depleting drugs such as reserpine may have an additive effect. Observe patient closely for evidence of hypotension and/or marked bradycardia. Vertigo, syncope, or postural hypotension may be present.

• May be used in combination with thiazide diuretics and also other antihypertensive agents.

• Digitalis slows A-V conduction as does metoprolol tartrate. Therefore, administer cautiously with frequent monitoring.

• May potentiate insulin-induced hypoglycemia.

OVERDOSAGE/ANTIDOTE:

• Overdosage is characterized by an exaggeration of the adverse effects.

• There is no antidote for metoprolol tartrate. Perform gastric lavage. If bradycardia occurs, administer atropine. If there is no response to vagal blockade, administer vasopressors cautiously. If hypotension occurs, administer vasopressors such as epinephrine or levarterenol. Bronchospasm may be treated with a beta 2-stimulating agent and/or a theophylline derivative. For cardiac failure, digitalis glycosides and diuretics are indicated.

Nitroprusside Sodium

GENERAL CLINICAL USES

Nitroprusside sodium, administered only by infusion with dextrose 5% in water, is indicated for the immediate reduction of blood pressure of patients in hypertensive crises. Concomitant oral antihypertensive medication should be started while the hypertensive emergency is being brought under control.

PHARMACOLOGY

Nitroprusside sodium is a potent, rapid-acting antihypertensive agent. The action is immediate and ends when the intravenous infusion is stopped. The antihypertensive effects are caused by peripheral vasodilatation as a result of direct action in the blood vessels independent of autonomic innervation. No relaxation is noted in the smooth muscle of the uterus. Nitroprusside sodium is metabolized to thiocyanate.

SPECIAL PRECAUTIONS

• Do not use in the treatment of compensatory hypertension, e.g., arteriovenous shunt or coarctation of the aorta.

• If excessive amounts are used, thiocyanate toxicity (tinnitus, blurred vision, delirium) may occur.

• Use with caution in patients with hypothyroidism or severe renal impairment; thiocyanate inhibits both the uptake and binding of iodine.

• Patients receiving antihypertensive agents are more sensitive to the effects of sodium nitroprusside, and dosage should be adjusted accordingly.

• Safe use in women who are or who may become pregnant has not been established.

• Safe use in children has not been established.

• Use with caution and, initially, with low doses in elderly patients.

ADVERSE EFFECTS

CNS EFFECTS: apprehension, headache, restlessness, dizziness

CARDIOVASCULAR EFFECTS: palpitations

AUTONOMIC EFFECTS: diaphoresis

GASTROINTESTINAL EFFECTS: nausea, retching, abdominal pain

METABOLIC AND ENDOCRINE EFFECTS: hypothroidism (1 case)

MUSCULOSKELETAL EFFECTS: muscle twitching, retrosternal discomfort.

CLINICAL GUIDELINES

ADMINISTRATION:

• Monitor blood pressure vigilantly; the effect is rapid.

• Administer only as an intravenous infusion with sterile 5% dextrose in water; *not* for direct injection.

• Infusion rates greater than 8 mcg/kg/min are rarely required.

• Solution deteriorates in the presence of light; wrap container.

• Do not keep solution longer than 4 hours.

• If solution is colored (blue, green, dark red), discard.

• Determine blood levels of thiocyanate if treatment is to be extended in patients with severe renal dysfunction. Blood thiocyanate levels should not exceed 10 mg/100 ml.

EFFECTS:

• The effect is rapid, and continuous infusion is required to maintain the hypotensive effect.

DRUG INTERACTIONS:

• The antihypertensive effect is augmented by ganglionic blocking agents.

• May be used simultaneously with oral antihypertensive medications.

OVERDOSAGE/ANTIDOTE:

• Overdosage is characterized by signs of thiocyanate toxicity, namely, tinnitus, blurred vision, delirium, progressing to intoxication.

• Peritoneal dialysis will reduce thiocyanate levels.

Pargyline Hydrochloride

GENERAL CLINICAL USES

Pargyline hydrochloride is useful in treating some types of essential and secondary hypertension. It may be used alone or concurrently with most other antihypertensive agents.

PHARMACOLOGY

Pargyline hydrochloride is an orally administered monoamine oxidase inhibitor which has a potent antihypertensive action. Its exact mode of action is unknown. Full therapeutic effect is reached in about 4 days to 3 weeks after initiation of therapy. Pargyline hydrochloride is excreted by the kidneys.

SPECIAL PRECAUTIONS

• Do not use in patients with pheochromocytoma, paranoid schizophrenia, hyperthyroidism, advanced renal failure, or malignant hypertension, or in children under 12 years of age.

• Caution patients to avoid use of any over-the-counter "cold preparation," antihistamines, and also tyramine-containing foods and alcoholic beverages.

• Patients with angina pectoris or coronary artery disease should be warned not to increase their physical activities in response to a diminution in anginal symptoms or an increase in well-being.

• Discontinue pargyline at least 2 weeks before elective surgery.

• Hypoglycemia may be induced; administer with caution to diabetic patients; adjust dosage if necessary.

• Administer with caution to patients with impaired renal function.

• Patients with impaired circulation to vital organs, angina pectoris, coronary artery disease, and cerebral arteriosclerosis should be observed for orthostatic hypotension; reduce dosage if hypotension occurs since cerebral or coronary vessel thrombosis may be precipitated.

• Since hypotensive effects may be augmented by febrile illness, withdraw drug during such diseases.

• Use with caution in patients with impaired renal function; since cumulation may occur.

• Use with caution in patients with hyperactive or hyperexcitable personalities; an undesirable increase in motor activity with restlessness, confusion, agitation, and disorientation may occur; severe psychotic symptoms may be unmasked.

• Use with caution in patients with parkinsonism; symptoms may be increased.

ADVERSE EFFECTS

CNS EFFECTS: dizziness, weakness, fainting, nightmares, hyperexcitability, extrapyramidal symptoms

CARDIOVASCULAR EFFECTS: hypotension, palpitation, congestive heart failure

AUTONOMIC EFFECTS: dry mouth, sweating

GASTROINTESTINAL EFFECTS: mild constipation, increased appetite, nausea, and vomiting

METABOLIC AND ENDOCRINE EFFECTS: fluid retention with or without edema, impotence, delayed ejaculation, gain in weight, decreased blood glucose

HEMATOLOGIC EFFECTS: purpura

ALLERGIC EFFECTS: drug fever

MUSCULOSKELETAL EFFECTS: arthralgia, muscle twitching

OPHTHALMIC EFFECTS: blurred vision

CLINICAL GUIDELINES

ADMINISTRATION:

• Measure liver function periodically, since other monoamine oxidase inhibitors have caused liver damage.

• Monitor renal function, since pargyline is excreted by the kidneys.

EFFECTS:

• Orthostatic hypotension may occur; advise patient.

DRUG INTERACTIONS:

• Do not administer meperidine to patients receiving pargyline.

• Response to all anesthetic agents may be exaggerated.

• The therapeutic response to a variety of drugs may be changed or exaggerated in patients receiving a monoamine oxidase inhibitor; drugs include caffeine, alcohol, antihistamines, barbiturates, chloral hydrate, hypnotics, sedatives, tranquilizers, and narcotics; dosage reduction may be necessary.

• Do not administer with centrally acting sympathomimetic amines such as amphetamine and its derivatives (including those in anorectic preparations) or with peripherally acting sympathomimetic drugs such as ephedrine and its derivatives (commonly found in decongestants, cold remedies, and hay fever preparations).

• Patients should be advised to avoid eating aged cheese (Cheddar, Camembert, and Stilton), processed cheese, beer and wine (particularly Chianti), and other foods which require the action of bacteria or molds for their preparation or preservation because of the presence of pressor substances such as tyramine.

• Patients should also avoid chocolate, yeast extract, avocado, pickled herring, pods of broad beans, ripened bananas, papaya products (including certain meat tenderizers), and chicken livers.

• Cream cheese, ricotta cheese, and cottage cheese may be eaten since they have a low tyramine content.

• Do not administer concurrently with guanethidine; hypertensive reaction may result; guanethidine and reserpine should not be given parenterally during and for at least 1 week following treatment with pargyline.

• Do not administer concurrently with imipramine, amitriptyline, desipramine, nortriptyline, protriptyline, doxepin, or their analogs; concurrent administration has resulted in vascular collapse and hyperthermia which may be fatal. A 2 week drug-free interval should separate therapy with use of these agents.

• Other monoamine oxidase inhibitors administered concurrently may augment the effects of pargyline.

• Methyldopa or dopamine administration in patients receiving pargyline may cause hyperexcitability.

• Pressor effects of pargyline may be potentiated by L-dopa. At least 1 month should separate therapy with these drugs.

OVERDOSAGE/ANTIDOTE:

• Tyramine ingestion may precipitate an abrupt rise in blood pressure which may be accompanied by the following: severe headache, chest pain, profuse sweating, palpitation, tachycardia or bradycardia, visual disturbances, stertorous breathing, coma, and intracranial bleeding which could be fatal.

• Overdosage is characterized by agitation, hallucinations, hyperreflexia, convulsions, and both hypotension and hypertension.

• Treat conservatively; maintain normal temperature, respiration, blood pressure, and fluid and electrolyte balance. Phentolamine may be administered parenterally for treatment of such an acute hypertensive reaction as occurs with ingestion of tyramine.

Phenoxybenzamine Hydrochloride

GENERAL CLINICAL USES

Phenoxybenzamine hydrochloride is used in patients with pheochromocytoma to control episodes of hypertension and sweating. It may also be effective in vasospastic peripheral vascular disease in which venospasm is prominent, such as Raynaud's syndrome, acroyanosis, and frostbite sequelae.

PHARMACOLOGY

Phenoxybenzamine hydrochloride is a long-acting alpha adrenergic receptor blocking agent which can produce and maintain "chemical sympathectomy" by oral administration. It increases blood flow to the skin, mucosa and abdominal viscera, and lowers both supine and erect blood pressure. It has no effect in the parasympathetic system.

SPECIAL PRECAUTIONS

• Do not use in conditions in which a fall in blood pressure may be undesirable.

• Administer with caution to patients with marked cerebral or coronary arteriosclerosis or renal damage.

• The adrenergic blocking effect may aggravate symptoms of respiratory infections.

• Do not use in diseases involving the larger blood vessels where direct-acting vasodilators are preferred therapy.

ADVERSE EFFECTS

RESPIRATORY EFFECTS: nasal congestion

CARDIOVASCULAR EFFECTS: postural hypotension, tachycardia
GASTROINTESTINAL EFFECTS: gastric irritation
METABOLIC AND ENDOCRINE EFFECTS: inhibition of ejaculation

CLINICAL GUIDELINES

ADMINISTRATION:
• Small initial doses should be increased slowly until the desired effect is obtained or the side effects from blockage become troublesome.

EFFECTS:
• After each increase, the patient should be observed at that level for at least 4 days before instituting another increase.

DRUG INTERACTIONS:
• Alcohol can cause an added decrease in blood pressure.
• Avoid concurrent use of epinephrine (and similar drugs used for asthma); may cause a dangerous drop in blood pressure.
• May cause increased effects of antihypertensive drugs, that is, lowering of blood pressure.

OVERDOSAGE/ANTIDOTE:
• The signs of overdosage, largely the result of block of the sympathetic nervous system and of circulating epinephrine, may include postural hypotension resulting in dizziness, faintness, tachycardia (particularly postural), vomiting, lethargy, and shock.
• Treatment consists of discontinuing the drug. Treatment of circulatory failure, if present, is a prime consideration. In cases of mild overdosage, recumbent position with the legs elevated usually restores cerebral circulation. In more severe cases, the usual measures to combat shock should be initiated. Usual pressor agents are not effective. Epinephrine is contraindicated because it stimulates both alpha and beta receptors; since alpha receptors are blocked, the net effect of epinephrine administration is vasodilation and a further drop in blood pressure. The patient may have to be kept supine for 24 hours or more in the case of overdose; the effect of this drug is prolonged. Leg bandages and an abdominal binder may shorten the period of disability. Intravenous infusion of levarterenol may be used to combat severe hypotensive reactions, because it stimulates alpha receptors primarily. Phenoxybenzamine hydrochloride is an alpha adrenergic blocking agent; a sufficient dose of levarterenol bitartrate will overcome this effect.

Phentolamine

GENERAL CLINICAL USES
Phentolamine, administered orally, is useful in preventing or controlling hypertensive episodes in a patient with pheochromocytoma resulting from stress or manipulation during preoperative preparation and surgical excision.

PHARMACOLOGY
Phentolamine, an alpha adrenergic blocking agent, produces a transient decrease in blood pressure. It also causes cardiac and gastrointestinal tract stimulation. Peripheral vasodilatation also occurs. Phentolamine causes a decrease in peripheral resistance and an increase in venous capacity. The dilatation is predominantly due to a direct action on vascular smooth muscle.

SPECIAL PRECAUTIONS
• Do not use in patients with myocardial infarction (recent or old), coronary insufficiency, angina and other evidence of coronary artery disease.
• Safe use in pregnancy and lactation has not been established; weigh benefits against potential hazards.

ADVERSE EFFECTS

CNS EFFECTS: weakness, dizziness, flushing
CARDIOVASCULAR EFFECTS: hypotension, tachycardia, arrhythmias, orthostatic hypotension
RESPIRATORY TRACT EFFECTS: nasal stuffiness
GASTROINTESTINAL EFFECTS: nausea, vomiting, diarrhea

CLINICAL GUIDELINES

ADMINISTRATION:
• Monitor patient continuously during diagnostic procedures.
EFFECTS:
• Tachycardia and cardiac arrhythmias may occur.
DRUG INTERACTIONS:
• Defer concomitant administration of cardiac glycosides until cardiac rhythm returns to normal if tachycardia and arrhythmias occur during administration.
OVERDOSAGE/ANTIDOTE:
• Overdosage may be characterized by a significant drop in blood pressure to dangerous levels resulting in a shocklike condition.
• Maintain blood pressure. Use supportive measures. Do NOT use epinephrine since paradoxical decrease in blood pressure may occur.

Prazosin Hydrochloride

GENERAL CLINICAL USES
Prazosin hydrochloride is indicated for treatment of hypertension; it may be used alone or with a diuretic and/or other antihypertensive drugs as needed.

PHARMACOLOGY
Prazosin hydrochloride, administered orally, acts predominantly as a smooth muscle relaxant; the exact mechanism of the antihypertensive action is unknown.

It does not appear to have alpha adrenergic receptor blocking activity. Blood pressure is lowered in both supine and standing position; the effect is most pronounced on the diastolic blood pressure. Prazosin hydrochloride is extensively metabolized in the liver and excreted mainly in the bile and feces.

SPECIAL PRECAUTIONS
• May cause syncope with sudden loss of consciousness; this is probably due to excessive postural hypotension.
• Syncopal episodes may be preceded by severe tachycardia with heart rates of 120 to 160 beats per minute.
• Hypotension may develop in patients who are also receiving a beta blocker such as propranolol.
• Safe use in pregnancy has not been established; use only if potential benefit outweighs the potential risk to mother and fetus.

ADVERSE EFFECTS
CNS EFFECTS: dizziness, headache, drowsiness, lack of energy, weakness, nervousness, vertigo, depression, paresthesia
RESPIRATORY EFFECTS: dyspnea, epistaxis, nasal congestion
CARDIOVASCULAR EFFECTS: palpitations, syncope, tachycardia
URINARY TRACT EFFECTS: frequency
AUTONOMIC EFFECTS: dry mouth, diaphoresis
GASTROINTESTINAL EFFECTS: nausea, vomiting, diarrhea, constipation, abdominal discomfort and/or pain
METABOLIC AND ENDOCRINE EFFECTS: edema, impotence
DERMATOLOGIC EFFECTS: rash, pruritus
OPHTHALMIC EFFECTS: blurred vision, reddened sclera, pigmentary mottling and serous retinopathy (1 case), cataract development or disappearance
OTIC EFFECTS: tinnitus

CLINICAL GUIDELINES

ADMINISTRATION:
• Caution patients about possible postural hypotension.

EFFECTS:
• Occurrences of dizziness and light-headedness are frequently indications of postural hypotension.

DRUG INTERACTIONS:
• Prazosin hydrochloride has been administered concomitantly, without any adverse effects, with digitalis, digoxin, insulin, chlorpropamide, phenformin, tolazamide, tolbutamide, chlordiazepoxide, diazepam, phenobarbital, and allopurinol. Also, with colchicine, probenecid, procainamide, propranolol, quinidine, propoxyphene, aspirin, indomethacin, and phenylbutazone.

OVERDOSAGE/ANTIDOTE:
• Overdosage may lead to hypotension.
• Accidental ingestion of at least 50 mg in a child 2 years old resulted in profound drowsiness and depressed reflexes. No decrease in blood pressure was noted. Recovery was uneventful.
• Treat hypotension supportively. Normalize heart rate. Keep patient supine. Volume expanders and vasopressors may be necessary.

Propranolol Hydrochloride

GENERAL CLINICAL USES

Propranolol hydrochloride is indicated in the management of hypertension. It is usually used in combination with other drugs, particularly a thiazide diuretic.

Propranolol hydrochloride is also indicated in selected patients with moderate to severe angina who have not responded to concomitant measures such as weight control, rest, cessation of smoking, use of sublingual nitroglycerin, and avoidance of precipitating circumstances.

It may also be used in supraventricular arrhythmias, ventricular tachycardia, tachyarrhythmias of digitalis intoxication, and resistant tachyarrhythmias due to excessive catecholamine action during anesthesia; hypertrophic subaortic stenosis.

PHARMACOLOGY

Propranolol hydrochloride is a beta adrenergic receptor blocking agent, possessing no other autonomic nervous system activity. It exerts its antiarrhythmic effect in concentrations associated with beta adrenergic blockage and this appears to be the mechanism of action. Propranolol hydrochloride decreases heart rate, cardiac output, and blood pressure. It is almost completely absorbed from the gastrointestinal tract; a portion is immediately bound by the liver. A peak effect is noted in 1 to 1½ hours. Propranolol hydrochloride is not significantly dialyzable.

SPECIAL PRECAUTIONS

• Do not use in patients with bronchial asthma; allergic rhinitis during the pollen season; sinus bradycardia and greater than first degree block; cardiogenic shock; right ventricular failure secondary to pulmonary hypertension; congestive heart failure unless the failure is secondary to a tachyarrhythmia treatable with propranolol; with adrenergic augmenting psychotropic drugs (including MAO-inhibitors), and during the second week withdrawal period from such drugs.
• In patients with no history of cardiac failure, continued depression of the myocardium over a period of time can, in some cases, lead to cardiac failure; it has been observed rarely with propranolol hydrochloride therapy.
• In patients with angina pectoris, there have been reports of exacerbation of angi-

na, and, is some cases, myocardial infarction following abrupt discontinuance of propranolol therapy. Always discontinue this drug gradually.

• In patients with thyrotoxicosis special consideration should be given to propranolol's potential for aggravating congestive heart failure.

• Propranolol may mask the clinical signs of developing or continuing hyperthyroidism or complications and give a false impression of improvement; abrupt withdrawal may be followed by an exacerbation of symptoms of hyperthyroidism, including thyroid storm; withdraw patient from propranolol slowly.

• In several patients with Wolff-Parkinson-White syndrome, the tachycardia was replaced by a severe bradycardia requiring a demand pacemaker; in one case this resulted after an initial dose of propranolol hydrochloride, 5 mg.

• In patients anesthetized with agents that require catecholamine release for maintenance of adequate function, beta blockade will impair the desired muscle contraction effect; propranolol should be titrated carefully when administered for arrhythmias occurring during anesthesia.

• In patients prone to nonallergic bronchospasm (e.g., chronic bronchitis, emphysema), propranolol should be administered with caution since it may block bronchodilatation produced by endogenous or exogenous catecholamine stimulation of beta receptors.

• Because of its beta adrenergic blocking activity, propranolol may prevent the appearance of premonitory signs and symptoms (pulse rate and pressure changes) of acute hypoglycemia in diabetics and patients subject to hypoglycemia; hypoglycemia attacks may be accompanied by a precipitous elevation of blood pressure.

• Safe use in pregnancy has not been established; weigh use in pregnancy or in women of childbearing potential against the possible risks to the mother and/or fetus.

ADVERSE EFFECTS

CNS EFFECTS: light-headedness; mental depression manifested by insomnia, lassitude, weakness, fatigue; reversible mental depression progressing to catatonia; visual disturbances; hallucinations; and an acute reversible syndrome characterized by disorientation for time and place, short-term memory loss, emotional lability, slightly clouded sensorium; decreased performance on neuropsychometrics, paresthesias of hands

RESPIRATORY EFFECTS: bronchospasm, pharyngitis

CARDIOVASCULAR EFFECTS: bradycardia, congestive heart failure, intensification of A-V block, hypotension, arterial insufficiency usually of the Raynaud type, thrombocytopenic purpura

GASTROINTESTINAL EFFECTS: nausea, vomiting, epigastric distress, abdominal cramping, diarrhea, constipation

HEMATOLOGIC EFFECTS: agranulocytosis, nonthrombocytopenic purpura, thrombocytopenic purpura

ALLERGIC EFFECTS: erythematous rash, fever combined with aching and sore throat; laryngospasm and respiratory distress

DERMATOLOGIC EFFECTS: reversible alopecia

CLINICAL GUIDELINES

ADMINISTRATION:

• In patients undergoing major surgery, beta blockage impairs the ability of the heart to respond to reflex stimuli; withdraw propranolol 48 hours prior to surgery.

• In cases of emergency surgery, since propranolol is a competitive inhibitor of beta receptor agonists, its effects can be reversed by administration of such agents, e.g., isoproterenol or levarterenol; such patients may be subject to protracted severe hypotension.

EFFECTS:

• Elevated BUN occurs in patients with severe heart disease.

• Elevated SGOT, alkaline phosphatase, and lactic dehydrogenase may occur.

DRUG INTERACTIONS:

• Propranolol hydrochloride and digitalis are additive in depressing A-V conduction, resulting in bradycardia.

• Patients receiving catecholamine-depleting drugs such as reserpine should be closely observed if propranolol is administered; hypotension may occur.

• Thyroid function tests are not distorted.

• The added catecholamine-blocking action of this drug may then produce an excessive reduction of the resting sympathetic nervous system; hypotension and/or marked bradycardia or orthostatic hypotension may occur.

OVERDOSAGE/ANTIDOTE:

• Overdosage is characterized by bradycardia, cardiac failure, hypotension, and bronchospasm.

• Treat bradycardia with atropine (0.25 to 1.0 mg); if there is no response to vagal blockage, administer isoproterenol cautiously. Treat cardiac failure with digitalization and diuretics. Treat hypotension with vasopresssors, e.g., levarterenol or epinephrine, and bronchospasm with isoproterenol and aminophylline.

Trimethaphan Camsylate

GENERAL CLINICAL USES

Trimethaphan camsylate is indicated for the production of controlled hypotension during surgery, for acute control of blood pressure in hypertensive emergencies, in the emergency treatment of pulmonary edema.

PHARMACOLOGY

Trimethaphan camsylate, administered intravenously, produces ganglionic blockade by occupying receptor sites on the ganglion cells and by stabilizing the postsynaptic membranes against the action of acetylcholine liberated from the presynaptic nerve endings.

Trimethaphan camsylate also exerts a direct peripheral vasodilator effect; the vasodilation results in the lowering of the blood pressure. This compound also liberates histamine.

A systolic blood pressure of 100 mm will usually be attained within 10 minutes after stopping administration.

SPECIAL PRECAUTIONS

• Do not use in those conditions in which hypotension may subject the patient to undue risk, e.g., uncorrected anemia, hypovolemia, shock, asphyxia, or uncorrected respiratory insufficiency.

• Inadequate availability of fluids and inability to replace blood for technical reasons may constitute a contraindication.

• Use in surgery or medical indications should be limited to physicians with proper training in this technique. Adequate monitoring equipment, oxygen, and personnel should be available.

CLINICAL GUIDELINES

ADMINISTRATION:

• Always dilute before use; prepare fresh; discard any unused portions.

• Dilute with 5% Dextrose Injection, USP; use of other dilutents is not reccommended since experience has not been reported.

- Position patient to avoid cerebral anoxia.
- Terminate administration in surgical use prior to wound closure in order to permit blood pressure to return to normal.

EFFECTS:

- This drug has a specific effect on the pupil; consequently, pupillary dilatation does not necessarily indicate anoxia or the depth of anesthesia.

DRUG INTERACTIONS:

- When administered concurrently with antihypertensive agents and anesthetics, especially spinal anesthetics, enhanced hypotension may occur.
- Diuretics may markedly enhance the responses evoked by ganglionic blocking drugs.

OVERDOSAGE/ANTIDOTE:

- Overdosage is characterized by enhanced pharmacologic effects, i.e., hypotension.
- Vasopressor agents may be used to correct undesirable low blood pressure. Phenylephrine hydrochloride or mephentermine sulfate should be tried initially; norepinephrine should be reserved for refractory cases.

Diuretic Agents

GENERAL CLINICAL USES

The diuretic agents are useful as adjunctive therapy for treating edema associated with congestive heart failure, hepatic cirrhosis, corticosteroid and estrogen therapies, and renal dysfunction.

The diuretic agents are classified according to their mechanism of action into the following groups:

1. Thiazides and related compounds
2. Carbonic anhydrase inhibitors
3. Mercurial compounds
4. Osmotic diuretics
5. Others (ethacrynate sodium, furosemide, spironolactone, triamterene)

Thiazides and Related Diuretic Agents

SPECIFIC PRODUCTS AND DOSAGES

Therapy should be individualized depending upon the patient's response. To obtain maximal therapeutic response, the dosage should be titrated. Excessive dosage may cause profound diuresis with resultant water and electrolyte depletion.

GENERIC NAME	TRADE NAME	ROUTE OF ADMIN.	USUAL DAILY DOSAGE	
			ADULTS	CHILDREN
bendroflumethiazide	NATURETIN RAUZIDE*	po	**Edema:** 5–20 mg od **Hypertension:** 5–20 mg/day	Not established
benzthiazide	(G)† AQUATAG EXNA	po	**Edema:** 50–200 mg od **Hypertension:** initially 50–200 mg/day, then 25 mg bid to 50 mg tid	1–4 mg/kg/day divided in 3 doses
chlorothiazide	(G) DIURIL	po	**Edema:** 0.5–1.0 gm od, bid **Hypertension:** 0.5–2 gm/day in divided doses	10–15 mg/lb/day divided in 2 doses
chlorothiazide sodium	DIURIL Intravenous Solution	iv	**Edema:** 0.5–1.0 gm od, bid	Not recommended
chlorthalidone	HYGROTON	po	**Edema:** 50–200 mg/day **Hypertension:** 25–100 mg/day	2 mg/kg 3 times/week
cyclothiazide	ANHYDRON	po	**Edema:** 1–2 mg/day **Hypertension:** 2 mg bid or tid	0.02–0.04 mg/kg/day
hydrochlorothiazide	(G) ESIDRIX ESIMIL* HYDRODIURIL ORETIC	po	**Edema:** 25–200 mg od **Hypertension:** 50–100 mg od, then 25–100 mg/day	1 mg/lb/day divided in 2 doses Less than 6 mos.: up to 1.5 mg/lb/day divided in 2 doses
hydroflumethiazide	DIUCARDIN SALURON	po	**Edema:** 25–200 mg/day **Hypertension:** 50–100 mg bid; max 200 mg/day	1 mg/kg/day as a single dose
methyclothiazide	AQUATENSEN ENDURON LEXXOR	po	**Edema:** 2.5–10 mg/day **Hypertension:** Not established	0.05–0.2 mg/kg/day as a single dose
metolazone	ZAROXOLYN	po	**Edema:** 5–20 mg/day **Hypertension:** 2.5–5 mg/day	Not established
polythiazide	RENESE	po	**Edema:** 1–4 mg/day **Hypertension:** 2–4 mg/day	0.02–0.08 mg/kg/day as a single dose

*Contains more than one active ingredient.
†(G) designates availability as a generic product.

(continued facing page)

GENERIC NAME	TRADE NAME	ROUTE OF ADMIN.	USUAL DAILY DOSAGE	
			ADULTS	CHILDREN
quinethazone	HYDROMOX	po	**Edema:** 50–100 mg/day **Hypertension:** 50–200 mg/day	Not established
trichlormethiazide	(G) METAHYDRIN NAQUA	po	**Edema:** 1–4 mg/day in 1 or 2 doses **Hypertension:** 2–4 mg/day in 1 or 2 doses	0.07 mg/kg/day as a single dose or divided in 1 or 2 doses

PHARMACOLOGY

The thiazides have both diuretic and antihypertensive activities. The mechanism of antidiuretic activity is by interference with electrolyte reabsorption in the renal tubules causing an increased excretion of sodium and chloride. This natriuresis causes a secondary loss of potassium and bicarbonate. The thiazides enhance the tubular reabsorption of uric acid. The onset of diuretic action is about 2 hours, the peak effect at 4–6 hours, and the action persists for approximately 6 to 12 hours. Following intravenous administration, diuresis occurs in about 15 minutes; maximal effect occurs in 30 minutes.

The exact mechanism of antihypertensive action of the thiazides may be due to a direct dilating action on the arterioles.

The thiazides appear in the milk of nursing mothers. They also cross the placental barrier and appear in cord blood.

SPECIAL PRECAUTIONS

• Diuresis should not be induced with any diuretic agent in patients with benign prostatic hypertrophy; distention of the bladder may precipitate obstruction.
• Determine serum electrolytes (Na, K, Cl), BUN, uric acid, and glucose periodically; this is particularly important if the patient is vomiting.

• Do not administer to patients with anuria or those hypersensitive to these drugs or sulfonamide-derived drugs.
• Safe use in pregnancy has not been established.
• Diuretics do not prevent development of toxemia of pregnancy.
• Administer cautiously in patients with severe renal disease, impaired hepatic function, or progressive liver disease.
• Hypokalemia may develop during brisk diuresis, particularly when severe cirrhosis is present or if ACTH or corticosteroids are used concomitantly.
• Hypokalemia can exaggerate response of heart to toxic effects of digitalis.
• Avoid hypokalemia by potassium supplements, dietary or otherwise.
• Do not use in patients who develop anuria or progressive renal dysfunction, including increasing oliguria and increasing azotemia or in patients who develop hyperkalemia.
• Do not use in patients with pre-existing elevated serum potassium, as may be seen in impaired renal function.
• Before using in pregnant patients, weigh benefits versus possible hazards to fetus. Hazards include fetal or neonatal jaundice, thrombocytopenia, and possibly other adverse reactions which have occurred in the adult.

ADVERSE EFFECTS

CNS EFFECTS: dizziness, vertigo, paresthesias, headache, xanthopsia

RESPIRATORY EFFECTS: respiratory distress including pneumonitis

CARDIOVASCULAR EFFECTS: orthostatic hypotension

GASTROINTESTINAL EFFECTS: anorexia, gastric irritation, nausea, vomiting, cramping, diarrhea, constipation, pancreatitis, sialadenitis

METABOLIC AND ENDOCRINE EFFECTS: hypoglycemia, glucosuria, hyperuricemia

HEPATIC EFFECTS: intrahepatic cholestatic jaundice

HEMATOLOGIC EFFECTS: leukopenia, agranulocytosis, thrombocytopenia, aplastic anemia

ALLERGIC EFFECTS: purpura, photosensitivity, rash, urticaria, necrotizing angiitis, fever, anaphylactic reactions

OPHTHALMIC EFFECTS: transient blurred vision

CLINICAL GUIDELINES

ADMINISTRATION:
• Administer thiazide diuretics in the morning to obtain diuresis during the day and avoid disturbing the patient's nighttime rest.
• Instruct patients to take food that is high in potassium (e.g., bananas, raisins, grapes).

EFFECTS:
• Observe patients for clinical signs of fluid or electrolyte imbalance, namely, hyponatremia, hypochloremic alkalosis, and hypokalemia.
• Calcium excretion is decreased by thiazides.
• Asymptomatic hyperuricemia may develop.

DRUG INTERACTIONS:
• Thiazides may potentiate the action of other antihypertensive drugs; potentiation occurs with ganglionic or peripheral adrenergic blocking agents. Dosage adjustment may be required.
• Lithium carbonate should not be given with diuretics because of a high risk of lithium toxicity.
• Insulin requirements in diabetic patients receiving thiazides may be changed.
• Thiazide drugs may increase patient's response to tubocurarine.
• Thiazides may decrease arterial responsiveness to norepinephrine. Thiazides may decrease serum PBI levels without signs of thyroid disturbances.

OVERDOSAGE/ANTIDOTE:
• Symptoms of overdosage include diuresis, lethargy which may progress to coma, depression of respiration and cardiovascular function; irritation and hypermotility may occur.
• No specific antidote is known. Use supportive therapy and restore electrolyte balance.

Carbonic Anhydrase Inhibiting Diuretics

SPECIFIC PRODUCTS AND DOSAGES

Therapy should be individualized depending upon the patient's response. To obtain maximal therapeutic response, the dosage should be titrated. Excessive dosage may cause profound diuresis with resultant water and electrolyte depletion. Careful medical supervision is required.

GENERIC NAME	TRADE NAME	ROUTE OF ADMIN.	USUAL DAILY DOSAGE FOR DIURESIS IN ADULTS
acetazolamide	(G)* DIAMOX HYDRAZOL	po	250–500 mg/day (5 mg/kg)
		ophth.	See Chapter 11, *Drugs Affecting the Eye,* page 451
acetazolamide sodium	DIAMOX Parenteral	iv	250–500 mg/day (5 mg/kg)
dichlorphenamide	DARANIDE ORATROL	po ophth.	75–200 mg/day See Chapter 11, *Drugs Affecting the Eye,* page 451
ethoxzolamide	CARDRASE ETHAMIDE	po ophth.	62.5–250 mg/day See Chapter 11, *Drugs Affecting the Eye,* page 451
methazolamide	NEPTAZANE	po ophth.	50–100 mg/day See Chapter 11, *Drugs Affecting the Eye,* page 451

*(G) designates availability as a generic product.

PHARMACOLOGY

Acetazolamide, dichlorphenamide ethoxzolamide, and methazolamide, potent anhydrase inhibitors, promote diuresis by inhibiting the enzyme which catalyzes the reversible reaction involving the hydration of carbon dioxide and the dehydration of carbonic acid in the kidney. The resulting diuresis also carries out sodium and potassium; urinary pH rises.

These drugs are also used to control fluid secretion in some types of glaucoma. For additional information, see Chapter 11, *Drugs Affecting the Eye,* page 451.

SPECIAL PRECAUTIONS

• Diuresis should not be induced with any diuretic agent in patients with benign prostatic hypertrophy; distention of the bladder may precipitate obstruction.
• Determine serum electrolytes (Na, K, Cl), BUN, uric acid, and glucose periodically; this is particularly important if the patient is vomiting.

• Do not administer to patients with anuria or to patients hypersensitive to this drug or related drugs.
• Safe use in pregnancy has not been established.
• Do not administer to patients with depressed sodium and/or potassium levels, with marked kidney or liver disease or dysfunction, adrenal failure, and hyperchloremic acidosis.
• Do not administer for a prolonged period to patients with glaucoma.

ADVERSE EFFECTS

CNS EFFECTS: paresthesias, tingling feeling in the extremities, drowsiness, confusion, convulsions, flaccid paralysis
RENAL EFFECTS: polyuria, hematuria, glucosuria
GASTROINTESTINAL EFFECTS: anorexia, acidotic state, melena
HEPATIC EFFECTS: hepatic insufficiency
HEMATOLOGIC EFFECTS: agranulocytosis, thrombocytopenia

ALLERGIC EFFECTS: urticaria
OPHTHALMIC EFFECTS: transient myopia

CLINICAL GUIDELINES

ADMINISTRATION:
• Increasing the dose does not increase diuresis but may increase drowsiness and/or paresthesias.
• For parenteral administration, the reconstituted drug will retain potency for 2 weeks, or, if refrigerated, 4 weeks.
• Since the product contains no preservative, use within 24 hours.

• Intramuscular administration may be employed but it is painful because of the alkaline pH of the solution.
EFFECTS:
• Note that since these drugs are sulfonamides, all adverse reactions and precautions relating to sulfonamides should be considered.
OVERDOSAGE/ANTIDOTE:
• Overdosage consists of an exaggeration of the adverse effects. Profound diuresis occurs.
• There is no known antidote. Treat supportively.

Osmotic Diuretics

SPECIFIC PRODUCTS AND DOSAGES
Therapy should be individualized depending upon the patient's response. To obtain maximal therapeutic response, the dosage should be titrated. Excessive dosage may cause profound diuresis with resultant water and electrolyte depletion. Careful medical supervision is required.

GENERIC NAME	TRADE NAME	ROUTE OF ADMIN.	USUAL DAILY DOSAGE FOR DIURESIS IN ADULTS
glycerin	(G)* GLYROL OSMOGLYN 50%	po	1–1.5 gm/kg 1–1.5 hr. prior to surgery; See Chapter 11, *Drugs Affecting the Eye*, page 452
mannitol	(G) OSMITROL	iv	50–200 gm infusion/24 hr.
urea	(G) UREAPHIL	iv	1–1.5 gm/kg **Children:** 0.5–1.5 gm/kg

*(G) designates availability as a generic product.

PHARMACOLOGY
Glycerin is an orally administered osmotic agent which reduces intraocular pressure. Both mannitol and urea also have this action.

Mannitol and urea, obligatory diuretics, induce diuresis by elevating the osmolarity of the glomerular filtrate and by hindering tubular reabsorption of water. Increased excretion of sodium and chloride also occurs.

SPECIAL PRECAUTIONS

• Diuresis should not be induced with any diuretic agent in patients with benign prostatic hypertrophy; distention of the bladder may precipitate obstruction.

• Determine serum electrolytes (Na, K, Cl), BUN, uric acid, and glucose periodically; this is particularly important if the patient is vomiting.

• Do not use in patients hypersensitive to these drugs or related drugs.

• Safe use in pregnancy has not been established.

• Urea is indicated only for reduction of intracranial pressure in control of cerebral edema and of intraocular pressure.

• Do not administer urea to patients with severely impaired renal function, active intracranial bleeding, or marked dehydration or frank liver failure.

• Urea may cause electrolyte depletion resulting in hyponatremia and hypokalemia.

• Use cautiously in patients with liver or renal impairment.

• With mannitol or urea infusion, renal function must be closely monitored; osmotic nephrosis, a reversible vacuolization of the tubules, may proceed to severe irreversible nephrosis.

• Prior to mannitol or urea infusion, carefully evaluate the cardiovascular status of the patient, since sudden expansion of the extracellular fluid may lead to fulminating congestive heart failure.

ADVERSE EFFECTS

CNS EFFECTS: glycerin—headache; urea—headache, syncope, disorientation; mannitol—headache, convulsions, chills, dizziness, fever

RESPIRATORY EFFECTS: mannitol—pulmonary congestion

CARDIOVASCULAR EFFECTS: mannitol—thrombophlebitis, hypotension, hypertension, tachycardia, anginalike chest pains

RENAL EFFECTS: mannitol—urinary retention

AUTONOMIC EFFECTS: mannitol—dry mouth

GASTROINTESTINAL EFFECTS: glycerin—occasional nausea, vomiting; urea—nausea, vomiting; mannitol—thirst, nausea, and vomiting

METABOLIC AND ENDOCRINE EFFECTS: mannitol—fluid and electrolyte imbalance, acidosis, electrolyte loss

ALLERGIC EFFECTS: mannitol—rhinitis

OPHTHALMIC EFFECTS: mannitol—blurred vision

CLINICAL GUIDELINES

ADMINISTRATION:

• Accidental extravasation may cause reactions ranging from mild irritation to tissue necrosis.

• With urea administration by infusion, increased capillary bleeding may occur if infusion rate exceeds 60 drops per minute.

• Do not administer urea through the same infusion set used for blood.

• Do not administer electrolyte-free mannitol solution conjointly with blood. If blood is given simultaneously, at least 20 mEq of sodium chloride should be added to each liter of mannitol solution to avoid pseudoagglutination.

• Insert an indwelling urethral catheter in comatose patients.

• When exposed to low temperatures, solutions of mannitol may crystallize; warm in 50°C water bath to recrystallize. Use filter with infusion of 20% mannitol solution since crystals may form.

EFFECTS:

• Use of hypothermia with urea infusion may increase the risk of venous thrombosis and hemoglobinuria.

• Mannitol infusion may lower serum sodium concentration and aggravate preexisting hyponatremia.

OVERDOSAGE/ANTIDOTE:
- Overdosage consists of an exaggeration
- of the clinical and adverse effects.
- There is no known antidote.

Mercurial Diuretics

SPECIFIC PRODUCTS AND DOSAGES
Therapy should be individualized depending upon the patient's response. To obtain maximal therapeutic response, the dosage should be titrated. Excessive dosage may cause profound diuresis with resultant water and electrolyte depletion. Careful medical supervision is required.

GENERIC NAME	TRADE NAME	ROUTE OF ADMIN.	USUAL DAILY DOSAGE FOR DIURESIS IN ADULTS
mercaptomerin sodium	MERCUHYDRIN THIOMERIN	im/sc	0.2–2 cc/day
merethoxylline procaine	DICURIN Procaine	im/sc	0.5–2 cc/day

PHARMACOLOGY
The mercurial diuretic agents depress the tubular reabsorption of sodium and chloride, and secondarily water. They usually increase potassium excretion. The mercurial compounds are rapidly absorbed and rapidly excreted by the kidneys.

SPECIAL PRECAUTIONS
- Diuresis should not be induced with any diuretic agent in patients with benign prostatic hypertrophy; distention of the bladder may precipitate obstruction.
- Determine serum electrolytes (Na, K, Cl), BUN, uric acid, and glucose periodically; this is particularly important if the patient is vomiting.
- Do not administer to patients with anuria or to patients hypersensitive to this drug or related drugs.
- Safe use in pregnancy has not been established.
- Do not administer to patients with acute nephritis or ulcerative colitis, or with evidence of dehydration or hypersensitivity to mercury.
- Do not use mercaptomerin sodium solution if it has color or a precipitate.
- Do not administer merethoxylline procaine to patients hypersensitive to mercury, procaine, or theophylline; do not administer to patients who are sensitive to other drugs containing the p-aminobenzoic acid group such as benzocaine, tetracaine, or butacaine.

ADVERSE EFFECTS
CNS EFFECTS: flushing face, chills, headache
GASTROINTESTINAL EFFECTS: gastrointestinal disturbances, nausea, vomiting, diarrhea
METABOLIC AND ENDOCRINE EFFECTS: rarely hyperuricemia

HEMATOLOGIC EFFECTS: neutropenia, agranulocytosis

ALLERGIC EFFECTS: urticaria, occasional anaphylactic reactions

DERMATOLOGIC EFFECTS: cutaneous eruptions, pruritus

LOCAL EFFECTS: ecchymoses, induration

CLINICAL GUIDELINES

ADMINISTRATION:

• Administer merethoxylline procaine with caution to patients receiving sulfonamides.

• Do not administer intravenously.

EFFECTS:

• Watch patient for salt deficiency, especially in hot weather, dietary sodium should be reduced but not severely restricted.

• Sodium deficiency may be indicated by leg muscle cramps.

• Watch elderly patients closely for signs of excessive dehydration, particularly if the patient has been treated for a prolonged time and has had salt restricted.

• If diuresis does not occur in patients previously responsive, call to physician's attention immediately.

OVERDOSAGE/ANTIDOTE:

• Overdosage with the mercurial compounds results in severe disturbances of electrolyte balance.

• Dimercaprol (BAL) has been shown to reduce the acute toxicity of the mercury ion; it may or may not be of aid when the concentration of mercury in the tissues is very low.

Other Diuretic Agents

SPECIFIC PRODUCTS AND DOSAGES

Therapy should be individualized depending upon the patient's response. To obtain maximal therapeutic response, the dosage should be titrated. Excessive dosage may cause profound diuresis with resultant water and electrolyte depletion. Careful medical supervision is required.

GENERIC NAME	TRADE NAME	ROUTE OF ADMIN.	USUAL DOSAGE	
			ADULTS	CHILDREN
ethacrynate sodium	EDECRIN Sodium	iv	50 mg/day or 0.5–1.0 mg/kg/day	Not established
ethacrynic acid	EDECRIN	po	50–200 mg/day	25 mg/day
furosemide	LASIX	po iv/im	20–80 mg/day 20–80 mg/day	2 mg/kg/day 1–2 mg/kg/day
spironolactone	ALDACTONE	po	25–200 mg/day divided doses	3.3 mg/kg/day in in divided doses
triamterene	DYRENIUM	po	100–300 mg/day in divided doses	Not established

Ethacrynate Sodium
Ethacrynic Acid

PHARMACOLOGY

Ethacrynic acid and the sodium salt act similarly to furosemide; they inhibit the reabsorption of sodium in the proximal tubules, distal tubules, and loop of Henle. Following oral administration, diuresis begins promptly, usually within 1 hour, and lasts as long as 8 hours. After intravenous administration, diuresis begins in 5 minutes and lasts approximately 2 hours.

SPECIAL PRECAUTIONS

• Diuresis should not be induced with any diuretic agent in patients with benign prostatic hypertrophy; distention of the bladder may precipitate obstruction.
• Determine serum electrolytes (Na, K, Cl), BUN, uric acid, and glucose periodically; this is particularly important if the patient is vomiting.
• Do not use in patients hypersensitive to this drug or related drugs.
• Safe use in pregnancy has not been established.
• Hypoproteinemia may reduce the effectiveness of ethacrynic acid.
• Do not administer to patients with anuria.

ADVERSE EFFECTS

CNS EFFECTS: vertigo, headache, fever, chills, fatigue, apprehension, confusion
RENAL EFFECTS: hyperuricemia, acute gout, hematuria
GASTROINTESTINAL EFFECTS: anorexia, abdominal discomfort or pain, dysphagia, nausea, vomiting, diarrhea, bleeding, pancreatitis rarely

METABOLIC AND ENDOCRINE EFFECTS: acute pancreatitis (rare), hypoglycemia with convulsions, hyperglycemia
HEPATIC EFFECTS: jaundice, abnormal liver function
HEMATOLOGIC EFFECTS: agranulocytosis, severe neutropenia, Henoch-Schonlein purpura
DERMATOLOGIC EFFECTS: skin rash
OPHTHALMIC EFFECTS: blurred vision
AUDITORY EFFECTS: deafness, tinnitus, fullness in ears, vertigo

CLINICAL GUIDELINES

ADMINISTRATION:
• Liberalize salt intake and supplementary potassium chloride as necessary.
EFFECTS:
• Note that excessive diuresis may result in dehydration and reduction in blood volume with circulatory collapse; thrombosis and embolism may occur, particularly in elderly patients.
• Ethacrynic acid has produced severe, watery diarrhea in a few patients; if this occurs, discontinue and do not readminister.
• Too vigorous a diuresis with ethacrynic acid may inducean acute hypotensive episode.
DRUG INTERACTIONS:
• Lithium should not be given with diuretics because they reduce renal clearance and add a high risk of lithium toxicity.
• Concomitant administration of ethacrynic acid and antihypertensive agents may require dosage adjustment of the antihypertensive agent; hypotension may occur.
OVERDOSAGE/ANTIDOTE:
• Overdosage is characterized by an exaggeration of the adverse and pharmacological effects.
• There is no known antidote. Discontinue therapy immediately. Treat supportively as indicated.

Furosemide

PHARMACOLOGY

Furosemide inhibits the reabsorption of sodium in the proximal tubules, distal tubules, and loop of Henle. Following oral administration of furosemide, diuresis usually begins in about 1 hour and lasts 6 to 8 hours. After intravenous administration, diuresis begins in about 5 minutes, reaches a peak within 30 minutes, and lasts approximately 2 hours.

SPECIAL PRECAUTIONS

• Diuresis should not be induced with any diuretic agent in patients with benign prostatic hypertrophy; distention of the bladder may precipitate obstruction.

• Determine serum electrolytes (Na, K, Cl), BUN, uric acid, and glucose periodically; this is particularly important if the patient is vomiting.

• Do not administer to patients with anuria.

• Safe use in pregnancy has not been established.

• Do not administer to patients hypersensitive to this drug or related drugs.

• Do not institute therapy in patients with hepatic coma or in states of electrolyte depression until basic condition is controlled.

ADVERSE EFFECTS

CNS EFFECTS: paresthesias, weakness, fatigue, light-headedness, dizziness
CARDIOVASCULAR EFFECTS: postural hypotension
RENAL EFFECTS: bladder spasm, urinary frequency, marked diuresis
AUTONOMIC EFFECTS: increased perspiration
GASTROINTESTINAL EFFECTS: nausea, vomiting, diarrhea
METABOLIC AND ENDOCRINE EFFECTS: edema, dehydration, hypoglycemia
HEMATOLOGIC EFFECTS: anemia, leukopenia, aplastic anemia, thrombocytopenia with purpura, rare agranulocytosis
DERMATOLOGIC EFFECTS: dermatitis including urticaria, exfoliative dermatitis, erythema multiforme
OPHTHALMIC EFFECTS: blurred vision
AUDITORY EFFECTS: reversible deafness and tinnitus

CLINICAL GUIDELINES

ADMINISTRATION:
• Parenteral administration should be reserved for patients where oral medication is not practical.
EFFECTS:
• Note that excessive diuresis may result in dehydration and reduction in blood volume with circulatory collapse; thrombosis and embolism may occur, particularly in elderly patients.
• Monitor patients receiving furosemide for occurrence of blood dyscrasias, liver damage, or other idiosyncratic reactions.
• Asymptomatic hyperuricemia can occur and gout can be precipitated.
• Since furosemide can cause excessive potassium loss, digitalis toxicity may be precipitated in patients receiving digitalis glycosides.
• Watch for potassium imbalance in patients receiving potassium-depleting steroids concomitantly with furosemide.
DRUG INTERACTIONS:
• Furosemide potentiates the hypotensive circulation, blood vessels, and blood effect of antihypertensive medications and may enhance the nephrotoxicity of cephaloridine.
• In patients receiving high doses of salicylates, as in rheumatic diseases, concurrent administration of furosemide may cause salicylate toxicity at low doses because of competitive renal excretion.

• Lithium should not be given with diuretics because they reduce renal clearance and add a high risk of lithium toxicity.

OVERDOSAGE/ANTIDOTE:

• Overdosage is characterized by an exaggeration of adverse and pharmacologic effects.

• There is no known antidote. Treat supportively as required.

Spironolactone

PHARMACOLOGY

Spironolactone, a physiological antagonist of aldosterone, acts in the distal convoluted renal tubules. Spironolactone does not appear to elevate uric acid or interfere with carbohydrate metabolism. The potassium-sparing action of spironolactone is outstanding. Maximal response may not occur for 2 or more weeks.

SPECIAL PRECAUTIONS

• Diuresis should not be induced with any diuretic agent in patients with benign prostatic hypertrophy; distention of the bladder may precipitate obstruction.

• Determine serum electrolytes (Na, K, Cl), BUN, uric acid, and glucose periodically; this is particularly important if the patient is vomiting.

• Do not use in patients hypersensitive to this drug or related drugs.

• Safe use in pregnancy has not been established.

• Spironolactone should not be administered to patients with acute renal insufficiency, rapidly progressing impairment of renal function, or hyperkalemia.

• Potassium supplementation in patients receiving spironolactone may cause hyperkalemia.

• Hyponatremia may be caused or aggravated by concomitant administration of spironolactone.

• BUN may increase in patients with pre-existing renal impairment.

• Contraindicated in patients with anuria.

ADVERSE EFFECTS

CNS EFFECTS: drowsiness, lethargy, mental confusion, headache, drug fever, ataxia

GASTROINTESTINAL EFFECTS: diarrhea

METABOLIC AND ENDOCRINE EFFECTS: gynecomastia, inability to achieve or maintain erection, mild andregenic manifestations

DERMATOLOGIC EFFECTS: maculopapular rash, erythematous cutaneous eruptions, urticaria

CLINICAL GUIDELINES

ADMINISTRATION:

• Maximal effects may not occur before 5 days, then adjust dosage to optimal maintenance level.

EFFECTS:

• Note that excessive diuresis may result in dehydration and reduction in blood volume with circulatory collapse; thrombosis and embolism may occur, particularly in elderly patients.

DRUG INTERACTIONS:

• Spironolactone when given with other diuretics may cause hyponatremia.

• Spironolactone potentiates the action of other antihypertensive drugs. Dosages of these drugs, particularly the ganglionic blocking drugs, should be reduced at least 50 percent when spironolactone is administered.

• Spironolactone and triamterene are usually not used concomitantly.

OVERDOSAGE/ANTIDOTE:
• Overdosage is characterized by exaggeration of the adverse and pharmacologic effects.
• There is no known antidote. Treat supportively as indicated.

Triamterene

PHARMACOLOGY

Triamterene inhibits the reabsorption of sodium ions in exchange for potassium and hydrogen ions in the distal renal tubules. This is a direct effect on the renal tubule and not by competitive aldosterone antagonism. Onset of action is 2 to 4 hours. However, maximal clinical response may not be seen for several days. Triamterene has potassium-sparing actions.

SPECIAL PRECAUTIONS

• Diuresis should not be induced with any diuretic agent in patients with benign prostatic hypertrophy; distention of the bladder may precipitate obstruction.
• Determine serum electrolytes (Na, K, Cl), BUN, uric acid, and glucose periodically; this is particularly important if the patient is vomiting.
• Do not use in patients hypersensitive to this drug or related drugs.
• Safe use in pregnancy has not been established.
• Potassium supplementation in patients receiving triamterene may cause hyperkalemia.
• Triamterene should not be given to patients with severe or progressive kidney disease except nephrosis, with severe hepatic disease, or patients with a pre-existing elevated serum potassium.

• Triamterene can cause mild nitrogen retention which is reversible.
• Triamterene conserves potassium; hyperkalemia may occur.
• Do not administer to patients with anuria.

ADVERSE EFFECTS
CNS EFFECTS: weakness, headache
HEPATIC EFFECTS: liver damage
AUTONOMIC EFFECTS: dry mouth
GASTROINTESTINAL EFFECTS: diarrhea, nausea, vomiting
ALLERGIC EFFECTS: anaphylaxis
DERMATOLOGIC EFFECTS: photosensitivity, rash

CLINICAL GUIDELINES
ADMINISTRATION:
• Patients should be observed regularly for possible occurrence of blood dyscrasias or liver damage.
EFFECTS:
• Note that excessive diuresis may result in dehydration and reduction in blood volume with circulatory collapse; thrombosis and embolism may occur, particularly in elderly patients.
• Blood pressure may decrease; concomitant use of antihypertensive drugs may have an additive effect.
DRUG INTERACTIONS:
• Triamterene and spironolactone are usually not used concomitantly.
• When triamterene is used concurrently with other antihypertensive drugs, reduce dosage of antihypertensive drugs, especially ganglionic blocking agents.
OVERDOSAGE/ANTIDOTE:
• Signs of overdosage include hyperkalemia, nausea, vomiting, and possibly hypotension.
• There is no specific antidote. Treat supportively.

Congestive Heart Failure Agents

GENERAL CLINICAL USES

The digitalis or cardiac glycosides (digitoxin, digoxin, lanatoside C, deslanoside, gitalin, and G-strophanthin) are indicated for use in congestive heart failure, atrial fibrilliation, atrial flutter, paroxysmal atrial tachycardia, cardiogenic shock, and supraventricular tachycardia.

Dobutamine hydrochloride is indicated when parenteral therapy is necessary for inotropic support in the short-term treatment of adults with cardiac decomposition due to depressed contractility.

SPECIFIC PRODUCTS AND DOSAGES

GENERIC NAME	TRADE NAME	ROUTE OF ADMIN.	USUAL DOSAGE FOR DIGITALIZING	
			ADULTS	CHILDREN
deslanoside	CEDILANID-D	im/iv	0.8–1.6 mg/day	Not established
digitalis	(G)* DIGIFORTIS	po	1.2–1.8 gm/day in divided doses	Not established
digitoxin	(G) CRYSTODIGIN	iv	1.2–1.6 mg/day	**Premature and newborn infants:** 0.022 mg/kg/day **Under 1 yr.:** 0.045 mg/kg/day **1–2 yrs.:** 0.04 mg/kg/day **Over 2 yrs.:** 0.03 mg/kg/day
		po	0.05–0.6 mg/day	Not established
digoxin	(G) LANOXIN	po	1.0–1.5 mg/day in divided doses; reduce dose in elderly	**Over 10 yrs.:** 1–1.5 mg/day **2–10 yrs.:** 40–60 mcg/kg/day **1 mo.–2 yrs.:** 60–80 mcg/kg/day **Newborn–1 mo.:** 40–60 mcg/kg/day
		iv/im	0.25–0.50 mg	**Over 10 yrs.:** 0.25–0.5 mg/day in divided doses **2–10 yrs.:** 25–40 mcg/kg/day in divided doses **2 wks.–2 yrs.:** 35–50 mcg/kg/day in divided doses **Premature and newborn:** 25–40 mcg/kg/day in divided doses

*(G) designates availability as a generic product.

(continued facing page)

GENERIC NAME	TRADE NAME	ROUTE OF ADMIN.	USUAL DOSAGE FOR DIGITALIZING	
			ADULTS	CHILDREN
dobutamine hydrochloride	DOBUTREX	iv infusion	2.5–10 mcg/kg/min.	Not established
gitalin	GITALIGIN	po	2.5–6 mg/day in divided doses	Not established
G-strophanthin (ouabain)	(G)	iv	0.25–0.5 mg/day in divided doses	Not established
lanatoside C	CEDILANID	po	10 mg/total in divided doses over 4–5 days	Not established

Digitalis Glycosides

PHARMACOLOGY

Qualitatively, the digitalis or cardiac glycosides have the same effects on the heart, namely, increased force of contraction, increased refractory period of the atrioventricular node; to a lesser degree they affect the sinoatrial node and conduction system via the parasympathetic and sympathetic nervous systems.

Formulations are available for oral, intravenous, and intramuscular administration. For rapid effect, deslanoside, G-strophanthin, digitoxin, and digoxin are available for intravenous and/or intramuscular administration. Following intravenous administration of digitoxin, an effect is noted in 25 minutes to 2 hours, with a maximal effect in 4 to 12 hours. Following oral administration, absorption is complete; effect is noted at a later time.

Digoxin administered intravenously produces an initial effect within 5 to 10 minutes, the action is maximal in 1 to 2 hours. With intramuscular administration, the onset of effect occurs within 30 minutes, the action is maximal in 4 to 6 hours.

Following oral administration the onset of therapeutic effect is 1 to 2 hours and the peak is 6 to 8 hours. Digoxin is excreted by the kidneys unmetabolized when there is significant renal failure. Digoxin is not effectively removed from the body by dialysis, exchange transfusions, or during cardiopulmonary bypass, primarily because of tissue binding.

Lanatoside C, following oral administration, is poorly absorbed. The results are variable.

Deslanoside has an onset of action of about 5 minutes after intravenous administration. The peak effect is noted in 2 to 4 hours. The therapeutic effect persists for 2 to 5 days.

Gitalin is well absorbed following oral administration. Its action is prompt and the rate of elimination or dissipation is relatively rapid.

G-strophanthin when administered intravenously acts more rapidly than any other cardiac glycoside now available. Full digitalis effect is obtained within 2 hours. It is eliminated rapidly and the duration of effect is shorter than that of the glycosides in either *Digitalis lanata* or *Digitalis pur-*

purea. Therefore, cumulation is less likely to occur. Administration is limited to intravenous use since absorption from the gastrointestinal tract is poor and irregular.

SPECIAL PRECAUTIONS

• Toxic effects induced by any digitalis preparation are an absolute contraindication to all other digitalis glycosides.
• Do not use in patients with a history of hypersensitivity to any digitalis preparation or with ventricular fibrillation or ventricular tachycardia unless congestive failure supervenes after a protracted episode not due to digitalis.
• Many of the arrhythmias for which digitalis is advised are identical with those reflecting digitalis intoxication.
• Potassium depletion sensitizes the myocardium to digitalis, and toxicity is apt to develop even with the usual dosage; hypokalemia also tends to reduce the positive inotropic effect of digitalis.
• Patients with acute myocardial infarction, severe pulmonary disease, or far advanced heart failure are apt to be more sensitive to digitalis and more prone to disturbances of rhythm.
• In patients with myxedema, digitalis requirements are less because the excretion rate is decreased and blood levels are significantly higher.
• Patients with incomplete A-V block, especially patients subject to Stokes-Adams attacks, may develop advanced to complete heart block.
• Chronic constrictive pericarditis is apt to respond unfavorably.
• Idiopathic hypertrophic subaortic stenosis must be managed extremely carefully; unless cardiac failure is severe, it is doubtful whether digitalis should be employed.
• Use in pregnancy and lactation only when the potential benefits outweigh the possible risks to fetus and mother. Adverse effects on the fetus have been reported.
• In patients with renal disease, excretion may be delayed; adjust to lower dosage accordingly.
• Electrical conversion of arrhythmias may require adjustment of digitalis dosage.
• Allergy, though rare, may occur. It may not extend to all preparations and another may be tried.
• Use great care if given to a patient who has frequent premature ventricular beats or who has received any preparation of digitalis during the preceding 3 weeks.

ADVERSE EFFECTS

LOCAL EFFECTS: in children, intramuscular administration may result in painful local reactions; adults may also experience pain following intramuscular administration.
CNS EFFECTS: headache, weakness, apathy
CARDIOVASCULAR EFFECTS: arrhythmias, premature ventricular beats, paroxysmal and nonparoxysmal nodal rhythms, A-V dissociation, paroxysmal atrial tachycardia, bradycardia, slowing of pulse
GASTROINTESTINAL EFFECTS: anorexia, nausea, vomiting, diarrhea
METABOLIC AND ENDOCRINE EFFECTS: gynecomastia, uncommon
ALLERGIC EFFECTS: urticaria, rash, rarely
OPHTHALMIC EFFECTS: blurring of vision, diplopia, halo effect, patient may see yellow or blue

CLINICAL GUIDELINES

ADMINISTRATION:
• Monitor ECG and serum potassium levels frequently; evidence of overdosage will generally appear on the ECG as paroxysmal atrial tachycardia or as premature ventricular contraction.
• Administer intravenous preparations

slowly and observe patient closely.

• Reduced dosage should be used in small or elderly patients and in those with renal insufficiency or certain metabolic and electrolyte abnormalities.

• Advise patient to keep drug out of reach of children.

EFFECTS:

• The adverse effects are usually caused by overdosage.

DRUG INTERACTIONS:

• Calcium may produce serious arrhythmias in digitalized patients.

• Drugs producing a potassium loss such as the glucocorticoids and thiazide diuretics may cause serious digitalis toxicity.

• Antacids may interfere with drug absorption.

• Phenobarbital and phenylbutazone increase elimination of digitalis compounds and reduce effectiveness.

OVERDOSAGE/ANTIDOTE:

• Overdosage is characterized by an exaggeration of the adverse effects. In the adult, the initial symptoms are nausea, vomiting, diarrhea, fatigue, excessive slowing of the pulse, (less than 60 beats/minute), A-V block of increased degree which may proceed to complete heart block. Nodular tachyarrhythmias and bigeminal PVC's may also be present. Overdosage in children is characterized initially by cardiac arrhythmias; nausea or vomiting are rare as initial signs.

• Discontinue drug. Therapy may include gastric lavage, if indicated, and administration of potassium chloride, saline cathartics, atropine, and nitroglycerin. Potassium chloride in divided doses totaling 4 to 6 gm are used for adults if renal function is adequate. Potassium may be administered intravenously as a solution in 5% dextrose in water, 40 to 100 mEq at a rate of 40 mEq/hr. Monitor ECG to avoid potassium intoxi-

cation. Chelating agents to bind calcium may be used to counteract the arrhythmic effect of digitalis intoxication. EDTA, 4 gm dissolved in 500 ml of 5% dextrose in water, may be used. Other counteracting agents include quinidine, procainamide, and adrenergic beta blocking agents.

Dobutamine Hydrochloride

PHARMACOLOGY

Dobutamine hydrochloride stimulates the beta receptors of the heart, increasing cardiac output but not markedly increasing heart rate. The cardiac stroke volume is usually increased.

Dobutamine hydrochloride produces an effect within 1 to 2 minutes, but 10 minutes may be required to obtain the peak effect. Dobutamine hydrochloride is excreted in the urine as conjugates of dobutamine and 3-O-methyl dobutamine.

SPECIAL PRECAUTIONS

• Be aware that a marked increase in heart rate or blood pressure, especially systolic pressure, may occur.

• Patients with atrial fibrillation are at risk of developing rapid ventricular response.

• Patients with pre-existing hypertension appear to face an increased risk of developing an exaggerated pressor response.

• Dobutamine hydrochloride may precipitate or exacerbate ventricular ectopic activity, but it rarely has caused ventricular tachycardia.

• Safety for use following acute myocardial infarction has not been established.

• Dobutamine hydrochloride has not been administered to pregnant women. Therefore, use only when the expected benefits clearly outweigh the potential risks to the fetus.

ADVERSE EFFECTS

CNS EFFECTS: headache
RESPIRATORY EFFECTS: shortness of breath
CARDIOVASCULAR EFFECTS: increased heart rate, blood pressure; ventricular ectopic activity, anginal pain, nonspecific chest pain, palpitations

CLINICAL GUIDELINES

ADMINISTRATION:
• Before administering dobutamine hydrochloride, make sure hypovolemia has been corrected with suitable volume expanders.
• ECG, blood pressure, and urine flow should be monitored continuously.
• Pulmonary wedge pressure and cardiac output should be monitored whenever possible.
EFFECTS:
• In the presence of marked mechanical obstruction, such as severe valvular aortic stenosis, no improvement may be observed.

DRUG INTERACTIONS:
• Concomitant use with nitroprusside results in a higher cardiac output and, usually, a lower pulmonary wedge pressure than when either drug is used alone.
• Dobutamine hydrochloride has been administered concurrently with digitalis preparations, furosemide, spironolactone, lidocaine, glyceryl trinitrate, isosorbide dinitrate, morphine, atropine, heparin, protamine, potassium chloride, folic acid, and acetaminophen; no evidence of drug interactions was noted.
• Dobutamine hydrochloride is incompatible with alkaline solutions and should not be mixed with products such as 5% Sodium Bicarbonate Injection.
OVERDOSAGE/ANTIDOTE:
• Overdosage is evidenced in patients by excessive alteration of blood pressure or by tachycardia.
• Reduce the rate of administration or temporarily discontinue dobutamine until patient's condition stabilizes. Because the duration of action of dobutamine is short, no additional remedial measures are usually necessary.

Electrolyte Solutions

For information on additional products affecting electrolyte balance, see Chapter 16, *Nutritional Agents,* page 586.

SPECIFIC PRODUCTS AND DOSAGES

GENERIC NAME	ROUTE OF ADMIN.
Balanced replacement electrolyte injection	iv
5% dextrose in maintenance electrolyte No. 56 injection	iv
Replacement electrolyte No. 148 injection	iv
5% dextrose in replacement electrolyte No. 148 injection	iv

Balanced Replacement Electrolyte Injection

GENERAL CLINICAL USES

Balanced replacement electrolyte injection is a replacement solution for parenteral therapy. Its use is suggested in surgical, medical, and pediatric patients where saline or other electrolyte solutions would ordinarily be given.

PHARMACOLOGY

Balanced replacement electrolyte solution contains sodium chloride, calcium, and magnesium in the same concentrations in which they are found in normal human plasma. Potassium, the chief intracellular ion, is present in twice the concentration found in normal plasma to facilitate intracellular replacement. Bicarbonate is also provided in twice the normal plasma concentration in the form of its physiological precursor, acetate, which is converted rapidly by the cells of the body to bicarbonate.

SPECIAL PRECAUTIONS

• Do not administer in diseases in which high serum potassium levels are frequently encountered. Such states include chronic nephritis, untreated diabetic acidosis, and Addison's disease.
• In patients with severe renal insufficiency or adrenal insufficiency, administration may cause potassium intoxication.
• Take precautions not to overload the circulatory system, especially in patients with cardiac or pulmonary disorders.
• Defer use until either the presence of adequate urinary flow is assured or it has been determined beyond question that carefully regulated potassium administration, in combination with the other substances provided in this solution, is indicated in spite of anuria or oliguria.

CLINICAL GUIDELINES

ADMINISTRATION:
• Administer by intravenous route only; do NOT administer by hypodermoclysis.
• Do not infuse rapidly.
• Discard any flask in which the contents are not clear or which lacks a vacuum.

EFFECTS:
• Elevation of plasma CO_2 without clinical manifestations concurrently may result from its use in excess.

OVERDOSAGE/ANTIDOTE:
• Overdosage is characterized by the signs and symptoms of potassium overdosage, namely, changes in ECG including peaking of T waves, loss of P wave, depression of S-T segment, and prolongation (widening and slurring) of the QT interval. Late manifestations include muscle paralysis and cardiovascular collapse from cardiac arrest.
• Discontinue infusion immediately; institute intensive corrective therapy to reduce potassium levels. Administer intravenously one molar sodium lactate, 150 ml; or 10% to 25% dextrose injection, USP, 300–500 ml with 10 units of crystalline insulin for 20 gm dextrose over 1 hour. Peritoneal dialysis or hemodialysis may be used. Cation exchange resin may be administered rectally.

5% Dextrose in Maintenance Electrolyte No. 56 Injection

GENERAL CLINICAL USES

Dextrose 5% in maintenance electrolyte No. 56 injection is ideal for maintaining water and electrolyte balance during routine intravenous therapy. It is useful in maintaining water and electrolyte balance during routine intravenous therapy and for hydrating the patient prior to and following surgery.

PHARMACOLOGY

Dextrose 5% in maintenance electrolyte No. 56 injection minimizes the possibility of unbalanced deficits of essential ions. Each liter of solution supplies the following milliequivalents:

cations:	anions:
sodium 40	chloride 40
potassium 13	acetate 16
magnesium 3	

It can be given in the presence of mild to moderate oliguria when the creatinine levels are less than 25 mg/100 ml.

SPECIAL PRECAUTIONS
• Avoid overloading the circulatory system, especially in cardiovascular or pulmonary disorders.

CLINICAL GUIDELINES
ADMINISTRATION:
• Administer only by the intravenous route.
• Not a replacement for whole blood, plasma, or volume expanders in the treatment of hemorrhage, plasma protein deficiency, or hypovolemia.
• Inspect each bottle before use; discard any flask if the contents are not clear or if it lacks a vacuum.
EFFECTS:
• May overcome potassium deficiencies prevalent in many hospitalized patients on intravenous fluids and resulting from increased urinary excretion of potassium due to stress.

Replacement Electrolyte No. 148 Injection; 5% Dextrose in Replacement Electrolyte No. 148 Injection

GENERAL CLINICAL USES
The replacement electrolyte No. 148 solutions are intended primarily for restoring extracellular fluid volume while maintaining normal electrolyte relationships. They are useful in trauma, surgery, burns or other conditions which result in electrolyte loss.

PHARMACOLOGY
Replacement electrolyte No. 148 injection contains the principal ions found in plasma. It is also available with carbohydrates. The composition is similar to that of plasma. Each liter of solution supplies the following milliequivalents:

cations:	anions:
sodium 140	chloride 98
potassium cation 5	acetate 27
magnesium 3	gluconate 23

SPECIAL PRECAUTIONS
• Avoid overloading the circulatory system, especially in cardiac or pulmonary disorders.

CLINICAL GUIDELINES
ADMINISTRATION:
• Administer only by the intravenous route.
• These products are not replacements for whole blood, plasma, or volume expanders in the treatment of hemorrhage, plasma protein deficiency, or hypovolemia.
• Inspect each bottle before use; discard any flask if the contents are not clear or if it lacks a vacuum.

EFFECTS:
• May overcome potassium deficiencies prevalent in many hospitalized patients on intravenous fluids and resulting from increased urinary excretion of potassium due to stress.

Hemostatic Agents

The hemostatic agents are used to control bleeding; they may be applied topically, ingested, or administered intravenously or intramuscularly. The clinical uses of each product will be discussed in detail, because each has specific applications.

SPECIFIC PRODUCTS AND DOSAGES

GENERIC NAME	TRADE NAME	ROUTE OF ADMIN.	USUAL DOSAGE
Topical Application: cellulose, oxidized	OXYCEL	topical	Apply minimal amount of an appropriate size to control bleeding; hold firmly against bleeding surface
collagen, microfibrillar hemostat	AVITENE	topical	Apply directly to source of bleeding
gelatin, absorbable	GELFOAM Powder GELFOAM Sponge Film	topical	Sprinkle on bleeding surface Place an appropriate sized piece on bleeding surface
negatol	NEGATAN	topical	Paint area or dip gauze into solution and apply to tissue surface
thrombin	(G)*	topical	100–2000 units/ml
Systemic Administration: aminocaproic acid	AMICAR	po iv infusion	5 gm, then 1–1.25 gm hourly; maximal dose 30 gm/24 hr 4–5 gm during first hr, then 1 gm/hr
antihemophilic factor (human)	(G)* HUMAFAC KOATE	iv	10–25 units/kg once daily as needed for bleeding; for surgery, 30–40 units/kg; for prophylaxis, 250–500 units/day

*(G) designates availability as a generic product.

(continued overleaf)

GENERIC NAME	TRADE NAME	ROUTE OF ADMIN.	USUAL DOSAGE
factor IX complex (human)	KONYNE PROPLEX	iv	2 units/kg
fibrinogen	(G)*	iv	2–8 gm
menadiol sodium diphosphate	KAPPADIONE SYNKAYVITE	po im/sc/iv	5–10 mg/day **Adults:** 5–15 mg od or bid **Children:** 5–10 mg od or bid
menadione	(G)*	po/im	2–10 mg/day
menadione sodium bisulfite	HYKINONE	sc/im iv	2.5–10 mg/day 50–100 mg for treating overdosage of oral anticoagulants
phytonadione	AQUAMEPHYTON KONAKION MEPHYTON	sc/im/iv po	5–20 mg 1–25 mg

*(G) designates availability as a generic product.

Hemostatic Agents, Topical

Cellulose, Oxidized

GENERAL CLINICAL USES

Oxidized cellulose is used adjunctively in surgical procedures to assist in the control of capillary, venous, and small arterial hemorrhage when ligation or other conventional methods of control are unproductive or ineffective.

PHARMACOLOGY

Oxidixed cellulose provides hemostatic action when applied to sites of bleeding. It is absorbed and swells on contact with blood; the resultant pressure adds to the hemostatic action. On contact with blood, it becomes a dark reddish-brown or almost black, tenacious, adhesive mass. After 24 to 48 hours it becomes gelatinous and can be removed, usually without causing additional bleeding.

SPECIAL PRECAUTIONS
• Do not use for packing or implantation in fractures or laminectomies because it interferes with bone regeneration and can cause cyst formation; in hemorrhage from large arteries; on nonhemorrhagic serous oozing surfaces, as it is ineffective in limiting serous exudates; as a wrap in vascular surgery because it has a stenotic effect; around the optic nerve and chiasm.
• Do not apply as wadding or packing as a hemostatic agent.
• Do not autoclave, as it causes a physical breakdown of the product; it is chemically sterilized.
• Oxidized cellulose is not meant as a substitute for careful surgery and the proper use of sutures and ligatures.

• In contaminated wounds, closure without drainage may lead to complications.
• Do not impregnate with anti-infective agents or thrombin, with other materials such as buffering or other hemostatic substances.
• Use only amount needed for hemostasis; remove excess prior to surgical closure to facilitate absorption and to minimize the possibility of foreign-body reaction.
• In urological cases, exercise care to prevent plugging of urethra, ureter, or a catheter.
• Do not precede use by the application of silver nitrate or any other escharotic material.

ADVERSE EFFECTS

LOCAL EFFECTS: foreign body reactions with or without infection; necrosis of nasal mucous membrane or perforation of nasal septum due to tight packing; intestinal obstruction due to transmigration of a bolus from gallbladder to terminal ileum or due to adhesions in a loop of denuded intestine to which it had been applied; urethral obstruction following retropubic prostatectomy and introduction of oxidized cellulose within enucleated prostatic capsule; sneezing in cases of epistaxis, stinging sensation, burning
SYSTEMIC EFFECTS: headache

CLINICAL GUIDELINES

ADMINISTRATION:
• The hemostatic effect is greater when it is applied dry; product should not be moistened with saline or water.
• Apply by loosely packing against bleeding surface; avoid wadding or packing tightly.
EFFECTS:
• It is advisable to remove the oxidized cellulose once hemostasis is achieved; it

may be left *in situ*.

Collagen, Microfibrillar Hemostat

GENERAL CLINICAL USES
Microfibrillar collagen hemostat is used as an adjunct to hemostasis when ligature or conventional procedures prove ineffective or impractical in controlling bleeding.

PHARMACOLOGY
Microfibrillar collagen is an absorbable topical hemostatic agent. In contact with a bleeding surface, it attracts platelets which adhere, resulting in formation of thrombi.

SPECIAL PRECAUTIONS
• Cannot control bleeding due to systemic coagulation disorders.
• Do not use in the closure of skin incisions; it may interfere with the healing of skin edges.
• May seal over exit sites and conceal underlying hematoma as in penetrating liver wounds.
• Moistening or wetting with saline or thrombin impairs its hemostatic efficacy.
• This product is inactivated by autoclaving.
• Use in contaminated wounds may enhance infection.
• Use only amount necessary to produce hemostasis; remove excess material after several minutes.
• Contains a low level of intercalated bovine serum protein which reacts immunologically, as does beef serum albumin.
• Avoid spillage on nonbleeding surfaces, particularly in abdominal or thoracic viscera.
• Use in pregnant women only when clearly needed.

ADVERSE EFFECTS

LOCAL EFFECTS: potentiation of infection (abscess formation, hematoma, wound dehiscence, mediastinitis,) foreign body reaction, subgaleal ceroma (1 case)

SYSTEMIC EFFECTS: allergic reaction

CLINICAL GUIDELINES

ADMINISTRATION:
- Use dry; discard any unused portion.
- Apply directly to bleeding source.
- Compress bleeding site with sponges immediately prior to application of dry product.
- This product will adhere to wet gloves, instruments, or tissue surfaces.

Gelatin, Absorbable

GENERAL CLINICAL USES

Absorbable gelatin, applied topically, is useful in controlling baccessible capillaries and small venules.

PHARMACOLOGY

Absorbable gelatin sponge is insoluble in water; it is absorbable and may be left in place after closure of a surgical wound. It is completely absorbed in 4 to 6 weeks without causing excessive scar tissue formation or cellular reaction.

SPECIAL PRECAUTIONS
- Use only the minimal amount required to control hemorrhage.

ADVERSE EFFECTS

ALLERGIC EFFECTS: hypersensitivity reactions

CLINICAL GUIDELINES

ADMINISTRATION:
- Moisten thoroughly with sterile sodium chloride.

EFFECTS:
- Eight days to six months may be required for absorption.

Negatol

GENERAL CLINICAL USES

Negatol is used as a styptic (astringent and hemostatic).

PHARMACOLOGY

Negatol has a powerful coagulant effect on protein. It is a highly acidic solution. It also has strong germicidal action in dilutions up to 1:100.

SPECIAL PRECAUTIONS
- Hypersensitivity reactions may occur.
- Use with caution and in 1:10 dilution when used initially in the vagina.

ADVERSE EFFECTS

LOCAL EFFECTS: slight irritation of the skin

CLINICAL GUIDELINES

ADMINISTRATION:
- Clean and dry area to be treated; paint with full strength or 1:10 dilution until hypersensitivity is disproved.
- Advise patient to wear a perineal pad to prevent soiling of clothing if treatment is intravaginal.
- If used on oral ulceration, apply to dried lesion with applicator for 1 minute.

EFFECTS:
- Treatment in the vagina usually produces a grayish membrane.

DRUG INTERACTIONS:
- A topical anesthetic may be used first; after treatment neutralize with copious amounts of water.

Thrombin

GENERAL CLINICAL USES

Thrombin, a topically administered product, is useful in controlling oozing blood from accessible capillaries and small venules. It is particularly useful where there is bleeding from parenchymatous tissues, cancellous bone, dental sockets, laryngeal and nasal surgery, and skin grafting procedures. It may also be used orally to control hemorrhage of the upper gastrointestinal tract.

PHARMACOLOGY

Thrombin clots the fibrinogen of the blood directly. It is of bovine origin. The speed with which thrombin clots blood is dependent upon its concentration.

Thrombin is antigenic and has caused sensitivity and allergic reactions when injected into animals.

SPECIAL PRECAUTIONS
- Do not use in patients with a history of hypersensitivity to any of its components and/or to material of bovine origin.
- Do not inject or otherwise allow to enter large blood vessels; extensive intravascular clotting and even death may result.

ADVERSE EFFECTS
ALLERGIC EFFECTS: febrile reactions, hypersensitivity reactions

CLINICAL GUIDELINES
ADMINISTRATION:
- Solutions may be prepared in sterile distilled water or isotonic saline.
- Solutions should be used the day they are prepared.
- If several hours are to elapse, the solution should be refrigerated.

DRUG INTERACTIONS:
- Dilute acids, alkalies, salts of heavy met-

als, and heat are detrimental to thrombin activity; therefore, stomach acids must be neutralized prior to oral administration.

Hemostatic Agents, Systemic

Aminocaproic Acid

GENERAL CLINICAL USES

Aminocaproic acid is useful in the treatment of excessive bleeding which results from systemic hyperfibrinolysis and urinary fibrinolysis.

PHARMACOLOGY

Aminocaproic acid is an effective inhibitor of fibrinolysis. It inhibits plasminogen activator substances and, to a lesser degree, antiplasmin activity. The drug is absorbed rapidly following oral administration. It is excreted largely unchanged in the urine.

SPECIAL PRECAUTIONS
- Do not use if there is evidence of an active intravascular clotting process.
- Safe use has not been established with respect to adverse effects upon fetal development.
- Do not administer without a definite diagnosis, and/or laboratory findings indicative of hyperfibrinolysis.
- Use with caution in patients with cardiac, hepatic, or renal disease.
- Avoid rapid intravenous administration since hypotension, bradycardia, and/or arrhythmia may be induced.

ADVERSE EFFECTS
CNS EFFECTS: dizziness, malaise, headache
RESPIRATORY EFFECTS: nasal stuffiness
CARDIOVASCULAR EFFECTS: thrombophlebitis

GASTROINTESTINAL EFFECTS: nausea, cramps, and diarrhea
DERMATOLOGIC EFFECTS: rash, pruritus, erythema
OPHTHALMIC EFFECTS: conjunctival suffusion
OTIC EFFECTS: tinnitus

CLINICAL GUIDELINES
ADMINISTRATION:
• Therapy should be accompanied by tests designed to determine the amount of fibrinolysis present.
• Do not administer rapidly.
• Reduce dosage in patients with renal disease or oliguria.
EFFECTS:
• Aminocaproic acid is of no value in controlling hemorrhage due to thrombocytopenia or most other coagulation defects.
DRUG INTERACTIONS:
• When given intravenously, sodium chloride injection, 5% dextrose injection, or Ringer's injection may be used to dilute aminocaproic acid.
OVERDOSAGE/ANTIDOTE:
• Overdosage is characterized by exaggeration of the adverse effects. Intravascular clotting may occur.
• There is no specific antidote. Transfusion of fresh whole blood counteracts the effect.

Antihemophilic Factor (Human)

GENERAL CLINICAL USES
Antihemophilic factor (human) is indicated for the treatment of classical hemophilia (hemophilia A) in which there is demonstrated deficiency of the plasma clotting factor, Factor VIII. It provides a means of temporarily replacing the missing clotting factor in order to correct or prevent bleeding episodes or in order to perform emergency and elective surgery.

PHARMACOLOGY
Antihemolytic factor (human) is a plasma protein which corrects the coagulation defect in patients with classical hemophilia. It is needed for the transformation of prothrombin to thrombin by the intrinsic pathway.

SPECIAL PRECAUTIONS
• May transmit viral hepatitis.
• Factor VIII deficiency should be proven prior to administering this product.
• Contains measurable levels of blood group isoagglutinins which are not clinically significant when controlling relatively minor bleeding episodes; when large or frequently repeated doses are required in patients of blood groups A, B, or AB, the possibility of intravascular hemolysis should be considered.

ADVERSE EFFECTS
CNS EFFECTS: transient dizziness
RESPIRATORY EFFECTS: chest discomfort, cough
HEMATOLOGIC EFFECTS: intravascular hemolysis
ALLERGIC EFFECTS: mild reactions

CLINICAL GUIDELINES
ADMINISTRATION:
• Store at temperature below 2° to 8° C (35° to 46° F) until reconstituted for use.
• After reconstitution administer promptly (within 3 hours); do not refrigerate.
• Administer only by intravenous route.
• Use filter prior to administering the reconstituted solution.

Factor IX Complex (Human) (Factors II, VII, IX, and X)

GENERAL CLINICAL USES

Factor IX complex is indicated whenever one or more of the specific coagulation factors, II, VII, IX, and X, must be elevated in order to correct or prevent a dangerous bleeding episode or in order to perform surgery, in patients with a Factor II, VII, IX, and X deficiency.

PHARMACOLOGY

Factor IX complex consists of factors II, VII, IX, and X, all essential factors in the coagulation schema. Factor IX complex may be safely used without typing or cross matching. Factor II is prothrombin; Factor VII, proconvertin; Factor IX, plasma thromboplastin component; and Factor X, Stuart-Prower factor. A deficiency of vitamin K results in a decreased quantity of these factors.

SPECIAL PRECAUTIONS
- May transmit viral hepatitis.
- When used in patients with liver disease, weigh the expected benefits against the potential hazard of superimposing a viral hepatitis on an already damaged liver.
- Do not use in cases of known liver disease where there is any suspicion of intravascular coagulation or fibrinolysis.
- Postoperative thrombosis has occurred following administration to a higher degree than usual during the postoperative period.
- Keep postoperative patients under close observation for signs and symptoms of intravascular coagulation.

ADVERSE EFFECTS
CNS EFFECTS: transient fever, chills, headache, flushing, tingling

CLINICAL GUIDELINES
ADMINISTRATION:
- Store below 8° C (46° F) until reconstituted for use; after reconstitution administer promptly.
- Administer only by intravenous route.
- Do not reconstitute and administer in a concentration greater than 50 units/ml.

DRUG INTERACTIONS:
- A deficiency of vitamin K results in a decreased quantity of Factor IX complex.

OVERDOSAGE/ANTIDOTE:
- Since Factor IX and Factor X have long postinfusion half-lives, repeated administration generally results in successively larger increases in blood levels. The risk of intravascular coagulation, therefore, increases.

Fibrinogen

GENERAL CLINICAL USES

Fibrinogen administered parenterally is indicated for the treatment of deficiency states associated with deposition of extravascular fibrin or extensive hemorrhage; also when there is a physiologic increase in fibrinolysis.

PHARMACOLOGY

Fibrinogen, a fraction of normal human plasma, is one of the normal clotting factors produced in the liver. When added to a solution containing thrombin, it is converted to insoluble fibrin.

SPECIAL PRECAUTIONS
- May transmit viral hepatitis if the fibrinogen is derived from pooled venous blood.

ADVERSE EFFECTS
CARDIOVASCULAR EFFECTS: tachycardia, cyanosis
HEMATOLOGIC EFFECTS: thrombosis

Menadiol Sodium Diphosphate
Menadione
Menadione Sodium Bisulfite
Phytonadione (Vitamin K$_1$)

GENERAL CLINICAL USES

The phytonadione derivatives are indicated in the treatment of hypoprothrombinemia secondary to factors limiting absorption or synthesis of vitamin K such as obstructive jaundice, biliary fistula, sprue, and ulcerative colitis, or in hemorrhagic disease of the newborn and hypoprothrombinemia due to oral antibacterial therapy.

These agents are also indicated in hypoprothrombinemia secondary to the administration of salicylates and other drugs.

PHARMACOLOGY

The phytonadione derivatives are synthetic, water-soluble forms of vitamin K. The salts are converted *in vivo* to vitamin K. Vitamin K is necessary for the synthesis in the liver of prothrombin (Factor II), proconvertin (Factor VII), thromboplastin (Factor IX), and Stuart-Prower factor (Factor X). The mechanism of action is not known. The activity is generally detectable within 1 to 2 hours. Hemorrhage is usually controlled within 3 to 6 hours after parenteral administration. The minimal daily requirements have been estimated as 1 to 5 mcg/kg for infants and 0.03 mcg/kg for adults.

SPECIAL PRECAUTIONS

• Do not administer to the mother during the last few weeks of pregnancy as a prophylactic measure against physiologic hypoprothrombinemia or hemolytic disease of the newborn.
• In the prophylaxis and treatment of hemorrhagic disease of the newborn, the vitamin K analogs are not as safe as phytonadione.
• These products will not counteract the anticoagulant effects of heparin.
• Safe use in pregnancy has not been established.
• If relatively large doses have been employed, it may be necessary, when reinstituting anticoagulant therapy, to use larger doses of the prothrombin-depressing anticoagulant, or use one which acts on a different principle such as heparin.
• Hypoprothrombinemia resulting from hepatocellular damage is not corrected by large doses of vitamin K.
• Repeated large doses of vitamin K are not warranted in liver disease if the response to the initial use of the vitamin is unsatisfactory.
• Failure to respond to vitamin K may indicate the presence of a coagulant defect or that the condition being treated is unresponsive to vitamin K.
• Do not use in patients with a history of hypersensitivity to the phytonadione derivatives.

ADVERSE EFFECTS

HEPATIC EFFECTS: BSP retention; increased bilirubinemia in infants, particularly premature babies; kernicterus; depressed liver function in patients with severe liver disease

HEMATOLOGIC EFFECTS: prolongation of prothrombin time; hemolysis in persons with a genetic deficiency of glucose-6-phosphate dehydrogenase

ALLERGIC EFFECTS: rash, urticaria, anaphylactoid reaction

LOCAL EFFECTS: pain, swelling, tenderness

CLINICAL GUIDELINES

ADMINISTRATION:
• Store in a dark place and protect from light at all times.

- Do not refrigerate.

EFFECTS:
- Temporary resistance to prothrombin-depressing anticoagulants may result, especially when large doses are used.

DRUG INTERACTIONS:
- Uptake of vitamin K is diminished when a patient receives prolonged oral antibiotic therapy, undergoes prolonged bowel cleansing for colonic surgery, or has a malabsorption syndrome.
- Competitive inhibition of vitamin K in the liver by antagonists such as the coumarin derivatives may result in hemorrhage.

OVERDOSAGE/ANTIDOTE:
- Overdosage is characterized by bruising and/or hemorrhage.
- Fresh plasma or blood transfusions may be required for severe blood loss or lack of response to vitamin K.

Thrombolytic Agents

SPECIFIC PRODUCTS AND DOSAGES

GENERIC NAME	TRADE NAME	ROUTE OF ADMIN.	USUAL DOSAGE
fibrinolysin	THROMBOLYSIN	iv	50,000–100,000 U/hr.
streptokinase	STREPTASE	iv	**Loading dose:** 250,000 IU/30 min. **Maintenance dose:** 100,000 IU/hr.
urokinase	ABBOKINASE	iv infusion	**Priming dose:** 4,400 IU/kg in 10 min. **Maintenance dose:** 4,400 IU/kg in 12 hr.

Fibrinolysin
Streptokinase
Urokinase

GENERAL CLINICAL USES
Fibrinolysin is indicated for use in phlebothrombosis, thrombophlebitis, pulmonary embolism, and thrombosis of arteries with the exclusion of thrombosis of coronary and cerebral arteries.

Streptokinase is indicated for the lysis of acute massive pulmonary emboli; embolization accompanied by unstable hemodynamics; lysis of acute, extensive thrombi of the deep veins; clearing of occluded arteriovenous cannulae. Streptokinase is not indicated for superficial thrombophlebitis.

Urokinase is indicated for lysis of acute passive pulmonary emboli.

PHARMACOLOGY

The thrombolytic agents act on the endogenous fibrinolytic system by converting plasminogen to the proteolytic enzyme plasmin (fibrinolysin). Plasmin degrades fibrin clots and also fibrinogen and other plasma proteins. Plasminogen present in the thrombus/embolus is activated.

SPECIAL PRECAUTIONS

- Because of the increased risk of bleeding, do not use within 10 days of surgery, liver or kidney biopsy, lumbar puncture, thoracentesis or paracentesis; extensive or multiple cutdowns, intra-arterial diagnostic procedures, ulcerative wounds, recent trauma with possibility of internal injuries, visceral or intracranial malignancy.
- Do not use in pregnant patients or within the first 10 postpartum days; with ulcerative colitis, diverticulitis or an actively bleeding lesion of the gastrointestinal or genitourinary tract; with severe hypertension, acute or chronic hepatic or renal insufficiency, uncontrolled hypocoagulable states, chronic lung disease with cavitation, subacute bacterial endocarditis or rheumatic valvular disease.
- Do not use in patients with recent cerebral embolism, thrombosis, or hemorrhage, or with any other condition in which bleeding might constitute a significant hazard.
- Use in septic thrombophlebitis or in an occluded arteriovenous cannula at an infected site may introduce the infection systemically.
- Use is contraindicated in patients with a history of a previous severe allergic reaction to the drug or those who present a significant risk of an allergic response.
- Avoid intramuscular administration because of the high risk of hematoma formation.
- Avoid arterial invasive procedures because of the possibility of bleeding.
- If serious bleeding occurs, discontinue therapy.
- In patients with atrial fibrillation or conditions putting patient at risk of cerebral embolism, there is the risk of bleeding into the infarcted area.
- Allow effects of heparin to diminish before starting therapy with a thrombolytic agent.
- Safe use in children has not been established.

ADVERSE EFFECTS

CNS EFFECTS: with streptokinase and fibrinolysin, fever

CARDIOVASCULAR EFFECTS: with streptokinase, transient lowering or elevation of blood pressure; with fibrinolysin, symptomatic hypertension, chest pain, tachycardia, hypotension

GASTROINTESTINAL   EFFECTS: abdominal pain, nausea, vomiting

DERMATOLOGIC EFFECTS: with fibrinolysin, facial flushing

ALLERGIC EFFECTS: with streptokinase, anaphylaxis including mild breathing difficulty to bronchospasm; periorbital swelling, or angioneurotic edema, urticaria, itching, flushing, nausea, headache, or musculoskeletal pain

LOCAL EFFECTS: with streptokinase, phlebitis

CLINICAL GUIDELINES

ADMINISTRATION:
- Unnecessary handling of the patient should be avoided; there is a great possibility of bruising during thrombolytic therapy.
- Make sure all venipunctures are performed carefully and as infrequently as possible.

EFFECTS:
- Rethrombosis has been observed after termination of treatment.

DRUG INTERACTIONS:
- Concurrent use of anticoagulants is not recommended and may be hazardous.
- Concurrent use of drugs altering plate-

let function (aspirin, indomethacin, phenylbutazone) should be avoided.
OVERDOSAGE/ANTIDOTE:
Not established.

Plasma Substitutes/Blood Extenders

GENERAL CLINICAL USES

The plasma extenders, dextran 40, dextran 70, and normal serum albumin (human), are used in treating shock or impending shock due to hemorrhage, burns, surgery, or other trauma.

Normal serum albumin is also used in treating hypoproteinemia, hyperbilirubinemia, and erythroblastosis fetalis.

Dextran 40 and dextran 70 are used for emergency treatment only when whole blood or blood products are not available, and must not be regarded as a substitute for whole blood or plasma proteins. Dextran 40 is also indicated for use as a priming fluid, either as sole primer or as an additive in pump oxygenators during extracorporeal circulation.

SPECIFIC PRODUCTS AND DOSAGES

GENERIC NAME	TRADE NAME	ROUTE OF ADMIN.	USUAL DOSAGE
albumin, normal serum (human)	(G)* PLASMANATE 5% and 25% ALBUSPAN 5% and 25% PLASMATEIN 5%	iv	25–50 gm; 200–500 ml; Normal serum albumin 25%: 1 ml/min; 5%, 4 ml/min
dextran 40	DEXTRAN 40 Injection LMD 10% RHEOMACRODEX	iv	**Adjunctive in shock:** 500 ml; do not exceed 20 ml/kg **Hemodiluent in extracorporeal circulation:** 10–20 ml/kg; do not exceed 20 ml/kg
dextran 70	DEXTRAN 70 Injection MACRODEX GENTRAN 75	iv	**Adults:** 500 ml; rate 20–40 ml/min **Children:** do not exceed 20 ml/kg

*(G) designates availability as a generic product.

Albumin, Normal Serum (Human)

PHARMACOLOGY

Normal serum albumin, highly active osmotically, is an important factor in the regulation of the volume of circulating blood. The albumin component normally constitutes approximately 60 percent of plasma protein, and because of its relatively low molecular weight, exerts 80 percent of the colloidal osmotic pressure of the blood.

Albumin is free of the danger of homologous serum hepatitis. It is stable at room temperature and quite soluble. It is available in 5% and 25% solutions.

SPECIAL PRECAUTIONS

- Do not use in patients with severe anemia or cardiac failure.
- Do not administer more than 250 gm in 48 hours; patients who require more than this amount probably need whole blood or plasma.
- Administer with caution to patients with low cardiac reserve or with no albumin deficiency because a rapid increase in plasma volume may cause circulatory embarrassment or pulmonary edema.
- Do not use any solution of normal albumin (human) if it appears turbid or if there is sediment in the bottle.
- Patients with marked dehydration require administration of additional fluids since drawing additional fluids from the tissues of a dehydrated patient is undesirable; fluid may be given by any route, including orally.

ADVERSE EFFECTS

CARDIOVASCULAR EFFECTS: circulatory embarrassment
RESPIRATORY EFFECTS: pulmonary edema
ALLERGIC EFFECTS: urticaria, fever, chills

CLINICAL GUIDELINES

ADMINISTRATION:
- Dilute 25% normal serum albumin with sodium chloride injection, 5% dextrose injection or other suitable fluids, in conditions other than nephrosis; use undiluted in patients with nephrosis.
- Dilution with dextrose is preferable in patients with edematous conditions.
- Use promptly after opening the bottle since normal albumin contains no preservatives.

EFFECTS:
- If administered rapidly, may result in vascular overload with resultant pulmonary edema.

DRUG INTERACTIONS:
- May be administered in combination with or through the same administration set with the usual intravenous solutions of carbohydrates or saline.
- Certain solutions containing protein hydrolysates or alcohol must not be infused through the same administration set in conjunction with normal serum albumin; precipitation may occur.

Dextran 40
Dextran 70

PHARMACOLOGY

Dextran has colloid properties approximating those of human albumin. Intravenous infusion of dextran 40 results in an expansion of plasma volume slightly in excess of the volume infused and decreases from this maximum over the succeeding 24 hours. This expansion improves the hemodynamic status for 24 hours or longer. Dextran molecules below 50,000 molecular weight are eliminated by renal excretion, with approximately 40 percent appearing in the urine in 24 hours. The remaining dextran is enzymatically degraded to glucose at a rate of about 70 to 90 mg/kg body weight/day.

SPECIAL PRECAUTIONS
• Do not use in patients with a history of hypersensitivity to dextran; with marked hemostatic defects of all types (thrombocytopenia, hypofibrinogenemia, etc.), including those induced by drugs; marked cardiac decompensation.
• Do not use in patients with renal disease with severe dysuria or anuria; decreased urinary output secondary to shock is not a contraindication unless there is no improvement in urine output after the initial dose of dextran 70.
• Safe use in pregnancy has not been established with respect to effects on fetal development.
• Although infrequent, severe and fatal anaphylactoid reactions consisting of marked hypotension and/or cardiac and respiratory arrest have been reported.
• May interfere with platelet function; use with caution in patients with thrombocytopenia.
• Take care to prevent a depression of hematocrit below 30 vol percent.
• The possibility of circulatory overload should be kept in mind.
• Use special care in patients with impaired renal clearance.
• When the risk of pulmonary edema and/or congestive heart failure may be increased, dextran should be used with caution.
• Use with caution in patients with active hemorrhage; additional blood loss may occur.

ADVERSE EFFECTS
CNS EFFECTS: fever
URINARY TRACT EFFECTS: renal failure, sometimes irreversible, has been reported with dextran 40
GASTROINTESTINAL EFFECTS: nausea, vomiting

ALLERGIC EFFECTS: urticaria, nasal congestion, wheezing, tightness in chest, mild hypotension
MUSCULOSKELETAL EFFECTS: joint pains

CLINICAL GUIDELINES
ADMINISTRATION:
• Draw blood samples before initiating infusion so suitable assays may be performed.
• Most anaphylactoid reactions occur in patients not previously exposed to dextran and in the early infusion period.
• Observe patients closely during early part of infusion period.
EFFECTS:
• Transient prolongation of bleeding time may occur with the administration of doses greater than 1000 ml.
• When large volumes of dextran are administered, plasma protein levels will be decreased.
• Dosages in the range of 15 ml/kg markedly decrease Factor VIII and decrease fibrinogen, Factor V, and Factor IX to a greater extent than should be expected to occur from hemodilution alone.
• Renal excretion of dextran produces an elevation in urine viscosity and specific gravity in proportion to the urine dextran concentration.
DRUG INTERACTIONS:
• In patients who have received dextran 70, blood sugar determinations that employ high concentrations of acid may result in hydrolysis of dextran yielding falsely elevated glucose assay results.
• In other laboratory tests, dextran may result in development of turbidity which can interfere with the assay (example, bilirubin, protein, blood sugar).
• Blood grouping and cross matching tests may be difficult to interpret after dextran infusion because of the tendency toward rouleau formations.

Sclerosing Agents

GENERAL CLINICAL USES
Morrhuate sodium and sodium tetradecyl sulfate are used for the obliteration of varicose veins in the lower extremities.

SPECIFIC PRODUCTS AND DOSAGES

GENERIC NAME	TRADE NAME	ROUTE OF ADMIN.	USUAL DOSAGE
morrhuate sodium	(G)*	iv	1–5 ml
sodium tetradecyl sulfate	SOTRADECOL Inj.	iv	0.5–2 ml for each injection

*(G) designates availability as a generic product.

Morrhuate Sodium

PHARMACOLOGY
Morrhuate sodium, a solution of the sodium salts of the fatty acids of cod liver oil, causes obliteration of varicose veins following administration. The injected vein promptly becomes hard and swollen for 2 to 4 inches, depending on the size of the vein and its response. The vein is firm and hard after 24 hours and not very tender to touch. Aching and stiffness may occur and last for 48 hours.

SPECIAL PRECAUTIONS
• Do not use in patients with a history of hypersensitivity to morrhuate sodium.
• Do not inject extensively in patients with advanced debility and senility.

• Any unusual local reaction at the injection site or any systemic reaction is a contraindication to the continued use of this medication.
• Persistent occlusion of deep veins definitely contraindicates obliteration of superficial veins.
• Treatment should be delayed if there is any acute local or systemic infection.
• Great care should be taken when therapy is reinstituted after a period of time has elapsed, because there have been reports of anaphylactoid reactions.
• Safe use in pregnancy has not been established.

ADVERSE EFFECTS
ALLERGIC EFFECTS: anaphylactoid reactions including dizziness, weakness, vascu-

lar collapse, respiratory depression, gastro-intestinal disturbances, and urticaria

CLINICAL GUIDELINES

ADMINISTRATION:
• May be administered in multiple injections at one time or in single doses repeated at intervals.
• Warm solution if cold.

EFFECTS:
• Bronzing of the skin about the injected vein occurs but disappears in a short time.

Sodium Tetradecyl Sulfate

PHARMACOLOGY

Sodium tetradecyl sulfate is a mild sclerosing agent which produces a penetrating but not diffuse intimal irritation.

SPECIAL PRECAUTIONS

• Do not use in acute superficial thrombophlebitis, underlying arterial disease, varicosities caused by abdominal and pelvic tumors, uncontrolled diabetes mellitus, thyrotoxicosis, tuberculosis, neoplasms, asthma, blood dyscrasias, acute respiratory or skin disease.
• Consider benefit-to-risk ratio in patients who are great surgical risks due to conditions such as old age.
• Do not undertake sclerotherapy if tests show significant valvular or deep venous incompetence.
• Safe use in pregnancy has not been established.
• Treatment should be delayed if there is any acute local or systemic infection.
• Do not use in bedridden patients.
• In patients receiving antiovulatory products, no well-controlled study data are available; one death has occurred.

ADVERSE EFFECTS

DERMATOLOGIC EFFECTS: sloughing, discoloration at injection site
ALLERGIC EFFECTS: anaphylactoid reactions

CLINICAL GUIDELINES

ADMINISTRATION:
• Inject slowly with a small amount (not over 2 ml).
• Since anaphylactoid reactions have occurred, have appropriate drugs and equipment ready for this emergency.
• Do not use solution if precipitated.

EFFECTS:
• Necrosis may occur following injection.

Vasodilating Agents/Antianginal Agents

The vasodilating agents are divided into three groups:
1. Coronary vasodilators/antianginal agents
2. Agents for peripheral vascular circulatory disease
3. Cerebral vasodilators

SPECIFIC PRODUCTS AND DOSAGES

GENERIC NAME	TRADE NAME	ROUTE OF ADMIN.	USUAL DOSAGE
Coronary/Antianginal Agents:			
For acute attacks			
amyl nitrite	(G)†	inhalation	0.18–0.3 ml as needed
nitroglycerin	(G)	subling.	0.15–0.6 mg
	NITROSTAT	subling.	0.15–0.6 mg
For prophylaxis and long-term treatment of attacks			
dipyridamole	PERSANTINE	po	50 mg tid
erythrityl tetranitrate	CARDILATE	po	5–10 mg tid
		subling.	5 mg before stress; increase as needed
	CARDILATE-P*	po	10 mg 3–6 x/day
isosorbide dinitrate	(G)	po	5–30 mg qid
	ISORDIL		
	SORBITRATE		
nitroglycerin	NITRO-BID 2.5 Plateau Cap.	po	2.5 mg bid or tid
	NITRO-BID 6.5	po	6.5 mg bid or tid
	NITROGLYN	po	1.3–6.5 mg tid or bid
	NITRO-BID Ointment	topical	apply every 3–4 hr. as needed
	NITROL Ointment	topical	apply every 3–4 hr. as needed
	NITRONG	po	2.6–6.5 mg bid or tid
	NITROSPAN	po	2.5 mg bid (sustained release); 2.5–6.5 bid or tid
	NITROBON	po	6.5 mg bid (sustained release)
pentaerythritol tetranitrate (P.E.T.N.)	(G)	po	10–40 mg bid to qid
	ANTORA		
	CARTRAX*		
	DUOTRATE Plateau Cap.		
	DUOTRATE 45 Plateau Cap.		
	MILTRATE*		
	NEO-COROVAS-30 TYMCAPS		
	NEO-COROVAS-80 TYMCAPS		
	PAPAVATRAL L.A.*		
	PENTRITOL		
	PERITRATE		
	SK-PETN		
General/Peripheral Vasodilators:			
cyclandelate	(G)	po	**Initial:** 1200–1600 mg/day in divided doses
	CYCLANFOR		**Maintenance:** 400–800 mg/day in divided doses
	CYCLOSPASMOL		

*Contains more than one active ingredient.
†(G) designates availability as a generic product.

(continued facing page)

GENERIC NAME	TRADE NAME	ROUTE OF ADMIN.	USUAL DOSAGE
ethaverine HCl	CEBRAL ETHAQUIN ISOVEX-100 PAPAVATRAL*	po	100–200 mg bid
isoxsuprine HCl	(G) VASODILAN	po im	30–80 mg/day in divided doses 10–30 mg/day in divided doses
nylidrin	(G) ARLIDIN	po	3–12 mg tid or qid
papaverine HCl	(G) CEREBID LAPAV Elixir PAVATRAN	po iv/im	60–300 mg 1–6 x/day 30–120 mg; repeat as indicated, every 3 hrs.
Cerebral Vasodilators:			
cyclandelate	(G) CYCLANFOR CYCLOSPASMOL	po	600–800 mg bid
dioxyline phosphate	PAVERIL Phosphate	po	100–400 mg tid or qid
ethaverine HCl	CEBRAL ETHAQUIN	po	100–200 mg tid
isoxsuprine HCl	(G) VASODILAN	po im	30–80 mg/day in divided doses 10–30 mg/day in divided doses
papaverine HCl	(G) CEREBID LAPAV PAVATRAN	po iv/im	60–300 mg 1–6 x/day 30–120 mg; repeat as indicated

*Contains more than one active ingredient.

Amyl Nitrite
Isosorbide Dinitrate
Nitroglycerin (Glyceryl Trinitrate)

GENERAL CLINICAL USES

These products are used for the relief of the acute attacks (pain) of angina pectoris. Amyl nitrite, an inhalant, is used for immediate relief, as is nitroglycerin. Nitroglycerin is also available for oral and topical administration for prophylaxis of angina. Isosorbide dinitrate is available in sublingual and chewable tablets for prophylaxis in situations likely to provoke attacks.

PHARMACOLOGY

These products relax smooth muscle principally in the smaller blood vessels and dilate the arteries and capillaries, especially in the coronary vasculature. The mechanism of action in relieving anginal attacks is unknown.

Amyl nitrite, an inhalant, has an effect within approximately 30 seconds and lasts about 3 to 5 minutes. Nitroglycerin administered sublingually has a similar effect; the sustained-release formulations produce a prolonged effect for up to 8 to 12 hours.

Nitroglycerin may also be administered as a topical ointment which produces a prolonged effect. Site of application is not important. Isosorbide dinitrate chewable and sublingual tablets produce an effect in 2 to 5 minutes; the oral tablets in 15 to 30 minutes. The duration of action for the chewable and sublingual tablets is 1 to 2 hours and for the oral tablet, approximately 4 to 6 hours.

SPECIAL PRECAUTIONS
• Do not use or use with great caution in patients with glaucoma, head trauma, or cerebral hemorrhage since these products may increase intraocular and intracranial pressures.
• Transient episodes of dizziness, weakness, or syncope or other signs of cerebral ischemia due to postural hypotension may develop following inhalation of amyl nitrite, particularly if patient is standing immobile.
• The formulations for oral or topical administration are not for immediate relief of anginal attacks.
• Tolerance may develop to amyl nitrite with repeated use.
• Cross tolerance may develop to other organic nitrates or nitrites.
• Do not use in patients with a history of hypersensitivity to these drugs.

ADVERSE EFFECTS
CNS EFFECTS: transient or severe persistent headache, restlessness, dizziness, weakness

CARDIOVASCULAR EFFECTS: tachycardia, hypotension, syncope, collapse
URINARY TRACT EFFECTS: involuntary passing of urine with amyl nitrite
GASTROINTESTINAL EFFECTS: nausea, vomiting
DERMATOLOGIC EFFECTS: flushing of face, pallor, cold sweat, rash, exfoliative dermatitis

CLINICAL GUIDELINES
ADMINISTRATION:
• With amyl nitrite, crush fragile glass container between fingers for release of inhalant.
• For best absorption, administer oral dose on an empty stomach.
• If vascular headache cannot be effectively controlled by ordinary measures, dosage may be taken with meals to minimize this side effect.
• With use of the ointment, occasionally an elderly patient may have no untoward symptoms while recumbent but may develop postural hypotension with faintness upon sudden arising.
EFFECTS:
• Tolerance may be minimized by starting with the smallest effective dose and by alternating amyl nitrite with other coronary vasodilators.
• An occasional individual exhibits marked sensitivity to the hypotensive effect of nitrates, and severe responses (nausea, vomiting, weakness, restlessness, pallor, perspiration, and collapse) can occur even with the usual therapeutic dose.
DRUG INTERACTIONS:
• When amyl nitrite is taken with antihypertensive agents or tricyclic antidepressants, the decrease in blood pressure may be enhanced.
• Propranolol may cause additional lowering of blood pressure.

• Alcohol enhances the adverse effects probably by increasing absorption from the gastrointestinal tract.

• May act as a physiological antagonist to norepinephrine, acetylcholine, histamine, and many other agents.

OVERDOSAGE/ANTIDOTE:

• Overdosage is initially characterized by headache, dizziness, and marked flushing of the skin. Larger overdoses may cause vomiting, weakness, sweating, fainting, shortness of breath and coma. Extended and excessively high doses may cause methemoglobinemia.

• Discontinue drug. Treat supportively and symptomatically.

Cyclandelate

GENERAL CLINICAL USES

Cyclandelate may be useful as adjunctive therapy in peripheral or cerebral vascular disease.

PHARMACOLOGY

Cyclandelate is a vasodilating agent, active when administered orally. It relaxes vascular smooth muscle by direct action, it has no significant adrenergic stimulating or blocking actions.

SPECIAL PRECAUTIONS

• Do not use in patients with a history of hypersensitivity to this drug.

• Use with extreme caution in patients with severe obliterative coronary artery or cerebral vascular disease since there is a possibility that these diseased areas may be compromised by the vasodilating effects of the drug elsewhere.

• Safe use in pregnancy or lactation has not been established.

• When administered to a patient with active bleeding or a bleeding tendency, be aware that the hazard of a prolonged bleeding time may occur.

• Use with caution in patients with glaucoma.

ADVERSE EFFECTS

CNS EFFECTS: headache, feeling of weakness

CARDIOVASCULAR EFFECTS: tachycardia

GASTROINTESTINAL EFFECTS: pyrosis, pain, eructation

DERMATOLOGIC EFFECTS: mild flush

CLINICAL GUIDELINES

ADMINISTRATION:

• Advise patient to take medication with meals or with concomitant use of antacids to minimize gastrointestinal distress.

EFFECTS:

• Although objective signs of therapeutic benefit may be rapid and dramatic, more often, this improvement comes gradually over weeks of therapy.

• Short-term use is rarely beneficial; prolonged use may be necessary.

OVERDOSAGE/ANTIDOTE:

• Overdosage is characterized by an exaggeration of the pharmacologic and adverse effects.

• Discontinue drug. Treat supportively.

Dioxyline Phosphate

GENERAL CLINICAL USES

Dioxyline phosphate may be useful for symptomatic treatment of angina pectoris and conditions in which there is reflex spasm of blood vessels in the arms, legs, or lungs.

PHARMACOLOGY

Dioxyline phosphate, a derivative of papaverine, has essentially the same pharmacologic activities. It relaxes smooth muscle of peripheral and coronary vessels.

SPECIAL PRECAUTIONS

• Do not use in patients with a history of hypersensitivity to dioxyline phosphate.
• Use with caution in patients with glaucoma.
• Safe use in pregnancy and lactation has not been established.

ADVERSE EFFECTS

CNS EFFECTS: dizziness, sedation
AUTONOMIC EFFECTS: sweating, flushing
GASTROINTESTINAL EFFECTS: nausea, abdominal cramps

CLINICAL GUIDELINES

OVERDOSAGE/ANTIDOTE:
• Overdosage is characterized by gastric irritation, vasodilatation, nausea, dizziness, sweating, flushing, and also by abdominal cramping.
• General management consists of symptomatic therapy, including gastric lavage.

Dipyridamole

GENERAL CLINICAL USES

Dipyridamole is useful for long-term therapy of chronic angina pectoris; the drug is not intended to abort the acute anginal attack.

PHARMACOLOGY

Dipyridamole increases coronary blood flow by a selective dilation of the coronary arteries. It produces no significant alteration of systemic blood pressure or blood flow in peripheral arteries. It increases coronary sinus oxygen saturation without significantly altering myocardial oxygen consumption.

SPECIAL PRECAUTIONS

• Use with caution in patients with hypotension since excessive doses can produce peripheral vasodilatation.
• Do not use in patients with a history of hypersensitivity or idiosyncrasy to dipyridamole.

ADVERSE EFFECTS

CNS EFFECTS: headache, dizziness, weakness, syncope
CARDIOVASCULAR EFFECTS: aggravation of angina pectoris, rarely
GASTROINTESTINAL EFFECTS: nausea, anorexia, vomiting
DERMATOLOGIC EFFECTS: rash, flushing

CLINICAL GUIDELINES

ADMINISTRATION:
• Administer at least 1 hour before meals.
EFFECTS:
• Side effects may increase with increased dosage.
• Clinical response may not be evident before the second or third month of continuous therapy.

Erythrityl Tetranitrate
Pentaerythritol Tetranitrate

GENERAL CLINICAL USES

Erythrityl tetranitrate and pentaerythritol tetranitrate are used for prophylaxis and long-term treatment of patients with frequent or recurrent anginal pain and reduced exercise tolerance associated with angina pectoris.

PHARMACOLOGY

The mechanism of action of these compounds in the relief of angina pectoris is unknown. Erythrityl tetranitrate and pentaerythritol tetranitrate both relax smooth muscle, particularly in the coronary vasculature.

SPECIAL PRECAUTIONS

• Use with caution since some fall in blood pressure may occur with large doses.
• Do not use in patients with increased intraocular pressure or glaucoma.
• Administer with caution to patients with a history of recent cerebral hemorrhage, because of the vasodilatation which occurs in the area.
• Do not use in patients with a history of hypersensitivity to these compounds.

ADVERSE EFFECTS

CNS EFFECTS: headache, dizziness, weakness
CARDIOVASCULAR EFFECTS: postural hypotension occasionally, cerebral ischemia
GASTROINTESTINAL EFFECTS: nausea, vomiting, anorexia

CLINICAL GUIDELINES

ADMINISTRATION:
• Administer on empty stomach.
• NOT for sublingual use.
EFFECTS:
• An occasional individual exhibits marked sensitivity to the hypotensive effects of nitrates, and severe responses (nausea, vomiting, weakness, restlessness, pallor, perspiration, and collapse) can occur, even with usual therapeutic doses.
• Cross tolerance and tolerance to other nitrites and nitrates may occur.
DRUG INTERACTIONS:
• See *Amyl Nitrite, Isosorbide Dinitrate,* and *Nitroglycerin,* page 286, for pertinent information.
OVERDOSAGE/ANTIDOTE:
• See *Amyl Nitrite, Isosorbide Dinitrate,* and *Nitroglycerin,* page 287, for pertinent information.

Ethaverine Hydrochloride

GENERAL CLINICAL USES

Ethaverine hydrochloride is used for the relief of cerebral and peripheral ischemia associated with arterial spasm. It may be used as a smooth muscle spasmolytic in spastic conditions of the gastrointestinal and genitourinary tracts.

PHARMACOLOGY

Ethaverine hydrochloride resembles papaverine in therapeutic activity but it is not an opium alkaloid as is papaverine. Ethaverine relaxes smooth muscle of the larger blood vessels, especially the coronary, systemic, peripheral, cerebral, and pulmonary arteries, also smooth muscle of the intestines, biliary tree, and ureter. This relaxation may be prominent if spasm exists. The muscle cell is not paralyzed but still responds to other drugs causing contraction. The antispasmodic effect is a direct one, and unrelated to muscle innervation. Ethaverine is devoid of central nervous system effects. It also, however, acts directly on heart muscle to depress conduction and prolong the refractory period.

SPECIAL PRECAUTIONS
- Do not use if complete atrioventricular dissociation is present.
- Use with caution in patients with glaucoma.
- If signs of hepatic hypersensitivity occur (gastrointestinal symptoms, jaundice, eosinophilia and altered liver function tests) discontinue drug.
- Safe use in pregnancy and lactation has not been established.

ADVERSE EFFECTS
CNS EFFECTS: malaise, drowsiness, vertigo, headache
RESPIRATORY EFFECTS: depression
CARDIOVASCULAR EFFECTS: hypotension, cardiac depression, arrhythmias
AUTONOMIC EFFECTS: sweating
GASTROINTESTINAL EFFECTS: nausea, abdominal distress, anorexia, constipation, diarrhea
DERMATOLOGIC EFFECTS: rash

Isoxsuprine Hydrochloride

GENERAL CLINICAL USES
Isoxsuprine hydrochloride may be useful in relief of symptoms associated with cerebral vascular insufficiency; and in peripheral vascular diseases such as arteriosclerosis obliterans, thromboangiitis obliterans, and Raynaud's disease.

PHARMACOLOGY
Isoxsuprine hydrochloride is a beta adrenergic stimulant. Following oral administration, it is well absorbed and appears to dilate the cerebral and peripheral blood vessels.

Isoxsuprine hydrochloride may also

be administered parenterally.

SPECIAL PRECAUTIONS
- Do not administer immediately postpartum or in the presence of arterial bleeding.
- Parenteral administration is not recommended in the presence of hypotension or tachycardia.
- Safe use in pregnancy and lactation has not been established.

ADVERSE EFFECTS
CNS EFFECTS: dizziness
CARDIOVASCULAR EFFECTS: hypotension, rarely; tachycardia
GASTROINTESTINAL EFFECTS: nausea, vomiting, abdominal distress
DERMATOLOGIC EFFECTS: severe rash

CLINICAL GUIDELINES
ADMINISTRATION:
- Administer intramuscularly only in severe or acute conditions.
EFFECTS:
- Administration of a single dose of 1 mg intramuscularly may result in hypotension and tachycardia.
- If rash appears, discontinue drug.
OVERDOSAGE/ANTIDOTE:
- Overdosage is characterized by hypotension, transient palpitation, or dizziness. Adverse effects are exaggerated.
- Overdosage is usually controlled by reducing the dose. There is no specific antidote.

Nylidrin Hydrochloride

GENERAL CLINICAL USES
Nylidrin hydrochloride is indicated for increasing the blood supply in vasospastic disorders such as peripheral vascular

disease and circulatory disturbances of the inner ear.

PHARMACOLOGY

Nylidrin hydrochloride acts predominantly by beta adrenergic receptor stimulation. It dilates arterioles in skeletal muscles and increases cardiac output.

SPECIAL PRECAUTIONS

- Do not use in patients with acute myocardial infarction, paroxysmal tachycardia, progressive angina pectoris, and thyrotoxicosis.
- In patients with cardiac disease such as tachyarrhythmias and uncompensated congestive heart failure, the benefit to risk ratio should be weighed prior to therapy and reconsidered at intervals during treatment.
- Safe use in pregnancy and lactation has not been established.

ADVERSE EFFECTS

CNS EFFECTS: trembling, nervousness, weakness, dizziness (not associated with labrynthine artery insufficiency)
CARDIOVASCULAR EFFECTS: palpitations
GASTROINTESTINAL EFFECTS: nausea, vomiting

CLINICAL GUIDELINES

ADMINISTRATION:
- Monitor the patient's cardiovascular response periodically.
EFFECTS:
- See pharmacology
DRUG INTERACTIONS:
- Not established
OVERDOSAGE/ANTIDOTE:
- Overdosage may result in palpitations, nausea, and vomiting.
- There is no specific antidote. Withdraw or reduce medication and treat supportively.

Papaverine Hydrochloride

GENERAL CLINICAL USES

Papaverine hydrochloride is indicated for relief of cerebral and peripheral ischemia associated with arterial spasm and myocardial ischemia complicated by arrhythmia.

PHARMACOLOGY

Papaverine hydrochloride relaxes the smooth muscle of larger blood vessels, especially coronary, systemic, peripheral, cerebral, and pulmonary arteries. The relaxation may be prominent if spasm exists. The muscle cell is not paralyzed but still responds to drugs and other stimuli causing contraction. Papaverine is practically devoid of central nervous system effects.

Papaverine also acts directly on heart muscle to depress conduction and prolong the refractory period. It may be administered orally or intravenously in an emergency to produce coronary vasodilation without depressing myocardial contraction or causing cinchonism.

An effect is noted in 30 to 60 minutes and persists for 4 to 6 hours.

SPECIAL PRECAUTIONS

- Use with caution in patients with glaucoma.
- If hepatic hypersensitivity (including gastrointestinal symptoms, jaundice, eosinophilia, and altered liver function tests) occurs, discontinue drug.
- Safe use in pregnancy and lactation has not been established.

ADVERSE EFFECTS

CNS EFFECTS: malaise, drowsiness, vertigo, headache
AUTONOMIC EFFECTS: sweating, dryness of mouth and throat
GASTROINTESTINAL EFFECTS: nausea, ab-

dominal distress, anorexia, constipation, diarrhea

HEPATIC EFFECTS: hepatitis, jaundice

CLINICAL GUIDELINES

ADMINISTRATION:

• Caution patient that drowsiness may occur; use caution in driving a motor vehicle or undertaking hazardous tasks.

• Watch for jaundice, frothy urine, clay-colored stools; these signs may indicate the development of drug-related hepatitis.

EFFECTS:

• May cause excessive sweating in hot environments.

DRUG INTERACTIONS:

• Effects of sedatives, tranquilizers, hypnotics, analgesics, and narcotics may be enhanced.

OVERDOSAGE/ANTIDOTE:

• Overdosage with moderate amounts of papaverine hydrochloride is characterized by nausea, vomiting, marked drowsiness, and possibly severe constipation. Larger amounts result in weakness, faintness, flushed and warm face, excessive sweating, stupor, and irregular pulse.

• Discontinue drug. Treat supportively.

Vasopressor Agents/Vasoconstrictor Agents

SPECIFIC PRODUCTS AND DOSAGES

GENERIC NAME	TRADE NAME	ROUTE OF ADMIN.	USUAL DOSAGE
dopamine hydrochloride	INTROPIN	iv	2–5 mcg/kg/min; increase to 20–50 mcg/kg/min.
epinephrine HCl	(G)* ADRENALIN GLUCON	im/sc	0.2–1 ml of 1:1000 solution
		iv	0.1–0.4 mg
		intracardiac	0.1–0.2 mg
isoproterenol hydrochloride	ISUPREL Hydrochloride	iv	0.01–0.2 mg as needed
		im	0.02–1 mg as needed
		sc	0.15–0.2 mg as needed
		intracardiac	0.02 mg
		po	30–180 mg/day
		sublingual	5–50 mg/day
		pr	5–15 mg/day

*(G) designates availability as a generic product.

(continued facing page)

GENERIC NAME	TRADE NAME	ROUTE OF ADMIN.	USUAL DOSAGE
levarterenol bitartrate	LEVOPHED	iv infusion	**Initial:** 2–3 ml/min. (8–12 mcg base) **Maintenance:** 0.5–1 ml/min. (2–4 mcg base)
metaraminol bitartrate	(G) ARAMINE	iv im sc iv infusion	0.5–5 mg followed by infusion 2–10 mg 2–10 mg 15–100 mg in 500 ml of sodium chloride injection, or 5% dextrose injection, USP
methoxamine hydrochloride	VASOXYL	im iv	10–15 mg 3–5 mg

Dopamine Hydrochloride

GENERAL CLINICAL USES

Dopamine hydrochloride is indicated for the correction of hemodynamic imbalances present in the shock syndrome due to myocardial infarction, trauma, endotoxic septicemia, open heart surgery, renal failure, and chronic cardiac decompensation as congestive failure.

PHARMACOLOGY

Dopamine hydrochloride exerts an inotropic effect on the myocardium resulting in an increased cardiac output. It produces less increase in myocardial oxygen consumption than isoproterenol and its use is usually not associated with a tachyarrhythmia.

SPECIAL PRECAUTIONS

• Do no use in patients with pheochromocytoma or uncorrected tachyarrhythmias or ventricular fibrillation.
• Safe use in children has not been established.
• Safe use in pregnancy has not been established; weigh the expected benefits against the potential risk to the fetus.
• Avoid hypovolemia.
• Monitor patients with a history of occlusive vascular disease for changes in color or temperature of the skin of the extremities; if a change occurs and is thought due to compromised circulation to the extremities, weigh benefits against the risk of possible necrosis.

ADVERSE EFFECTS

CNS EFFECTS: headache
RESPIRATORY EFFECTS: dyspnea
CARDIOVASCULAR EFFECTS: ectopic beats, tachycardia, anginal pain, palpitations, hypotension, vasoconstriction, aberrant conduction, bradycardia, elevated blood pressure, widened QRS complex
GASTROINTESTINAL EFFECTS: nausea, vomiting
METABOLIC AND ENDOCRINE EFFECTS: azotemia
DERMATOLOGIC EFFECTS: piloerection

CLINICAL GUIDELINES

ADMINISTRATION:
• Dilute before use; Sodium Chloride Injection, USP, Dextrose 5% Injection, USP,

Sodium Chloride (0.9%) Injection, USP; 5% Dextrose in 0.45% Sodium Chloride Solution; Dextrose (5%) in Lactated Ringer's Solution; Sodium Lactate (1/6 molar) Injection, USP; Lactated Ringer's Injection, USP may be used.

• Infuse into a large vein whenever possible to prevent the possibility of extravasation into tissue adjacent to the infusion site; extravasation may cause necrosis and sloughing of surrounding tissue.

• Large veins of the antecubital fossa are preferred to veins in the dorsum of the hand or ankle.

• Monitor infusion site continuously for free flow.

EFFECTS:

• If a disproportionate rise in diastolic pressure is observed in patients receiving dopamine, the infusion rate should be decreased and the patient observed for further evidence of dominant vasoconstrictor activity, unless such an effect is desired.

DRUG INTERACTIONS:

• Do not add to any alkaline diluent solution, since such solutions inactivate the drug.

• Dopamine is metabolized by monoamine oxidase. Inhibition of this enzyme prolongs and potentiates the effect of dopamine hydrochloride. Patients who have received MAO-inhibitors prior to administration of dopamine should have a starting dose reduced to at least 1/10 of the usual dose.

• Avoid cyclopropane or halogenated hydrocarbon anesthetics since they may increase cardiac autonomic irritability and therefore sensitize the myocardium to the action of certain intravenously administered catecholamines.

OVERDOSAGE/ANTIDOTE:

• Overdosage is characterized by an excessive elevation in blood pressure.

• Reduce rate of administration or temporarily discontinue the drug until the patient's cardiac condition stabilizes. Since the duration of action is quite short, no additional measures are usually necessary. Short-acting alpha adrenergic blocking agents such as phentolamine may be considered.

Epinephrine Hydrochloride

GENERAL CLINICAL USES

Epinephrine is useful in acute attacks of ventricular standstill; physical measures should be applied initially. When external cardiac compression and attempts to restore the circulation by electrical defibrillation or use of a pacemaker fail, intracardiac punctures and intramyocardial injection may be effective.

Epinephrine is used to relieve respiratory distress due to bronchospasm, to provide rapid relief of hypersensitivity reactions, and to prolong the action of infiltration anesthetic agents. Its cardiac effects may be of use in restoring cardiac rhythm in cardiac arrest but it should not be used in cardiac failure or in hemorrhagic, traumatic, or cardiogenic shock.

PHARMACOLOGY

Epinephrine acts on both alpha and beta receptor sites of the sympathetic effector cells. When administered by rapid intravenous injection, it produces a rapid rise in blood pressure, mainly systolic, by directly stimulating the cardiac muscle and increasing the heart rate. Arterioles of the skin, mucosa, and splanchnic areas are constricted. When administered slowly (intravenously) it produces only a moderate rise in systolic blood pressure and a fall in diastolic pressure.

Epinephrine is inactivated rapidly in

the body. It is degraded by enzymes in the liver and other tissues. A large portion is excreted in the urine as inactivated compounds, and the remainder as partly unchanged or conjugated.

SPECIAL PRECAUTIONS

• Do not use in patients with narrow-angle (congestive) glaucoma, shock, during general anesthesia with halogenated hydrocarbons or cyclopropane; in patients with organic brain damage.

• Do not use with local anesthetics in certain areas such as toes, fingers because of the danger of vasoconstriction producing sloughing of tissue.

• Use in labor is not recommended since it may cause delay in the second stage.

• Use is contraindicated in cardiac dilatation and coronary insufficiency, and in patients with ventricular fibrillation.

• Administer with caution to elderly people, those with cardiovascular disease, hypertension, diabetes, hyperthyroidism, in psychoneurotic patients, and in pregnancy.

• Administer with extreme caution in patients with long-standing bronchial asthma and emphysema who have developed degenerative heart disease.

• Intravenous epinephrine must be used judiciously with extreme caution in patients with prefibrillatory rhythm because of its excitatory action on the heart.

• Epinephrine may convert asystole to ventricular fibrillation if used in the treatment of anesthetic cardiac accidents.

ADVERSE EFFECTS

CNS EFFECTS: anxiety (minor and transient), fear, restlessness, weakness, dizziness, throbbing headache

RESPIRATORY EFFECTS: breathing difficulty

CARDIOVASCULAR EFFECTS: palpitations, cerebral hemorrhage, hemiplegia, subarachnoid hemorrhage, anginal pain in patients with angina pectoris

DERMATOLOGIC EFFECTS: pallor

CLINICAL GUIDELINES

ADMINISTRATION:

• Epinephrine injection should be protected from exposure to light; do not use if solution is brown in color or contains a precipitate.

EFFECTS:

• If a sharp rise in blood pressure occurs, rapid-acting vasodilators (nitrites, or alpha adrenergic blocking agents) can be given to counteract the effect.

DRUG INTERACTIONS:

• Do not administer concurrently with excessive doses of digitalis, mercurial diuretics, or other drugs that sensitize the heart to arrhythmias.

• Effect is markedly potentiated in patients receiving MAO-inhibitors.

• Effect may be potentiated by tricyclic antidepressants, certain antihistamines (diphenhydramine, tripelennamine, d-chlorpheniramine) and sodium l-thyroxine.

• Epinephrine is rapidly destroyed by alkalies and oxidizing agents (oxygen, chlorine, bromine, iodine, permanganates, chromates, nitrites, iron).

• Do not use concurrently with isoproterenol; the combined effect may cause serious arrhythmias.

OVERDOSAGE/ANTIDOTE:

• Acute overdosage or rapid administration is characterized by increased ventricular contraction, increased heart rate, and constriction of the arterioles of the skin, mucosa and splanchnic areas of circulation. Adverse effects may be accentuated.

• There is no recommended specific antidote. Treat supportively as indicated by patient's condition.

Isoproterenol Hydrochloride

GENERAL CLINICAL USES

Isoproterenol hydrochloride is indicated as an adjunct in the management of shock (hypoperfusion syndrome), in the treatment of cardiac standstill or onset; in cardiac sinus hypersensitivity; in Adams-Stokes syndrome; and in ventricular tachycardia and ventricular arrhythmias that require increased inotropic cardiac activity for therapy.

It may also be used in the management of bronchospasm during anesthesia.

PHARMACOLOGY

Isoproterenol hydrochloride acts primarily on the heart and on smooth muscle of bronchi, skeletal muscle vasculature, and alimentary tract. It increases cardiac output and venous return to the heart; it also lowers peripheral vascular resistance; consequently, the diastolic pressure may be expected to fall in normal individuals.

Isoproterenol hydrochloride relaxes most smooth muscle, particularly in the bronchi and gastrointestinal tract.

SPECIAL PRECAUTIONS

• Use with caution and adjust dosage carefully in patients with coronary insufficiency, diabetes, or hyperthyroidism, and in patients sensitive to sympathomimetic amines.
• Correct hypovolemia by suitable volume expanders before treatment with isoproterenol hydrochloride.
• Observe patients in shock carefully during isoproterenol treatment.
• Safe use in pregnancy has not been established; weigh expected benefits of drug against possible risk to mother or child.
• Do not administer to patients with tachycardia caused by digitalis intoxication.
• Isoproterenol may produce an increase in myocardial work and oxygen consumption; these effects may be detrimental to myocardial metabolism and functioning in patients who are in cardiogenic shock secondary to coronary artery occlusion and myocardial infarction.

ADVERSE EFFECTS

CNS EFFECTS: mild tremors, nervousness, headache
RESPIRATORY EFFECTS: pulmonary edema
CARDIOVASCULAR EFFECTS: tachycardia with palpitations
AUTONOMIC EFFECTS: sweating
DERMATOLOGIC EFFECTS: flushing of face

CLINICAL GUIDELINES

ADMINISTRATION:
• If heart rate exceeds 110 beats per minute, it may be advisable to decrease the infusion rate or temporarily discontinue the infusion.
• Dilute in 5% Dextrose Injection, USP, before administering to patients in shock.
• May administer intracardiac to patient *in extremis.*
EFFECTS:
• Doses of isoproterenol sufficient to increase the heart rate to more than 130 beats/minute may induce ventricular arrhythmia.
DRUG INTERACTIONS:
• Isoproterenol hydrochloride and epinephrine should not be administered simultaneously, since both drugs are direct cardiac stimulants and their combined effects may induce serious arrhythmias.
OVERDOSAGE/ANTIDOTE:
• Overdosage is characterized by an exaggeration of the adverse and pharmacologic effects.
• Discontinue drug and treat symptomatically.

Levarterenol Bitartrate

GENERAL CLINICAL USES

Levarterenol bitartrate is used for the restoration of blood pressure in controlling certain acute hypotensive states (e.g., pheochromocytomectomy, sympathectomy, poliomyelitis, spinal anesthesia, myocardial infarction, septicemia, blood transfusion, and blood reactions).

It is also used adjunctively in the treatment of cardiac arrest and profound hypotension.

PHARMACOLOGY

Levarterenol bitartrate is a powerful peripheral vasoconstrictor (alpha adrenergic action) and a powerful inotropic stimulator of the heart and dilator of coronary arteries (beta adrenergic action). These actions result in an increase in systemic blood pressure and coronary artery blood flow.

SPECIAL PRECAUTIONS

• Do not use in patients who are hypotensive from blood volume deficits except as an emergency measure to maintain coronary and cerebral artery perfusion until blood volume replacement therapy can be completed.

• Do not give to patients with mesenteric or peripheral vascular thrombosis (because of the risk of increasing ischemia and extending the area of infarction) unless, in the opinion of the attending physician, the administration of levarterenol bitartrate is necessary as a lifesaving procedure.

• Use with extreme caution in patients receiving monoamine oxidase (MAO) inhibitors or antidepressants of the tryptyline or imipramine types; prolonged severe hypotension may result.

• Avoid hypertension.

• Avoid using veins of the leg in elderly patients or in those suffering from occlu-

sive vascular disorders; gangrene has been reported in a lower extremity when an ankle vein was used.

ADVERSE EFFECTS
CARDIOVASCULAR EFFECTS: bradycardia, plasma volume depletion

CLINICAL GUIDELINES
ADMINISTRATION:
• Record blood pressure every 2 minutes from the time administration is started until the desired blood pressure is obtained, then every 5 minutes if administration is to be continued.

• Watch rate of flow constantly; never leave patient unattended.

• Give in a large vein (antecubital) to minimize risk of necrosis of overlying skin from peripheral vasoconstriction.

• Avoid catheter tie-in technique.

• The infusion site should be checked frequently for free flow.

EFFECTS:
• Extravasation may cause local necrosis due to the vasoconstrictive action of the drug.

DRUG INTERACTIONS:
• Cyclopropane and halothane anesthesias increase cardiac autonomic irritability and therefore seem to sensitize the myocardium to the action of intravenously administered epinephrine or levarterenol; therefore do NOT use levarterenol bitartrate during cyclopropane or halothane anesthesia because of the risk of producing ventricular tachycardia or fibrillation. The same types of cardiac arrhythmias may result from the use of levarterenol bitartrate in patients with profound hypoxia or hypercarbia.

• Administer in 5% dextrose in saline solution.

• Administration in saline solution alone is not recommended.

• When whole blood or plasma, if indicated to increase blood volume, is administered, it should be administered separately and in individual flasks if given simultaneously.

OVERDOSAGE/ANTIDOTE:

• Overdosage is characterized by headache which may be a symptom of hypertension due to overdosage. Extreme hypertension, reflex bradycardia, marked increase in peripheral resistance, and decreased cardiac output may occur.

• Antidote for extravasation ischemia: To prevent sloughing and necrosis in areas in which extravasation has taken place, the area should be infiltrated as soon as possible with 10 to 15 ml saline solution containing 5 to 10 mg phentolamine, an adrenergic blocking agent.

• Discontinue medication; treat supportively.

Metaraminol Bitartrate

GENERAL CLINICAL USES

Metaraminol bitartrate is indicated for prevention and treatment of the acute hypotensive state during spinal anesthesia; adjunctive treatment of hypotension due to hemorrhage; reactions to medications; surgical complications; and shock associated with brain damage due to trauma or to tumor.

PHARMACOLOGY

Metaraminol bitartrate is a potent sympathomimetic amine that increases both systolic and diastolic blood pressure. The pressor effect begins in 1 to 2 minutes after intravenous infusion; in about 1 minute after intramuscular injection; and in 5 to 20 minutes after subcutaneous injection. The effect lasts about 20 to 60 minutes. Metaraminol bitartrate has a positive inotropic effect on the heart and a peripheral vasoconstrictor action.

SPECIAL PRECAUTIONS

• Use caution to avoid excessive blood pressure response; rapidly induced hypertensive responses have caused acute pulmonary edema, arrhythmias, and cardiac arrest.

• Use with caution in digitalized patients, since the combination of digitalis and sympathomimetic amines is capable of causing ectopic arrhythmias.

• Use with caution in patients with cirrhosis; restore electrolytes if diuresis ensues.

• Use with caution in patients with heart or thyroid disease, with hypertension, or with diabetes.

• Sympathomimetic amines may provoke a relapse in patients with a history of malaria.

ADVERSE EFFECTS

CARDIOVASCULAR EFFECTS: sinus or ventricular tachycardia, or other arrhythmias, especially in patients with myocardial infarction.

LOCAL EFFECTS: abscess formation, tissue necrosis or sloughing, rarely

CLINICAL GUIDELINES

ADMINISTRATION:

• The larger veins of the antecubital fossa or the thigh are preferred to the veins in the dorsum of the hand or the ankle veins, particularly in patients with peripheral vascular disease, diabetes mellitus, Buerger's disease, or conditions with coexistent hypercoagulability.

• Allow 10 minutes to elapse before increasing the dose because the maximal effect is not immediately apparent.

EFFECTS:
• A cumulative effect is possible with the prolonged action of metaraminol bitartrate; with an excessive vasopressor response, there may be a prolonged elevation of blood pressure even with discontinuation of therapy.
• When vasopressor amines are used for prolonged periods, the resulting vasoconstriction may prevent adequate expansion of circulating volume and may cause perpetuation of the shock state.

DRUG INTERACTIONS:
• The pressor effect of metaraminol bitartrate is decreased but not reversed by adrenolytic agents.
• Do not use with cyclopropane or halothane anesthesia.
• Monoamine oxidase inhibitors may potentiate the action of sympathomimetic amines.
• For dilution use only Sodium Chloride Injection or 5% Dextrose Injection when administering intravenously.

OVERDOSAGE/ANTIDOTE:
• Overdosage is characterized by increases in both systolic and diastolic blood pressure; and cardiac arrhythmias may also occur.
• Discontinue drug; treat symptomatically and supportively.

Methoxamine Hydrochloride

GENERAL CLINICAL USES
Methoxamine hydrochloride is used for terminating some episodes of paroxysmal supraventricular tachycardia. It is also indicated for supporting, restoring or maintaining blood pressure during anesthesia (including cyclopropane anesthesia).

PHARMACOLOGY
Methoxamine hydrochloride is a vasopressor agent which produces a prompt and prolonged rise in blood pressure following parenteral administration. It is especially useful for maintaining blood pressure when surgery is performed under general or spinal anesthesia. The pressor action of methoxamine hydrochloride appears to be due primarily to peripheral vasoconstriction. Unlike most pressor amines, there is no increase in cardiac rate; rather, a reflex decrease in rate develops on occasion as the blood pressure increases.

SPECIAL PRECAUTIONS
• Do not use in combination with local anesthetics to prolong their action at local sites.
• Methoxamine hydrochloride is not a substitute for the replacement of blood, plasma, fluids, and electrolytes which should promptly be restored when loss has occurred.
• Caution should be exercised to avoid overdosage so that undesirably high blood pressure or excessive bradycardia will not occur.
• Use with caution in patients with hyperthyroidism or severe hypertension.
• The increase in peripheral resistance may possibly produce or exacerbate heart failure associated with a diseased myocardium, due to the increased work load.

ADVERSE EFFECTS
CARDIOVASCULAR EFFECTS: excessive blood pressure increase with severe headache, pilomotor response
URINARY TRACT EFFECTS: a desire to void
GASTROINTESTINAL EFFECTS: projectile vomiting

CLINICAL GUIDELINES

ADMINISTRATION:

• Intravenous administration should be reserved for emergencies when a strong immediate pressor response is imperative, in which case not more than 5 mg should be given slowly.

EFFECTS:

• Intramuscular administration produces a more prolonged effect than intravenous administration.

DRUG INTERACTIONS:

• When used closely following parenteral injection of oxytocic drugs, an excessive rise in blood pressure may occur.

OVERDOSAGE/ANTIDOTE:

• Overdosage is characterized by an exaggeration of the adverse effects.

• Treat supportively.

Drugs affecting the respiratory tract

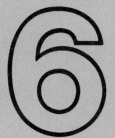

INTRODUCTION

Because of the complexity and frequency of disorders of the respiratory tract, numerous drugs are needed for either therapeutic or prophylactic use. Information concerning the many drugs used for respiratory tract disorders is organized by therapeutic use into several groups. The information presented, however may be limited because the drug is discussed elsewhere in the text in detail.

SPECIFIC THERAPEUTIC CLASSIFICATION

The drugs affecting the respiratory tract are grouped as follows:

1. Antiallergy/Anti-Inflammatory Agents: antihistamines and corticosteroids
2. Anti-infective Agents: see Chapter 2, page 10, *Anti-Infective Agents*, for detailed information

3. Antitussive Agents: narcotic and non-narcotic agents
4. Bronchodilators/Antiasthma Agents: theophylline and related compounds and adrenergic (sympathomimetic) agents
5. Expectorants
6. Nasal Decongestants: adrenergic agents and imidazolines; antihista-mines and corticosteroids used in combination products
7. Respiratory Stimulants: medullary stimulants; narcotic antagonists which act as respiratory stimulants are included in Chapter 20, *Drug Overdosage, Intoxication, Abuse—Narcotic Antagonists*, page 695.
8. Therapeutic Gases

Antiallergy Agents

Antihistamines

GENERAL CLINICAL USES

Antihistamines are used to suppress the symptoms produced by allergens such as those accompanying pollenosis, perennial rhinitis, urticaria, angio-edema, allergic rhinitis, rhinorrhea, and bronchial asthma. The antihista-mines modify or prevent the allergic manifestations such as sneezing, lacri-mation, rhinorrhea, and itching. Many drug formulations are available which contain an antihistamine in addition to other active ingredients. Only the an-tihistaminic component will be included in this section. Information about other active ingredients may be found in the appropriate section.

PHARMACOLOGY

The antihistamines relieve or suppress the symptoms caused by the release of histamine by preventing its effect on receptor cells. They also may sup-press nausea due to motion, induce sedation, decrease capillary permeability, produce mild local anesthesia, and have anticholinergic properties.

The antihistamines are divided into groups based on their chemical struc-ture, namely (1) the ethanolamines—including carbinoxamine maleate, dex-chlorpheniramine maleate, dimethindene maleate, diphenhydramine hydro-chloride, doxylamine succinate, and triprolidine HCl; (2) the ethylenediamines—methapyrilene hydrochloride, pyrilamine maleate and tripelennamine hydrochloride; (3) the alkylamines—including brompheniramine maleate, chlorpheniramine maleate, and dexbrompheniramine maleate; (4) the pheno-thiazines—including methdilazine hydrochloride, promethazine hydrochloride, and trimeprazine tartrate; (5) others—azatadine maleate, clemastine fumarate, and cyproheptadine hydrochloride.

SPECIFIC PRODUCTS AND DOSAGES

GENERIC NAME	TRADE NAME	ROUTE OF ADMIN.	USUAL DOSAGE
Alkylamines:			
brompheniramine maleate	(G)† DIMETANE	po	**Adults:** 4–8 mg tid or qid **Children over 6 yrs.:** 2–4 mg tid or qid **Children under 6 yrs.:** 0.5 mg/kg/day divided in 3 or 4 doses
	DIMETANE–10	im/sc/iv	**Adults:** 5–20 mg od or bid **Children:** 0.5 mg/kg/day divided in 3 or 4 doses
chlorpheniramine maleate	(G) CHLOR- TRIMETON HISTASPAN TELDRIN	po	**Adults:** 2–4 mg tid to qid **Children 6–12 yrs.:** 2 mg tid or qid **Children 2–6 yrs.:** 1 mg tid or qid
	(G)	im/iv/sc	**Adults:** 5–20 mg single dose **Children:** 0.35 mg/kg/day divided in 4 doses
dexbrompheniramine maleate	DISOPHROL* DRIXORAL*	po	**Adults:** 2–6 mg bid **Children:** not established
dexchlorpheniramine maleate	POLARAMINE	po	**Adults:** 2 mg tid or qid **Children:** 0.15 mg/kg/day divided in 4 doses
Ethanolamines:			
carbinoxamine maleate	CLISTIN	po	**Adults:** 4–8 mg tid to qid **Children:** 0.2 mg/kg/day divided in 3 or 4 doses
dimethindene maleate	FORHISTAL TRITEN	po	**Adults:** 2.5 mg od or bid **Children over 6 yrs.:** 2.5 mg od or bid **Children under 6 yrs.:** not established
diphenhydramine hydrochloride	(G) BENADRYL	po	**Adults:** 25–50 mg tid to qid **Children under 12 yrs.:** 5 mg/kg/day divided in 4 doses
		iv/im	**Adults:** 10–50 mg tid; maximum: 400 mg/day **Children under 12 yrs.:** 5 mg/kg/day divided in 4 doses
doxylamine succinate	DECAPRYN	po	**Adults:** 12.5–25 mg tid or qid **Children:** 2 mg/kg/day divided in 4 to 6 doses

*Contains more than one active ingredient.
†(G) designates availability as a generic product.

(continued overleaf)

GENERIC NAME	TRADE NAME	ROUTE OF ADMIN.	USUAL DOSAGE
triprolidine hydrochloride	ACTIDIL	po	**Adults:** 2.5 mg bid to tid **Children over 2 yrs.:** 2.5 mg divided in 3–4 doses **Children under 2 yrs.:** 1.25 mg divided in 3–4 doses
Ethylenediamines: methapyrilene hydrochloride	(G)† SURFADIL*	po im/sc	**Adults:** 25–100 mg tid or qid **Children:** 4–6 mg/10 lb every 4–6 hr. **Adults:** 1/4 to 1/3 of oral dose **Children:** not established
pyrilamine maleate	(G) ALLERTOC TRIAMINIC*	po	**Adults:** 25–50 mg tid–qid **Children:** 12.5–25 mg qid
tripelennamine hydrochloride	(G) PBZ PBZ–SR PYRIBENZAMINE	po	**Adults:** 25–50 mg tid or qid **Children:** 5 mg/kg/day divided in 4–6 doses **Infants:** 5 mg/kg/day divided in 4–6 doses
Phenothiazines: methdilazine hydrochloride	TACARYL	po	**Adults:** 8 mg bid to tid **Children:** 0.3 mg/kg/day divided in 2 doses
promethazine hydrochloride	(G) PHENERGAN	po im/iv	**Adults:** 12.5–25 bid or tid **Children:** 0.13 mg/kg in a.m. and 0.5 mg/kg at bedtime
trimeprazine tartrate	TEMARIL	po	**Adults:** 2.5 mg qid **Children under 2 yrs.:** 3.75 mg daily divided in 3 doses **Children 3–12 yrs.:** 7.5 mg divided in 3 doses
Others: azatadine maleate	OPTIMINE	po	**Adults:** 2 mg bid **Children under 12 yrs.:** not recommended
clemastine fumarate	TAVIST	po	**Adults:** 2.68 mg tid; maximum: 8.04 mg/day **Children under 12 yrs.:** not recommended
cyproheptadine	PERIACTIN	po	**Adults:** 4–20 mg/day divided in 3 to 4 doses; do not exceed 0.5 mg/kg/day **Children 7–14 yrs.:** 4 mg bid or tid; maximum: 16 mg/day **Children 2–6 yrs.:** 2 mg bid to tid; maximum: 12 mg/day

*Contains more than one active ingredient.
†(G) designates availability as a generic product.

Alkylamines

Brompheniramine Maleate
Chlorpheniramine Maleate
Dexbrompheniramine Maleate
Dexchlorpheniramine Maleate

Ethanolamines

Carbinoxamine
Dimethindene Maleate
Diphenhydramine Hydrochloride
Doxylamine Succinate
Triprolidine Hydrochloride

Ethylenediamines

Methapyrilamine Hydrochloride
Pyrilamine Maleate
Tripelannamine Hydrochloride

SPECIAL PRECAUTIONS

• If condition persists or irritation develops with use of the topical preparations, discontinue use and consult physician.
• Do not use topical preparations in the eyes.
• Do not use in patients with a history of hypersensitivity to these compounds.
• Safe use in pregnancy and lactation has not been established.
• Do not use in patients with narrow-angle glaucoma, stenosing peptic ulcer, symptomatic prostatic hypertrophy, bladder neck obstruction, pyloroduodenal obstruction, lower respiratory tract symptoms (including asthma).
• Antihistamines may produce excitation, particularly in children.
• Use with caution in patients with hyperthyroidism, increased intraocular pressure, cardiovascular disease, hypertension, or a history of bronchial asthma because of atropinelike effects.

ADVERSE EFFECTS

CNS EFFECTS: sedation, drowsiness, fatigue, confusion, restlessness, excitation, nervousness, vertigo, headache
RESPIRATORY EFFECTS: thickening of bronchial secretions, wheezing
CARDIOVASCULAR EFFECTS: hypotension, tightness in chest, palpitations, tachycardia
URINARY TRACT EFFECTS: dysuria, frequency, retention
AUTONOMIC EFFECTS: nasal stuffiness, dry mouth, nose, and throat
GASTROINTESTINAL EFFECTS: nausea, vomiting, diarrhea, constipation, epigastric distress
ALLERGIC EFFECTS: urticaria, anaphylactic shock
DERMATOLOGIC EFFECTS: rash, photosensitivity
OPHTHALMIC EFFECTS: blurring of vision, dyplopia
OTIC EFFECTS: tinnitus

CLINICAL GUIDELINES

ADMINISTRATION:
• Caution patients that drowsiness may occur which possibly will interfere with driving a car or operating machinery.
• Antihistamines are more likely to cause dizziness, sedation, and hypotension in elderly than in young patients.
EFFECTS:
• May cause inhibition of lactation.
DRUG INTERACTIONS:
• Concomitant use of alcohol or other CNS depressants such as hypnotics, sedatives, tranquilizers, and antianxiety agents may have an additive effect.
• Do not administer concurrently with

MAO inhibitors.

OVERDOSAGE/ANTIDOTE:
- Overdosage may cause convulsions and/or death in infants and children.
- In adults, overdosage is usually characterized by CNS depression.
- There is no specific antidote. Stimulants should *not* be used. Levarterenol bitartrate may be used for hypotension.

Phenothiazines

Methdilazine Hydrochloride
Promethazine Hydrochloride
Trimeprazine Tartrate

For additional information about phenothiazines, see Chapter 3, page 116.

SPECIAL PRECAUTIONS
- Do not use in patients with a history of hypersensitivity to the phenothiazines or related compounds.
- Do not use in patients with jaundice or a history of jaundice.
- Do not use in patients with asthmatic attacks, narrow-angle glaucoma, prostatic hypertrophy, stenosing peptic ulcer, pyloroduodenal obstruction, bladder neck obstruction.
- Do not use in premature or newborn infants.
- Do not use in acutely ill or dehydrated children because there is a greater susceptibility to dystonias in this group than others.
- If neuromuscular reactions occur, terminate therapy and do not reinstitute.
- Consider potential atropinelike effects before prescribing, particularly in patients with inactive asthma.
- Note that antiemetics such as the phenothiazines may mask symptoms of an unrecognized disease.
- Safe use in pregnancy has not been established.
- Use cautiously in patients with acute or chronic respiratory impairment, particularly in children.
- Development of photosensitization is a contraindication to further treatment with promethazine.

ADVERSE EFFECTS
Adverse effects characteristic of the phenothiazines may occur. Since lower doses are used for antihistaminic effects than for psychotropic effects, fewer adverse effects may occur; however, all of the following adverse effects have been reported with phenothiazines.

For additional information, see Chapter 3, *Psychotherapeutic Agents,* page 99.

CNS EFFECTS: syncope, toxic confusional states, extrapyramidal signs including parkinsonism, sedation, akathisia, persistant dyskinesia, drowsiness, dizziness, jitteriness, headache

CARDIOVASCULAR EFFECTS: postural hypotension, hypertension, reflex tachycardia, bradycardia, cardiac arrhythmias

URINARY TRACT EFFECTS: urinary frequency, dysuria

AUTONOMIC EFFECTS: dry mucous membranes

GASTROINTESTINAL EFFECTS: anorexia, nausea, vomiting, constipation, epigastric distress

HEPATIC EFFECTS: cholestatic jaundice

HEMATOLOGIC EFFECTS: agranulocytosis, leukopenia rarely

ALLERGIC EFFECTS: urticaria, dermatitis, asthma, laryngeal edema, angioedema, anaphylactoid reactions

DERMATOLOGIC EFFECTS: photosensitivity rare, rash

MUSCULOSKELETAL EFFECTS: painful constriction of skeletal muscles

OPHTHALMIC EFFECTS: blurring of vision

CLINICAL GUIDELINES
ADMINISTRATION:
• Warn patient that drowsiness may occur which can interfere with driving a car or operating machinery.
EFFECTS:
• Elderly patients are more prone to develop adverse effects than younger patients.
• Jaundice and prolonged extrapyramidal symptoms have occurred in infants whose mothers have received phenothiazines during pregnancy.
• The cough reflex may be suppressed.
DRUG INTERACTIONS:
• Do not use, or reduce dosage by at least one half when administered concomitantly with barbiturates, alcohol, narcotics, and analgesics; the sedative effects are additive.
• Do not use concomitantly with other phenothiazines or with other antihistamines.
• Do not use concomitantly with MAO-inhibitors.
OVERDOSAGE/ANTIDOTE:
• Overdosage in children may produce convulsions and death. The usual signs of overdosage in adults and children include CNS depression such as deep sedation or coma.
• There is no specific antidote. Do NOT induce emesis. Aspiration of vomitus may occur. Treat supportively.

Azatadine Maleate
Cyproheptadine Hydrochloride

SPECIAL PRECAUTIONS
• Do not use in newborn or premature infants or in nursing mothers.
• Do not use to treat lower respiratory tract symptoms including asthma.

• Do not use in patients with a history of hypersensitivity to cyproheptadine hydrochloride, azatadine maleate, or related compounds.
• Administer with considerable caution to patients with angle-closure glaucoma, stenosing peptic ulcer, symptomatic prostatic hypertrophy, bladder neck obstruction, pyloroduodenal obstruction, and elderly and debilitated patients.
• Safe use in pregnancy has not been established.
• Use with caution in patients with a history of bronchial asthma or with increased intraocular pressure, hyperthyroidism, cardiovascular disease or hypertension.
• Prolonged therapy may rarely cause blood dyscrasias.

ADVERSE EFFECTS
CNS EFFECTS: sedation, sleepiness, dizziness, disturbed coordination, fatigue, confusion, restlessness, excitation, nervousness, hallucinations, insomnia, euphoria, faintness, vertigo, headache, tremor, irritability, paresthesias hysteria, convulsions
RESPIRATORY EFFECTS: thickening of bronchial secretions, tightness of chest, wheezing, nasal stuffiness
CARDIOVASCULAR EFFECTS: hypotension, palpitations, extrasystoles
URINARY TRACT EFFECTS: frequency, difficulty urinating, retention
AUTONOMIC EFFECTS: dry mouth, nose, and throat, excessive perspiration, chills
GASTROINTESTINAL EFFECTS: epigastric distress, anorexia, nausea, vomiting, diarrhea, constipation
HEMATOLOGIC EFFECTS: hemolytic anemia, thrombocytopenia, leukopenia, agranulocytosis
ALLERGIC EFFECTS: urticaria, drug rash, anaphylactic shock, photosensitivity
OPHTHALMIC EFFECTS: blurred vision, dyplopia

OTIC EFFECTS: tinnitus, acute labyrinthitis

CLINICAL GUIDELINES

ADMINISTRATION:
• Caution patients that drowsiness may occur which may interfere with driving a car or operating equipment.

EFFECTS:
• Drowsiness may decrease with continued administration.

DRUG INTERACTIONS:
• Do not administer to patients receiving MAO inhibitors; the MAO inhibitors may prolong and intensify the anticholinergic effect of antihistamines.
• An additive effect may be noted with concomitant administration of other CNS depressants, such as hypnotics, sedatives, tranquilizers, and antianxiety agents.

OVERDOSAGE/ANTIDOTE:
• CNS stimulation, hallucinations, convulsions, and death may occur in children with overdosage. In adults overdosage may cause CNS depression. Atropinelike signs and symptoms (dry mouth, fixed dilated pupils, flushing, etc.) as well as gastrointestinal symptoms may occur.
• There is no specific antidote. Treat supportively.

Clemastine Fumarate

SPECIAL PRECAUTIONS
• Antihistamine therapy is contraindicated in nursing mothers because of the high risk of antihistamines generally, and for newborns and prematures in particular.
• Do not use antihistamines to treat lower respiratory tract symptoms including asthma.
• Do not use in patients with a history of hypersensitivity to clemastine fumarate.
• Use with considerable caution in patients with narrow-angle glaucoma, sten-osing peptic ulcer, pyloroduodenal obstruction, symptomatic prostatic hypertrophy, or bladder neck obstruction.
• Safe use in pregnancy has not been established.
• Use with caution in patients with a history of bronchial asthma, increased intraocular pressure, hyperthyroidism, cardiovascular disease, or hypertension.

ADVERSE EFFECTS
CNS EFFECTS: drowsiness, sedation, sleepiness, dizziness, disturbed coordination, fatigue, confusion, restlessness, excitation, nervousness, tremor, irritability, insomnia, euphoria, paresthesias, hysteria, neuritis, convulsions, headache
RESPIRATORY EFFECTS: thickening of bronchial secretions, tightness of chest and wheezing, nasal stuffiness
CARDIOVASCULAR EFFECTS: hypotension, palpitations, tachycardia, extrasystoles
GASTROINTESTINAL EFFECTS: epigastric distress, anorexia, nausea, vomiting, diarrhea, constipation
AUTONOMIC EFFECTS: excessive perspiration, dryness of mouth, nose, and throat
URINARY TRACT EFFECTS: frequency, difficult urination, urinary retention
HEMATOLOGIC EFFECTS: hemolytic anemia, thrombocytopenia, agranulocytosis
METABOLIC AND ENDOCRINE EFFECTS: early menses
DERMATOLOGIC EFFECTS: drug rash, photosensitivity
ALLERGIC EFFECTS: urticaria, anaphylactic shock

CLINICAL GUIDELINES
ADMINISTRATION:
• Caution patients that drowsiness may interfere with activities requiring alertness

such as driving a car or operating appliances and machinery

EFFECTS:

- Antihistamines are more likely to cause dizziness, sedation, and hypotension in elderly patients than in young patients.

DRUG INTERACTIONS:

- MAO-inhibitors prolong and intensify the drying effects of antihistamines.
- When used concurrently with alcohol, barbiturates, sedatives, tranquilizers, and other CNS depressants, the CNS depressant effects will be additive.

OVERDOSAGE/ANTIDOTE:

- In children, overdosage is most frequently characterized by stimulation. However, overdosage in general causes CNS depression. Atropinelike effects (fixed, dilated pupils; flushing; gastrointestinal effects) are noted also.
- There is no specific antidote. If vomiting has not occurred, induce the conscious patient to vomit. Gastric lavage is indicated if ingestion has ocurred within 3 hours. Saline cathartics (milk of magnesia) are useful because they draw water into the bowel and dilute the contents.
- Do not use stimulants. Treat supportively as indicated.

Anti-Inflammatory Agents

Corticosteroids (Glucocorticoids)

The anti-inflammatory corticosteroids (glucocorticoids), major drugs used in the treatment of allergies, are discussed in detail in Chapter 15, *Endocrine and Other Drugs Affecting Metabolism,* page 535.

Anti-inflammatory corticosteroids administered by inhalation are discussed separately in the following pages because of their therapeutic significance.

GENERAL CLINICAL USES

The anti-inflammatory corticosteroids for inhalation are indicated for use in patients with bronchial asthma and related bronchiostatic states who usually require chronic treatment with corticosteroids for control of symptoms.

These products are not for use in patients who require relief from an occasional, mild, or isolated attack of asthma.

SPECIFIC PRODUCTS AND DOSAGES—Refer to table, page 310.

Beclomethasone Dipropionate

PHARMACOLOGY

Beclomethasone, chemically related to prednisolone, is a potent anti-inflammatory agent. When administered as an aerosol, absorption occurs from all respiratory tissues as indicated in isotope studies in animals. The mechanisms responsible for the anti-inflammatory and respiratory tract actions are unknown.

GENERIC NAME	TRADE NAME	ROUTE OF ADMIN.	USUAL DAILY DOSAGE
beclomethasone dipropionate	VANCERIL	inhalation	**Adults:** 2 inhalations (100 mcg) tid or qid; maximum: 20 inhalations **Children 6–12 yrs.:** 1–2 inhalations tid or qid; maximum: 10 inhalations/day **Children under 6 yrs.:** not established
dexamethasone sodium phosphate	DECADRON Phosphate respihaler	inhalation	**Adults:** 3 inhalations tid or qid; maximum: 12 inhalations/day **Children:** 2 inhalations tid or qid; maximum: 8 inhalations/day

SPECIAL PRECAUTIONS

• Do not use as primary treatment of status asthmaticus or other acute episodes when intensive measures are required.

• Do not use in patients hypersensitive to any component.

• Deaths have occurred due to adrenal insufficiency in asthmatic patients during and after transfer from systemic corticosteroids to aerosol beclomethasone.

• Long-term effects, local or systemic, are still unknown.

• Use in pregnancy requires that the possible benefits be weighed against potential hazards.

ADVERSE EFFECTS

LOCAL EFFECTS: hoarseness, dry mouth
SYSTEMIC EFFECTS: depression of HPA function (reduction of early morning cortisol levels); death

CLINICAL GUIDELINES

ADMINISTRATION:

• During periods of stress or during a severe asthma attack, transfer patients will require supplementary treatment with systemic steroids.

• After approximately 1 week of therapy, gradual withdrawal of the patient's systemic steroid dosage should be initiated; reduce very slowly.

EFFECTS:

• Localized infections with *Candida albicans* or *Aspergillus niger* have occurred in the mouth and larynx of patients treated with beclomethasone.

Dexamethasone Sodium Phosphate

PHARMACOLOGY

Dexamethasone sodium phosphate is a highly water-soluble anti-inflammatory corticostoid. Consequently the aerosolized particles dissolve in the bronchiolar secretions and mucous membranes resulting in a greater local therapeutic effect than obtained with the same dose ingested. The mechanism of action in relief of asthmatic attacks and in the anti-inflammatory activity is unknown.

SPECIAL PRECAUTIONS

• Do not use in patients with systemic fungal disease, hypersensitivity to any component, or with persistently postive sputum cultures for *Candida albicans*.

ADVERSE EFFECTS

LOCAL EFFECTS: laryngeal and pharyngeal fungal infections rarely; coughing, hoarseness, throat irritation.

Anti-Infective Agents

GENERAL CLINICAL USES

Infections of the respiratory tract are frequent and vary in severity. Consequently, a wide variety of anti-infective agents are available for treating the bacterial and fungal infections of the respiratory tract. Although frequently the initial selection of an anti-infective agent is empiric, appropriate susceptibility tests and microbial identification should be performed prior to the administration of the anti-infective agent.

For information concerning the drugs appropriate for treating respiratory tract infections, see Chapter 2, *Anti-Infective Agents*, page 10.

Antitussive Agents

GENERAL CLINICAL USES

The antitussive agents suppress the cough but have no direct effect on the underlying disease. Suppressive therapy may be adequate to permit rest, facilitate sleep, and reduce the irritation which may make the cough self-perpetuating.

SPECIFIC PRODUCTS AND DOSAGES—Refer to table, page 312.

Benzonatate

PHARMACOLOGY

Benzonatate has both a central and a peripheral pharmacologic action. It is a non-narcotic antitussive agent; the antitussive effect begins within 15 to 20 minutes after administration and lasts for 3 to 8 hours. It has no inhibitory effect on the respiratory center in the recommended dosages.

	GENERIC NAME	TRADE NAME	ROUTE OF ADMIN.	USUAL DAILY DOSAGE	
				ADULTS	**CHILDREN**
	benzonatate	TESSALON*	po	100 mg tid; maximum: 600 mg/day	**Over 10 yrs.:** 100 mg tid
CII†	codeine/codeine phosphate/ codeine sulfate	(G)††	po	10–20 mg q 4–6 hr.; maximum: 120 mg/day	**6–12 yrs.:** 5–10 mg q 4–6 hr.; maximum: 60 mg/24 hr. **2–6 yrs.:** 2.5–5 mg q 4–6 hr.; maximum: 30 mg/24 hr.
	dextromethorphan hydrobromide	CODIMAL* DIMACOL* ROMILAR	po	15–30 mg tid or qid	**6–12 yrs.:** 10–15 mg tid or qid **2–6 yrs.:** 5–7.5 mg tid or qid
CII	hydrocodone bitartrate	CODONE EXPECTIO*	po	5–10 mg tid or qid	0.6 mg/kg/day divided in 3–4 doses
	levopropoxyphene napsylate	NOVRAD	po	50–100 mg q 4 hr.; maximum: 600 mg/day	0.5 mg/lb q 4 hr.; maximum: 25 lbs—75 mg/ day, 50 lbs—150 mg, 75 lbs—200 mg/day
	noscapine	ACTOL* CONAR* THEO-NAR TUSSCAPINE	po	15–30 mg tid or qid; maximum: 120 mg/day	**6–12 yrs.:** 15 mg tid or qid; maximum: 60 mg/day **2–6 yrs.:** 7.5–15 mg tid or qid **Under 2 yrs.:** Not established

*Contains more than one active ingredient.
†C denotes schedule listing under the Controlled Substances Act.
††(G) designates availability as a generic product.

SPECIAL PRECAUTIONS

• Safe use in pregnancy has not been established.
• Do not use in patients with a history of hypersensitivity to benzonatate or related compounds.
• Benzonatate may cause temporary local anesthesia of the oral mucosa.

ADVERSE EFFECTS

CNS EFFECTS: sedation, headache, mild dizziness
RESPIRATORY EFFECTS: nasal congestion, numbness in the chest
GASTROINTESTINAL EFFECTS: gastrointestinal upset
ALLERGIC EFFECTS: hypersensitivity

DERMATOLOGIC EFFECTS: pruritus, skin eruption
OPHTHALMIC EFFECTS: sensation of burning in the eyes

CLINICAL GUIDELINES
ADMINISTRATION:
• Drug is administered as perles. Warn patients if chewed or dissolved oropharyngeal anesthesia will develop rapidly.
OVERDOSAGE/ANTIDOTE:
• Benzonatate is chemically related to tetracaine and other topical anesthetics and shares their toxicity and pharmacology. CNS stimulation may cause restlessness and tremors. Clonic convulsions followed by CNS depression may occur with overdosage. Cough and gag reflexes may be depressed; caution against aspiration of gastric contents.
• There is no specific antidote. Do *not* use CNS stimulants. Treat supportively.

Codeine, Codeine Phosphate, Codeine Sulfate

PHARMACOLOGY
Codeine and its salts inhibit the cough reflex in the medullary center. For additional information see Chapter 4, *Drugs Affecting the Brain and Spinal Cord*, page 127. Information concerning special precautions, adverse reactions, and guidelines for nurses of significance when codeine is used in dosages adequate for an antitussive effect is included herein.

Codeine has a drying effect on the mucosa of the respiratory tract which may be advantageous when excessive mucus is present. Codeine is absorbed rapidly and the effect is noticeable within 15 minutes. Codeine phosphate is more soluble in water than is the sulfate; it acts more rapidly than the sulfate.

SPECIAL PRECAUTIONS
• Do not use in patients with a history of hypersensitivity to codeine and related compounds.
• Codeine and its salts are narcotic agents; tolerance and addiction may occur.
• Safe use in pregnancy has not been established.

ADVERSE EFFECTS
CNS EFFECTS: addiction, dizziness, mental clouding, dysphoria, delirium and insomnia rarely, drowsiness, agitation
RESPIRATORY EFFECTS: depression
CARDIOVASCULAR EFFECTS: palpitation
AUTONOMIC EFFECTS: hyperhydrosis
GASTROINTESTINAL EFFECTS: nausea, constipation, vomiting
ALLERGIC EFFECTS: allergic reactions, urticaria
DERMATOLOGIC EFFECTS: pruritus, dermatitis
OPHTHALMIC EFFECTS: miosis

CLINICAL GUIDELINES
ADMINISTRATION:
• Any medication administered to a patient before meals, that is, with an empty stomach, is absorbed more rapidly than if administered during or after meals, resulting in a more rapid relief of discomfort than might otherwise be obtained.
EFFECTS:
• Repeated daily use causes eventual tolerance to therapeutic effects.
DRUG INTERACTIONS:
• The depressant effect of codeine may be exaggerated by phenothiazines, MAO inhibitors, imipramine, and other tricyclic antidepressants.

- Methaqualone potentiates codeine as an antitussive agent.
- When codeine and aspirin are administered concomitantly, there is a significant supra-additive analgesic effect.

OVERDOSAGE/ANTIDOTE:
- Symptoms of overdosage of codeine include coma and respiratory depression with hypoxia. Overdosage can also cause convulsions of spinal origin, particularly in children.
- To overcome codeine-induced respiratory depression, use a narcotic antagonist (e.g., naloxone). See Chapter 20, page 695, for information concerning use of the narcotic antagonists.

Dextromethorphan Hydrobromide

PHARMACOLOGY

Dextromethorphan, a non-narcotic antitussive agent, exerts its activity by increasing the threshold of the medullary cough center. A clinical effect is noted within 1 hour and the duration of action ranges from 8 to 12 hours. No tolerance or addiction has been noted. Dextromethorphan hydrobromide has no depressant effect on respiration.

SPECIAL PRECAUTIONS
- Safe use in pregnancy has not been established.
- Do not use in patients with a history of hypersensitivity to dextromethorphan hydrobromide or related compounds.

ADVERSE EFFECTS
CNS EFFECTS: slight drowsiness, dizziness
GASTROINTESTINAL EFFECTS: nausea, constipation, gastrointestinal upset

CLINICAL GUIDELINES
OVERDOSAGE/ANTIDOTE:
- Doses as high as 300 to 1500 mg have resulted in a state resembling intoxication accompanied by euphoria, stuporousness, and disturbances in gait. After emesis recovery was rapid.
- Empty stomach. Treat supportively.

Hydrocodone Bitartrate

PHARMACOLOGY

Hydrocodone bitartrate is an effective antitussive agent derived from codeine. Pharmacologically it is more active than codeine. The antitussive activity is 3 to 10 times that of codeine on a weight basis. Hydrocodone bitartrate causes suppression of the cough reflex by a direct effect on the cough center of the medulla. When administered orally it is rapidly absorbed and the duration of action is approximately 4 hours.

SPECIAL PRECAUTIONS
- Tolerance and/or addiction may occur.
- Do not use in patients with a history of hypersensitivity to hydrocodone bitartrate or related compounds.
- Safe use in pregnancy has not been established.

ADVERSE EFFECTS
CNS EFFECTS: addiction, dizziness, mental clouding, dysphoria, delirium and insomnia rarely, drowsiness, agitation
RESPIRATORY EFFECTS: depression
CARDIOVASCULAR EFFECTS: palpitation
AUTONOMIC EFFECTS: hyperhydrosis
GASTROINTESTINAL EFFECTS: nausea, constipation, vomiting

HEPATIC EFFECTS: increased pressure in the biliary tract

ALLERGIC EFFECTS: allergic reactions, urticaria

DERMATOLOGIC EFFECTS: pruritus, dermatitis

OPHTHALMIC EFFECTS: miosis

CLINICAL GUIDELINES

ADMINISTRATION:
- Caution patients that drowsiness may occur which may interfere with tasks requiring alertness or physical coordination.

EFFECTS:
- Repeated daily use causes eventual tolerance to therapeutic effects.

DRUG INTERACTIONS:
- The depressant effect may be exaggerated by phenothiazines, MAO inhibitors, imipramine, and other tricyclic antidepressants.
- Methaqualone potentiates codeine and might also potentiate hydrocodone bitartrate.

OVERDOSAGE/ANTIDOTE:
- Symptoms of overdosage include coma and respiratory depression with hypoxia. Overdosage can also cause convulsions of spinal origin, particularly in children.
- To overcome the respiratory depression, use a narcotic antagonist (e.g., naloxone). See Chapter 20, page 695, for information concerning use of the narcotic antagonists.

Levopropoxyphene Napsylate

PHARMACOLOGY
Levopropoxyphene napsylate administered orally controls cough effectively for approximately 4 hours. Both intensity and frequency of cough are reduced. Levopropoxyphene napsylate has no analgesic properties and does not alter the respiratory tract fluid.

SPECIAL PRECAUTIONS
- Do not administer to patients with a history of hypersensitivity to levopropoxyphene napsylate or related compounds.
- Safe use in pregnancy has not been established.
- If symptoms of CNS stimulation or sedation develop, the dosage should be reduced or medication discontinued.

ADVERSE EFFECTS
CNS EFFECTS: drowsiness, dizziness, nervousness

GASTROINTESTINAL EFFECTS: nausea, epigastric burning

ALLERGIC EFFECTS: urticaria

DERMATOLOGIC EFFECTS: rash

CLINICAL GUIDELINES
DRUG INTERACTIONS:
- Nalorphine is contraindicated in treatment of overdosage according to animal data.

OVERDOSAGE/ANTIDOTE:
- Overdosage is characterized by symptoms such as uncontrollable muscle tremor, agitation, and vomiting, followed by sedation.
- There is no specific antidote. Treat supportively.

Noscapine

PHARMACOLOGY
Noscapine, a non-narcotic antitussive agent, is well absorbed after oral administration. The potency is equivalent to codeine.

No tolerance was noted with doses as high as 90 mg daily for 4 to 6 weeks. It has no addictive liability and no analgesic property.

SPECIAL PRECAUTIONS

• Persons with high fever or persistent cough should not use this preparation unless directed by a physician.
• Safe use in pregnancy has not been established.
• Do not use in patients with a history of hypersensitivity to noscapine or related compounds.

ADVERSE EFFECTS

CNS EFFECTS: drowsiness
GASTROINTESTINAL EFFECTS: nausea

CLINICAL GUIDELINES

ADMINISTRATION:
• Do not exceed 4 doses per day.
• Do not administer to children less than 2 years of age.

EFFECTS:
• Antitussive agents do not obviate the need for expectorants and the administration of fluids for asthmatics in whom excess mucus production or mucus plugging is suspected.

OVERDOSAGE/ANTIDOTE:
• Noscapine has no effect on respiration in doses as high as 90 mg. Overdosage is characterized by an exaggeration of the adverse effects.
• There is no specific antidote. Treat supportively.

Bronchodilators/Antiasthma Agents

GENERAL CLINICAL USES

The bronchodilators are useful for symptomatic treatment of acute and chronic bronchial asthma and other pulmonary diseases with bronchospasm such as bronchitis and emphysema. The bronchodilators may be divided into two groups: the theophylline group of xanthine derivatives and the adrenergic agents. Drugs in the latter group are more effective than the xanthine derivatives in relieving bronchospasm.

The bronchodilator formulated as an elixir is useful in acute conditions whereas the capsule, tablet, or sustained or delayed release formulation is useful in chronic conditions as a preventive agent. Although many products contain more than a single ingredient, only the bronchodilating agents will be discussed herein. Information about the other active ingredients, will be found elsewhere, e.g., in the discussion of expectorants.

Cromolyn sodium, an antiasthma drug, is not a bronchodilator but is used adjunctively to bronchodilators to decrease the frequency of allergy-oriented asthma attacks; it is *not* of use in acute asthma attacks.

The anti-inflammatory corticosteroids (glucocorticoids), major drugs used in the treatment of asthma, are discussed in detail in Chapter 15, page 535.

SPECIFIC PRODUCTS AND DOSAGES

| GENERIC NAME | TRADE NAME | ROUTE OF ADMIN. | USUAL DAILY DOSAGE | |
			ADULTS	CHILDREN
Xanthine Derivatives: aminophylline	(G)† LIXAMINOL SOMOPHYLLIN	po im iv infusion pr	200–315 mg tid to qid 500 mg as needed 0.9–5.6 mg/kg/hr. 300 mg od to tid	3–6 mg/kg tid to qid Not recommended Not established 5 mg/kg qid
dyphylline	AIRET	po im	200–400 mg tid or qid 250–500 mg; repeat if necessary; do not exceed 600 mg/day	20–35 mg/day in divided doses Not recommended
oxtriphylline	BRONDECON* CHOLEDYL	po	200 mg qid	**2–12 yrs.:** 100 mg/60 lb qid
theophylline	(G) BRONKODYL ELIXOPHYLLIN QUIBRON* THEODUR	po pr	200–250 mg qid 250–500 mg bid or tid	100 mg qid 10 mg/kg/24 hr. in divided doses
theophylline monoethyanolamine	FLEET THEO-PHYLLINE	pr	250–500 mg bid; maximum: 2 doses/day	Not established
theophylline sodium glycinate	(G) ASBRON* THEOBID	po	330–660 mg tid or qid	**6–12 yrs.:** 220–330 mg tid or qid **Under 6 yrs.:** 83–165 mg/10 lbs tid or qid
Adrenergic Agents: ephedrine HCl	(G) VEREQUAD*	po	24–48 mg tid or qid	**6–12 yrs.:** 12–24 mg tid **Under 6 yrs.:** proportionately less
epinephrine	(G) MICRONEPHRINE VAPONEFRIN	aerosol nebulizer	1/100—0.2–0.4 ml diluted; may be repeated every 3–4 hr.	Not established
epinephrine bitartrate	E-CARPINE* MEDIHALER EPI	inhalation	1–2 inhalations; may be repeated	Not established
epinephrine HCl	(G) ADRENALIN GLUCON	im/sc	0.2–1.0 ml; repeat if necessary	0.01 ml/kg; repeat in 4 hr. if required
ethylnorepinephrine HCl	BRONKEPHRINE	im/sc	0.5–1.0 ml; repeat if necessary	0.1–0.5 ml; repeat if necessary

*Contains more than one active ingredient.
†(G) designates availability as a generic product.

(continued overleaf)

GENERIC NAME	TRADE NAME	ROUTE OF ADMIN.	USUAL DAILY DOSAGE	
			ADULTS	**CHILDREN**
isoetharine HCl	BRONKOMETER BRONKOSOL	inhalation	1–2 inhalations; repeat every 4 hr.; see labeling	Not established
isoproterenol HCl	(G) ISUPREL HCl MEDIHALER-ISO ISUPREL	inhalation	1–2 inhalations 4–6 times daily	Not established
		sublinqual	15–20 mg qid; maximum: 60 mg/day	5–10 mg; do not exceed 30 mg in one day
metaproterenol sulfate	ALUPENT METAPREL	po	20 mg tid or qid	**Over 60 lbs.:** 20 mg tid to qid **Under 60 lbs.:** 10 mg tid to qid **Under 6 yrs.:** Not recommended
		inhalation	1.30–1.95 mg (2–3 inhalations); do not exceed 7.8 mg (12 inhalations)	Not recommended
protokylol HCl	VENTAIRE	po	2–4 mg qid	Not established
terbutaline sulfate	BRETHINE	po	2.5–5 mg tid; maximum: 15 mg/day	**12–15 yrs.:** 2.5 mg tid; maximum: 7.5 mg/day **Under 12 yrs.:** Not recommended
		sc	0.25–0.5 mg as 1 or 2 doses	**Under 12 yrs.:** Not recommended
cromolyn sodium	INTAL	inhalation	20 mg qid	**Over 5 yrs.:** 20 mg qid **Under 5 yrs.:** Not established

Xanthine Derivatives

Aminophylline
Dyphylline
Theophylline
Theophylline Monoethanolamine
Theophylline Sodium Glycinate

Aminophylline, theophylline, and related drugs are potent xanthine bronchodilators which relieve bronchospasm and increase the vital capacity and forced expiratory volume. Theophylline is absorbed rapidly after oral administration and produces minimal gastrointestinal irritation.

Dyphylline, a molecular modification of theophylline, is a bronchodilating agent which apparently is well tolerated and causes minimal gastric irritation. The neutral pH of dyphylline prevents precipitation by gastric or intestinal juices. It is readily absorbed after oral administration and it has all the pharmacologic effects of theophylline; it also may be administered intramuscularly.

The sustained release formulations are absorbed in the bowel after bypassing the stomach thereby reducing gastric irritation. The elixir is useful in acute attacks, primarily because of its rapid absorption and effect.

Theophylline monoethanolamine is effective when administered rectally and thereby minimizes the undesirable gastro-intestinal reactions associated with oral administration. Clinically effective plasma levels are usually obtained within one half hour following rectal administration.

Theophylline calcium salicylate is a well tolerated theophylline sale with bronchodilator activity similar to theophylline and its other salts.

SPECIAL PRECAUTIONS
• Use with extreme caution, if at all, in patients with peptic ulcer, glaucoma, gout, coronary artery disease, angina pectoris, or hypertension.
• Do not use in patients with a history of hypersensitivity to theophylline or related compounds.
• Do not use in patients with severe cardiac, renal, or liver impairment.
• Use theophylline calcium salicylate cautiously in patients sensitive to salicylates.
• Safe use in pregnancy has not been established.
• Use cautiously in children.

ADVERSE EFFECTS
CNS EFFECTS: headache, dizziness, nervousness, insomnia
CARDIOVASCULAR EFFECTS: palpitation, precordial pain, decrease in blood pressure
URINARY TRACT EFFECTS: albuminuria, diuresis, kidney irritation
GASTROINTESTINAL EFFECTS: nausea, vomiting, epigastric pain, intestinal bleeding, reactivation of peptic ulcer
LOCAL EFFECTS: with dyphylline, irritation, pain

CLINICAL GUIDELINES
ADMINISTRATION:
• Administer to patients with an empty stomach; however, if gastric irritation occurs, advise patient to take with or after meals to eliminate or reduce this discomfort.
• Rapid intravenous administration may cause sudden and profound hypotension.
• Administer dyphylline intramuscularly slowly; do NOT give intravenously.
• Intravenous administration should be slow and cautious, especially in patients with myocardial ischemia.
EFFECTS:
• Prolonged use of suppositories may cause irritation to the rectal mucosa.
DRUG INTERACTIONS:
• Avoid concurrent administration with other theophylline preparations such as cough preparations.
• In children avoid concomitant administration with sympathomimetic drugs unless accompanied by sufficient sedation to prevent undue stimulation.
OVERDOSAGE/ANTIDOTE:
• Deaths have occurred from overdosage in adults and also following rectal administration of adult doses to children. Overdosage may cause peripheral vascular collapse.
• Symptoms of acute toxicity may include fever, delirium, agitation, convulsions, hematemesis, bloody diarrhea, shock, dehydration, and even death.
• There is no specific antidote. Treat supportively.

Oxtriphylline

PHARMACOLOGY
Oxtriphylline, the choline salt of the-ophylline, is a bronchodilating agent less ir-

ritating to the gastric mucosa than aminophylline. It is readily absorbed from the gastrointestinal tract.

SPECIAL PRECAUTIONS
• Do not use in patients with a history of hypersensitivity to oxtriphylline or related compounds.
• Safe use in pregnancy has not been established.
• Use with extreme caution, if at all, in patients with peptic ulcer, gout, coronary artery disease, angina pectoris, or hypertension.
• Do not use in patients with severe renal or liver impairment.

ADVERSE EFFECTS
CNS EFFECTS: stimulation
CARDIOVASCULAR EFFECTS: palpitation
GASTROINTESTINAL EFFECTS: gastric distress

CLINICAL GUIDELINES
ADMINISTRATION:
• Administer after meals to minimize gastric discomfort.
EFFECTS:
• If adverse reactions occur, discontinue oxtriphylline and institute the appropriate therapy.
DRUG INTERACTIONS:
• Do not use other xanthine-containing preparations or other CNS stimulants concurrently.
OVERDOSAGE/ANTIDOTE:
• Overdosage is characterized by an exaggeration of the adverse effects, particularly cardiovascular effects.
• There is no specific antidote. Treat supportively.

Ephedrine Hydrochloride

PHARMACOLOGY
Pharmacologically ephedrine and epinephrine are similar. Ephedrine, an adrenergic agent, stimulates both alpha and beta receptors. Therefore, it has both vasoconstrictor properties resulting in reduction of mucosal and submucosal edema and bronchodilator properties resulting in reduction of airway smooth muscle spasm. Ephedrine differs from epinephrine in that it is effective after oral administration, has more pronounced central actions, and is less potent. The duration of bronchodilating action is more prolonged than with epinephrine.

SPECIAL PRECAUTIONS
• Do not use in patients with a history of hypersensitivity to ephedrine or related compounds.
• Excessive dosage may result in severe and serious tachyarrhythmias.
• Use with caution in elderly male patients or those with known prostatic hypertrophy.
• Safe use in pregnancy has not been established.
• Do not use in patients with hyperthyroidism, cardiovascular disease, and hypertension.

ADVERSE EFFECTS
CNS EFFECTS: headache, insomnia, excitation, tremulousness, nervousness, vertigo
CARDIOVASCULAR EFFECTS: increased heart rate, palpitations, tachycardia, precordial pain, cardiac arrhythmias
URINARY TRACT EFFECTS: urinary hesitation, occasionally acute urinary retention
AUTONOMIC EFFECTS: sweating, warmth, dry nose and throat
GASTROINTESTINAL EFFECTS: nausea

CLINICAL GUIDELINES

ADMINISTRATION:
• Administer with or after meals to reduce gastric irritation.
EFFECTS:
• Repeat administration is usually not needed more often than every 3 to 4 hours; more frequent therapy such as every 2 hours may be required in severe situations.
DRUG INTERACTIONS:
• Administer only one adrenergic drug at a time because these drugs act additively.
• Concomitant use of an adrenergic agent and theophylline may provide bronchodilator action superior to that obtained with either drug administered alone.
OVERDOSAGE/ANTIDOTE:
• Overdosage may be characterized by tachycardia, palpitations, nausea, and headache.
• There is no specific antidote. Treat supportively.

Adrenergic (Sympathomimetic Agents)

Epinephrine
Epinephrine Bitartrate
Epinephrine HCl
Ethylnorepinephrine Hydrochloride

PHARMACOLOGY

Following oral administration, epinephrine is inactivated in the gastrointestinal tract. Consequently, administration is usually parenterally or by inhalation. After intramuscular or subcutaneous administration, adsorption is rapid. With aerosol administration, the actions are generally limited to the respiratory tract, although systemic reactions may occur. Aerosol administration relieves temporarily the acute paroxysms of bronchial asthma by its short-acting sympathomimetic activity.

Ethylnorepinephrine hydrochloride has actions similar to epinephrine but is without significant pressor effects. The bronchodilator effect of ethylnorepinephrine hydrochloride is less than that of epinephrine.

SPECIAL PRECAUTIONS

• Do not use in patients with hypertension, cardiovascular disease, diabetes, hyperthyroidism, coronary insufficiency, cardiac arrhythmias, and with any history of hypersensitivity to sympathomimetic drugs.
• Refractoriness may occur after too frequent administration.

ADVERSE EFFECTS

CNS EFFECTS: nervousness, anxiety, dizziness, restlessness, insomnia, headache, tremulousness
RESPIRATORY EFFECTS: bronchial irritation, respiratory weakness, rebound bronchospasm
CARDIOVASCULAR EFFECTS: changes in blood pressure or pulse rate, palpitations, tachycardia
GASTROINTESTINAL EFFECTS: nausea
DERMATOLOGIC EFFECTS: pallor

CLINICAL GUIDELINES

ADMINISTRATION:
• Take care that intramuscular preparations are not inadvertently administered intravenously.
• Advise patients in proper cleaning of nebulizer to minimize bacterial contamination.
EFFECTS:
• Isoproterenol and epinephrine may be used interchangeably if the patient becomes unresponsive to one or the other; do not use concurrently.

• Four hours should elapse before changing medications.

• Too frequent administration may cause irritation and dryness of mucous membranes and cause retention of mucus plugs in the bronchioles.

• Inhalation may cause a severe, prolonged attack of asthma.

DRUG INTERACTIONS:

• Administer only one adrenergic agent at a time because these drugs act additively.

• Concomitant use of an adrenergic agent and theophylline may provide bronchodilator action superior to either drug administered alone.

Isoetharine Hydrochloride

PHARMACOLOGY

Isoetharine hydrochloride is a sympathomimetic amine which has a preferential affinity for beta 2 adrenergic receptor sites of the bronchial and cardiac arteriolar musculature. It relieves symptoms of bronchospasm rapidly and relief is of long duration.

SPECIAL PRECAUTIONS

• Do not use in patients with a history of hypersensitivity to isoetharine or related compounds.

• Safe use in pregnancy has not been established.

• Discourage excessive use of an adrenergic aerosol since it may lose its effectiveness.

• Severe paradoxical airway resistance may develop with repeated excessive uses of the adrenergic aerosol.

• Administer with caution and adjust dos-age carefully in patients with hyperthyroidism, hypertension, acute coronary disease, cardiac asthma, and limited cardiac reserve.

• Use with caution in patients with prostatic hypertrophy; urinary retention may occur.

ADVERSE EFFECTS

CNS EFFECTS: headache, anxiety, tension, restlessness, insomnia, tremor, weakness, dizziness, excitement

CARDIOVASCULAR EFFECTS: tachycardia, palpitations, changes in blood pressure

URINARY TRACT EFFECTS: urinary retention

GASTROINTESTINAL EFFECTS: nausea

CLINICAL GUIDELINES

ADMINISTRATION:

• Caution patients to avoid excessive use of an adrenergic aerosol since it may lose its effectiveness.

EFFECTS:

• Paradoxical airway resistance may develop with repeated and excessive use of the adrenergic aerosol.

DRUG INTERACTIONS:

• Administer only one adrenergic agent at a time because these drugs act additively.

• Concomitant use of an adrenergic agent and theophylline may provide bronchodilator action superior to that obtained with either drug administered alone.

• Isoethararine hydrochloride may be administered simultaneously with other therapeutic agents such as antibiotics or wetting agents.

OVERDOSAGE/ANTIDOTE:

• Signs of overdosage include tachycardia, palpitations, nausea, headache, or epinephrinelike side effects. Cardiac arrest has occurred.

• There is no specific antidote. Treat supportively.

Isoproterenol

PHARMACOLOGY

Isoproterenol, a short acting sympathomimetic drug, will prevent or overcome histamine-induced asthma. It is a potent bronchodilator which acts primarily on the beta receptors and has almost no action on the alpha receptors. Isoproterenol also has a cardioaccelerator effect and vasoconstricting action. It is readily absorbed following inhalation and parenteral administration. The duration of action is short and similar to epinephrine.

SPECIAL PRECAUTIONS

• Do not use in patients with pre-existing cardiac arrhythmias associated with tachycardia.

• Do not use in patients with a history of hypersensitivity to isoproterenol or related compounds.

• Note that cardiac arrest has occured in patients receiving isoproterenol.

• Safe use in pregnancy has not been established.

• Use with caution in patients with cardiovascular disorders including coronary insufficiency, diabetes, or hyperthyroidism.

ADVERSE EFFECTS

CNS EFFECTS: tremulousness, dizziness, weakness, tremor, restlessness, headache, sleepiness, vertigo, insomnia, CNS excitement

RESPIRATORY EFFECTS: with aerosol, throat irritation; bronchial edema and inflammation

CARDIOVASCULAR EFFECTS: palpitations, tachycardia, angina-type pain, elevation of blood pressure, precordial pain, arrhythmias

AUTONOMIC EFFECTS: sweating, flushing

GASTROINTESTINAL EFFECTS: nausea, vomiting

METABOLIC AND ENDOCRINE EFFECTS: hyperglycemia

OTIC EFFECTS: tinnitus

CLINICAL GUIDELINES

ADMINISTRATION:

• Do not use solutions if discolored (brownish) or if a precipitate is present.

• Advise patients in hygienic care of nebulizers and aerosol equipment to minimize bacterial contamination.

EFFECTS:

• No cumulative effects have been reported.

• Excessive inhalation may cause refractory bronchial obstruction.

• Excessive use of an adrenergic aerosol may result in loss of effectiveness.

DRUG INTERACTIONS:

• Do not administer concurrently with epinephrine since both drugs are direct cardiac stimulants and may result in serious arrhythmias.

• Isoproterenol and epinephrine may be used interchangeably if the patient becomes unresponsive to one or the other.

OVERDOSAGE/ANTIDOTE:

• Deaths have occurred with overdosage. Cardiac arrest has occurred. Overdosage can produce palpitations, tachycardia, tremulousness, flushing, angina-type pain, arrhythmias, nausea, dizziness, weakness, sweating, and vomiting.

- There is no specific antidote. Treat supportively.

Metaproterenol Sulfate

PHARMACOLOGY
Metaproterenol is a potent beta adrenergic stimulator which has a rapid onset of bronchodilating action following oral administration or inhalation. It is absorbed rapidly after both inhalation and oral administration; it is excreted primarily in the urine as glucuronic acid conjugate. The mean duration of effect may be as long as 4 hours.

SPECIAL PRECAUTIONS
- Do not use in patients with cardiac arrhythmias associated with tachycardia.
- Do not use in patients with a history of hypersensitivity to metaproterenol sulfate or related drugs.
- Paradoxical bronchoconstriction with repeated excessive administration has occurred with other sympathomimetic agents, and therefore may occur with metaproterenol sulfate.
- A sufficient time should elapse prior to administration of another sympathomimetic agent.
- Use with great caution in patients with hypertension, coronary artery disease, congestive heart failure, hyperthyroidism, and diabetes.
- Safe use in pregnancy has not been established.

ADVERSE EFFECTS
CNS EFFECTS: nervousness, tremor
CARDIOVASCULAR EFFECTS: tachycardia, hypertension, palpitations
GASTROINTESTINAL EFFECTS: nausea, vomiting, bad taste

CLINICAL GUIDELINES
ADMINISTRATION:
- Advise patients to contact physician if they do not respond to the usual dose of drug.

EFFECTS:
- Excessive use of adrenergic aerosols may result in loss of effectiveness and is potentially dangerous.

DRUG INTERACTIONS:
- If metaproterenol sulfate is administered before or after other sympathomimetic bronchodilators, potentiation of adrenergic effects is possible and cardiac arrhythmias may occur.

OVERDOSAGE/ANTIDOTE:
- The symptoms of overdosage consist of an exaggeration of the adverse (pharmacologic) effects. Cardiac arrest has occurred with excessive use.
- There is no specific antidote. Treat supportively and symptomatically.

Protokylol Hydrochloride

PHARMACOLOGY
Protokylol hydrochloride, a sympathomimetic amine, is a long-acting bronchodilator. It is a derivative of isoproterenol and similarly stimulates selectively the beta receptors. After oral administration the onset of action is within 30 to 90 minutes and the effects persist for 3 to 4 hours.

SPECIAL PRECAUTIONS
- Do not use in patients with cardiac arrhythmias or insufficiency of coronary circulation, diabetes, hyperthyroidism, pro-

static hypertrophy or glaucoma.

• Do not use in patients with a history of hypersensitivity to protokylol hydrochloride or related compounds.

• Use cautiously in patients who have received the sympathomimetic amines prior to protokylol hydrochloride.

• Safe use in pregnancy has not been established.

ADVERSE EFFECTS

CNS EFFECTS: tremulousness, tension, insomnia, dizziness, weakness

CARDIOVASCULAR EFFECTS: tachycardia, palpitations, increased blood pressure

URINARY TRACT EFFECTS: difficulty in voiding

GASTROINTESTINAL EFFECT: nausea

CLINICAL GUIDELINES

ADMINISTRATION:

• Caution patients that this bronchodilator is long acting.

EFFECTS:

• Effects persist for 3 to 4 hours.

DRUG INTERACTIONS:

• Use cautiously in patients who have received other sympathomimetic amines prior to protokylol hydrochloride.

OVERDOSAGE/ANTIDOTE:

• Overdosage is characterized by an exaggeration of the adverse (pharmacologic) effects.

• There is no specific antidote. Treat supportively.

Terbutaline Sulfate

PHARMACOLOGY

Terbutaline sulfate, a sympathomimetic amine, is a beta adrenergic receptor agonist exerting a preferential effect on beta 2 adrenergic receptors in bronchial smooth muscle. When administered orally, terbutaline sulfate relieves bronchospasm, producing a clinically significant decrease in airway and pulmonary resistance for at least 4 or more hours. The onset of action is approximately 30 minutes with significant clinical improvement noted in 1 to 2 hours.

SPECIAL PRECAUTIONS

• Do not use in patients with a history of hypersensitivity to terbutaline sulfate or other sympathomimetic amines.

• Safe use in pregnancy and lactation, or in children below 2 years of age, has not been established.

• Use with caution in patients with diabetes, hypertension, and hyperthyroidism.

• Administer with caution to cardiac patients, especially those with associated arrhythmias.

ADVERSE EFFECTS

CNS EFFECTS: nervousness, tremor, headache, drowsiness

CARDIOVASCULAR EFFECTS: tachycardia, palpitations

AUTONOMIC EFFECTS: sweating

GASTROINTESTINAL EFFECTS: nausea, vomiting

CLINICAL GUIDELINES

ADMINISTRATION:

• The frequency of undesirable effects appears to diminish with continued drug administration.

• Reduce dosage if undesirable effects are disturbing to patient.

DRUG INTERACTIONS:

• Administration concomitantly with other sympathomimetic agents is not recommended.

• Aerosol bronchodilators of the adrenergic stimulant type for relief of acute bronchospasm may be used.

OVERDOSAGE/ANTIDOTE:
• Overdosage is characterized by an exaggeration of the adverse effects.
• There is no specific antidote. Treat supportively.

Cromolyn Sodium

PHARMACOLOGY
Cromolyn sodium inhibits the release of histamine and the slow-reacting substance of anaphylaxis. Cromolyn sodium has no intrinsic bronchodilator, antihistaminic, or anti-inflammatory activity. Its action is prophylactic and consequently it is of no use in an acute attack of asthma.

After oral administration cromolyn sodium is poorly absorbed; however, after inhalation it is absorbed from the lungs and is excreted rapidly and unchanged in the bile and urine.

If clinical improvement occurs with cromolyn sodium, it usually occurs within the first 2 to 4 weeks of administration and is characterized by a decrease in severity and clinical symptoms, and/or in need for concomitant therapy.

SPECIAL PRECAUTIONS
• Do not use in patients with a history of hypersensitivity to cromolyn sodium.
• Use with caution in patients with impaired renal or hepatic function.
• Discontinue therapy if eosinophilic pneumonia occurs.
• Safe use in pregnancy has not been established.
• Note that occasionally patients may experience cough and/or brochospasm following cromolyn inhalation.
• If dosage is reduced below that recommended, symptoms of asthma may recur.

ADVERSE EFFECTS
RESPIRATORY EFFECTS: hoarseness, cough, bronchospasm
ALLERGIC EFFECTS: maculopapular rash, eosinophilic pneumonia, polymyositis, urticaria, angioedema, anaphylaxis

CLINICAL GUIDELINES
ADMINISTRATION:
• Cromolyn sodium *must* be inhaled; capsules are not absorbed if ingested and drug is ineffective.
• Cromolyn sodium is adjunctive therapy only in asthma.

EFFECTS:
• Symptoms of asthma may recur if dosage is below recommended levels or reduced.
• Improvement will ordinarily occur within the first 2 to 4 weeks of administration as manifested by a decrease in severity of asthmatic symptoms.

DRUG INTERACTIONS:
• Corticosteroids and bronchodilators have been administered concomitantly with cromolyn.
• Cromolyn sodium permits better management of patients who have intolerable side effects to sympathomimetic agents or methyl xanthines.

OVERDOSAGE/ANTIDOTE:
• Overdosage is characterized by an exaggeration of the adverse (pharmacologic) effects.
• There is no specific antidote. Treat supportively.

Expectorants

GENERAL CLINICAL USES

The expectorants are usually used in combination with antitussive agents and/or bronchodilators. They may aid in removing viscid mucus obstructing the bronchioles and soothe the mucous membrane inflammation by stimulation of the protective secretions. Dry, unproductive coughs become less frequent but more productive.

The expectorants are useful in treating the cough associated with respiratory disorders such as the common cold and bronchitis; chronic asthma; severe, chronic, and allergic bronchitis; chronic obstructive pulmonary emphysema.

SPECIFIC PRODUCTS AND DOSAGES

GENERIC NAME	TRADE NAME	ROUTE OF ADMIN.	USUAL DAILY DOSAGE
ammonium chloride	BENYLIN* Cough Syrup TRIAMINICOL* Cough Syrup	po	**Adults:** 250–500 mg qid **Children 6–12 yrs.:** 125–250 mg every 4–6 hr. **Children 2–6 yrs.:** 62.5–125 mg every 4–6 hr.
guaifenesin (glyceryl guaiacolate)	EXPECTRAN GLYCOTUSS	po	**Adults and children over 12 yrs.:** 100–200 mg q 3–4 hr. **Children 6–12 yrs.:** 100 mg q 3–4 hr. **Children 3–6 yrs.:** 50 mg q 3–4 hr.
potassium guaiacolsulfonate	CODIMAL* DH/DM/ EXP/PH PHENERGAN* Expectorant with Codeine PHENERGAN* VC Expectorant with Codeine	po	**Adults:** 100–200 mg qid **Children 6–12 yrs.:** 100 mg qid **Children 3–6 yrs.:** 50 mg qid
potassium iodide	(G)† ELIXOPHYLLIN-KI* MUDRANE* Tab PIMA Syrup QUADRINAL* Tab/Susp	po	**Adults:** 300–600 mg every 4–6 hrs. **Children:** 50–300 mg every 4–6 hrs.

*Contains more than one active ingredient.
†(G) designates availability as a generic product.

Ammonium Chloride

PHARMACOLOGY

Ammonium chloride increases the amount of mucus in the respiratory tract by reflex stimulation of the gastric mucosa.

SPECIAL PRECAUTIONS

- Use cautiously in patients with hepatic, renal, or pulmonary insufficiency.
- Safe use in pregnancy has not been established.
- Do not use in patients with a history of hypersensitivity to ammonium chloride or related compounds.

ADVERSE EFFECTS

- Not established.

CLINICAL GUIDELINES

ADMINISTRATION:
- Enteric coated tablets are ineffective as an expectorant.
- Efficacy of this product is questionable.

OVERDOSAGE/ANTIDOTE:
- Overdosage may result in metabolic acidosis.
- Empty stomach. Treat metabolic acidosis with alkali therapy.

Guaifenesin (Glyceryl Guiacolate) Potassium Guaicolsulfonate

PHARMACOLOGY

Guaifenesin and potassium guaicolsulfonate increase the secretion and decrease the viscosity of fluids in the respiratory tract. The increased fluids lubricate the inflamed mucous membranes and help the patient expel viscid mucus.

Guaifenesin has a relatively long action and is an effective stimulant of the respiratory tract fluid.

Potassium guaicolsulfonate is a derivative of guaifenesin which is thought to be converted in the body to the active expectorant, guaiacol.

SPECIAL PRECAUTIONS

- Do not use in patients with a history of hypersensitivity to either product.
- Do not administer for treatment of chronic or recurrent cough.

ADVERSE EFFECTS

CNS EFFECTS: drowsiness rarely
GASTROINTESTINAL EFFECTS: nausea, gastrointestinal upset, vomiting rarely

CLINICAL GUIDELINES

ADMINISTRATION:
- Administer after meals to minimize gastric irritation.

EFFECTS:
- A color interference with certain laboratory determinations of 5-hydroxyindole acetic acid (5-HIAA) and vanilmandelic acid (VMA) may occur.

DRUG INTERACTIONS:
- Guaifenesin is usually administered in combination with decongestants, antitussives, bronchodilators, and other expectorants.

OVERDOSAGE/ANTIDOTE:
- Overdosage usually results in nausea and vomiting.
- Terminate drug. Drug effects are usually self-limiting.

Potassium Iodide

PHARMACOLOGY

Potassium iodide aids in liquifying thick, tenacious mucus by increasing bronchial secretion by reflex stimulation of the gastric mucosa.

Potassium iodide crosses the placental barrier and large doses may produce thyroid enlargement in the fetus.

SPECIAL PRECAUTIONS
• Do not use in patients with a history of hypersensitivity to potassium iodide or related compounds.
• Do not use in patients with hyperthyroidism.
• Prolonged use of iodides has resulted in hypothyroidism.
• Do not administer potassium iodide alone in patients with acute bronchitis.
• Small bowel lesions may occur with administration of enteric coated potassium tablets.
• Use with caution, if at all, in pregnant patients.

ADVERSE EFFECTS
RESPIRATORY EFFECTS: laryngeal edema.
GASTROINTESTINAL EFFECTS: gastrointestinal upset, metallic taste, nausea, vomiting, epigastric pain
METABOLIC AND ENDOCRINE EFFECTS: thyroid adenoma, goiter, myxedema
HEMATOLOGIC EFFECTS: eosinophilia
ALLERGIC EFFECTS: angioneurotic edema, cutaneous and mucocutaneous hemorrhage, fever, arthralgia, lymph node enlargement, anaphylaxis
DERMATOLOGIC EFFECTS: eruption

CLINICAL GUIDELINES
ADMINISTRATION:
• If lacrimal and nasal secretions occur, reduce dosage.
• Use of potassium iodide will interfere with interpretation of thyroid function tests.
EFFECTS:
• Discontinue use if nausea, abdominal pain, distention, vomiting, and gastrointestinal bleeding occur.
OVERDOSAGE/ANTIDOTE:
• Overdosage is characterized by an exaggeration of the adverse effects.
• There is no specific antidote. Treat supportively.

Nasal Decongestants

GENERAL CLINICAL USES
The nasal decongestants whether applied topically or administered systemically relieve temporarily the symptoms of nasal congestion associated with the common cold, acute upper respiratory tract infections, sinusitis, and hay fever and other upper respiratory tract allergies. Eustachian tube congestion may also be relieved.

The nasal decongestants are grouped as adrenergic agents or imidazolines.

SPECIFIC PRODUCTS AND DOSAGES

GENERIC NAME	TRADE NAME	ROUTE OF ADMIN.	USUAL DOSAGE
Adrenergic Agents:			
ephedrine, ephedrine hydrochloride, ephedrine sulfate	(G)† ISOPROTERENOL HCl	topical po	Apply as needed **Adults:** 25–50 mg every 3–4 hr. **Children:** 3 mg/kg divided in 4–6 doses
epinephrine hydrochloride	(G) ADRENALIN GLUCON	topical	Apply as needed 1–2 drops in each nostril every 4 to 6 hr.
phenylephrine	(G) NEO-SYNEPHRINE	topical	**Adults and older children:** 0.25–1% solution needed q 3 to 4 hr. **Children over 6 yrs.:** 0.25% solution in each nostril q 3–4 hr.
	ISOPHRIN DIMETANE* Exp.	po	**Adults:** 10 mg tid **Children 6–12 yrs.:** 5 mg tid
phenylpropanolamine	(G) ALLEREST* DIMETANE* NALDECON* PROPADRINE PROTRIM	po	**Adults:** 25 mg every 3–4 hr. **Children 6–12 yrs.:** 12.5 mg q 4 hr. **Children 2–6 yrs.:** 6.25 mg q 4 hr.
propylhexedrine	BENZEDREX	topical	2 inhalations (0.6–0.8 mg) as needed
pseudoephedrine hydrochloride	(G) NOVAFED SINACET* SUDABID SUDAFED	po	**Adults and children over 12 yrs.:** 60 mg q 4 hr. **Children 6–12 yrs.:** 30 mg q 4 hr. **Children 2–5 yrs.:** 15 mg q 4 hr. **Children under 2 yrs.:** not established
tuaminoheptane	TUAMINE	inhalation	1–2 inhalations; repeat hourly if necessary
tuaminoheptane sulfate	TUAMINE Sulfate	topical	**Adults and children over 6 yrs.:** 4–5 drops every 3 or 4 hr. **Children 1–6 yrs.:** 2–3 drops; not more than 4–5 times daily
Imidazolines: naphazoline hydrochloride	(G) PRIVINE 0.05%	solution	2 drops in each nostril no more than every 3 hr.

*Contains more than one active ingredient.
†(G) designates availability as a generic product.

(continued facing page)

GENERIC NAME	TRADE NAME	ROUTE OF ADMIN.	USUAL DOSAGE
oxymetazoline hydrochloride	AFRIN DURATION	spray drops	**Adults:** 2–3 sprays bid usually adequate **Adults:** 2–4 drops bid
tetrahydrozoline hydrochloride	TYZINE 0.1%, 0.05%	drops	**Adults:** 2–4 drops not more than every 3 hr. (0.1% solution) **Children 2–6 yrs.:** 2–3 drops as needed, not more than every 3 hr. (0.05% solution)
xylometazoline hydrochloride	OTRIVIN 0.1%, 0.05% 0.05%	spray solution solution	**Adults:** 1–2 sprays every 4–6 hr. **Adults:** 2–3 drops every 2–6 hr. (0.1% solution) **Children under 12 yrs.:** 2–3 drops every 4–6 hr. (0.05% solution) **Children under 6 mos.:** 1 drop every 6 hr. (0.05% solution).

Adrenergic Agents:

Ephedrine
Epinephrine HCl
Phenylephrine
Phenylpropanolamine
Propylhexedrine
Pseudoephedrine
Tuaminoheptane

PHARMACOLOGY

The adrenergic agents which are effective nasal decongestants produce this effect by stimulating the alpha adrenergic receptors of the vascular smooth muscle. Constriction of the dilated arterioles within the nasal mucosa and reduction of blood flow are produced. The adrenergic agents may be administered orally or topically. With orally administered agents the relief provided may be more prolonged than with topically administered products.

The differences among these decongestant agents is primarily in the onset and duration of action. The topically applied products, namely, ephedrine, epinephrine, and phenylephrine, act rapidly and in general have a short duration of action. Several products are administered by inhalation exclusively; these products include those containing propylhexadrine and tuaminoheptane.

Oral administration of the adrenergic decongestant agents results in slower action than obtained with topically administered products but the duration of action is more prolonged and the effect more complete. Agents in this group are ephedrine, pseudoephedrine and phenylpropanolamine; of these, phenylpropanolamine is administered only by the oral route.

These agents have been detected in the milk of nursing mothers.

SPECIAL PRECAUTIONS
- Do not use in patients with severe hypertension, severe coronary artery disease, and in patients receiving MAO-inhibitors.

- Note that patient idiosyncrasy to adrenergic agents may be manifested by isomnia, dizziness, weakness, tremor, or arrythmias.
- Do not use in nursing mothers since these agents have been detected in mother's milk.
- Do not use in patients with a history of hypersensitivity to any of these or other sympathomimetic amines.
- Use with caution in patients with hypertension, diabetes mellitus, ischemic heart disease, increased intraocular pressure, hyperthyroidism, and prostatic hypertrophy.
- Safe use in pregnancy has not been established.
- Use with extreme caution in adults over 60 years of age since they are more likely to experience adverse reactions than younger patients.
- Sympathomimetic amines may produce CNS stimulation with convulsions or cardiovascular collapse with accompanying hypertension.

ADVERSE EFFECTS
LOCAL EFFECTS: stinging, burning, dryness of mucosa, interference with nasal ciliary action

CNS EFFECTS: headache, dizziness, fear, anxiety, tenseness, restlessness, tremor, weakness, pallor, insomnia

RESPIRATORY EFFECTS: dyspnea

CARDIOVASCULAR EFFECTS: tachycardia, palpitations, arrhythmias, cardiovascular collapse with hypotension

GASTROINTESTINAL EFFECTS: nausea

URINARY TRACT EFFECTS: dysuria

CLINICAL GUIDELINES
ADMINISTRATION:
- Advise patients in proper hygienic procedures in caring for dropper or spray tip to minimize contamination.

EFFECTS:
- Repeated administration of the high concentration topical preparations may cause irritation and swelling of the nasal mucosa.
- In general, topical administration procedures few or minimal adverse effects.
- Repeated administration of oral preparations does not result in reduced effectiveness.

DRUG INTERACTIONS:
- MAO-inhibitors and other beta adrenergic blockers may increase the effect of the decongestant administered.
- The antihypertensive effects of methyldopa, mecamylamine, reserpine, and veratrum alkaloids may be reduced.
- Do not administer concurrently with MAO-inhibitors.

OVERDOSAGE/ANTIDOTE:
- Overdosage of the orally administered products is characterized by an exaggeration of the adverse effects; hallucinations, convulsions, CNS depression, and death may ocurr. Hypertension followed by rebound hypotenson has occurred.
- There is no specific antidote. Treat supportively.
- Topical overdosage may result in systemic absorption which is characterized by transient hypertension, nervousness, nausea, and dizziness.
- There is no specific antidote.

Imidazolines

Naphazoline HCl
Oxymetazoline HCl
Tetrahydrozoline HCl
Xylometazoline HCl

PHARMACOLOGY
The imidazolines, sympathomimetic amines, constrict the smaller arterioles of the nasal passages producing a decongestant effect. Oxymetazoline HCl has a long

duration of action. Tetrahydrozoline HCl produces clinical relief lasting from 4 to 8 hours.

SPECIAL PRECAUTIONS
- Do not use in patients with a history of hypersensitivity to these drugs.
- Safe use in pregnancy has not been established.
- Use cautiously in patients with coronary artery disease, hypertension, hyperthyroidism, or diabetes mellitus.

ADVERSE EFFECTS
LOCAL EFFECTS: burning, stinging, sneezing, swelling, anosmia, rebound congestion, paralysis of nasal cilia, smarting
CNS EFFECTS: drowsiness, headache, insomnia, light-headedness, weakness, tremors
RESPIRATORY EFFECTS: with tetrahydrozoline HCl, chronic swelling of the nasal mucosa with prolonged use
CARDIOVASCULAR EFFECTS: arrhythmias, hypertension, bradycardia, palpitations, rebound hypotension

OPHTHALMIC EFFECTS: with xylometazoline HCl, blurred vision

CLINICAL GUIDELINES
ADMINISTRATION:
- Use sparingly, particularly in young children and in patients with angina.
- Advise patients in hygienic procedures to avoid bacterial contamination of applicator (dropper or spray tip).
EFFECTS:
- Prolonged use causes tolerance and decreased duration of action.
DRUG INTERACTIONS:
- Do not use in atomizers containing any parts made of aluminum.
- Do not administer the imidazolines and MAO-inhibitors concurrently; severe hypertensive crises may occur.
OVERDOSAGE/ANTIDOTE:
- In adults, overdosage may result in cardiac arrhythmias, sweating, drowsiness, deep sleep, coma, with hypotension and bradycardia. In children, results are similar.
- There is no specific antidote. Treat supportively. Drug effects usually are self-limiting.

Respiratory Stimulants

GENERAL CLINICAL USES
The respiratory stimulants, doxapram and nikethamide, are used as supportive treatment of respiratory depression, usually associated with drug-induced coma (not due to overdosage of inhalation anesthetics).

Naloxone and levallorphan are used in stimulating respiration in drug (narcotic) induced respiratory depression. They are classified as narcotic antagonists; detailed information may be found in Chapter 20, page 695.

SPECIFIC PRODUCTS AND DOSAGES

GENERIC NAME	TRADE NAME	ROUTE OF ADMIN.	USUAL DOSAGE
doxapram HCl	DOPRAM	iv infusion	**Adults:** 0.5–4 mg/kg at rate of 5 mg/min; then 1–3 mg/min; maximal dose 3 gm **Children:** not recommended
levallorphan tartrate	LORFAN	iv	**Adults:** 1 mg, then 0.5 mg twice at 5 to 10 min intervals; max 3 mg/day **Children:** 0.02 mg/kg **Neonates:** 0.05–1 mg in umbilical vein
naloxone HCl	NARCAN NARCAN Neonatal	im/iv/sc iv	**Adults:** 0.1–0.4 mg, repeat in 2–3 minutes **Children:** 0.01 mg/kg **Neonates:** 0.01 mg/kg in umbilical vein
nikethamide	CORAMINE	iv im/sc po	2–20 ml 2–15 ml 3–5 ml tid or qid

Doxapram Hydrochloride

PHARMACOLOGY

Doxapram hydrochloride is a direct stimulant of the central (medulla) respiratory center. The onset of respiratory stimulation usually occurs in 20 to 40 seconds; the peak effect is reached in 1 to 2 minutes and usually lasts 5 to 12 minutes. An increase in the tidal volume and a moderate increase in respiratory rate occurs. Blood pressure and pulse rate also may increase.

SPECIAL PRECAUTIONS

• Do not administer to patients with epilepsy or other convulsive states, severe hypertension, or cerebrovascular accidents.
• Do not use in patients taking MAO-inhibitors or adrenergic agents.
• Do not use in patients with a history of hypersensitivity to doxapram or related compounds.

• Safe use in pregnancy has not been established.
• Do not use in compromised ventilatory mechanism due to muscle paresis, flail chest, pneumothorax, airway obstruction, and extreme dyspnea.
• Use with caution in patients with cerebral edema, bronchial asthma, severe tachycardia, cardiac arrhythmia, cardiac disease, hyperthyroidism, and pheochromocytoma.

ADVERSE EFFECTS

CNS EFFECTS: hyperactivity, muscle tremor, clonus, increased deep tendon reflexes, dizziness, muscle spasticity, confusion, paresthesias, headache, bilateral Babinski, fasciculation and carpopedal spasm, grand mal seizures in epileptic patients
RESPIRATORY EFFECTS: cough, dyspnea, laryngospasm, bronchospasm, hiccups
CARDIOVASCULAR EFFECTS: hypertension, sinus tachycardia, bradycardia, extrasys-

toles, lowered T-waves, premature ventricular contraction, irregular heart rhythm, tightness in chest, hypertension
URINARY TRACT EFFECTS: urinary retention, stimulation of urinary bladder with spontaneous voiding, albuminuria, increased BUN
AUTONOMIC EFFECTS: feeling of warmth, sweating, pupillary dilatation, pyrexia, pilomotor erection
GASTROINTESTINAL EFFECTS: nausea, vomiting, salivation, stimulation of lower bowel, sour taste
HEMATOLOGIC EFFECTS: decreased hemoglobin, hematocrit, erythrocytes; increased leukopenia in patients having leukopenia
DERMATOLOGIC EFFECTS: pruritus
LOCAL EFFECTS: thrombophlebitis

CLINICAL GUIDELINES
ADMINISTRATION:
• Monitor blood gases.
• Evaluate deep tendon reflexes, pulse, and blood pressure periodically to avoid overdosage.
EFFECTS:
• Narcosis may reoccur after stimulation with doxapram.
DRUG INTERACTIONS:
• Do not mix with alkaline solutions such as thiopental sodium because doxapram is acidic.
• Administer oxygen concomitantly when indicated.
OVERDOSAGE/ANTIDOTE:
• Overdosage is characterized by exaggeration of the adverse effects such as excessive pressor effects, tachycardia, skeletal muscle hyperactivity and enhanced deep tendon reflexes.
• There is no specific antidote; however, intravenously administered short-acting barbiturates, oxygen, and resuscitation equipment should be available if needed.

Treat supportively.

Levallorphan Tartrate
Naloxone Hydrochloride

For detailed information, see Chapter 20, page 695.

Nikethamide

PHARMACOLOGY
Nikethamide is a central nervous system stimulant with a direct medullary effect. Secondary indirect stimulation of peripheral chemoreceptors may also occur.

SPECIAL PRECAUTIONS
• Do not use in patients known to be hypersensitive to niketamide or related compounds.
• Do not inject intra-arterially; spasm and thrombosis may result.
• Safe use in pregnancy has not been established. Therefore use in pregnant patients only when, in the judgment of the physician, its use is deemed essential to the welfare of the patient.

ADVERSE EFFECTS
CNS EFFECTS: generalized restlessness, fear, convulsions
CARDIOVASCULAR EFFECTS: tachycardia, elevated blood pressure
RESPIRATORY TRACT EFFECTS: burning or itching at back of nose, sneezing, coughing, changing depth and frequency of respiration
AUTONOMIC EFFECTS: flushing, sweating
GASTROINTESTINAL EFFECTS: nausea, vomiting
MUSCULOSKELETAL EFFECTS: muscle twitching (especially facial)

CLINICAL GUIDELINES

ADMINISTRATION:
• May be administered po, sc, im, or iv; it is most effective by iv administration.

OVERDOSAGE/ANTIDOTE:
• Overdosage is characterized by coughing, sneezing, hyperpnia, and muscle tremors. Cardiac rate and blood pressure are usually elevated. With severe overdosage, generalized muscle spasms and convulsive seizures occur.
• Treatment is usually not required except in severe overdosage. The muscle spasms and convulsions can be controlled by short-acting barbiturates. Treat supportively as required.

Therapeutic Gases

GENERAL CLINICAL USES
Of the gases used therapeutically, the general inhalation anesthetics are discussed in Chapter 4, *Drugs Affecting the Brain and Spinal Cord,* page 153. Oxygen and carbon dioxide and also the inert gases, nitrogen and helium, will be included herein.

Carbon dioxide is used to stimulate respiratory depression, to increase the speed of induction and emergence from anesthesia, to outline the kidney, heart and other organs for delineating in x-rays, to enter the fallopian tubes to determine patency, and to produce pneumoperitoneum for peritoneoscopy.

Helium, an inert gas, is used in inhalation therapy as a substitute for nitrogen. Its usefulness is due exclusively to its physical properties. Since mixtures of oxygen and helium have reduced specific gravity in comparison with air, the work of breathing is reduced, which is desirable in patients with obstructive pulmonary disease. It is of value in patients with respiratory obstruction.

Nitrogen, an inert gas, has little therapeutic usefulness. It serves as a diluent for pure oxygen.

Oxygen is used to form mixtures with inhalation anesthetics and also to relieve hypoxemia.

SPECIFIC PRODUCTS AND
IDENTIFICATION

GENERIC NAME	IDENTIFICATION
carbon dioxide	gray cylinders
helium	brown cylinders
nitrogen	black cylinders
oxygen	green cylinders

Carbon Dioxide

PHARMACOLOGY
Carbon dioxide is used therapeutically to stimulate the respiratory system, in-

crease cerebral blood flow, and maintain the acid-base balance. Also, it is added to oxygen to prevent reduction of carbon dioxide tension in the blood. Carbon dioxide, a potent respiratory stimulator, increases both rate and depth of ventilation.

SPECIAL PRECAUTIONS
• When concentrations approach 30 percent, the respiratory center may be depressed.
• Since carbon dioxide is a potent cerebrovascular dilator, do not use in patients with increased intracranial pressure, intracranial bleeding, expanding lesions, head injury, or those in coma.
• Do not use in an attempt to resuscitate patients in cases of drowning, electric shock, or asphyxiation.
• An acidotic state may be aggravated by carbon dioxide.
• Do not use to treat overdosage of central nervous system depressants because the medullary chemoreceptors are depressed and do not respond.

ADVERSE EFFECTS
CNS EFFECTS: headache, convulsions, coma, restlessness, paresthesias, feeling of discomfort
RESPIRATORY EFFECTS: depression
CARDIOVASCULAR EFFECTS: elevated blood pressure, tachycardia, possible arrhythmias

SPECIAL PRECAUTIONS
• Hypoxia may occur if adequate oxygen is not present in the mixture administered.

CLINICAL GUIDELINES
ADMINISTRATION:
• Helium decreases inflammability when used to dilute anesthetics containing cyclopropane and oxygen.
• Adequate amounts of oxygen must be administered concurrently.
EFFECTS:
• Positive pressure respiration adminis-

tered intermittantly may contribute to efficacy in respiratory obstruction.
OVERDOSAGE/ANTIDOTE:
• Overdosage is characterized by apnea. Administer oxygen.

Helium

PHARMACOLOGY
Helium, an inert gas, is used as a diluent for medicinal gases. Its pharmacologic actions are due exclusively to its physical properties. Because of its lightness, it is used to create artificial air which alleviates difficult breathing.

SPECIAL PRECAUTIONS
• Do not administer in concentrations over 60 to 80 percent.

CLINICAL GUIDELINES
ADMINISTRATION:
• Adequate amounts of oxygen (20 percent) must be administered concurrently with helium.
OVERDOSAGE/ANTIDOTE:
• Overdosage is characterized by apnea.
• Administer oxygen.

Nitrogen

PHARMACOLOGY
Nitrogen, an inert gas, has little therapeutic usefulness. It is used as a diluent for pure oxygen for which diagnostic procedures of hollow body cavities because it is absorbed slowly. Nitrogen administered under hyperbaric conditions dissolves in the blood and lipid tissues in proportion to the increased inhaled partial pressure.

SPECIAL PRECAUTIONS
• Nitrogen must be administered by inhalation with sufficient oxygen when used as a gas diluent.

- Rapid decompression if used under hyperbaric conditions may lead to embolization ("bends").

ADVERSE EFFECTS
Embolization (bends) occurs on rapid decompression.

CLINICAL GUIDELINES
ADMINISTRATION:
- Adequate amounts of oxygen must be administered concurrently.

EFFECTS:
- Since nitrogen dissolves in the blood and lipid tissues, decompression must take place slowly.

OVERDOSAGE/ANTIDOTE:
- Nitrogen narcosis occurs with overdosage. Administer oxygen.

Oxygen

PHARMACOLOGY
Oxygen is used therapeutically in hypoxia and in treating pulmonary hypertension. Oxygen, inhalation appears to relax the pulmonary vasculature. It can be a lifesaving stopgap until the existing condition can be corrected. "Hyperbaric oxygen" is also used in certain circulatory disturbances and respiratory difficulties; in treating anaerobic infections; in carbon monoxide poisoning; and in tumor therapy and surgery.

SPECIAL PRECAUTIONS
- Concentrations above 40 percent may cause retrolental fibroplasia and permanent blindness in premature infants.
- Watch for signs of carbon dioxide retention.
- Prolonged administration of high concentrations causes pulmonary irritation characterized by pneumonitis, congestion, and a decrease in vital capacity.

- Use humidification apparatus to eliminate or reduce dehydration of mucous membranes.
- Inhalation of 100 percent oxygen may result in mild respiratory depression.
- Use caution to avoid contamination of reservoir nebulizer with Pseudomonas and other bacteria.

ADVERSE EFFECTS
Pulmonary irritation manifested by substernal pain has occurred. Inhalation of 80 percent oxygen for more than 12 hours can cause irritation of the respiratory tract characterized by decreased vital capacity, coughing, nasal stuffiness, sore throat, and substernal distress; this does not occur with 50 percent oxygen. Inhalation of pure oxygen at pressures greater than 2 atmospheres may result in muscular twitching, nausea, vertigo, mood changes, paresthesias, eventual loss of consciousness, and generalized convulsions.

CLINICAL GUIDELINES
ADMINISTRATION:
- Note that the risk of fire or explosion is directly proportional to the concentration of oxygen in the mixture being supplied.
- The risk of fire is particularly great with oxygen tents.
- Never use electrical appliances and never allow smoking in areas close to oxygen use.
- Sterilize reservoir nebulizers and other inhalation equipment to avoid bacterial contamination.

EFFECTS:
- Respiratory depression may occur with high concentrations.
- Oxygen poisoning can occur with inhalation of concentrations of 80 percent or more for about 12 hours.

OVERDOSAGE/ANTIDOTE:
- Oxygen apnea may occur. Remove supply of oxygen or administer artificial respiration.

Drugs affecting the urinary tract

7

INTRODUCTION

The urinary tract is subject to many disorders and diseases, some directly concerned with the renal excretory mechanism, others having a primary locus elsewhere in the body but indirectly affecting the renal mechanism. The drugs used for treating urinary tract disorders have been grouped according to use regardless of the mechanism of the disorder.

SPECIFIC THERAPEUTIC CLASSIFICATION

The therapeutic agents of value in treating disorders affecting the urinary tract may be grouped into several categories, as follows:

1. Acidifying agents
2. Analgesic agents
3. Alkalinizing agents
4. Antienuretic agents
5. Anti-infective agents

6. Antispasmodic/Anticholinergic agents
7. Antiseptic agents
8. Diuretics (see Chapter 5, page 249.)
9. Irrigants

10. Stimulants/Cholinergic agents

Each group may be subdivided further depending upon the chemical and pharmacologic relationships of the individual drugs.

Acidifying Agents

GENERAL CLINICAL USES

The urinary acidifying agents aid in keeping calcium in urine in solution, thereby preventing formation of renal calculi. Consequently, patients who recurrently form calcium oxalate stones or stones due to calcium carbonate, calcium phosphate, and/or magnesium ammonium phosphate (struvite calculi) may be aided. A urine-acidifying agent will aid effectiveness of antibacterial agents such as methenamine. The urinary acidifying agents are also useful in controlling urine odor and the dermatitis and ulcerations caused by alkaline urine in the incontinent patient.

SPECIFIC PRODUCTS AND DOSAGES

Both single and multiple ingredient agents are marketed presently. Only single ingredient products will be listed.

GENERIC NAME	TRADE NAME	ROUTE OF ADMIN.	USUAL DOSAGE
ammonium chloride	(G)*	po	**Adults:** 500 mg qid
methionine	PEDAMETH URACID URANAP	po	**Adults:** 200 mg tid or qid **Infants (2–6 mos.:)** 75 mg tid **(6–14 mos.:)** 75 mg qid
methylene blue	UROLENE BLUE	po	**Adults:** 65–130 mg tid
potassium acid phosphate	K-PHOS	po	**Adults:** 1000 mg qid
sodium acid phosphate	(G)	po	**Adults:** 600 mg qid
vitamin C (ascorbic acid)	(G)	po	**Adults:** 500 mg tid to qid

*(G) designates availability as a generic product.

Ammonium Chloride
Methionine
Methylene Blue
Potassium Acid Phosphate
Vitamin C (Ascorbic Acid)

PHARMACOLOGY

The acidifying agents, by various mechanisms, change the urine pH from basic to acidic. The acidification of urine increases the solubility of the calcium salts. Methylene blue may inhibit growth of struvite calculi (magnesium-ammonium phosphate stones); it has resulted in stone dissolution.

SPECIAL PRECAUTIONS

• Potassium acid phosphate should not be administered to patients with hepatic disease, Addison's disease or renal insufficiency.

• Small bowel lesions consisting of stenosis, with or without ulceration, have been associated with use of enteric coated potassium salts.
• Do not administer methionine to patients with a history of liver disease.
• Use methylene blue cautiously in patients with renal impairment.

ADVERSE EFFECTS

RENAL EFFECTS: methylene blue—occasional irritation of bladder
GASTROINTESTINAL EFFECTS: potassium acid phosphate, sodium acid phosphate—mild laxative effect, hyperacidity, nausea

CLINICAL GUIDELINES

ADMINISTRATION:
• Advise patients to maintain an adequate fluid intake.
EFFECTS:
• Advise patients taking potassium salts to report any gastrointestinal symptoms.

Analgesic Agents

GENERAL CLINICAL USES

Urinary tract analgesics provide prompt relief of pain, and they alleviate dysuria, frequency, and urgency. Analgesics used for urinary tract pain are usually combined with antibacterial agents, antiseptics, and antispasmodic agents.

The narcotics, morphine and meperidine, are the only drugs adequate in the urological conditions associated with severe pain such as urolithiasis, infection, renal colic, and tumor. For more detailed information on the systemic analgesic agents, see Chapter 4, page 128.

Phenazopyridine HCl is an effective urinary tract analgesic which is usually formulated with other active drugs such as the sulfonamides.

SPECIFIC PRODUCTS AND DOSAGES

The dosage of these drugs, as with many medications, should be individualized on the basis of the patient's relief of discomfort.

GENERIC NAME	TRADE NAME	ROUTE OF ADMIN.	USUAL DOSAGE
CII† meperidine HCl	(G)* DEMEROL HCl	im/sc/po	**Adults:** 50–100 mg every 4 hrs. **Children:** 0.5–0.8 mg/lb every 3–4 hrs.
CII morphine sulfate	(G)	im/iv/sc/ po	**Adults:** 2–20 mg every 4 hrs. **Children:** 0.1–0.2 mg/kg/ dose
phenazopyridine hydrochloride	(G) AZODINE PYRIDIUM	po	**Adults:** 50–200 mg tid or qid **Children:** 4 mg/kg tid

*(G) designates availability as a generic product.
†designates schedule listing under Controlled Substances Act.

Meperidine Hydrochloride, Morphine Sulfate

For detailed information, see Chapter 4, pages 137 and 139, respectively.

Phenazopyridine Hydrochloride

PHARMACOLOGY
Phenazopyridine hydrochloride is rapidly absorbed from the gastrointestinal tract producing prompt and effective local anesthesia in the urinary tract. The rapid excretion in the urine produces a topical analgesia on the urinary tract mucosa. It produces no general sedation or narcosis.

SPECIAL PRECAUTIONS
• Do not administer to patients with glomerulonephritis, severe hepatitis, uremia, or pyelonephritis, or to pregnant patients.
• Do not use in patients hypersensitive to phenazopyridine hydrochloride or related compounds.

ADVERSE EFFECTS
CNS EFFECTS: headache
GASTROINTESTINAL EFFECTS: gastrointestinal upset
HEMATOLOGIC EFFECTS: methemoglobinemia with large doses, hemolytic anemia
OPHTHALMIC EFFECTS: yellowish tinge to sclerae.

CLINICAL GUIDELINES
ADMINISTRATION:
• Warn patients that phenazopyridine hydrochloride will impart an orange-red color of the urine soon after administration.
• The orange-red color of the urine may interfere with urinalysis.
• Administer after meals to avoid gastric discomfort.
OVERDOSAGE/ANTIDOTE:
• Overdosage or prolonged dosing may result in a yellowish tinge to the skin or sclerae.
• There is no known antidote.

Alkalinizing Agents

GENERAL CLINICAL USES

The alkalinizing agents are used in conditions when long-term maintenance of an alkaline urine is desirable such as in patients with uric acid and cystine calculi of the urinary tract. The alkalinizing agents are also of value in gout therapy as adjunctive agents to uricosuric drugs to prevent urates from crystallizing out of an acid urine. The alkalinizing agents are also effective in correcting the acidosis of renal tubular disorders.

SPECIFIC PRODUCTS AND DOSAGES

GENERIC NAME	TRADE NAME	USUAL DOSAGE
oral citrate mixture (citric acid, sodium citrate, potassium citrate)	POLYCITRA Syrup	**Adults:** 3–6 tsp qid **Children:** 1–4 tsp qid
potassium citrate	(G)	**Adults:** 7.5 gm/day in divided doses
sodium bicarbonate	(G)*	**Adults:** 3–15 gm/day in divided doses
sodium lactate	(G)	**Adults:** 1/6 molar solution iv 500 ml

*(G) designates availability as a generic product.

Oral Citrate Mixture
Potassium Citrate
Sodium Bicarbonate
Sodium Lactate

PHARMACOLOGY

The alkalinizing agents are administered orally, absorbed from the gastrointestinal tract, and excreted into the urine, producing an alkaline urine. The alkaline urine prevents formation of urate deposits in the urinary tract, for example, when sulfonamides are administered.

SPECIAL PRECAUTIONS

• Determine serum electrolytes periodically to avoid hyperkalemia and alkalosis.
• Do not use sodium lactate in patients with severe hepatic disease.
• Patients receiving sodium citrate should be on a low calcium diet, since alkaline urine may precipitate calcium.

ADVERSE EFFECTS

METABOLIC AND ENDOCRINE EFFECTS: hyperkalemia, alkalosis

CLINICAL GUIDELINES

ADMINISTRATION:
- Administer after meals and before bedtime.

EFFECTS:
- Maintain a urinary pH of 6.5 to 7.4.

OVERDOSAGE/ANTIDOTE:
- Signs of overdosage include hyperkalemia and alkalosis.
- There are no specific antidotes. Maintain fluid and electrolyte balance.

Antienuretic Agent

GENERAL CLINICAL USES

Enuresis, characterized by inappropriate voiding, has been treated with imipramine hydrochloride, a tricyclic antidepressant (see Chapter 3, *Psychotherapeutic Agents,* for additional information concerning this effect).

SPECIFIC PRODUCTS AND DOSAGES

The dosage of this drug, as with many medications, should be individualized on the basis of the patient's response. Periodic treatment is usually indicated.

GENERIC NAME	TRADE NAME	USUAL DAILY DOSAGE
imipramine hydrochloride	TOFRANIL	**Children 6–12 yrs.:** 25–50 mg at bedtime **Adolescents:** 50 mg at bedtime

Imipramine Hydrochloride

PHARMACOLOGY, SPECIAL PRECAUTIONS, ADVERSE EFFECTS, CLINICAL GUIDELINES

For detailed information, see the discussion of tricyclic antidepressants in Chapter 3, page 108.

Anti-Infective Agents

GENERAL CLINICAL USES

The systemically administered anti-infective agents used to treat urinary tract infections include chemotherapeutic agents and antibiotics to which the following organisms are susceptible: *Escherichia coli, Klebsiella-Enterobacter-Serratia* species, *Proteus mirabilis* and other *Proteus* species, *Streptococcus faecalis, Staphylococci,* coagulase-positive and negative, *Alcaligenes* species, *Acinetobacter (Herellea)* species, *Haemophilus* species, *Beta hemolytic streptococci,* usually Groups B and D, *Neisseria gonorrhoeae, Mycobacterium tuberculosis, Salmonella* and *Shigella* species. Other species of organisms may be involved in urinary tract infections but to a lesser extent than those listed.

Prior to initiation of therapy, ideally clinical isolates should be obtained for identification of the infecting organism or organisms and susceptibility testing to antimicrobial agents. Cultures are usually obtained, but therapy is initiated on an empirical basis. Because of the changing patterns of resistance and susceptibility among bacteria, it is essential that urine specimens be cultured initially and at appropriate intervals during therapy, particularly if the patient does not respond to therapy.

Dimethyl sulfoxide is indicated for symptomatic relief of interstitial cystitis. There is no evidence of its effectiveness in bacterial infections of the urinary tract.

SPECIFIC PRODUCTS AND DOSAGES

The dosages of the anti-infective agents used to treat urinary tract infections will vary with the infecting organism and severity of the infection. The status of renal function should be evaluated prior to therapy and periodically thereafter, paticularly with anti-infective agents which are potentially nephrotoxic.

| GENERIC NAME | TRADE NAME | ROUTE OF ADMIN. | USUAL DAILY DOSAGE | |
			ADULTS	INFANTS AND CHILDREN
Sulfonamides: sulfacytine	RENOQUID	po	500 mg, then 250 mg qid	Not established
				(continued overleaf)

GENERIC NAME	TRADE NAME	ROUTE OF ADMIN.	USUAL DAILY DOSAGE	
			ADULTS	INFANTS AND CHILDREN
sulfamethoxazole	BACTRIM* GANTANOL	po	2 gm, then 1 gm bid or tid	50–60 mg/kg, then 30 mg/kg bid
sulfisoxazole	GANTRISIN SK-SOXAZOLE SOXOMIDE	po	2–4 gm, then 4–8 gm q 4–6 hr.	60–75 mg/kg, then 150 mg/kg in divided doses
sulfisoxazole diolamine	GANTRISIN	iv/sc/im	**Initial dose:** 1/2 of 24 hr. dose **Maintenance dose:** 100 mg/kg/24 hr.	**Initial dose:** 1/2 of 24 hr. dose **Maintenance dose:** 100 mg/kg/24 hr.
Nitrofurans: nitrofurantoin	(G)† FURADANTIN MACRODANTIN	po	50–100 mg tid	5–7 mg/kg in divided doses qid
Penicillins: ampicillin	AMCILL POLYCILLIN	po	250–500 mg qid	100 mg in divided doses every 6–8 hrs.
carbenicillin disodium	GEOPEN PYOPEN	im/iv	200 mg/kg/day in divided doses	50–200 mg/kg in divided doses qid
carbenicillin indanyl sodium	GEOCILLIN	po	382–764 mg qid	Not established
methicillin sodium	AZAPEN STAPHCILLIN	iv im	1 gm every 6 hr. 1 gm every 4–6 hr.	Not established 25 mg/kg every 4–6 hr.
Cephalosporins: cefadroxil monohydrate	DURICEF	po	0.5–1 bid	Not established
cefazolin sodium	ANCEF KEFZOL	im/iv	0.5–1 gm bid	25–50 mg/kg/day divided in 3–4 equal doses; may increase to 100 mg/kg/day
cephalexin	KEFLEX	po	250 mg–1 gm qid	25–50 mg/kg divided in 4 doses
cephaloglycin	KAFOCIN	po	250–500 mg qid	25–50 mg/kg qid
cephaloridine	LORIDINE	im	0.5–1 gm 3 to 4 times daily	30–50 mg/kg divided in equal doses
cephalothin sodium	KEFLIN	im/iv	0.5–2 gm every 4–6 hr.	60–100 mg/kg divided in equal doses

*Contains more than one active ingredient.
†(G) designates availability as a generic product.

(continued facing page)

GENERIC NAME	TRADE NAME	ROUTE OF ADMIN.	USUAL DAILY DOSAGE	
			ADULTS	INFANTS AND CHILDREN
cephapirin sodium	CEFADYL	im/iv	0.5–1 gm every 4–6 hr.	40–80 mg/kg divided in 4 equal doses
cephradine	ANSPOR VELOSEF	im/iv po	0.5–1 gm qid 0.25–1 gm qid	50–100 mg/kg divided in 4 equal doses
Aminoglycosides: gentamicin sulfate	GARAMYCIN	im/iv	3 mg/kg divided in 3 equal doses	5–7.5 mg/kg divided in 3 or 4 doses
kanamycin sulfate	KANTREX	im iv	Up to 7.5–15 mg/kg q 12 hr Up to 15 mg/kg/day	Up to 7.5 mg/kg q 12 hr Not established
Polymyxins: colistimethate sodium	COLY-MYCIN M	iv/im	2.5–5 mg/kg divided in 2–4 doses	Same as adult
polymyxin B sulfate	(G) AEROSPORIN	im iv	15,000–25,000 U/kg/ day in divided doses 15,000–25,000 U/kg/ day q 12 hr. **Maximum:** 25000 U/ day	Not established Same as adult
Tetracyclines: tetracycline (hydrochloride)	(G) ACHROMYCIN PANMYCIN SUMYCIN TETRACYN TETREX-S	po im iv	250–500 mg qid 100–250 mg bid to tid 250–500 mg qid; maximum: 2 gm/day	25–50 mg/kg divided in 4 doses 15–25 mg/kg in 2 or 3 divided doses 12 mg/kg divided in 2 doses
Erythromycins: erythromycin	(G) E-MYCIN ERYTHROCIN ILOTYCIN	po	250–500 mg qid	30–50 mg/kg in divided doses
Cycloserine	SEROMYCIN	po	0.5–1 gm in divided doses; maximum: 1 gm	Not established
Others: nalidixic acid	NEG GRAM	po	1 gm qid	**3 mos.–12 yrs.:** 55 mg/kg/ day divided in 4 doses
oxolinic acic	UTIBID	po	750 mg bid	Not recommended
dimethyl sulfoxide (DMSO)	RIMSO-50	intra– vesicle	50 ml for 15 min.	Not recommended

PHARMACOLOGY, SPECIAL
PRECAUTIONS, ADVERSE EFFECTS,
CLINICAL GUIDELINES

See Chapter 2, *Anti-Infective Agents,*
for detailed information, page 10.

Detailed information follows for nalidixic and oxolinic acids, since they are used
exclusively for urinary tract infections, and
for dimethyl sulfoxide.

Nalidixic Acid
Oxolinic Acid

PHARMACOLOGY

Nalidixic acid and oxolinic acid are
effective against susceptible gram negative
bacteria including the majority of *Proteus*
strains, *Klebsiella, Enterobacter,* and *Escherichia coli.*

Following oral administration, nalidixic acid and oxolinic acid are rapidly
absorbed from the gastrointestinal tract.
They are partially metabolized in the liver
and rapidly excreted by the kidneys as
unchanged drug and active metabolite.
With nalidixic acid, peak serum levels occur in 1 to 2 hours after oral administration; peak levels in urine occur in 3 to 4
hours. With oxolinic acid, a bactericidal
concentration is obtained and maintained
in the urine for 4 and 12 hours, respectively. Nalidixic and oxolinic acids have been
found in infants of mothers who had received the drug during the last trimester of
pregnancy.

Oxolinic acid has CNS-stimulating
properties, which appear more frequently
than those occurring with nalidixic acid.

SPECIAL PRECAUTIONS

• Do not use in patients with a history of
hypersensitivity to these drugs, those with
convulsive disorders, or those with urinary
tract obstruction.

• Safe use in pregnancy has not been
established; the drugs have been used during the last two trimesters without apparent ill effects to the mother or child.

• Periodically perform blood counts and
liver and kidney function tests if treatment
is continued more than 2 weeks.

• Use with caution in patients with severe
renal failure.

• If photosensitivity occurs, discontinue
therapy.

• If bacterial resistance occurs, it usually
does so within 48 hours; change antibiotics.

• Do not administer to nursing mothers,
children, or infants.

• The stimulant properties of oxolinic
acid appear to increase in elderly patients.

ADVERSE EFFECTS

CNS EFFECTS: brief convulsions, rarely; increased intracranial pressure, toxic psychosis, rarely; drowsiness, weakness, headache,
dizziness, vertigo, paresthesias, insomnia,
agitation, feelings of disorientation

GASTROINTESTINAL EFFECTS: abdominal
pain, nausea, vomiting, diarrhea

METABOLIC AND ENDOCRINE EFFECTS:
with oxolinic acid, metabolic acidosis

HEPATIC EFFECTS: cholestasis; elevation of
liver function tests

HEMATOLOGIC EFFECTS: thrombocytopenia, leukopenia, hemolytic anemia

ALLERGIC EFFECTS: rash, pruritus, urticaria, angioedema, eosinophilia, arthralgia
with joint stiffness and swelling, anaphylactic reaction (rarely), photosensitivity

OPHTHALMIC EFFECTS: overbrightness of
lights, changes in color perception, difficulty in focusing, decrease in visual acuity,
double vision

CLINICAL GUIDELINES

EFFECTS:

• In infants and children, increased intraocular pressure with bulging anterior fonta-

nels, papilledema, and headache has occurred.

- With oxolinic acid, patient adherence to dosage regimen may be affected by CNS effects; weigh advantages against compliance.

DRUG INTERACTIONS:

- Concurrent administration with oral anticoagulants, warfarin or bishydroxycoumarin, may result in an enhanced effect of these drugs.
- A false positive glucose test (with Benedicts' of Fehling's solutions) may be obtained in patients receiving nalidixic acid.
- Incorrect values may be obtained for urinary 17-keto and ketogenic steroids because of an interaction between the drug and the m-dinitrobenzene used in the test; use of Porter-Silber test is advised.
- Safety of concomitant use of oxolinic acid and other CNS-stimulant drugs has not been established.

OVERDOSAGE/ANTIDOTE:

- Overdosage is characterized by toxic psychosis, convulsions, increased intracranial pressure, and metabolic acidosis. Nausea, vomiting, and lethargy may also occur.
- Reactions are short-lived, 2–3 hours, because the drugs are excreted rapidly. If noted early, empty stomach (gastric lavage). Treat symptomatically.

Dimethyl Sulfoxide (DMSO)

PHARMACOLOGY

Dimethyl sulfoxide has several pharmacologic activities: anti-inflammatory, nerve blockage, diuresis, cholesterase inhibition, vasodilation, and muscle relaxation.

DMSO is metabolized and excreted in the urine, feces, breath, and skin. The characteristic garlic odor is noted in patients treated with DMSO. Following topical application, DMSO is absorbed and generally distributed throughout the body fluids and tissues. After intravesicle installation, it can persist in the serum for longer than 2 weeks.

SPECIAL PRECAUTIONS

- Be aware that hypersensitivity reactions have occurred with topical administration although it has not been reported with intravesicle administration.
- Safe use in the human fetus has not been established.
- Mothers receiving DMSO should not nurse their infants.
- Intravesicle administration may be harmful in patients with urinary tract malignancy because of the DMSO–induced vasodilation.

ADVERSE EFFECTS

GASTROINTESTINAL EFFECTS: garliclike taste

LOCAL EFFECTS: transient chemical cystitis

CLINICAL GUIDELINES

ADMINISTRATION:

- Full eye evaluations including slit lamp examinations should be performed prior to and periodically during treatment. Changes in the refractive index and lens opacities have been seen in monkeys.
- Hepatic and renal function, and blood picture should be monitored prior to and periodically during treatment.
- Instill by catheter or aseptic syringe.
- Use of an analgesic lubricant gel on the urethra prior to catheterizaton may prevent spasm.
- Oral administration of an analgesic or use of suppositories containing belladonna and opium prior to instillation can reduce bladder spasm.

Antispasmodic/Anticholinergic Agents

GENERAL CLINICAL USES

The antispasmodic/anticholinergic agents, atropine sulfate, hyoscyamine sulfate, oxybutynin chloride, ethaverine hydrochloride, and flavoxate hydrochloride are used alone or in combination with other drugs for the management of spastic disorders of the lower urinary tract such as ureteral colic or vesicle spasm. The antispasmodic/anticholinergic agents are commonly used in combination with sedative or analgesic agents.

Both single ingredient and combination ingredient products are available. Only the active single ingredients will be included herein.

SPECIFIC PRODUCTS AND DOSAGES

GENERIC NAME	TRADE NAME	ROUTE OF ADMIN.	USUAL DAILY DOSAGE	
			ADULTS	CHILDREN
atropine sulfate	(G)*	im	0.4–0.6 mg	0.1–0.6 mg
ethaverine hydrochloride	ETHAQUIN	po	100–200 mg tid	Not specified
flavoxate hydrochloride	URISPAS	po	100–200 mg tid or qid	Not specified
hyoscyamine	ANASPAZ CYSTOPAZ	po	0.125–0.25 mg tid or qid	Reduce dosage in proportion to age and weight
hyoscyamine sulfate	CYSTOPAZ-M (sustained release)	po	0.375 mg bid	Not specified
oxybutynin chloride	DITROPAN	po	5 mg bid or tid maximum: 5 mg tid	**Over 5 yrs.:** 5 mg bid; maximum: 5 mg tid dn,15

*(G) designates availability as a generic product.

Atropine Sulfate
Ethaverine Hydrochloride
Flavoxate Hydrochloride
Hyoscyamine
Hyoscyamine Sulfate
Oxybutynin Chloride

PHARMACOLOGY

The anticholinergic agents, atropine sulfate, hyoscyamine sulfate, and oxybutynin chloride, exert their therapeutic action by inhibiting smooth muscle innervated by postganglionic cholinergic nerves. Atropine sulfate also has central nervous system effects which may be stimulating or depressing, depending on the dose. Atropine sulfate is absorbed rapidly and excreted in the urine, 50 percent within 24 hours.

Ethaverine hydrochloride is a spasmolytic agent similar to papaverine; it causes direct smooth muscle relaxation independent of innervation. The mechanism of action is unknown.

Flavoxate hydrochloride counteracts smooth muscle spasm of the urinary tract. The mechanism of action is unknown.

Oxybutynin chloride exerts a direct antispasmodic effect on smooth muscle by inhibiting the muscarinic action of acetylcholine.

SPECIAL PRECAUTIONS
• Do not administer anticholinergic agents to patients with glaucoma, asthma, urinary bladder neck or pyloric obstruction, severe colitis, duodenal obstruction, paralytic ileus, cardiac disease, or cardiospasm; also, to patients with adhesions between the iris and lens of the eye.
• Doses of atropine, 0.5 to 1.0 mg, are CNS-stimulating; larger doses may produce mental disturbances.
• Safe use in pregnancy has not been established.
• Anticholinergic agents should be administered cautiously to patients with hiatal hernia associated with reflux esophagitis.
• Use anticholinergic agents cautiously in elderly patients and in all patients with autonomic neuropathy or hepatic or renal disease.
• The anticholinergic agents may aggravate symptoms of hyperthyroidism, coronary heart disease, congestive heart failure, cardiac arrythmias, tachycardia, hypertension, and prostatic hypertrophy.
• Flavoxate is not to be used in patients with pyloric or duodenal obstruction, obstructive uropathies of the lower tract, gastrointestinal hemorrhage, obstructive intestinal lesions or ileus.

ADVERSE EFFECTS
CNS EFFECTS: atropine sulfate—headache, restlessness with asthenia (5 mg), ataxia, excitement, disorientation, hallucinations, delirium, coma (10 mg); hyoscyamine—drowsiness; oxybutynin—dizziness, drowsiness, sweating; ethaverine—malaise, lassitude, drowsiness, flushing, vertigo, headache

RESPIRATORY EFFECTS: atropine sulfate—dry mouth and nose (0.5 mg); ethaverine—respiratory depression

CARDIOVASCULAR EFFECTS: atropine sulfate—bradycardia, acceleration of heart (1 mg), tachycardia with palpitation (2 mg); oxybutynin—tachycardia, palpitations; ethaverine—hypotension, cardiac depression, arrhythmia; flavoxate—tachycardia, palpitation

RENAL EFFECTS: oxybutynin—urinary hesitance and retention; flavoxate—dysuria

AUTONOMIC EFFECTS: flavoxate—dry mouth; ethaverine—sweating

GASTROINTESTINAL EFFECTS: flavoxate—nausea, vomiting; hyoscyamine—dry mouth, constipation; oxybutynin—dry mouth, nausea, vomiting, constipation, bloated feeling; ethaverine—nausea, abdominal distress, anorexia, dry throat

METABOLIC AND ENDOCRINE EFFECTS: oxybutynin—impotence, suppression of lactation

HEMATOLOGIC EFFECTS: flavoxate—eosinophilia, leukopenia (1 case, reversible)

ALLERGIC EFFECTS: oxybutynin—urticaria, severe allergic reaction; flavoxate—urticaria and other dermatoses

DERMATOLOGIC EFFECTS: atropine sulfate—flushed, dry skin (2 mg), scarlatiniform rash

OPHTHALMIC EFFECTS: atropine sulfate—slight mydriasis (1 mg), mydriasis (2 mg), slight blurring of near vision (2 mg); hyoscyamine—photophobia; and oxybutynin—blurred vision, dilation of pupil, cycloplegia; flavoxate—blurred vision, increased ocular tension, disturbances in eye accommodation

CLINICAL GUIDELINES
ADMINISTRATION:
• Toxic effects from overdosage are com-

mon, especially in children.

• Administer cautiously to patients with known idiosyncracy to atropinelike compounds.

• Warn patients that slight dryness of the mouth may occur, also drowsiness and/or blurred vision which may interfere with driving a car or operating machinery.

• When administered in the presence of high environmental temperatures, heat prostration can occur.

• Administration to patients with ulcerative colitis may suppress intestinal motility, result in paralytic ileus, and precipitate megacolon.

EFFECTS:

• Discontinue if rapid pulse, dizziness, or blurring of vision occurs.

• In patients who have prostatic hypertrophy, acute urinary retention may be precipitated.

DRUG INTERACTIONS:

• Flavoxate is compatible with drugs used for treatment of urinary tract infections.

OVERDOSAGE/ANTIDOTE:

• Overdosage is characterized by an intensification of the adverse effects. Death may occur due to paralysis of the medullary centers.

• Pilocarpine is sometimes administered as an antidote to atropine but is of limited value. Physostigmine, 0.5 to 2 mg, administered intravenously, has been used as an antidote for oxybutynin; repeat if necessary.

Antiseptic Agents

GENERAL CLINICAL USES

Acute, recurrent, and chronic urinary tract infections, primarily pyelonephritis, pyelitis, cystitis, and urethritis caused by susceptible organisms, may be successfully treated with the urinary tract antiseptics.

The urinary tract antiseptics, methenamine and its various salts, and methylene blue, are used alone or in combination with analgesic agents for longterm treatment of infections. Regardless of whether these drugs are administered orally or parenterally, they are excreted rapidly and in high concentrations in the urine.

SPECIFIC PRODUCTS AND DOSAGES

The dosages of these drugs, as with many medications, should be individualized on the basis of the patient's response and the results of urine cultures. Treatment should not be prolonged without full diagnostic investigation.

GENERIC NAME	TRADE NAME	ROUTE OF ADMIN.	USUAL DAILY DOSAGE	
			ADULTS	**CHILDREN**
methenamine	(G)† TRAC TABS* URISED*	po	1 gm qid	**6–12 yrs.:** 500 mg qid **Under 6 yrs.:** 50 mg/kg/ day divided in 3 doses
	URISTAT*	po	100 mg qid	50 mg qid
	URO-PHOSPHATE*	po	300–600 mg 4–6 times/day	Not established
methenamine hippurate	HIPREX UREX	po	1 gm bid	**6–12 yrs.:** 0.5–1.0 gm bid **Under 6 yrs.:** Not established
methenamine mandelate	AZO-MANDELAMINE* DONNA SEP* MANDELAMINE UROQID-ACID	po	1 gm qid	**6–12 yrs.:** 0.5 gm qid **Under 6 yrs.:** 250 mg/30 lb qid
methenamine sulfosalicylate	HEXALET	po	1 gm qid	**6–12 yrs.:** 0.5 gm qid **Under 6 yrs.:** Not established
methylene blue	M-B Tab UROLENE BLUE	po	65–130 mg tid	Not established

*Contains more than one active ingredient.
†(G) designates availability as a generic product.

Methenamine
Methenamine Hippurate
Methenamine Mandelate
Methenamine Sulfosalicylate
Methylene Blue

PHARMACOLOGY

The antiseptic agents used for treating urinary tract infections have various modes of action. Following oral administration, methenamine, methenamine sulfosalicylate, methenamine hippurate, and methenamine mandelate are absorbed rapidly. They are excreted in the urine. The antibacterial action is based on the formaldehyde produced by hydrolysis of the salt; an acid urine is necessary for hydrolysis. Methenamine and its salts are effective against both gram-negative and gram-positive pathogens causing urinary tract infections.

Methylene blue has an oxidation-reduction action in addition to the bactericidal properties. The mechanism of the bactericidal activity is unclear.

SPECIAL PRECAUTIONS
• Do not administer any of the urinary tract antiseptics to patients with renal insufficiency, severe hepatic insufficiency, or severe dehydration.
• Do not use methenamine or its salts as the sole therapeutic agent in patients with

acute parenchymal infections causing systemic symptoms.
• Do not use a drug in patients hypersensitive to that drug or related drugs.
• Safe use in pregnancy has not been established.
• Note that superinfections may occur.

ADVERSE EFFECTS

URINARY TRACT EFFECTS: with methenamine, dysuria; with large doses, bladder irritation, painful and frequent micturition, albuminuria with gross hematuria
GASTROINTESTINAL EFFECTS: with methenamine, upset stomach; with methylene blue, nausea, vomiting, diarrhea
METABOLIC AND ENDOCRINE EFFECTS: with methenamine, metabolic acidosis

HEMATOLOGIC EFFECTS: with methylene blue, marked anemia

CLINICAL GUIDELINES

ADMINISTRATION:
• Urine must be acidic during methenamine therapy.
• Warn patients treated with methylene blue that the urine and sometimes the stool will turn blue-green.
EFFECTS:
• Methylene blue may cause marked anemia due to accelerated destruction of erythrocytes.
OVERDOSAGE/ANTIDOTE:
• Overdosage of methenamine salts or methylene blue is characterized by an exaggeration of the adverse reactions.
• No antidotes are known. Treat supportively.

Diuretics

For detailed information, see Chapter 5, page 249.

Irrigants

GENERAL CLINICAL USES

The urological irrigating fluids are used for removing calcifications and deposits from indwelling urethral catheters and from the urinary bladder, for irrigation following transurethral prostatic resection or other transurethral surgical procedures.

SPECIFIC PRODUCTS AND DOSAGES

GENERIC NAME	TRADE NAME	COMPOSITION	USUAL DOSAGE
potassium citrate	(G)	7.5 gm daily	Depends on procedure; administer as 10% solution in sterile water
sorbitol irrigant	(G) †	3% solution	As needed
sodium bicarbonate	(G)	3.0–7.5 gm daily	Depends on procedure; may be administered as 10% solution in sterile water
urological irrigating fluid	RENACIDIN*	citric acid, anhydrous 156–171 gm D-gluconic acid 21–30 gm purified magnesium hydroxy-carbonate 75–87 gm magnesium acid citrate 9–15 gm calcium carbonate 2–6 gm water, combined and fixed, 17–21 gm	30–60 ml of 10% solution bid or tid

*Contains more than one active ingredient.
†(G) designates availability as a generic product.

Potassium Citrate
Sodium Bicarbonate
Sorbitol Irrigant
Urological Irrigating Fluid

PHARMACOLOGY

The urological irrigating fluid contains citric acid and D-gluconic acid, which dissolve or prevent formation of deposits and calcifications through control of pH.

SPECIAL PRECAUTIONS

• Do not use in patients with anuria or for intravenous administration.
• Do not use for therapy or preventive therapy for conditions above the ureteral-vesical junction.
• If a burning sensation occurs, discontinue use.
• Use with caution in patients with significant cardiopulmonary or renal dysfunction.
• Use sorbitol with caution in patients with diabetes mellitus; alterations in serum glucose may occur.

ADVERSE EFFECTS

LOCAL EFFECTS: pain, transient; burning

CLINICAL GUIDELINES

ADMINISTRATION:
• Do not use sorbitol for nephrostomy or

pyelostomy tubes or renal lavage for dissolving calculi.

EFFECTS:
- If a patient experiences burning or transient pain, discontinue use.

Smooth Muscle Stimulants (Cholinergic Agents)

GENERAL CLINICAL USES

The smooth muscle stimulants (cholinergic agents) are useful in the treatment of nonobstructive urinary retention and atony of the bladder. They stimulate the smooth muscle of the urinary tract, and thereby restore normal micturition. These agents also stimulate the smooth muscles of the gastrointestinal tract (see Chapter 8, *Drugs Affecting the Gastrointestinal Tract* for additional information, page 405).

Acute postoperative and postpartum functional urinary retention and neurogenic atony may be reversed with use of the smooth muscle stimulant agents. Neostigmine bromide may be used to prevent urinary retention.

SPECIFIC PRODUCTS AND DOSAGES

The dosage of these drugs, as with many medications, should be individualized on the basis of the patient's response.

GENERIC NAME	TRADE NAME	ROUTE OF ADMIN.	USUAL DAILY DOSAGE	
			ADULTS	CHILDREN
bethanechol chloride	(G)* MYOTONACHOL URECHOLINE	sc po	2.5–5 mg; repeat if necessary 5–30 mg tid or qid	0.15–0.2 mg/kg in divided doses 0.6 mg/kg divided in 3 doses
neostigmine bromide	PROSTIGMIN Bromide	im/iv	0.5–2.0 mg	Not established
neostigmine methylsulfate	PROSTIGMIN Methylsulfate	sc/im	0.25–0.50 mg tid or qid	Not established
physostigmine salicylate	(G) ANTILIRIUM	im/iv	0.5–2.0 mg	Not established

*(G) designates availability as a generic product.

Bethanechol Chloride
Neostigmine Methylsulfate
Neostigmine Bromide
Physostigmine Salicylate

PHARMACOLOGY

Bethanechol, physostigmine, and neostigmine stimulate the cholinergic receptors, producing actions similar to acetylcholine, the naturally occurring cholinergic agent which stimulates smooth muscle. Bethanechol has a more prolonged effect than acetylcholine.

Oral administration results in a drug effect in 30 to 90 minutes; the effect lasts about 1 hour. Subcutaneous administration usually results in a drug effect in 5 to 15 minutes.

SPECIAL PRECAUTIONS

• Do not administer if mechanical obstruction is present or if the integrity of the bladder is questionable.
• Do not administer to patients with asthma, hyperthyroidism, coronary occlusion, bradycardia, atrioventricular conduction defects, vasomotor instability, hypotension, hypertension, coronary artery disease, epilepsy, parkinsonism.
• Because of the possibility of hypersensitivity, atropine and antihistamine medications should always be available.
• Safe use in pregnancy has not been established.

ADVERSE EFFECTS

RESPIRATORY EFFECTS: asthmatic attacks, especially in asthmatic patients, dyspnea, increased bronchial secretions
CARDIOVASCULAR EFFECTS: substernal pressure or pain, myocardial hypoxia, transient syncope with cardiac arrest, heart block, orthostatic hypotension, atrial fibrillation in hyperthyroid patients

AUTONOMIC EFFECTS: sweating
GASTROINTESTINAL EFFECTS: abdominal cramps, salivation, nausea, vomiting, involuntary defecation after large doses, diarrhea
DERMATOLOGIC EFFECTS: flushing of skin
OCULAR EFFECTS: with use of neostigmine, miosis
MUSCULOSKELETAL EFFECTS: with neostigmine, muscle cramps, fasciculations, weakness

CLINICAL GUIDELINES

ADMINISTRATION:
• Administer bethanecol with meals because it increases gastric volume and also acidity.
• Note that neostigmine bromide administered orally acts more slowly than the parenterally administered drug; intensity of action is more uniform.
• Neostigmine bromide is usually used primarily for symptomatic control in myasthenia gravis.
DRUG INTERACTIONS:
• Antagonism may occur with quinidine and procainamide.
• Additive effects may occur with cholinesterase inhibitors.
• Patients receiving ganglionic blocking agents may experience a critical fall in blood pressure, preceded by severe abdominal pains.
OVERDOSAGE/ANTIDOTE:
• Signs of an overdosage of bethanechol include nausea, vomiting, and sweating; orthostatic hypotension may occur. Overdosage of neostigmine may result in cholinergic crises, characterized by increasing muscle weakness which may involve the respiratory muscles.
• Atropine is a specific antidote. A dose of 0.5 to 1.0 mg (1/100 grain to 1/50 grain) intramuscularly or intravenously may counteract the severe toxic cardiovascular or bronchoconstrictor effects.

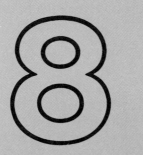

Drugs affecting the gastrointestinal tract

INTRODUCTION

The gastrointestinal tract is subject to a variety of disorders, and consequently a multitude of drugs are available for treatment of these conditions. The drugs are available both by prescription and over-the-counter. Many of the products are combinations of more than one active ingredient. The information presented herein will deal with the properties of each active ingredient; marketed products containing this ingredient will be listed and designated if they contain additional active ingredients.

SPECIFIC THERAPEUTIC CLASSIFICATION

Drugs affecting the gastrointestinal tract or used to treat gastrointestinal tract disorders are grouped as follows:

1. Adsorbents

2. Anorectic/Antiobesity agents
3. Antacids
4. Antidiarrheals
5. Antiflatulents
6. Antihemorrhoidal preparations
7. Anti-infective agents
8. Anti-inflammatory agents
9. Antinauseants/Antiemetics/Antivertigo agents / Antimotion - sickness agents
10. Antispasmodics/Direct smooth muscle relaxants
11. Antiulcer agents
12. Cathartics
13. Choleretics/Hydrocholeretics
14. Digestive enzymes
15. Emetics
16. Gastric acidifiers
17. Smooth muscle stimulants
18. Hepatic coma and precoma agent

Adsorbents

GENERAL CLINICAL USES

Adsorbents such as activated charcoal, kaolin, pectin, and magnesium trisilicate, administered orally, protect the gastrointestinal mucosa in conditions such as ulcers, enteritis, diarrhea, dysentery, and ulcerative colitis; they are also useful in poisonings.

GENERIC NAME	TRADE NAME	ROUTE OF ADMIN.	USUAL DOSAGE
bismuth salts (subcarbonate, subgallate, subsalicylate, subnitrate)	DIAVAL* KOBAC* ROMACH*	po	1–4 gm every 2–4 hr.
charcoal, activated	(G)†	po	1–10 gm
kaolin (hydrated aluminum silicate)	DONNAGEL* KAOPECTATE* PAREPECTOLIN*	po	30 ml of 20% suspension
magnesium trisilicate	KAMADROX	po	0.5–1 gm tid or qid
pectin	PAREPECTOLIN* PECTO-KALIN* KAOPECTATE*	po	60–90 mg for 3 or 4 doses

*Contains more than one active ingredient.
†(G) designates availability as a generic product.

Bismuth Salts

Bismuth Subcarbonate
Bismuth Subgallate
Bismuth Subsalicylate
Bismuth Subnitrate

PHARMACOLOGY

The bismuth salts act as astringents, protective agents, and adsorbents. They coat ulcer craters providing mechanical protection. They also adsorb noxious substances such as gases, toxins, and bacteria.

SPECIAL PRECAUTIONS

- Do not use in patients with obstruction of the bowel.
- Bismuth salts may be constipating.

ADVERSE EFFECTS
GASTROINTESTINAL EFFECTS: constipation

Charcoal, Activated

PHARMACOLOGY

Activated charcoal, a fine black powder, adsorbs gases and, importantly, certain drugs and chemicals (e.g., mercuric chloride, sulfonamides, strychine nitrate, morphine hydrochloride, atropine sulfate, nicotine, salicylic acid, phenol, phenobarbital, alcohol). In poisoning it is not a substitute for gastric lavage; however, it may be used in the lavage fluid.

SPECIAL PRECAUTIONS

- Do not use in patients with obstruction of the bowel.

Kaolin (Hydrated Aluminum Silicate)

PHARMACOLOGY

Kaolin may adsorb bacteria and toxins, principally in the stomach and small intestine. It also coats ulcers, providing mechanical protection.

SPECIAL PRECAUTIONS

- Do not use in patients with obstruction of the bowel.
- Do not use concurrently with lincomycin.

Magnesium Trisilicate

PHARMACOLOGY

Magnesium trisilicate, a weak antacid, is also an effective adsorbent. When combined with the gastric contents, gelatinous silicon dioxide is formed which may protect ulcerated mucosal surfaces.

SPECIAL PRECAUTIONS

- Do not use in patients with obstruction of the bowel.

Pectin

PHARMACOLOGY

Pectin is a purified carbohydrate derived from the rind of fruit. It may act in the bowel as an adsorbent and protective agent. It is decomposed in the colon by bacterial action.

SPECIAL PRECAUTIONS

- Do not use in patients with obstruction of the bowel.

Anorectic/Antiobesity Agents

GENERAL CLINICAL USES

The anorectic agents are used adjunctively in weight reduction programs, particularly in patients in whom alternative therapy has been ineffective.

SPECIFIC PRODUCTS AND DOSAGES

	GENERIC NAME	TRADE NAME	ROUTE OF ADMIN.	USUAL ADULT DOSAGE
	Amphetamines:			
CII†	amphetamine	(G)††	po	5–30 mg/day in divided doses
CII	amphetamine resin complex	BIPHETAMINE	po	1 capsule daily (7.5–20 mg amphetamine)
CII	amphetamine sulfate	(G) BENZEDRINE	po	5–30 mg/day in divided doses
CIII	benzphetamine	DIDREX	po	25–50 mg od to tid
CII	dextroamphetamine HCl	(G) DARO	po	5–30 mg/day in divided doses
CII	dextroamphetamine sulfate	(G) DEXAMPEX	po	5–30 mg/day in divided doses
CII	dextroamphetamine tannate	OBOTAN	po	5–30 mg/day in divided doses
CII	methamphetamine HCl	DESOXYN	po	2.5–5 mg tid
	Nonamphetamines:			
CIII	chlorphentermine HCl	(G) PRE-STATE	po	65 mg/day single dose
CIII	clortermine HCl	VORANIL	po	50 mg/day single dose
CIV	diethylpropion HCl	(G) TENUATE	po	25 mg tid

†C designates schedule listing under the Controlled Substances Act.
††(G) designates availability as a generic product.

(continued overleaf)

	GENERIC NAME	TRADE NAME	ROUTE OF ADMIN.	USUAL ADULT DOSAGE
CIII	phendimetrazine tartrate	(G) ADPHEN PLEGINE	po	35 mg bid or tid
CII	phenmetrazine HCl	PRELUDIN	po	50–75 mg bid or tid
CIV*	phentermine HCl	(G)† ADIPEX FASTIN	po	8 mg tid
	Others:			
CIV	fenfluramine HCl	PONDIMIN	po	20 mg tid
CIII	mazindol	SANOREX	po	1 mg tid or 2 mg/day
	phenylpropanolamine	ANOREXIN‡ APPEDRINE‡ COFFEE-BREAK	po	25 mg tid

*C designates schedule listing under the Controlled Substances Act.
†(G) designates availability as a generic product.
‡Contains more than one active ingredient.

Amphetamine
Amphetamine Resin Complex
Amphetamine Sulfate
Benzphetamine
Dextroamphetamine Hydrochloride
Dextroamphetamine Sulfate
Dextroamphetamine Tannate
Methamphetamine Hydrochloride

PHARMACOLOGY

The amphetamines are sympathomimetic amines. Following oral administration the effects are primarily central nervous system stimulation and increased blood pressure (systolic and diastolic). The anorectic effect may be due to appetite suppression or other central nervous system and metabolic effects. The amphetamines also have weak bronchodilator and respiratory stimulant actions.

For additional information, see the discussion of psychostimulants in Chapter 3, page 123.

SPECIAL PRECAUTIONS

• Do not use in patients with advanced arteriosclerosis, symptomatic cardiovascular disease, moderate to severe hypertension, hyperthyroidism, history of hypersensitivity to sympathomimetic amines, agitated states, and in patients with a history of drug abuse.

• Abrupt cessation following prolonged high doses results in extreme fatigue and mental depression; changes are also noted in the sleep EEG.

• Safe use in pregnancy has not been established.

• Safe use in children less than 12 years of age has not been established.

- The amphetamines may be abused.
- Tolerance may occur within several weeks.

ADVERSE EFFECTS

CNS EFFECTS: nervousness, restlessness, dizziness, insomnia, tremor, headache; psychotic episodes rarely; depression following withdrawal

CARDIOVASCULAR EFFECTS: palpitations, tachycardia, hypertension

AUTONOMIC EFFECTS: sweating, dry mouth.

GASTROINTESTINAL EFFECTS: disturbances of gastrointestinal tract, nausea, vomiting, unpleasant taste.

METABOLIC AND ENDOCRINE EFFECTS: changes in libido

ALLERGIC EFFECTS: urticaria

CLINICAL GUIDELINES

ADMINISTRATION:
- The amphetamines are drugs of abuse, and prescription is governed by Federal Narcotics Regulations, Controlled Substances Act.
- Watch patient for insomnia and nervousness.

EFFECTS:
- Discontinuance may result in extreme fatigue and depression.
- When discontinued in drug abusers, mental depression, asthenia, tremors, gastrointestinal disturbances may result.
- Psychologic disturbances have been reported in patients receiving an anorectic drug together with dietary restrictions.

DRUG INTERACTIONS:
- When sympathomimetic amines have been used concurrently or within 14 days following use of monoamine oxidase inhibitors, hypertensive crises have resulted.
- Do not use in patients receiving guanethidine.
- Do not administer concurrently with other central nervous system stimulants.
- Insulin requirements in patients with diabetes mellitus may be altered with use of anorectic agents and concomitant dietary restrictions.

OVERDOSAGE/ANTIDOTE:
- Chronic intoxication is manifested by severe dermatoses, marked insomnia, irritability, hyperactivity, and personality changes. The most severe manifestation of chronic intoxication is psychosis, often clinically indistinguishable from schizophrenia.
- Acute overdosage is characterized by restlessness, tremor, hyperreflexia, rapid respiration, confusion, assaultiveness, hallucinations, panic states. Fatigue and depression usually follow central stimulation. Cardiovascular effects include arrhythmias, hypertension, hypotension, and circulatory collapse. Gastrointestinal symptoms include nausea, vomiting, diarrhea, and abdominal cramps. Fatal poisoning usually terminates in convulsions and coma.
- There is no specific antidote. Treatment is symptomatic. Empty stomach by lavage or vomiting; sedate with a barbiturate. If hypertension is marked, the use of a nitrite or rapidly acting alpha receptor blocking agent should be considered.

Chlorphentermine Hydrochloride
Chlortermine Hydrochloride
Diethylpropion Hydrochloride
Phendimetrazine Tartrate
Phenmetrazine
Phentermine Hydrochloride

PHARMACOLOGY

Chlorphentermine HCl, chlortermine HCl, diethylpropion HCl, phendimetrazine tartrate, phentermine HCl, and phenmetrazine are related chemically and have pharmacologic properties similar to the amphetamines, namely, central nervous system stimulation and elevation of blood pressure. Tachyphylaxis and tolerance have also been demonstrated. Although they are classified as anorectic agents, their action in treating obesity may not be appetite suppression but other central nervous system and metabolic effects.

SPECIAL PRECAUTIONS
- Do not use in patients with advanced arteriosclerosis, symptomatic cardiovascular disease, moderate to severe hypertension, hyperthyroidism, history of hypersensitivity or idiosyncrasy to the sympathomimetic amines, or glaucoma.
- Do not use in patients in agitated states or with a history of drug abuse.
- Safe use in pregnancy or in children less than 12 years of age has not been established.
- Use with caution in patients with even mild hypertension.

ADVERSE EFFECT
CNS EFFECTS: overstimulation, restlessness, dizziness, insomnia, euphoria, dysphoria, tremor, headache; psychotic episodes rarely; with diethylpropion hydrochloride, increase in convulsions in epileptic patients
RESPIRATORY EFFECTS: with diethylpropion hydrochloride, dyspnea
CARDIOVASCULAR EFFECTS: palpitation, tachycardia, elevation of blood pressure; with diethylpropion hydrochloride, precordial pain, arrhythmias
AUTONOMIC EFFECTS: dry mouth, increased sweating
GASTROINTESTINAL EFFECTS: unpleasant taste, diarrhea, constipation, other gastrointestinal disturbances
METABOLIC AND ENDOCRINE EFFECTS: impotence, changes in libido; with diethylpropion hydrochloride, gynecomastia, menstrual upset

HEMATOLOGIC EFFECTS: with diethylpropion hydrochloride, bone marrow depression, agranulocytosis, leukopenia
ALLERGIC EFFECTS: urticaria; with diethylpropion, rash, ecchymoses, erythema
DERMATOLOGIC EFFECTS: with diethylpropion, hair loss
OPHTHALMIC EFFECTS: with diethylpropion, mydriasis
MUSCULOSKELETAL EFFECTS: with diethylpropion, muscle pain

CLINICAL GUIDELINES
ADMINISTRATION:
- Caution patients that these drugs may impair the ability to engage in potentially hazardous activities such as operating machinery or driving a motor vehicle.
EFFECTS:
- Tolerance to the anorectic effect usually develops within a few weeks; discontinue drug rather than increase dosage.
- Abrupt cessation of prolonged high doses may result in extreme fatigue and mental depression; also, changes in the sleep EEG may be noted.
DRUG INTERACTIONS:
- With chlorphentermine hydrochloride there have been reports of pulmonary hypertension in patients who receive related drugs.
- Do not use in patients during or within 14 days following the administration of monoamine oxidase inhibitors; hypertensive crises may result.
- Insulin requirements in patients with diabetes mellitus may be altered in association with the use of the anorectic agents and the concomitant dietary regimen.
- May decrease the hypotensive effect of guanethidine.
OVERDOSAGE/ANTIDOTE:
- Acute overdosage is characterized by restlessness, tremor, hyperreflexia, rapid respiration, confusion, assaultive behavior,

hallucinations, panic states. Fatigue and depression usually follow the central nervous system stimulation. Cardiovascular effects include arrhythmias, hypertension or hypotension and circulatory collapse. Gastrointestinal symptoms include nausea, vomiting, diarrhea, and abdominal cramps. In fatal poisoning, death is usually preceded by convulsions and coma.

• Chronic intoxication is characterized by severe dermatoses, marked insomnia, irritability, hyperactivity, and personality changes. The most severe manifestation is psychosis, which is often indistinguishable from schizophrenia.

• There is no specific antidote. Management is largely symptomatic and includes gastric lavage and sedation with a barbiturate. Acidification of the urine may increase excretion. Intravenously administered phentolamine (REGITINE) has been suggested for possible acute, severe hypertension if this complicates overdosage.

Fenfluramine Hydrochloride

PHARMACOLOGY
Fenfluramine hydrochloride differs pharmacologically somewhat from the amphetamines although it is chemically similar. Fenfluramine abuse (80 to 400 mg) is associated with euphoria, derealization, and perceptual changes; it does not produce signs of dependence in animals and appears to produce sedation more often than central nervous stimulation.

SPECIAL PRECAUTIONS
• Safety and efficacy in pregnancy, lactation or in children less than 12 years of age has not been established.

• Use with caution in patients with hypertension; monitor blood pressure.

• Do not use in severely hypertensive patients or in patients with symptomatic cardiovascular disease including arrhythmias.

• Use with caution in patients with a history of mental depression; further depression of mood may become evident while the patient is on fenfluramine or following withdrawal of fenfluramine.

• Do not use in patients with a history of hypersensitivity to fenfluramine hydrochloride.

ADVERSE EFFECTS
CNS EFFECTS: drowsiness, dizziness, confusion, incoordination, headache, elevated mood, depression, anxiety, nervousness or tension, insomnia, weakness or fatigue, agitation, fever

CARDIOVASCULAR EFFECTS: palpitation, hypotension, hypertension, fainting, chest pain

URINARY TRACT EFFECTS: dysuria, and urinary frequency

AUTONOMIC EFFECTS: dry mouth, sweating, chills, blurred vision

GASTROINTESTINAL EFFECTS: diarrhea, constipation, abdominal pain, nausea, bad taste

METABOLIC AND ENDOCRINE EFFECTS: increased or decreased libido

ALLERGIC EFFECTS: urticaria

DERMATOLOGIC EFFECTS: rash, burning sensation

OPHTHALMIC EFFECTS: irritation

MUSCULOSKELETAL EFFECTS: dysarthria, myalgia

CLINICAL GUIDELINES
DRUG INTERACTIONS:
• Other central nervous system depressant drugs should be used with caution in patients taking fenfluramine; the results may be additive.

• Fenfluramine may increase slightly the effect of antihypertensive drugs, e.g., guanethidine, methyldopa, reserpine.

OVERDOSAGE/ANTIDOTE:

• Overdosage is characterized by agitation and drowsiness, confusion, flushing, tremor (or shivering), fever, sweating, abdominal pain, hyperventilation, and dilated nonreactive pupils. Reflexes may be either exaggerated or depressed and some patients may have rotary nystagmus. Tachycardia may be present, but blood pressure may be normal or only slightly elevated. Convulsions, coma, and ventricular extrasystoles, cumulating in ventricular fibrillation, may occur at higher dosage.

• In a small child the lowest reported fatal dose was a few hundred milligrams. In an adult, the highest reported nonfatal dose was 1800 mg.

• There is no specific antidote. Treatment consists of supportive measures, if possible with cardiac monitoring. In more severe cases, forced diuresis with acidification of the urine may be beneficial to hasten excretion. Although hypertension has not been a feature of overdosage with fenfluramine, if it should occur, the use of intravenously administered phentolamine (REGITINE) has been suggested.

Mazindol

PHARMACOLOGY

Mazindol, although similar pharmacologically in many ways to the amphetamines, differs in that it appears to exert its primary effects on the limbic system; however, it causes central nervous system stimulation similar to the amphetamines.

SPECIAL PRECAUTIONS

• Do not use in patients with glaucoma, agitated states, a history of hypersensitivity or idiosyncrasy to mazindol or related compounds, or a history of drug abuse.

• Tolerance to the anorectic effects may occur within a few weeks; discontinue drug; do not increase dosage.

• Safe use in pregnancy has not been established.

• Safe use in children less than 12 years of age has not been established.

• Use with caution in patients with hypertension; monitor blood pressure.

• Do not use in severely hypertensive patients.

• Do not use in patients with symptomatic cardiovascular disease, including arrhythmias.

ADVERSE EFFECTS

CNS EFFECTS: nervousness, insomnia, overstimulation, restlessness, dizziness, dysphoria, tremor, headache, depression, drowsiness, weakness

CARDIOVASCULAR EFFECTS: tachycardia, palpitations

AUTONOMIC EFFECTS: dry mouth, excessive sweating

GASTROINTESTINAL EFFECTS: constipation, unpleasant taste, diarrhea, nausea, other gastrointestinal disturbances

METABOLIC AND ENDOCRINE EFFECTS: impotence, changes in libido

DERMATOLOGIC EFFECTS: rash, and clamminess

CLINICAL GUIDELINES

ADMINISTRATION:

• Caution patients that the ability to engage in potentially hazardous activities such as operating machinery or driving a motor vehicle may be impaired.

DRUG INTERACTIONS:

• Do not use during or within 14 days following the administration of monoamine oxidase inhibitors; hypertensive crises may result.

• May decrease the hypotensive effect of

guanethidine; monitor blood pressure.
• May potentiate the pressor effect of exogenous catecholamines. If it should be necessary to give a pressor amine (e.g., levarterenol or isoproterenol) to a patient in shock (e.g., from a myocardial infarction) who has recently been taking mazindol, monitor blood pressure at frequent intervals and with extreme care; initiate pressor therapy with a low initial dose and titrate carefully.
• Insulin requirements in patients with diabetes mellitus may be altered in association with use of mazindol and concomitant dietary regimen.

OVERDOSAGE/ANTIDOTE:
• Symptoms of overdosage are similar to those seen with the amphetamines and related substances, namely, restlessness, tremor, rapid respiration, dizziness. Fatigue and depression may follow the stimulatory phase of overdosage. Cardiovascular effects include tachycardia, hypertension, and circulatory collapse. Gastrointestinal symptoms include nausea and vomiting, and abdominal cramps.
• There is no specific antidote. Management of overdosage is symptomatic. Mazindol is poorly excreted except at very acid pH.

Phenylpropanolamine

PHARMACOLOGY
Phenylpropanolamine is a sympathomimetic amine which may depress the appetite. The mechanism of action is unknown.

SPECIAL PRECAUTIONS
• Use with caution in patients with thyroid disease, diabetes mellitus, symptomatic cardiovascular disease, moderate to severe hypertension, known sensitivity or idiosyncrasy to phenylpropanolamine or similar drugs, renal disorders, glaucoma.
• Do not exceed recommended dosage.
• Discontinue use if rapid pulse, dizziness, or palpitations occur.
• Safe use in pregnancy and in children less than 18 years of age has not been established.

ADVERSE EFFECTS
CNS EFFECTS: dizziness
CARDIOVASCULAR EFFECTS: rapid pulse, palpitations
URINARY TRACT EFFECTS: diuresis
GASTROINTESTINAL EFFECTS: nausea occasionally

Antacids

GENERAL CLINICAL USES
The antacids alleviate the symptoms of heartburn, sour stomach, and/or acid indigestion associated with disorders of the gastrointestinal tract such as hyperacidity.

TRADE NAME	aluminum hydroxide	calcium carbonate	dihydroxyaluminum aminoacetate	magaldrate	magnesium carbonate	magnesium hydroxide	magnesium trisilicate	potassium bicarbonate	sodium bicarbonate
ALKA-SELTZER Effervescent Antacid	—	—	—	—	—	—	—	x	x
ALKA-2 Chewable Antacid Tablet	—	x	—	—	—	—	—	—	—
ALUDROX Oral Suspension	x	—	—	—	—	x	—	—	—
ALUREX	x	—	—	—	—	—	—	—	—
AMPHOJEL Suspension,	x	—	—	—	—	—	—	—	—
Tablet	x	—	—	—	—	—	—	—	—
CAMALOX	x	x	—	—	—	x	—	—	—
DELCID	x	—	—	—	—	—	—	—	—
DICARBOSIL	—	x	—	—	—	—	—	—	—
EQUILET	—	x	—	—	—	—	—	—	—
ESCOT CAPSULES	x	—	—	—	—	—	x	—	—
GAVISCON	x	—	—	—	—	—	x	—	x
GELUSIL	x	—	—	—	—	—	—	—	—
GELUSIL- M	x	—	—	—	—	x	—	—	—
KOLANTYL	x	—	—	—	—	x	—	—	—
KUDROX Suspension,	x	—	—	—	—	x	—	—	—
Tablet	x	—	—	—	x	—	—	—	—
MAALOX	x	—	—	—	—	x	—	—	—
MAGNATRIL Suspension,	x	—	—	—	—	x	x	—	—
Tablet	x	—	—	—	—	x	x	—	—
MARBLEN	—	x	—	—	x	—	—	—	—
NEUTRALOX Suspension,	x	—	—	—	—	x	—	—	—
Tablet	x	—	—	—	—	x	—	—	—
RIOPAN	—	—	—	x	—	—	—	—	—
ROBALATE	—	—	x	—	—	—	—	—	—
ROMACH	—	—	—	—	x	—	—	—	x
TITRALAC	—	x	—	—	—	—	—	—	—
TRISOGEL	x	—	—	—	—	—	x	—	—

PHARMACOLOGY

The antacids reduce the amount of acid in the stomach. They are combinations of aluminum hydroxide, calcium carbonate, magaldrate, magnesium carbonate, magnesium hydroxide, magnesium trisilicate, dihydroaluminum monoacetate, potassium bicarbonate, and sodium bicarbonate. The neutralizing capacity varies among the components and products.

Aluminum hydroxide, a nonabsorbable antacid, has a slow onset of action and a low neutralizing capacity. It is also a demulcent, adsorbent and astringent.

Calcium carbonate, an antacid with a high neutralizing capacity, has a rapid onset and relatively prolonged duration of action.

Dihydroxyaluminum aminoacetate, also a nonabsorbable antacid, has a greater neutralizing capacity than dried aluminum hydroxide gel.

Magaldrate, a chemically bonded aluminum and magnesium hydroxide, may be absorbed in a limited amount. It has a low sodium content.

Magnesium carbonate is an antacid with high neutralizing capacity. It is a common ingredient in antacid mixtures.

Magnesium hydroxide has a rapid onset of action and a high neutralizing capacity. The duration of action is longer than that of sodium bicarbonate.

Magnesium trisilicate, a relatively poor antacid-buffer, has a delayed onset of action and reacts with hydrochloric acid to form hydrated silica dioxide.

Sodium and potassium bicarbonate, highly soluble antacids, provide immediate and pronounced neutralizing effects. The duration of action, however, is brief.

SPECIAL PRECAUTIONS
• Note that some products contain large amounts of sodium; therefore use with caution in patients requiring sodium restriction.
• Do not use in patients receiving any form of tetracycline antibiotic; absorption of tetracycline may be prevented.
• Use with caution in patients with hypercalcemia, renal disease, or concurrent administration with large amounts of milk.
• Use products containing magnesium salts with caution in patients with renal insufficiency.
• Do not exceed maximal dose recommended by manufacturer in package insert.
• Certain products may cause constipation or may have a laxative effect.

ADVERSE EFFECTS
CNS EFFECTS: dizziness
GASTROINTESTINAL EFFECTS: laxative effect, constipation, vomiting, nausea, stomatitis, abdominal discomfort
DERMATOLOGIC EFFECTS: rash

Antidiarrheal Agents

GENERAL CLINICAL USES
The antidiarrheal agents are indicated to reverse abnormal frequency and liquidity of fecal discharges. The anticholinergic agents, commonly used, reduce motility and secretion of the gastrointestinal tract; the Lactobacillus group of microorganisms restore and stabilize normal intestinal flora; and paragoric and diphenoxylate hydrochloride used adjunctively slow motility and reduce discomfort from cramps and intestinal colic.

	GENERIC NAME	TRADE NAME	ROUTE OF ADMIN.	USUAL DOSAGE
	Anticholinergic Agents:			
	homatropine methylbromide	(G)†† MATROPINAL* RU-SPAS NO.2	po	**Adults:** 2.5–10 mg qid **Children:** 3–6 mg tid **Infants:** 0.3 mg 5–6 x/day
	hyoscyamine sulfate, atropine sulfate, hyoscine hydrobromide	DONNAGEL*	po	**Adults:** 2 tbs; repeat 1–2 tbs after each stool **Children:** 30 lb, 1–2 tsp. 20 lb, 1 tsp; 10 lb, 1/2 tsp
		ANASPAZ LEVSIN	po	**Adults:** 0.125–0.25 mg tid or qid **Children 2–10 yrs.:** 1/2 adult dose **Infants:** 1/4 adult dose
	Lactobacillus Group:			
	Lactobacillus acidophilus	BACID Caps DOFUS LACTINEX* Tablets NOVAFLOR*	po po po po	2 caps bid or qid 1 tab tid 3–4 tabs tid or qid 4 caps qid
	Lactobacillus bulgaricus	LACTINEX* Tablets NOVAFLOR* Capsules	po po	3–4 tabs tid or qid 4 caps qid
	Miscellaneous Drugs:			
CIII†	paregoric	(G)†† PAREPECTOLIN	po	**Adults:** 5–10 ml od to qid **Children:** 0.25–0.5 mg/kg od to qid
CV	diphenoxylate hydrochloride	LOMOTIL* Liquid, Tablets	po	**Adults:** 5–20 mg daily divided in 4 equal doses **Children 2–12 yrs.:** 0.3–0.4 mg/ kg/day in divided doses **Children 8–12 yrs.:** 2 mg 5 times daily **Children 5–8 yrs.:** 2 mg qid **Children 2–5 yrs.:** 2 mg tid
CV	loperamide	IMODIUM	po	**Adults:** 4 mg initial, then 2 mg after each loose bowel movement; maximum: 16 mg/day **Children:** not recommended

*Contains more than one active ingredient.
†C denotes schedule listing under the Controlled Substances Act.
††(G) designates availability as a generic product.

Anticholinergic Agents

Atropine Sulfate
Homatropine Methylbromide
Hyoscyamine Hydrobromide
Hyoscyamine Sulfate

PHARMACOLOGY
The anticholinergic agents slow intestinal motility and reduce gastrointestinal secretions.

SPECIAL PRECAUTIONS, ADVERSE EFFECTS, GUIDELINES FOR NURSES
See the section *Antispasmodic Agents/Smooth Muscle Relaxants* in this chapter.

Lactobacillus Acidophilus
Lactobacillus Bulgaricus

PHARMACOLOGY
Lactobacillus acidophilus and *L. bulgaricus* aid in restoring and stabilizing normal intestinal flora by restoring normal intestinal pH.

SPECIAL PRECAUTIONS
• Do not use for more than 2 days or in the presence of a high fever.
• Do not use in infants or children less than 3 years old.

ADVERSE EFFECTS
GASTROINTESTINAL EFFECTS: increased frequency of bowel movements

Paregoric

PHARMACOLOGY
Paregoric relieves gastrointestinal cramps and reduces motility accompanying diarrhea. It is a 4-percent opium tincture in which there is also benzoic acid, camphor, and anise oil. Paregoric is readily absorbed from the gastrointestinal tract and is metabolized in the liver.

SPECIAL PRECAUTIONS
• Do not use in patients with a history of hypersensitivity to paregoric.
• Use with caution in patients with impaired renal function.
• Do not use in diarrhea caused by poisoning until toxic material is removed from the gastrointestinal tract.

ADVERSE EFFECTS
GASTROINTESTINAL EFFECTS: nausea

Diphenoxylate Hydrochloride

PHARMACOLOGY
Diphenoxylate hydrochloride slows intestinal motility. It is chemically related to the narcotic, meperidine. Following oral administration it is rapidly absorbed, and effects are noted within 1 hour. Diphenoxylate hydrochloride is excreted in breast milk.

SPECIAL PRECAUTIONS
• Do not use in children less than 2 years old.
• Do not use in patients with a history of hypersensitivity to diphenoxylate hydrochloride, or in jaundiced patients.
• Do not use to treat diarrhea associated with pseudomembranous enterocolitis which may occur during or up to several weeks following treatment with antibiotics such as clindamycin (CLEOCIN) or lincomycin (LINCOCIN).

• Use with extreme caution in patients with cirrhosis and other advanced hepatic disease, and in all patients with abnormal liver function tests; hepatic coma may be precipitated.
• Safe use in pregnancy has not been established.
• Addiction to (dependency on) diphenoxylate hydrochloride is theoretically possible at high dosage.
• Use with caution in patients who are receiving addicting drugs, in individuals known to be addiction prone, or in those whose histories suggest they may increase the dosage on their own initiative.

ADVERSE EFFECTS

CNS EFFECTS: drowsiness, restlessness, sedation, headache, dizziness, depression, malaise, coma, lethargy, euphoria
RESPIRATORY EFFECTS: respiratory depression
GASTROINTESTINAL EFFECTS: abdominal discomfort, swelling of gums, paralytic ileus, toxic megacolon, nausea, vomiting, anorexia
METABOLIC AND ENDOCRINE EFFECTS: angioneurotic edema
ALLERGIC EFFECTS: giant urticaria
DERMATOLOGIC EFFECTS: pruritus, rash

CLINICAL GUIDELINES

EFFECTS:
• If abnormal distention occurs, particularly in patients with acute ulcerative colitis, discontinue drug immediately.
• Effects in young children may be extremely variable.
• Dehydration, particularly in younger children, may further influence the variable response to this drug and may predispose to delayed diphenoxylate intoxication.
DRUG INTERACTIONS:
• Concurrent use with monoamine oxidase inhibitors may, in theory, precipitate hypertensive crisis.
• May potentiate the action of barbiturates, tranquilizers, and alcohol.
OVERDOSAGE/ANTIDOTE:
• Initial signs of overdosage include dry skin and mucous membranes, flushing, hyperthermia, and tachycardia followed by lethargy or coma, hypotonic reflexes, nystagmus, pinpoint pupils and respiratory depression. Respiratory depression may occur from 12 to 30 hours after drug ingestion.
• Establish a patent airway and assist respiration mechanically if needed. The narcotic antagonist NARCAN (naloxone hydrochloride), may be used. When administered intravenously, the onset of action is generally apparent within 2 minutes. Note that the action of diphenoxylate hydrocloride is longer than that of naloxone hydrochloride.

Loperamide

GENERAL CLINICAL USES

Loperamide is useful in treating acute nonspecific diarrhea, chronic diarrhea associated with inflammatory bowel disease, and also for reducing the volume of discharge from ileostomies.

PHARMACOLOGY

Loperamide, a phenylpiperidine derivative, inhibits gastrointestinal motility in mice. In humans systemic absorption is slow. About 10 percent of the drug is recovered in the urine and 42 percent is excreted in the feces. The biological half-life ranges from 7 to 14 hours.

SPECIAL PRECAUTIONS

• Safe use has not been established in

children, pregnant women, or nursing mothers.

ADVERSE EFFECTS
CNS EFFECTS: drowsiness, dizziness, and tiredness
GASTROINTESTINAL EFFECTS: constipation, abdominal discomfort, nausea, vomiting, dry mouth
DERMATOLOGIC EFFECTS: rash

CLINICAL GUIDELINES
OVERDOSAGE/ANTIDOTE:
- Overdosage is characterized by CNS depression.
- There is no specific antidote. Treat with gastric lavage and activated charcoal. CNS depression can be treated with narcotic antagonists such as naloxone (NARCAN). For detailed information see Chapter 20, page 696.

Antiflatulents

GENERAL CLINICAL USES
The antiflatulent simethicone is useful for the relief of the painful symptoms of excess gas in the digestive tract in conditions such as postoperative gaseous distention, air swallowing, functional dyspepsia, peptic ulcer, spastic or irritable colon, and diverticulitis.

GENERIC NAME	TRADE NAME	ROUTE OF ADMIN.	USUAL DOSAGE
simethicone	MYLICON PHAZYME* SIDONNA* SIMECO*	po	40–100 mg qid; maximal daily dose 500 mg

*Contains more than one active ingredient.

PHARMACOLOGY
Simethicone, a silicone which reduces surface tension, disperses and prevents the formation of mucus-surrounded gas pockets in the gastrointestinal tract.

Simethicone is formulated in combination with antispasmodic/anticholinergic agents, enzymes, barbiturates, and antacids. Significant amounts of simethicone are not absorbed from the gastrointestinal tract. It does not appear to be active pharmacologically.

SPECIAL PRECAUTIONS
• Tablet must be chewed thoroughly.

Antihemorrhoidal Preparations

GENERAL CLINICAL USES
The various products available for treating hemorrhoids and other anorectal conditions relieve the symptoms of pain, inflammation, swelling, and itching; they also provide lubrication to facilitate evacuation and minimize irritation.

The antihemorrhoidal preparations contain local anesthetic agents, anti-inflammatory agents, and emollients/lubricants.

SPECIFIC PRODUCTS AND DOSAGES

GENERIC NAME	TRADE NAME	SUGGESTED DAILY DOSAGE
Local Anesthetic Agents:		
benzocaine	AMERICAINE*	Apply liberally in morning and after bowel movements
dibucaine hydrochloride	NUPERCAINAL	Apply small amounts as needed
lidocaine hydrochloride	XYLOCAINE	Apply small amounts as needed
pramoxine hydrochloride	ANUGESIC* PERIFOAM*	Apply small amounts as needed
Anti-Inflammatory Agents:		
hydrocortisone/hydrocortisone acetate	CORT-DOME	1 suppository bid to tid
	ANUSOL-HC* PROCTOFOAM-HC* Rectal MEDICONE-HC*	1 suppository tid or bid 1 applicatorful bid to tid 1 suppository tid or bid
Emollients/Lubricants:		
peruvian balsam	ANUGESIC*	apply small amounts as needed
polyethylene glycol	AMERICAINE*	apply liberally in morning and after bowel movements

*Contains more than one active ingredient.

Local Anesthetics

PHARMACOLOGY, SPECIAL PRECAUTIONS, ADVERSE EFFECTS, CLINICAL GUIDELINES

For detailed information, see Chapter 9, *Drugs Affecting the Skin* (page 410).

Anti-Inflammatory Agents

PHARMACOLOGY

Hydrocortisone acetate reduces the signs of inflammation, swelling, hyperemia, pruritus, and pain. The exact mechanism of action is unknown. For additional information, see the discussion of adrenocortical hormones in Chapter 15, page 535.

SPECIAL PRECAUTIONS (pertaining to rectal use)

• Do not use in patients with a history of hypersensitivity to any component.
• If rectal bleeding, rash, irritation, or other signs of sensitivity develop, discontinue immediately.
• Do not use for a prolonged time.
• Use cautiously in patients with drug sensitivities.

Anti-Infective Agents

GENERAL CLINICAL USES

The anti-infective agents are used to treat infections within the gastrointestinal tract caused by a wide variety of microorganisms (bacteria and parasites); these agents are also used to eliminate naturally occurring microorganisms prior to surgery on the gastrointestinal tract. The anti-infective agents used for these indications act locally within the lumen and are absorbed to a limited extent, if at all.

GENERIC NAME	TRADE NAME	INDICATION	SUGGESTED DOSAGE	
			ADULTS	CHILDREN
ampicillin	AMCILL OMNIPEN	Gastrointestinal infections due to strains of *Shigella, Salmonella* (including *S. typhosa*), *E. coli, H. influenzae, P. mirabilis,* and *N. gonorrhoeae*	Over 20 kg (44 lb): 500 mg qid	Under 20 kg (44 lb): 100 mg/kg/day divided in equal doses in 6- to 8-hr. intervals

(continued overleaf)

GENERIC NAME	TRADE NAME	INDICATION	SUGGESTED DOSAGE	
			ADULTS	**CHILDREN**
colistin sulfate	COLY-MYCIN S	Diarrhea in infants and children caused by *E. coli;* gastroenteritis caused by *Shigella* organisms	Not indicated	5–15 mg/kg/day divided in 3 doses
furazolidone	FUROXONE	Amebiasis	100 mg qid	5–8.8 mg/kg/day divided in 4 equal doses
gentamicin sulfate	GARAMYCIN	Infections of GI tract such as peritonitis caused by *Ps. aeruginosa, E. coli, Proteus* species, *Klebsiella-Enterobacter-Serratia* species, *Citrobacter, Staph.*	3–5 mg/kg/day divided in 3 equal doses	6–7.5 mg/kg/day divided in 3 equal doses **Infants and neonates:** 7.5 mg/kg/day administered in 3 equal doses (Use GARAMYCIN Pediatric Injectable) **Premature or full-term neonates:** 5 mg/kg/day divided in 2 equal doses
kanamycin sulfate	KANTREX	Suppression of intestinal bacteria prior to surgery	1 gm every 4–6 hr.	Not established
metronidazole	FLAGYL	Amebiasis	500–750 mg tid	35–50 mg/kg/day divided in 3 doses
neomycin sulfate	(G)* MYCIFRADIN Sulfate	Suppression of intestinal bacteria; diarrhea due to enteropathogenic *E. coli*	40–50 mg/kg/day in divided doses	40–50 mg/kg/day in divided doses
paromomycin sulfate	HUMATIN	Intestinal amebiasis, acute and chronic; adjunctive therapy in hepatic coma	25–35 mg/kg/day divided in 3 doses	25–35 mg/kg/day divided in 3 doses
sulfasalazine	AZULFIDINE S.A.S.-500	Mild to moderate ulcerative colitis; adjunctive therapy in severe ulcerative colitis	3–4 gm/day in equally divided doses	40–60 mg/kg/day divided in 3–6 doses
tetracycline	(G) ACHROMYCIN	Amebiasis	1–2 gm divided in 2–4 doses	25–50 mg/kg/day divided in 2–4 equal doses
vancomycin HCl	VANCOCIN	Staphylococcal entero-colitis	500 mg qid or 1 gm bid	20 mg/lb/day in divided doses

*(G) designates availability as a generic product.

PHARMACOLOGY, SPECIAL
PRECAUTIONS, ADVERSE
EFFECTS, CLINICAL GUIDELINES
For detailed information, see Chapter 2, page 10.

Anti-Inflammatory Agents (Glucocorticoids)

GENERAL CLINICAL USES

The anti-inflammatory steroids, glucocorticoids, have been used in retention enemas for the adjunctive treatment of ulcerative colitis; for the temporary relief of anorectal inflammation, pruritus, pain and swelling associated with hemorrhoids, proctitis, cryptitis, fissures, postoperative pain and pruritus ani, and pain and swelling associated with episiotomy.

The glucocorticoids may be useful when administered systemically to tide the patient over a critical period, as in ulcerative colitis or regional enteritis. For information concerning systemic use of the glucocorticoids, see Chapter 15, page 535.

Topically applied glucocorticoids are useful in relieving the symptoms associated with anorectal conditions such as hemorrhoids and proctitis. For additional information concerning this use, please refer to the discussion of antihemorrhoidal preparations in this chapter.

SPECIFIC PRODUCTS AND DOSAGES

GENERIC NAME	TRADE NAME	ROUTE OF ADMIN.	USUAL DOSAGE
hydrocortisone	CORTENEMA RECTOID	retention enema	100 mg nightly
hydrocortisone acetate	ANUSOL-HC CORTIFOAM PROCTOFOAM-HC*	topical, intra-anally	1 applicatorful 2–3 times daily and after each bowel evacuation
methylprednisolone acetate	MEDROL ENPAK	retention enema	40 mg 3 to 7 times weekly

*Contains more than one active ingredient.

Hydrocortisone
Hydrocortisone Acetate
Methylprednisolone Acetate

PHARMACOLOGY

Hydrocortisone and methylprednisolone acetate administered in a retention enema provide potent anti-inflammatory effects. They may be absorbed from the colon, thus providing a combined topical and systemic effect.

SPECIAL PRECAUTIONS
• Do not use in patients with systemic fungal infections.
• Do not use during the immediate or

early postoperative period of ileocolostomy.
• In severe ulcerative colitis, it is hazardous to delay needed surgery while awaiting response to medical treatment.
• Damage to the rectal wall can result from careless or improper insertion of an enema tip.
• In patients on corticosteroid therapy who are subjected to unusual stress, an increased dosage of rapidly acting corticosteroids before, during, or after the stressful situation is indicated.
• Corticosteroids may mask some signs of infection, and new infections may appear during their use.
• There may be decreased resistance and inability to localize infection when corticosteroids are used.
• Prolonged use of corticosteroids may produce posterior subcapsular cataracts or glaucoma with possible damage to the optic nerves, and may enhance the establishment of secondary ocular infections due to fungi or viruses.
• Safe use in pregnancy has not been established.
• While on corticosteroid therapy, patients should not be vaccinated against smallpox; other immunization procedures should not be undertaken because of possible hazards of neurological complications and lack of antibody response.
• Hydrocortisone retention enema should be used with caution where there is a probability of impending perforation, abscess or other pyogenic infection; fresh intestinal anastomoses; obstruction; or extensive fistulas.
• Use with caution in the presence of active or latent peptic ulcer; diverticulitis; renal insufficiency; hypertension; osteoporosis; or myasthenia gravis.
• Steroid therapy might impair prognosis in surgery by increasing the hazard of infection; if infection is suspected, appropriate antibiotic therapy must be administered, usually in larger than ordinary doses.

• Drug-induced secondary adrenocortical insufficiency may occur with prolonged hydrocortisone retention enema therapy, and this is minimized by a gradual reduction of dosage.
• Use with caution in patients with ocular herpes simplex because of possible corneal perforation.

ADVERSE EFFECTS

LOCAL EFFECTS: local pain or burning, rectal bleeding, and apparent exacerbations of the disease or sensitivity reactions may occur in rare instances.

SYSTEMIC EFFECTS: see the discussion of adrenocortical hormones in Chapter 15, page 534.

CLINICAL GUIDELINES

ADMINISTRATION:
• The use of hydrocortisone retention enema should complement the concomitant use of other measures such as dietary control, sedatives, antidiarrheal agents, antibacterial therapy, blood replacement.
• Clinical symptoms usually subside promptly within 3 to 5 days; however, difficult cases may require as long as 2 or 3 months.
• Discontinue therapy gradually by reducing administration to every other night for 2 or 3 weeks.
• If clinical or proctologic improvement fails to occur within 2 or 3 weeks after starting treatment, discontinue use.

EFFECTS:
• Average and large doses of hydrocortisone can cause elevation of blood pressure, salt and water retention, and increased excertion of potassium; dietary salt restriction and potassium supplementation may be necessary.
• All corticosteroids increase calcium excretion.
• There is an enhanced effect of corticosteroids on patients with hypothyroidism and in those with cirrhosis.

• Psychic derangement may appear when corticosteroids are used, ranging from euphoria, insomnia, mood swings, personality changes, and severe depression to frank psychotic manifestations; also, existing emotional instability or psychotic tendencies may be aggravated by corticosteroids.

• Symptomatic improvement, evidenced by decreased diarrhea and bleeding, weight gain, improved appetite, lessened fever and decrease in leukocytosis may be misleading and should not be used as the sole criterion in judging efficacy. A sigmoidoscopic examination and x-ray visualization are essential for adequate monitoring.

DRUG INTERACTIONS:

• Aspirin should be used cautiously in conjunction with corticosteroids in patients with hypoprothrombinemia.

Antinauseants/Antiemetics/Antivertigo Agents/Antimotion-Sickness Agents

GENERAL CLINICAL USES

The antinauseants/antiemetic agents are used for prophylaxis and symptomatic treatment of nausea and vomiting associated with motion. Certain products have been used in treating postoperative vomiting and that associated with certain other pharmacologically active compounds. For example, benzquinamide hydrochloride is indicated for the prevention and treatment of nausea and vomiting associated with anesthesia and surgery. The phenothiazines such as prochlorperazine are indicated for control of severe nausea and vomiting.

Diphenidol, an antivertigo agent, is indicated for the control of nausea and vomiting encountered in postoperative states, malignant, neoplasms, and lakyrinthine disturbances such as inner ear surgery and Meniere's disease. Use is limited to hospitalized patients.

SPECIFIC PRODUCTS AND DOSAGES

GENERIC NAME	TRADE NAME	ROUTE OF ADMIN.	USUAL DOSAGE	
			ADULTS	CHILDREN
Antihistamines (for additional information, see Chapter 6, page 302.):				
benzquinamide HCl	EMETE-CON	im	50 mg (0.5–1.0 mg/kg); repeat in 1–4 hr.	Not recommended
		iv	25 mg (0.2–0.4 mg/kg)	Not recommended
buclizine HCl	BUCLADIN-S	po	50 mg bid; maximum 200 mg/day	Not established

(continued overleaf)

GENERIC NAME	TRADE NAME	ROUTE OF ADMIN.	USUAL DOSAGE	
			ADULTS	CHILDREN
cyclizine HCl	MAREZINE	im	50 mg q 4–6 hr. bid	Not established
		po	50 mg q 4–6 hr; maximum: 200 mg/day	**6–10 yrs.:** 25 mg q 4–6 hr; maximum: 75 mg/day
dimenhydrinate	(G)* DRAMAMINE	iv/im	50 mg	Reduce dosage
		po	50 mg q 4 hr.	**8–12 yrs.:** 25–50 mg tid **Younger children:** reduce dosage
		pr	100 mg od or bid	Not established
diphenhydramine	(G) BENADRYL	po	25–50 mg tid or qid	**Over 20 lb:** 12.5–25 mg tid or qid; maximum: 300 mg/day
		im/iv	10–50 mg; maximum: 400 mg	**Infants and children up to 20 lb:** 6.3–12.5 mg tid or qid 5 mg/kg/day divided in 4 doses; maximum: 300 mg
hydroxyzine HCl	(G) ATARAX	po	25–100 mg tid or qid	**6–16 yrs.:** 50 –100 mg/day in divided doses **Under 6 yrs.:** 50 mg/day in divided doses
hydroxyzine pamoate	VISTARIL	im	25–100 mg	0.5 mg/lb
		po	25–100 mg tid or qid	**Under 6 yrs.:** 50 mg in divided doses **Over 6 yrs.:** 50–100 mg in divided doses
meclizine HCl	(G) ANTIVERT BONINE	po	25–100 mg; may repeat in 24 hr.	Not recommended
pyrilamine maleate	EME-NIL†	pr	———	**Infants over 6 mos. and children up to 6 yrs.:** 25 mg; repeat 3–6 hr.
	MATROPINAL†	pr	1 or 2 q 3–4 hr.	1 or 2 q 4–6 hr. **Infants:** 1 or 2 q 4–6 hr. (12 mg/kg/day)
	WANS†	pr	50 mg q 4–6 hr.	**Under 2 yrs.:** 1/2 dose **2–12 yrs.:** 25 mg tid to qid
Phenothiazines: chlorpromazine	(G) THORAZINE	po	10–25 mg q 4–6 hr.	0.25 mg/lb q 4–6 hr. **Under 6 mos.:** not recommended
		pr	50–100 mg q 6–8 hr.	0.5 mg/lb q 6–8 hr. (1/2 25-mg suppository q 6–8 hr.)
		im	25 mg; may repeat	**Maximum:** 0.25 mg/lb q 6–8 hr. **up to 5 yrs.:** 40 mg/day; **5–12 yrs.:** 75 mg/day

*(G) designates availability as a generic product.
†Contains more than one active ingredient.

(continued facing page)

GENERIC NAME	TRADE NAME	ROUTE OF ADMIN.	USUAL DOSAGE	
			ADULTS	CHILDREN
perphenazine	TRILAFON	po	8–16 mg in divided doses	**Over 12 yrs.:** lowest adult dose
		im	5 mg q 6 hr.	Not established
prochlorperazine	COMPAZINE	po	5–10 mg tid or qid; maximum: 40 mg/day	**Under 20 lb:** not recommended **20–29 lb:** 2.5 mg od to bid; maximum: 7.5 mg **30–39 lb:** 2.5 mg bid or tid; maximum: 10 mg/day **40–85 lb:** 2.5 mg tid or 5 mg bid; maximum: 15 mg/day
		im	5–10 mg tid or qid; maximum: 40 mg/day	0.06 mg/lb
		pr	25 mg bid	Same as po
promethazine HCl	(G) PHENERGAN	po im pr	25 mg bid to qid 12.5–25 mg q 4 hr. 12.5–25 mg bid to qid	12.5–25 mg bid to qid 12.5–25 mg bid to qid Adjust for age and weight of patient and severity of condition
thiethylperazine	TORECAN	po pr im	10 mg od to tid 10 mg od to tid 10 mg od to tid	Not established Not established Not established
triflupromazine HCl	VESPRIN	po	20–30 mg in divided doses; maximum: 30 mg/day	0.2 mg/kg/day; maximum: 10 mg/day
		im	2.5–15 mg qid: maximum: 60 mg/day	0.2–0.25 mg/kg/day; maximum 10 mg/day
		iv	1–3 mg q 4–6 hr.	Not recommended
Others: diphenidol	VONTROL	po	25–50 mg q 4 hr.	0.4 mg/lb not more often than every 4 hr; maximum: 2.5 mg/lb/24 hr.
		im	20–40 mg; repeat in 1 hr; then q 4 hr.	0.2 mg/lb not more often than q 4 hr; maximum: 1.5 mg/lb/24 hr.
		iv	Hospitalized: 20 mg; may repeat	Not established
trimethobenzamide HCl	TIGAN	po	250 mg tid or qid	**30–90 lb:** 100–200 mg tid or qid
		pr	200 mg tid or qid	**Under 30 lb:** 100 mg tid or qid **30–90 lb:** 100–200 mg tid or qid
		im	200 mg tid or qid	Not recommended

Benzquinamide Hydrochloride

PHARMACOLOGY

Benzquinamide hydrochloride, an antihistamine, is an effective antiemetic agent. The onset of action following parenteral administration (im/iv) occurs within 15 minutes. The mechanism of action in humans is unknown. The drug is metabolized in the liver and excreted in the urine.

SPECIAL PRECAUTIONS
- Do not use in patients with a history of hypersensitivity to the drug.
- Safe use in pregnancy and children has not been established.
- Do not administer intravenously to patients with cardiovascular disease or to those receiving preanesthetic and/or concomitant cardiovascular drugs.
- May mask the signs of overdosage of toxic drugs or may obscure diagnosis of such conditions as intestinal obstruction and brain tumor.

ADVERSE EFFECTS

CNS EFFECTS: drowsiness, insomnia, restlessness, headache, excitement, nervousness, fatigue, chills, increased temperature.

CARDIOVASCULAR EFFECTS: hypertension, hypotension, dizziness, atrial fibrillation, premature auricular and ventricular contractions, transient arrhythmias

AUTONOMIC EFFECTS: dry mouth, shivering, sweating, hiccups, flushing, salivation, blurred vision

GASTROINTESTINAL EFFECTS: anorexia, nausea

ALLERGIC EFFECTS: pyrexia, urticaria

DERMATOLOGIC EFFECTS: rash

MUSCULOSKELETAL EFFECTS: twitching, shaking, tremors, weakness

CLINICAL GUIDELINES

ADMINISTRATION:
- Intravenous administration should be restricted to patients without cardiovascular disease.
- If administered intravenously to elderly or debilitated patients, use lower dose range.
- For intravenous administration, reconstitute with sterile water for injection diluted drug maintains its potency for 14 days at room temperature.

- When administering intramuscularly, avoid inadvertent intravascular injection.

EFFECTS:
- Following intravenous administration, sudden increase in blood pressure and transient arrhythmias (premature ventricular and auricular contractions) have occurred.

DRUG INTERACTIONS:
- Concurrent use with other CNS depressants such as hypnotics, sedatives, tranquilizers and alcohol may result in additive depressant effects.

OVERDOSAGE/ANTIDOTE:
- Overdosage is characterized by a combination of central nervous system stimulant and depressant effects.
- There is no specific antidote. General supportive measures should be instituted. Atropine may be helpful. Although there has been no direct experience with dialysis, it is not likely to be of value since benzquinamide is extensively bound to plasma protein.

Buclizine HCl
Cyclizine HCl
Meclizine HCl

PHARMACOLOGY

Buclizine hydrochloride, cyclizine hydrochloride, and meclizine hydrochloride, antihistamines, are rapidly absorbed following oral administration. The site and mode of action are unknown. Both stimulant and depressant effects on the central nervous system have been observed.

SPECIAL PRECAUTIONS
- Do not use in patients with a history of hypersensitivity to these drugs.
- Safe use in pregnancy or lactation has not been established.
- Use with caution in patients with glau-

coma, or with obstructive diseases of the gastrointestinal or genitourinary tracts.

ADVERSE EFFECTS
CNS EFFECTS: drowsiness, headache, jitteriness, nervousness
AUTONOMIC EFFECTS: dry mouth, nose, and throat
HEPATIC EFFECTS: with cyclizine, cholestatic jaundice
DERMATOLOGIC EFFECTS: rash
OPHTHALMIC EFFECTS: blurred vision, diplopia

CLINICAL GUIDELINES
ADMINISTRATION:
• Caution patients that since drowsiness may occur, driving or performing tasks requiring alertness may be hazardous.
• May be taken without swallowing water. Patient can place tablet in mouth and allow to dissolve, or chew or swallow whole.
• Caution patients to avoid drinking alcoholic beverages with these drugs.
DRUG INTERACTIONS:
• May have additive effects with alcohol, hypnotics, sedatives, tranquilizers, antianxiety agents, or other CNS-depressant drugs.
OVERDOSAGE/ANTIDOTE
• Massive overdosage may cause convulsions whereas with moderate dosage hyperexcitability may alternate with drowsiness.
• There is no specific antidote. Empty stomach by gastric lavage or by inducing vomiting. Treat supportively. Do not use morphine or other respiratory depressants.

Dimenhydrinate

PHARMACOLOGY
Dimenhydrinate, an antihistamine which may be administered orally, intramuscularly, intravenously, or rectally, has a depressant effect on hyperstimulated labyrinthine function. The precise mode of antiemetic action is unknown. Following oral administration, dimenhydrinate is absorbed readily from the gastrointestinal tract. Effects are noted within 30 minutes. Nausea and vomiting may be controlled for approximately 4 hours.

SPECIAL PRECAUTIONS
• Since dimenhydrinate may mask the symptoms of vestibular ototoxicity, use caution when administering with certain antibiotics known to cause ototoxicity.
• Safe use in pregnancy has not been established.

ADVERSE EFFECTS
CNS EFFECTS: drowsiness

CLINICAL GUIDELINES
ADMINISTRATION:
• Caution patients that drowsiness may interfere with tasks which require alertness, such as driving.
DRUG INTERACTIONS:
• Concurrent use of alcohol-containing beverages or other CNS-depressants will enhance drowsiness.
OVERDOSAGE/ANTIDOTE:
• Overdosage is characterized by profound drowsiness.
• There is no specific antidote. Empty stomach by gastric lavage and treat supportively.

Diphenhydramine Hydrochloride

PHARMACOLOGY
Diphenhydramine hydrochloride, a potent antihistamine, also possesses anticholinergic (antispasmodic), antitussive,

antiemetic, and sedative properties. Following oral administration it is absorbed efficiently and the maximal effect occurs in approximately 1 hour. The duration of action is from 4 to 6 hours. Diphenhydramine hydrochloride inhibits lactation.

SPECIAL PRECAUTIONS, ADVERSE EFFECTS, CLINICAL GUIDELINES

For detailed information, see the discussion of antihistamines in Chapter 6, page 302.

Hydroxyzine Hydrochloride
Hydroxyzine Pamoate

PHARMACOLOGY

Hydroxyzine hydrochloride and hydroxyzine pamoate, sedative antihistamines and antianxiety agents, also have antiemetic activity. Following oral administration, absorption from the gastrointestinal tract is rapid and effects are noted within 15 to 30 minutes. The mechanism of action is unknown.

SPECIAL PRECAUTIONS, ADVERSE EFFECTS, CLINICAL GUIDELINES

For additional information, see the discussion of antianxiety agents in Chapter 3, page 106.

Phenothiazines:

Chlorpromazine
Perphenazine
Prochlorperazine
Promethazine Hydrochloride
Thiethylperazine
Triflupromazine Hydrochloride

PHARMACOLOGY

The phenothiazines have a direct effect on the chemoreceptor trigger zone, the vomiting center, or both. They are metabolized in the liver. The exact mechanism of action is unknown.

SPECIAL PRECAUTIONS

For complete cautionary information pertinent to all phenothiazines, see Chapter 3, page 117. Special precautions pertinent to use of the phenothiazines as antiemetic agents are included herein.
• Do not use in the presence of central nervous system depression and comatose states.
• Do not use in patients with a history of hypersensitivity to the compound.
• Do not administer intravenously because hypotension may occur.
• Safe use in pregnancy and lactation has not been established.
• Restlessness and postoperative central nervous system depression during anesthesia recovery may occur.
• After an initial injection, postural hypotension may occur.

ADVERSE EFFECTS

For a complete inventory of adverse effects which may occur with the phenothiazines, see Chapter 3, page 118.
CNS EFFECTS: extrapyramidal effects including dystonia, torticollis, dysphasia, oculogyric crises, akathesia, convulsions, dizziness, headache, fever, restlessness, ataxia, drowsiness, trigeminal neuralgia
CARDIOVASCULAR EFFECTS: cerebral vascular spasm
AUTONOMIC EFFECTS: dry mouth and nose; blurred vision, tinnitus, sialorrhea
METABOLIC AND ENDOCRINE EFFECTS: peripheral edema of arms, hands, and face
HEPATIC EFFECTS: cholestatic jaundice occasionally

CLINICAL GUIDELINES

ADMINISTRATION:
• When drug is administered intravenously or intramuscularly, patient should be in the recumbent position.
EFFECTS:
• May impair mental and/or physical abil-

ity required for the performance of potentially hazardous tasks such as driving a car or operating machinery; caution patients.

DRUG INTERACTIONS:

• Avoid administration of epinephrine in the treatment of drug-induced hypotension; phenothiazines may induce a reversed epinephrine effect on occasion.

• Should a vasoconstrictive agent be required, the most suitable are levarterenol and phenylephrine.

• Phenothiazines are capable of potentiating CNS depressants (e.g., anesthetics, opiates, alcohol), as well as atropine and phosphorus insecticides.

OVERDOSAGE/ANTIDOTE:

• Overdosage is characterized by an exaggeration of the central nervous system depressant effects.

• There is no specific antidote. Evacuate stomach by inducing vomiting or gastric lavage. Use general supportive therapy.

Promethazine Hydrochloride

PHARMACOLOGY

Promethazine hydrochloride, a phenothiazine derivative, has several pharmacologic actions: antiemetic, sedative, and antihistaminic effects. The latter may be prolonged and potent. It may be administered by intravenous, intramuscular, oral, and rectal routes.

SPECIAL PRECAUTIONS, ADVERSE EFFECTS, CLINICAL GUIDELINES

For additional information, see Chapter 6, page 306.

Pyrilamine Maleate

PHARMACOLOGY

Pyrilamine maleate, an antihistamine, is formulated for oral and rectal ad-

ministration. When administered rectally, absorption is rapid and effective between evacuations, even when diarrhea is present. Oral administration also results in a rapid effect.

SPECIAL PRECAUTIONS, ADVERSE EFFECTS, CLINICAL GUIDELINES

For additional information, see Chapter 6, page 305.

Diphenidol

PHARMACOLOGY

Diphenidol, an antivertigo agent, is not related to other antiemetic or antivertigo agents. It exerts its antivertigo effect on the vestibular apparatus and inhibits the chemoreceptor trigger zone which controls nausea and vomiting. It also has weak peripheral anticholinergic action. Following oral administration, peak blood levels occur in 1.5 to 3.0 hours. It is excreted by the kidneys.

SPECIAL PRECAUTIONS

• Do not use in patients with a history of hypersensitivity to diphenidol.

• Do not use in patients with anuria.

• Use only in hospitalized patients since hallucinations, disorientation, or confusion may occur.

• Use with caution in patients with glaucoma, obstructive lesions of the gastrointestinal and genitourinary tracts such as stenosing peptic ulcer, prostatic hypertrophy, pyloric and duodenal obstruction, and organic cardiospasm.

• Do not administer intravenously to patients with a history of sinus tachycardia; an attack may be initiated.

ADVERSE EFFECTS

CNS EFFECTS: auditory and visual hallucinations, disorientation, confusion; drowsiness, overstimulation, depression, sleep disturbances, slight dizziness, malaise, headache

CARDIOVASCULAR EFFECTS: slight, transient lowering of blood pressure

AUTONOMIC EFFECTS: dry mouth, blurred vision

GASTROINTESTINAL EFFECTS: nausea, indigestion, heartburn

HEPATIC EFFECTS: jaundice (questionable relationship)

DERMATOLOGIC EFFECTS: rash

CLINICAL GUIDELINES

ADMINISTRATION:
• Auditory and visual hallucinations, disorientation and confusion occur occasionally within 3 days after initial drug use; these reactions usually subside spontaneously within 3 days after discontinuing drug.
• Monitor blood pressure since hypotension has occurred following parenteral administration.
• Avoid subcutaneous or perivenous infiltration.

EFFECTS:
• The antiemetic effect may mask signs of drug overdose (e.g., digitalis) or may obscure diagnosis of conditions such as intestinal obstruction and brain tumors.

OVERDOSAGE/ANTIDOTE:
• Overdosage is characterized by an exaggeration of the adverse effects.
• Treatment is symptomatic; monitor blood pressure and respiration. With oral overdosage, early gastric lavage may be indicated.

Trimethobenzamide Hydrochloride

PHARMACOLOGY
Trimethobenzamide hydrochloride, an antiemetic agent, may act by stimulating the chemoreceptor trigger zone through which impulses are conveyed to the vomiting center. The exact mechanism of action is obscure.

SPECIAL PRECAUTIONS
• Do not use in patients with a history of hypersensitivity to trimethobenzamide hydrochloride.
• Since the suppositories contain benzocaine, they should not be used in patients known to be sensitive to this or similar local anesthetics.
• Use with caution in children; antiemetics are not recommended for treatment of uncomplicated vomiting in children, and their use should be limited to prolonged vomiting of known etiology.
• There has been some suspicion that centrally acting antiemetics in combination with viral illnesses (a possible cause of vomiting in children) is implicated in the development of Reye's syndrome, a potentially fatal acute childhood encephalopathy with visceral fatty degeneration, especially involving the liver.
• The extrapyramidal symptoms which can occur secondary to trimethobenzamide hydrochloride may be confused with central nervous system signs of an undiagnosed primary disease responsible for the vomiting, e.g., Reye's syndrome or other encephalopathy.
• Drugs with hepatotoxic potential such as trimethobenzamide hydrochloride may unfavorably alter the course of Reye's syndrome; such drugs should be avoided in children whose signs and symptoms (vomiting) could represent Reye's syndrome.
• Safe use in pregnancy or lactation has not been established.
• Severe emesis should not be treated with an antiemetic drug alone; when possible, the cause of vomiting should be established.

• The antiemetic effects may render diagnosis more difficult in such conditions as appendicitis and obscure signs of toxicity due to overdosage of other drugs.

ADVERSE EFFECTS

CNS EFFECTS: parkinsonian symptoms, coma, convulsions, depression of mood, disorientation, dizziness, drowsiness, headache
CARDIOVASCULAR EFFECTS: hypotension following parenteral administration, particularly in surgical patients
AUTONOMIC EFFECTS: blurring of vision
GASTROINTESTINAL EFFECTS: diarrhea
HEPATIC EFFECTS: jaundice
HEMATOLOGIC EFFECTS: blood dyscrasias
ALLERGIC EFFECTS: hypersensitivity reactions; skin reactions
MUSCULOSKELETAL EFFECTS: muscle cramps, opisthotonus
LOCAL EFFECTS (im administration): pain, burning, stinging, redness, swelling

CLINICAL GUIDELINES

ADMINISTRATION:
• Warn patients that trimethobenzamide

hydrochloride may cause drowsiness which may interfere with driving a motor vehicle or operating hazardous machinery.
EFFECTS:
• During the course of acute febrile illness, encephalitides, gastroenteritis, and dehydration with electrolyte imbalance, especially in children and the elderly or debilitated; central nervous system reactions such as opisthotonus, convulsions, coma, extrapyramidal symptoms have been reported with and without use of trimethobenzamide hydrochloride.
DRUG INTERACTIONS:
• Concurrent administration of trimethobenzamide hydrochloride and other CNS-acting drugs (phenothiazines, barbiturates, belladonna derivatives, alcohol) may be additive or may mask or enhance CNS effects.
OVERDOSAGE/ANTIDOTE:
• Overdosage is characterized by an exaggeration of the adverse effects.
• There is no specific antidote. Treat symptomatically. Empty stomach by inducing emesis or gastric lavage.

Antispasmodic Agents/Direct Smooth Muscle Relaxants

GENERAL CLINICAL USES
The antispasmodics/direct smooth muscle relaxants are used primarily to relieve the frequency and force of smooth muscle contractions of the gastrointestinal tract and adjunctively in the treatment of functional bowel disorders such as irritable colon, mild dysentery, diverticulitis, and pancreatitis. The antispasmodics may also relieve ureteral and biliary spasms.

The antispasmodics are grouped as anticholinergic agents (belladonna drugs and synthetic substitutes) and direct smooth muscle relaxants. For detailed information, see this discussion of vasodilating agents in Chapter 5, page 283.

GENERIC NAME	TRADE NAME	ROUTE OF ADMIN.	USUAL DOSAGE	
			ADULTS	CHILDREN
Belladonna Alkaloids:				
atropine sulfate	(G)†	po/im/ iv/sc	0.4–0.6 mg q 4–6 hr.	**7–16 lb:** 0.1 mg **17–24 lb:** 0.15 mg **24–40 lb:** 0.2 mg **40–65 lb:** 0.3 mg **65–90 lb:** 0.4 mg **Over 90 lb:** 0.4– 0.6 mg
atropine methyl, nitrate	FESTALAN*	po	1–2 mg tid	———
belladonna extract	(G) BELAP DOLATRIN*	po	10.8–21.6 mg tid or qid	———
belladonna preparations	(G) BELLADENAL* DONNAGEL* SIDONNA*	po	0.5–1.0 mg q 12 hr.	———
homatropine methylbromide	RU-SPAS No.2	po	10 mg qid	———
hyoscyamine/hyoscyamine sulfate	ANASPAZ* ARCO-LASE PLUS* CYSTOSPAZ DONPHEN* KUTRASE* LEVSIN*	po	0.125–0.25 mg tid or qid	**2–10 yrs.:** 1/2 adult dose **Up to 2 yrs:** 1/4 adult dose
scopolamine hydrobromide	(G)	po im/sc	0.4–0.8 mg 0.32–0.65 mg	——— **6 mos.–3 yrs.:** 0.1 –0.15 mg. **3–6 yrs.:** 0.15–0.2 mg **6–12 yrs.:** 0.2–0.3 mg
Synthetic Substitutes:				
anisotropine methylbromide	VALPIN 50	po	50 mg tid	———
clidinium bromide	LIBRAX* QUARZAN	po	2.5–5.0 mg tid or qid **Geriatric or debilitated:** 2.5 mg tid	———
dicyclomine HCl	(G) BENTYL	po	10–20 mg tid or qid	10 mg tid or qid **Infants:** 5 mg tid or qid
		im	20 mg q 4–6 hr.	———

*Contains more than one active ingredient.
†(G) designates availability as a generic product.

(continued facing page)

GENERIC NAME	TRADE NAME	ROUTE OF ADMIN.	USUAL DOSAGE	
			ADULTS	CHILDREN
diphemanil methylsulfate	PRANTAL	po	50–200 mg tid or qid	Not established
glycopyrrolate	ROBINUL	po im/sc/iv	1–2 mg tid 0.1 mg tid or qid	Not established Not established
hexocyclium methylsulfate	TRAL	po	25 mg tid to qid	———
isopropamide iodide	DARBID	po	5–10 mg bid	Not recommended in children under 12 yrs.
mepenzolate bromide	CANTIL	po	25–50 mg tid or qid	———
methantheline bromide	BANTHINE	po	50–100 mg qid	**Newborns:** 12.5 mg bid, then tid **Infants 1–12 mos:** 12.5–25 mg qid **Children over 1 yr.:** 12.5–50 mg qid
		im	50–100 mg	———
methixene HCl	TREST	po	1–2 mg tid	Not established
oxyphencyclimine HCl	DARICON VISTRAX*	po	10 mg bid	Not for use in children under 12 yrs.
oxyphenonium bromide	ANTRENYL	po	10 mg qid	Not recommended
propantheline bromide	(G) PRO-BANTHINE	po im/iv	15 mg qid 30 mg qid	Not established Not established
thiphenamil HCl	TROCINATE	po	400 mg q 4 hr.	Not established
tridihexethyl chloride	PATHIBAMATE* PATHILON	po im/iv/sc	25–50 mg tid or qid 10–20 mg qid	——— ———
Smooth Muscle Relaxants: dioxyline phosphate	PAVERIL Phosphate	po	100–400 mg tid or qid	———
ethaverine HCl	CIRCUBID ETHAQUIN	po	300–600 mg daily in divided doses	———
papaverine HCl	(G) LAPAV PAVATRAN	im/iv po	30–120 mg; repeat 3 hr. 60–300 mg 1–5 times daily	——— ———

*Contains more than one active ingredient.

Belladonna Alkaloids

Atropine Sulfate and Methyl Nitrate
Belladonna Extracts and Preparations
Homatropine Methyl Bromide
Hyoscyamine and Sulfate
Scopolamine Preparations

PHARMACOLOGY

The belladonna alkaloids, anticholinergic agents, block wholly or partly, the action of acetylcholine at postganglionic parasympathetic sites. These drugs reduce motility and secretory activity of the gastrointestinal system. They also have central nervous system (CNS) activity which is dose-related.

SPECIAL PRECAUTIONS

• Do not use in patients with glaucoma, adhesions (synechiae) between the iris and lens of the eye, or asthma.
• Use with caution when administering atropine sulfate since the effects are dose-related; low doses are mild stimulants to the central nervous system; large doses may be depressants.
• Do not use in patients with a history of hypersensitivity to the belladonna alkaloids.
• Use with caution in patients with renal or hepatic disease, or with pyloric obstruction.

ADVERSE EFFECTS

CNS EFFECTS: drowsiness; with large doses, ataxia, excitement, disorientation, hallucinations, delirium, coma, restlessness
CARDIOVASCULAR EFFECTS: tachycardia
URINARY TRACT EFFECTS: retention, and dysuria
AUTONOMIC EFFECTS: dry nose and mouth, slight mydriasis; flushed, dry skin; fever, particularly in children
GASTROINTESTINAL EFFECTS: constipation
DERMATOLOGIC EFFECTS: scarlatiniform rash

OPHTHALMIC EFFECTS: photophobia, blurred vision

CLINICAL GUIDELINES
EFFECTS:
• Discontinue if excessively rapid pulse, dry throat, or blurring of vision occurs.
DRUG INTERACTIONS:
• Concomitant administration of other drugs with anticholinergic action which would increase the anticholinergic effects should be avoided.
OVERDOSAGE/ANTIDOTE:
• Overdosage is characterized by an exaggeration of the adverse effects, particularly the CNS effects. Death, although rare, is usually due to paralysis of the medullary centers. Although large doses of atropine may cause an alarming condition, recovery is usual.
• To treat overdosage, empty stomach. In the treatment of atropine poisoning, respiratory assistance and symptomatic support are indicated. Pilocarpine is sometimes given but its value is limited and questionable.

Synthetic Substitutes

Anisotropine Methylbromide
Clidinium Bromide
Dicyclomine Hydrochloride
Diphemanil Methylsulfate
Glycopyrrolate
Hexocyclium Methylsulfate
Isopropamide Iodide
Mepenzolate Bromide
Methantheline Bromide
Methixene Hydrochloride
Oxyphencyclimine Hydrochloride
Oxyphenonium Bromide
Propantheline Bromide
Thiphenamil Hydrochloride
Tridihexethyl Chloride

PHARMACOLOGY

The synthetic substitutes for the belladonna alkaloids reduce spasm of the gastrointestinal tract, thereby relieving pain. They also have an inhibiting effect on lactation and characteristic atropine effects on the biliary tract, uterus, ureters, salivary glands, eyes, and cardiovascular system.

SPECIAL PRECAUTIONS

• Do not use in patients with glaucoma, obstructive uropathy (for example, bladder neck obstruction due to prostatic hypertrophy), obstructive disease of the gastrointestinal tract (as in achalasia, paralytic ileus, pyloroduodenal stenosis), intestinal atony of the elderly or debilitated patient, unstable cardiovascular state, acute hemorrhage, severe ulcerative colitis, toxic megacolon complicating ulcerative colitis, myasthenia gravis, and reflux esophagitis.

• Do not use in patients with acute intermittent porphyria.

• Safe use in pregnancy, lactation, women of childbearing potential, and children has not been established.

• In the presence of high environmental temperatures, heat prostration can occur with drug use (fever and heat stroke due to decreased sweating).

• In the treatment of gastric ulcer, the use of anticholinergic drugs may produce a delay in gastric emptying and may complicate therapy (antral stasis).

• Use with caution in patients with autonomic neuropathy, hepatic or renal disease, early evidence of ileus as in peritonitis, ulcerative colitis; large doses may suppress intestinal motility to the point of producing a paralytic ileus; toxic megacolon may be precipitated or aggravated.

• Use cautiously in debilitated patients with chronic lung disease because reduction in bronchial secretions can lead to inspissation and formation of bronchial plugs.

• These drugs are inappropriate in patients with diarrhea due to incomplete intestinal obstruction, especially those with ileostomy or colostomy.

• Use with caution in patients with hyperthyroidism, coronary artery disease, congestive heart failure, cardiac arrhythmias, hypertension, nonobstructing prostatic hypertrophy, hepatic or renal disease.

• Use with caution in patients with hiatal hernia associated with reflux esophagitis since anticholinergic drugs may aggravate this condition.

• Do not rely on use of these drugs in the presence of complications of biliary tract disease.

ADVERSE EFFECTS

CNS EFFECTS: headache, nervousness, drowsiness, weakness, dizziness, insomnia; mental confusion and/or excitement, especially in the elderly

CARDIOVASCULAR EFFECTS: tachycardia, palpitations

URINARY TRACT EFFECTS: hesitancy, retention

AUTONOMIC EFFECTS: decreased sweating, dry mouth

GASTROINTESTINAL EFFECTS: loss of taste, nausea, vomiting, constipation, bloated feeling, salivary secretion

METABOLIC AND ENDOCRINE EFFECTS: impotence, suppression of lactation

ALLERGIC EFFECTS: anaphylaxis, urticaria, dermatitis

DERMATOLOGIC EFFECTS: with isopronamide iodide, iodine skin rash, rarely

OPHTHALMIC EFFECTS: mydriasis, dilatation of pupil, cycloplegia, increased ocular tension, blurred vision

CLINICAL GUIDELINES

ADMINISTRATION:

• Warn patient that drowsiness and blurred vision may occur which may interfere with activities requiring alertness such as driving a motor vehicle or operating machinery.

DRUG INTERACTIONS:
• Concomitant administration of anticholinergic drugs and other drugs which would increase the anticholinergic effects should be avoided.

OVERDOSAGE/ANTIDOTE:
• With overdosage a curarelike effect may occur.
• Treat symptomatically as for atropine overdosage; empty the stomach by inducing emesis or gastric lavage. An activated charcoal slurry may be instilled in the stomach and removed by lavage. Physostigmine or other reversible anticholinesterases may be necessary. Use supportive therapy as necessary.

Direct Smooth Muscle Relaxants

Dioxyline Phosphate
Ethaverine Hydrochloride
Papaverine Hydrochloride

For detailed information, see Chapter 5, page 283.

Antiulcer Agents

SPECIFIC PRODUCTS AND DOSAGES

GENERIC NAME	TRADE NAME	ROUTE OF ADMIN.	USUAL ADULT DAILY DOSAGE
cimetidine	TAGAMET	po	300 mg qid
cimetidine hydrochloride	TAGAMET	iv	300 mg qid

Also see *Antispasmodic Agents/Direct Smooth Muscle Relaxants*, page 387.

Cimetidine
Cimetidine HCl

GENERAL CLINICAL USES

Cimetidine is useful in short-term treatment (up to 3 weeks) of duodenal ulcer and treatment of hypersecretory conditions such as Zollinger-Ellison syndrome, systemic mastocytosis, and multiple endocrine adenomas.

PHARMACOLOGY

Cimetidine may be administered orally or parenterally. It is an antisecretory agent, decreasing gastric acid production. It is classified as an antihistamine H2-antagonist drug.

When administered orally, cimetidine is absorbed rapidly. The half-life is approximately 2 hours. It is excreted primarily in the urine.

SPECIAL PRECAUTIONS

• Do not use in patients with a history of hypersensitivity to cimetidine.
• Safe use in pregnancy, children, or during lactation has not been established.
• There are no known contraindications to cimetidine.

ADVERSE EFFECTS

CNS EFFECTS: dizziness, confusional states
URINARY TRACT EFFECTS: small increases in plasma creatinine, increases in serum transaminase
GASTROINTESTINAL EFFECTS: diarrhea
METABOLIC AND ENDOCRINE EFFECTS: gynecomastia
HEMATOLOGIC EFFECTS: neutropenia
DERMATOLOGIC EFFESTS: rash
MUSCULOSKELETAL EFFECTS: muscular pain

CLINICAL GUIDELINES

ADMINISTRATION:
• Administer with meals and at bedtime.

• Concomitant antacids should be given as needed for relief of pain.
• Monitor prothrombia time closely if patient is receiving anticoagulants.
EFFECTS:
• Reduce dosage to 300 mg bid in patients with impaired renal function.
DRUG INTERACTIONS:
• The intravenous preparation may be diluted with Sodium Chloride Injection (0.9%), Dextrose Injection (5%).
• Antacids may be administered concomitantly.
• Effects of warfarin-type anticoagulants have been potentiated.
OVERDOSAGE/ANTIDOTE:
• Overdosage may be associated with respiratory failure and tachycardia.
• There is no specific antidote. Empty stomach by gastric lavage. Use assisted respiration and necessary supportive cardiac care. Doses up to 10 gm have not been associated with untoward effects.

Cathartics (Bowel Evacuants, Laxatives)

GENERAL CLINICAL USES

The cathartics are used to facilitate defecation by relieving constipation, softening the stool, and emptying the gastrointestinal tract of its contents prior to surgery or radiographic examination or after accidental or intentional poisoning. The cathartics are also useful in avoiding hazardous increases in blood pressure produced by straining, particularly in patients with hypertensive, cerebral, coronary, or other arterial disease.

The cathartics are grouped according to their mechanism of action as (1) lubricant cathartics, (2) stimulant cathartics, (3) saline cathartics, and (4) bulk-forming cathartics.

SPECIFIC PRODUCTS AND DOSAGES

GENERIC NAME	TRADE NAME	ROUTE OF ADMIN.	USUAL DOSAGE
Lubricant Cathartics: dioctyl sodium sulfosuccinate	(G)† BU-LAX PLUS* COLACE COMFOLAX DIALOSE* DILAX-100 SURFAX*	po	**Adults:** 50–240 mg daily **Children 6–12 yrs.:** 40–120 mg daily **Children 3–6 yrs.:** 20–60 mg daily **Children under 3 yrs.:** 10–40 mg daily
mineral oil	AGORAL HALEY'S M-O*	po	**Adults:** 1–2 tbsp (15–30 ml) at bedtime **Children 7–12 yrs.:** 2–4 tsp **Children 3–6 yrs.:** 1–2 tsp
	FLEET Mineral Oil Enema	pr	4 1/2 fl oz
Stimulant Cathartics: bisacodyl	(G)	pr	**Adults:** 10 mg daily **Infants and children under 2 yrs.:** 5 mg/daily **Children over 2 yrs.:** 10 mg daily
	(G) BON-O-LAX DULCOLAX	po	**Adults:** 10–15 mg **Children:** 5–10 mg
casanthranol	DIALOSE PLUS* PERI-COLACE* STIMULAX*	po	**Adults:** 30–60 mg daily
cascara sagrada	(G)	po	**Adults:** 325 mg at bedtime **Children:** Not established
castor oil, emulsified	(G) NEOLOID	po	**Adults:** 2–4 tbsp (30–60 ml) **Children:** adjust between adult and infant dose (7.5–30 ml) **Infant:** 0.5–1.5 tsp (2.5–7.5 ml)
danthron	ANAVAC DORBANE MODANE	po	**Adults:** 150 mg with p.m. meal **Children 6–12 yrs.:** 325 mg 37.5 mg **1–6 yrs.:** 37.5 mg **6–12 mos.:** 7–9 mg with pm. meal
phenolphthalein white	AGORAL* EVAC-Q-KIT	po	**Adults:** 60–200 mg daily at bedtime **Children over 6 yrs:** 30–60 mg daily **Children 2–5 yrs:** 15–20 mg daily
phenolphthalein yellow	(G)† EVAC-U-GEN SAROLAX* EX-LAX	po	**Adults:** 30–270 mg, preferably at bedtime **Children over 6 yrs.:** 30–60 mg

*Contains more than one active ingredient.
†(G) designates availability as a generic product.

(continued facing page)

GENERIC NAME	TRADE NAME	ROUTE OF ADMIN.	USUAL DOSAGE
senna concentrate	SENOKOT	po	**Adults:** 10–15 ml at bedtime **Children 5–15 yrs.:** 5–10 ml before or after meals **Children 1–5 yrs.:** 2.5–5 ml before or after meals
Saline Cathartics: milk of magnesia	(G)† HALEY'S M-O*	po	**Adults:** 2 tbsp a.m. and p.m. (15–30 ml) **Children 3–6 yrs.:** 1–2 tsp (5–15 ml) **Children 7–12 yrs.:** 2–4 tsp (15–30 ml)
sodium biphosphate/sodium phosphate	PHOSPHO-SODA*	po	**Adults:** 4–8 tsp (20–40 ml) **Children 10 yrs. and older:** 1/2 adult dose **Children 5–10 yrs.:** 1/4 adult dose
	FLEET Enema	pr	**Adults:** 4 1/2 fl oz **Children 2 yrs. and older:** 2 fl oz
	VACUETTS* Evacuant Supp.	pr	**Adults:** 1 daily **Children:** not recommended
	TUCKS Phosphate Enema	pr	**Adults:** 4 1/2 fl oz **Children and infants:** 2 oz **Infants under 2 yrs.:** not recommended
Bulk-forming Cathartics: barley malt extract, nondiastatic	MALTSUPEX	po	**Adults:** 1–2 tbsp liquid daily; 2–3 tab qid **Children:** 1–2 tsp liquid daily
plantago seed husks	SYLLAMALT	po	**Adults:** 1 rounded tsp tid **Children over 6 yrs:** 1/2 tsp tid
psyllium hydrocolloid	EFFERSYLLIUM	po	**Adults (over 12 yrs):** 1 rounded Tsp. 1–3 times daily **Children (6–12 yrs):** 1/2 the adult dosage
psyllium hydrophilic mucilloid	KONSYL METAMUCIL MODANE BULK	po	**Adults:** 7 gm od to tid **Children:** not established
methylcellulose	(G) COLOGEL	po	**Adults:** 1 gm 1–4 times/day **Children:** 500 mg bid or qid
carboxymethylcellulose sodium	(G) DIALOSE*	po	**Adults:** 1.5 gm bid or qid **Children:** 500 mg bid or tid

*Contains more than one active ingredient.
†(G) designates availability as a generic product.

Lubricant Cathartics

Dioctyl Sodium Sulfosuccinate

PHARMACOLOGY

Dioctyl sodium sulfosuccinate, an anionic surface active agent, softens fecal matter by facilitating the uptake of water by the feces; there is no stimulation of peristalsis. The carthartic effect is usually apparent 1 to 3 days after the first capsule is taken.

SPECIAL PRECAUTIONS
- Do not use when abdominal pain, nausea, or vomiting is present.
- Frequent or prolonged use may result in dependence on laxatives.

CLINICAL GUIDELINES
ADMINISTRATION:
- Give dioctyl sodium sulfosuccinate in a glass of milk or fruit juice or in infant formula to mask the bitter taste.
EFFECTS:
- Does not irritate the gastrointestinal tract or produce peristalsis.
- May be given in enemas; add 50 to 100 mg to a retention or flushing enema.
OVERDOSAGE/ANTIDOTE:
- In infants, doses as large as 50 mg/kg have not produced adverse effects.

Mineral Oil

PHARMACOLOGY

Mineral oil relieves constipation by lubricating and softening hard stools, causing the passage of feces without irritating the mucosa. It is indigestible and is absorbed only to a limited extent. When administered rectally, mineral oil eases the passage of impacted fecal material.

SPECIAL PRECAUTIONS
- Frequent or prolonged use may result in dependence on laxatives.
- Do not administer to infants or young children
- Do not use if abdominal pain, nausea, and vomiting is present.
- May interfere with the absorption of essential fat-soluble substances.
- May interfere with the healing of postoperative wounds in the anorectal region.

CLINICAL GUIDELINES
ADMINISTRATION:
- Administer on an empty stomach at bedtime.

Stimulant Cathartics

Bisacodyl

PHARMACOLOGY

Bisacodyl is a contact laxative which acts directly on the colonic mucosa to produce normal peristalsis throughout the large intestine. It may be administered orally or rectally. After oral administration, an effect is noted in approximately 6 hours. When administered rectally, bisacodyl is effective in 15 minutes to 1 hour. Bisacodyl is not absorbed from the gastrointestinal tract; systemic effects have not been reported.

SPECIAL PRECAUTIONS
- Do not use if nausea, vomiting, or abdominal pain is present.
- Do not take tablets within 1 hour of antacids or milk.
- Do not use in patients with a history of hypersensitivity to bisacodyl.
- Frequent or prolonged use may result in dependence on laxatives.

ADVERSE EFFECTS

GASTROINTESTINAL   EFFECTS: abnormal cramps, mild rectal irritation

Casanthranol

PHARMACOLOGY

Following oral administration, casanthrenol stimulates peristalsis producing copious watery evacuations in approximately 2 to 6 hours.

SPECIAL PRECAUTIONS
• Do not use when abdominal pain, nausea, or vomiting is present.
• Frequent or prolonged use may result in dependence on laxatives.
• Do not use in patients with a history of hypersensitivity to casanthranol.

ADVERSE EFFECTS

GASTROINTESTINAL EFFECTS: nausea, abdominal cramps or discomfort, diarrhea
DERMATOLOGIC EFFECTS: rash

CLINICAL GUIDELINES

• Overdosage is characterized by diarrhea, abdominal cramps, and nausea.
• There is no specific antidote. Treat symptomatically.

Cascara Sagrada

PHARMACOLOGY

Cascara sagrada acts primarily in the large bowel by increasing peristalsis. An effect is obtained approximately 8 hours after oral administration. The active principle may appear in milk during lactation.

SPECIAL PRECAUTIONS
• Do not use when nausea, vomiting, or abdominal pain is present.

• Frequent or prolonged use may result in dependence on laxatives.
• Caution patients that urine may be yellowish brown (if acid) or reddish (if alkaline).
• Use with caution in nursing mothers since the active component may appear in mother's milk.

ADVERSE EFFECTS

GASTROINTESTINAL   EFFECTS: abdominal cramps, gripping

Castor Oil, Emulsified

PHARMACOLOGY

Castor oil is a stimulant laxative having a lipolytic action, primarily in the small intestine. Catharsis is produced within 3 hours. The intensity of cathartic effect is proportional to the dosage.

SPECIAL PRECAUTIONS
• Do not use if abdominal pain, nausea, or vomiting is present.
• Frequent or continued use of the product may result in dependence on laxatives.

ADVERSE EFFECTS

GASTROINTESTINAL EFFECTS: diarrhea, cramps

CLINICAL GUIDELINES

OVERDOSAGE/ANTIDOTE:
• Overdosage results in severe diarrhea.
• Discontinue drug; treat symptomatically. There is no specific antidote.

Danthron

PHARMACOLOGY

Danthron is a mild peristaltic stimulant which acts mainly on the lower bowel and produces a soft or semisoft stool in 6 to 8 hours. Danthron is excreted in the milk of lactating mothers.

SPECIAL PRECAUTIONS
• Do not use in patients with abdominal pain, nausea, or vomiting.
• Frequent or prolonged use of this preparation may result in dependence on laxatives.
• Do not use in patients with a history of hypersensitivity to danthron or other anthraquinone derivatives.
• Do not use in lactating mothers.
• Caution patient that urine may be discolored pink or orange (if alkaline).

Senna Concentrate

PHARMACOLOGY
Senna concentrate when administered orally stimulates peristalsis, thereby emptying the gastrointestinal tract. The effect is noted approximately 6 hours after ingestion. The mechanism of action is unknown; the motor activity of the large bowel primarily is increased and excessively fluid feces are produced. The drug appears in the milk during lactation in sufficient amounts to affect the nursing infant.

SPECIAL PRECAUTIONS
• Do not use when nausea, vomiting, or abdominal pain is present.
• Frequent or prolonged use may result in dependence on laxatives.
• Administer with caution to diabetic patients since the sugar content of some formulations is high (X-PREP Liquid contains 30 grams of sugar per 2 1/2 fl oz dose).

ADVERSE EFFECTS
GASTROINTESTINAL EFFECTS: abdominal discomfort, nausea, vomiting rarely

Phenophthalein, white/yellow

PHARMACOLOGY
Following oral administration, phenophthalein stimulates the motor activity of the lower gastrointestinal tract, primarily the colon. Yellow phenophthalein is incompletely purified but is more active than white phenophthalein as a cathartic.

SPECIAL PRECAUTIONS
• Frequent or prolonged use may result in dependence on laxatives.
• Do not use in patients with a history of hypersensitivity to phenophthalein.
• Do not use if nausea, vomiting, or abdominal pain is present.
• Caution patient that urine may be pink or red if sufficiently alkaline.
• If feces are made alkaline by a soapsuds enema, they may be colored red.

ADVERSE EFFECTS
URINARY TRACT EFFECTS: urine may be red or pink if alkaline
ALLERGIC EFFECTS: hypersensitivity reactions; fixed drug eruptions colored pink to purple; itching, burning, vesiculation, ulceration
DERMATOLOGIC EFFECTS: rash

CLINICAL GUIDELINES
OVERDOSAGE/ANTIDOTE:
• Overdosage results in an excessive cathartic effect.
• Phenophthalein has been ingested in large amounts by children without untoward effects. The major effect of overdosage is fluid and electrolyte deficits resulting from the excessive cathartic effect. Treatment is symptomatic. Deaths have occurred due to hypersensitivity.

Saline Cathartics

Milk of Magnesia

PHARMACOLOGY

The magnesium salts, magnesium hydroxide and magnesium sulfate, are saline cathartics. They are absorbed slowly from the gastrointestinal tract, the majority, however, remains within the gastrointestinal tract. Catharsis is produced and evacuation of semifluid or watery feces occurs within 3 to 6 hours. Catharsis is due to the osmotic effect of salt remaining in the intestinal lumen.

Milk of magnesia is a suspension of magnesium hydroxide.

SPECIAL PRECAUTIONS

- Do not use when nausea, vomiting, or abdominal pain is present.
- Frequent or prolonged use may result in dependence on laxatives.
- Use with caution in patients with impaired renal function; sufficient magnesium may be absorbed to cause magnesium intoxication.
- Do not use in patients who are receiving neomycin.

ADVERSE EFFECTS

GASTROINTESTINAL EFFECTS: nausea
METABOLIC AND ENDOCRINE EFFECTS: magnesium intoxication

CLINICAL GUIDELINES

OVERDOSE/ANTIDOTE:
- Overdosage of magnesium salts results in severe diarrhea. In patients with impaired renal function, hypermagnesemia may occur. This is characterized by a decrease in blood pressure and respiratory paralysis.
- Treat symptomatically. Artificial respiration may be required. Intravenous administration of calcium salts will combat the effects of magnesium intoxication.

Sodium Biphosphate
Sodium Phosphate

PHARMACOLOGY

Sodium biphosphate and sodium phosphate, saline cathartics, act by their osmotic effect, that is retention of a large volume of water within the gastrointestinal tract. This bulk serves as a mechanical stimulus which increases intestinal motility.

In the suppository, the water-soluble base disintegrates and the released salts react to form carbon dioxide. The pressure from this gas stimulates normal peristalsis and defecation reflexes in the lower bowel.

SPECIAL PRECAUTIONS

- Do not use if nausea, vomiting, or abdominal pain is present.
- Frequent or prolonged use may result in dependence on laxatives.
- Do not use in patients with megacolon; hypernatremic dehydration may occur.
- Use with caution in patients with impaired renal function; hyperphosphatemia and hypocalcemia may occur.
- Do not use in cardiac patients with edema or evidence of congestive heart failure or in patients on a low sodium diet.

Bulk-forming Cathartics

Barley Malt Extract, nondiastatic
Carboxymethylcellulose Sodium
Methylcellulose
Plantago Seed Husks
Psyllium Hydrochloride
Psyllium Hydrophilic Mucilloid

PHARMACOLOGY

The bulk-forming cathartics are in general hydrophilic colloids and indigestible fibers. They promote defecation without subjecting the bowel to the undesirable action of irritating drugs. These laxatives dissolve or swell in the intestinal fluid, forming emollient gels which stimulate peristalsis and facilitate passage of the intestinal contents.

SPECIAL PRECAUTIONS

• Do not use in patients with intestinal obstruction, ulcerations, or stenosis; disabling adhesions, or difficulty in swallowing.
• Caution patients not to take if prescription drugs or salicylate-containing drugs are also being taken.

CLINICAL GUIDELINES

ADMINISTRATION:
• Caution patients to take with a full glass of water.
DRUG INTERACTIONS:
• These drugs may interact and combine with other drugs, including salicylates and digitalis glycosides.

Choleretics/Hydrocholeretics

GENERAL CLINICAL USES

Dehydrocholic acid is indicated for its hydrocholeretic effect in biliary tract conditions such as recurring noncalculous cholangitis, biliary dyskinesia, chronic partial obstruction of the common bile duct, sclerosing choledochitis, and in conditions in which it is desirable to stimulate secretory activity of the liver.

Intravenous administration of dehydrocholic acid is used to measure circulation time since it produces a bitter taste when it reaches the tongue.

SPECIAL PRODUCTS AND DOSAGES

GENERIC NAME	TRADE NAME	ROUTE OF ADMIN.	USUAL DOSAGE
dehydrocholic acid	(G)*		
	HEPAHYDRIN Tablet	po	250–500 mg tid
	DECHOLIN		
	DECHOLIN Sodium	iv	3–5 ml of 20% solution

*(G) designates availability as a generic product.

Dehydrocholic Acid

PHARMACOLOGY

Dehydrocholic acid is a potent hydrocholeretic agent and a mild laxative. The mechanism of action by which it increases the frequency of bowel movements is unknown. Hydrocholeretic agents stimulate the liver to increase the output of bile of low specific gravity.

SPECIAL PRECAUTIONS

• Do not use in patients with biliary tract obstruction, acute hepatitis, or sensitivity to any of the ingredients.
• Examine periodically to prevent fluid and electrolyte deficiency due to excessive laxative effects or inadequate fluid intake.
• Do not use if abdominal pain, nausea, or vomiting is present.
• Frequent use may result in dependence on laxatives.
• If administered into the perivascular tissues, there may be a moderate local reaction

ADVERSE EFFECTS
WITH INTRAVENOUS ADMINISTRATION:
CNS EFFECTS: faintness, headache
RESPIRATORY EFFECTS: dyspnea
CARDIOVASCULAR   EFFECTS: tachycardia, hypotension
AUTONOMIC EFFECTS: sweating, chills, and fever
GASTROINTESTINAL EFFECTS: nausea, vomiting, diarrhea, abdominal discomfort
ALLERGIC   EFFECTS: anaphylactoid reactions, uncommon; urticaria
DERMATOLOGIC EFFECTS: erythema, pruritus
LOCAL EFFECTS: pain, redness, swelling with perivascular administration

Digestive Enzymes

GENERAL CLINICAL USES
The digestive enzymes, available primarily as combination products in variable dosages, may be useful in the relief of gastrointestinal symptoms such as flatulence, gas and bloating, dyspepsia, distention, and heartburn caused by deficiency states or disorders of digestion.

The enzymes, proteolytic, amylolytic, lipolytic, and cellulolytic, are frequently combined with anticholinergic agents, bile salts, antiflatulents, sedatives, and/or analgesics.

The efficacy of these products is undergoing review by the Federal Food and Drug Administration.

SPECIFIC PRODUCTS

GENERIC NAME	TRADE NAME	GENERIC NAME	TRADE NAME
Products Containing Amylolytic Enzymes: *		protease	FESTAL†
amylase	ARCO-LASE†		GUSTASE†
	FESTAL†	proteolytic enzymes	ARCO-LASE†
	GUSTASE†		KUTRASE†
	MALLENZYME†		
	PENTAZYME†	*Products Containing Cellulolytic Enzymes:*	
		cellulase	KANULASE†
			PENTAZYME†
Containing Proteolytic Enzymes:			
pancreatin	(G)‡	cellulolytic enzymes	ARCO-LASE†
	DIGOLASE†		GUSTASE†
	DONNAZYME†		KUTRASE†
	ENTOZYME†		MALLENZYME†
	ENZYPAN†		FESTAL†
	KANULASE†		
	PHAZYME†	*Products Containing Lipolytic Agents:*	
pepsin	ENTOZYME†	lipase	ARCO-LASE†
	MURIPSIN†		ILOZYME†
	PENTAZYME†		FESTAL†
			KUTRASE†
prolase	TRI-CONE†		PENTAZYME†

*Because of variations in enzyme activity in different formulations, usual dosage information
is not included. The labeling of each product should be consulted prior to use.
†Contains more than one active ingredient.
‡(G) designates availability as a generic product.

PHARMACOLOGY

The amylolytic enzymes are responsible for the digestion of starch.

The cellulolytic enzymes digest cellulose, specifically the fiber in vegetables such as corn and cabbage.

The lipases are the enzymes responsible for the breakdown of lipids (fats).

The proteolytic enzymes are responsible for the digestion of protein and are usually obtained from the hog pancreas. They consist of pepsin, pancreatin, proteases, prolase, trypsin, chymotrypsin, and combinations considered "proteolytic enzymes."

SPECIAL PRECAUTIONS

• Do not use in patients hypersensitive to any ingredient.

• Pancreatic exocrine replacement therapy should not delay or supplant treatment of the primary disorder.

• Maintain proper balance between fat, protein, and carbohydrate intake to avoid indigestion.

ADVERSE EFFECTS

GASTROINTESTINAL EFFECTS: indigestion, nausea, diarrhea

Emetics

GENERAL CLINICAL USES

The emetics, apomorphine hydrochloride and ipecac syrup, are used to induce emesis (vomiting).

SPECIFIC PRODUCTS AND DOSAGES

GENERIC NAME	TRADE NAME	ROUTE OF ADMIN.	USUAL DOSAGE
apomorphine HCl	(G)*	sc	**Adults:** 2–10 mg; do not repeat **Children:** use with caution **Debilitated patients:** use with caution
ipecac syrup	(G)	po	**Persons over 1 yr.:** 1 tbsp (3 tsp or 15 ml) **Children under 1 yr.:** 2 tsp (5–10 ml)

*(G) designates availability as a generic product.

Apomorphine Hydrochloride

PHARMACOLOGY

Apomorphine hydrochloride acts centrally by stimulating the chemoreceptor trigger zone in the medulla. Vomiting is usually induced within 5 to 10 minutes after subcutaneous administration. It acts more efficiently when the stomach is full.

SPECIAL PRECAUTIONS

• Do not use in patients with corrosive poisoning; in narcosis due to opiates, barbiturates, alcohol, or other central nervous system depressants; in patients too inebriated to stand unaided; or those in shock.

• Use with caution in children, debilitated individuals, those with cardiac decompensation, persons predisposed to nausea and vomiting, or those with central nervous system depression.

• Do not use in patients with a history of hypersensitivity to morphine.

ADVERSE EFFECTS

CNS EFFECTS: depression, euphoria, restlessness, tremor

RESPIRATORY EFFECTS: polypnea

CARDIOVASCULAR EFFECTS: peripheral vascular collapse

CLINICAL GUIDELINES

ADMINISTRATION:
- If solution is green or brown, discard; apomorphine is not stable.

EFFECTS:
- The emetic effect is usually preceded by nausea and salivation.
- Respiratory depression may be produced.

OVERDOSAGE/ANTIDOTE:
- Excessive dosage may cause violent emesis, cardiac depression, and death.
- The depressant effects may be reversed by use of a narcotic antagonist (naloxone 0.05 mg/kg; levallorphan 0.02 mg/kg). Use supportive therapy as indicated. See Chapter 20, page 695, for detailed information.

Ipecac Syrup

PHARMACOLOGY

Ipecac syrup induces emesis, usually within 30 to 60 minutes after ingestion. The active ingredient is emetine, which acts both centrally and locally in the gastrointestinal tract. The drug is not useful in emergencies.

SPECIAL PRECAUTIONS
- May not be effective in patients in whom the ingested material is an antiemetic agent.
- Can exert a cardiotoxic effect if it is not vomited but absorbed.
- Do not use to induce vomiting when such substances such as petroleum distillates (kerosene, gasoline, coal oil, fuel oil, paint thinner, cleaning fluid), strong alkali (lye), or strychnine are ingested.
- Do not use in patients who are unconscious, semiconscious, severely inebriated, or in shock.
- Do not administer activated charcoal concomitantly; it nullified the effect of ipecac syrup.

CLINICAL GUIDELINES

ADMINISTRATION:
- Give with adequate amounts of water.

DRUG INTERACTIONS:
- Activated charcoal will absorb ipecac syrup.

OVERDOSAGE/ANTIDOTE
- Overdosage is characterized by excessive vomiting.
- If patient does not vomit, the ipecac syrup should be removed by lavage because of the potential cardiotoxicity.
- Treat supportively. There is no specific antidote.

Gastric Acidifiers (Hydrochloric Acid Substitutes/Replacements)

GENERAL CLINICAL USES
Gastric achlorhydria, usually associated with pernicious anemia, gastric carcinoma, congenital achlorhydria, and allergy, may be ameliorated by ingestion of glutamic acid hydrochloride.

SPECIFIC PRODUCTS AND DOSAGES

GENERIC NAME	TRADE NAME	ROUTE OF ADMIN.	USUAL DAILY DOSAGE
glutamic acid hydrochloride	ACIDULIN GLUTASYN* MURIPSIN*	po	1–3 tablets daily before meals

*Contains more than one active ingredient.

Glutamic Acid Hydrochloride

PHARMACOLOGY
Glutamic acid hydrochloride provides the equivalent of hydrochloric acid in a palatable form which does not injure the mucous membranes and teeth.

SPECIAL PRECAUTIONS
• Do not use in patients with gastric hyperacidity or peptic ulcer.
• Do not use in patients with a history of hypersensitivity to glutamic acid hydrochloride.

CLINICAL GUIDELINES
ADMINISTRATION:
• Oral administration in capsules prevents exposure of dental enamel to acid.
EFFECTS:
• Avoids uncontrolled acid release.
OVERDOSAGE/ANTIDOTE:
• Massive overdosage may produce systemic acidosis.
• Treat with alkalies such as sodium bicarbonate or sodium lactate solution, one molar (to be diluted).

Smooth Muscle Stimulants

GENERAL CLINICAL USES
The smooth muscle stimulants, dexpanthenol and physostigmine salicylate are used to assist peristalsis in postoperative intestinal atony; postpartum or postoperative retention of flatus; or paralytic ileus.

Metoclopamide hydrochloride stimulates gastric emptying and facilitates radiologic examination and passage of small bowel biopsy tubes.

SPECIFIC PRODUCTS AND DOSAGES

GENERIC NAME	TRADE NAME	ROUTE OF ADMIN.	USUAL ADULT DOSAGE
dexpanthenol	(G)* ILOPAN	im/iv	250–500 mg; repeat as necessary
metoclopramide hydrochloride	REGLAN	iv	**Adults:** 10 mg **Children (6–14 yrs):** 2.5–5 mg **Children (under 6 yrs):** 0.1 mg/kg
physostigmine salicylate	(G) ANTILIRIUM	im/iv	0.5–2.0 mg; repeat as necessary

*(G) designates availability as a generic product.

Dexpanthenol

PHARMACOLOGY

Dexpanthenol is a coenzyme-A precursor. Administered prophylactically immediately after major abdominal surgery, it minimizes the possibility of paralytic ileus.

SPECIAL PRECAUTIONS
• Wait 12 hours after neostigmine or other enterokinetic drugs and wait 1 hour after succinylcholine before administering dexpanthenol.
• Do not administer if ileus is caused by mechanical obstruction. Assure that patient is not hypokalemic.
• Do not discontinue prematurely.
• Do not use in children or in patients with hemophilia.

CLINICAL GUIDELINES
ADMINISTRATION:
• Administration of full-strength solution directly into the vein is not advised.
DRUG INTERACTIONS:
• Concomitant use of this drug and other drugs such as antibiotics, narcotics, and barbiturates has resulted in rare instances of allergic reaction of unknown cause.
• May be mixed with intravenous bulk solutions such as glucose or lactose-Ringer's and slowly infused by intravenous drip.

Physostigmine Salicylate

For detailed information, see Chapter 7, page 356.

Metoclopramide Hydrochloride

GENERAL CLINICAL USES
Metoclopramide hydrochloride is used to facilitate passage of small bowel biopsy tubes in patients where the tube does not pass the pylorus with conventional measures. It is also used for stimulation of gastric emptying of barium in cases where delayed emptying interferes with radiological examination of the stomach and small intestines.

PHARMACOLOGY

• Metoclopramide hydrochloride is a stimulant of the upper gastrointestinal tract without stimulating gastric, biliary, or pancreatic secretions. The effect can be abolished by atropine.

ADVERSE EFFECTS

CNS EFFECTS: sedation, extrapyramidal symptoms occur more frequently in children and young adults; involuntary movements of limbs and facial grimacing; rarely torticollis, oculogyric crisis, rhythmic protrusion of tongue, bulbar type of speech or trismus, one dystonic reaction resembling tetanus has been reported.

CLINICAL GUIDELINES

ADMINISTRATION:
• Administer slowly, over 1 to 2 minutes.
EFFECTS:
• With rapid administration, a transient but intense feeling of anxiety and restlessness followed by drowsiness may occur.

DRUG INTERACTIONS

• Sedative effects can occur when metoclopramide hydrochloride is administered with alcohol, sedatives, hypnotics, narcotics, or tranquilizers.

Hepatic Coma and Precoma Agent

SPECIFIC PRODUCTS AND DOSAGES

GENERIC NAME	TRADE NAME	ROUTE OF ADMIN.	USUAL DOSAGE
lactulose	CEPHULAC DUPHALAC	po	30–45 ml tid or qid

Lactulose

GENERAL CLINICAL USES

Lactulose is indicated for the prevention and treatment of portalsystemic encephalopathy, including the stages of hepatic pre-edema and coma.

PHARMACOLOGY

Lactulose causes a decrease in blood ammonia concentration and reduces the degree of portal-systemic encephalopathy. Lactulose is degraded by the colonic bacteria, resulting in acidification of colonic contents. This acidification results in the retention of ammonia as the ammonium ion in the colon. The acid contents of the colon convert NH_3 to the ammonium ion (NH_4^+), trapping it and preventing its absorption. The laxative effect of the metabolites of lactulose then facilitate expulsion of the intestinal contents, including the ammonium ion. Lactulose therapy reduces the blood ammonia levels by 25 to 50 percent.

SPECIAL PRECAUTIONS
• Lactulose is contraindicated in patients who require a low galactose diet.
• Safe use in pregnancy has not been established.
• Use with caution in diabetics. Lactulose syrup contains galactose and lactose.

ADVERSE EFFECTS
GASTROINTESTINAL EFFECTS: flatulence, belching, abdominal discomfort, cramping, diarrhea, nausea, vomiting

CLINICAL GUIDELINES
DRUG INTERACTIONS:
• Concomitant use of lactulose and neomycin and other antibiotics which affect colonic bacteria has not been clarified. Anti-infective agents may interfere with the desired degradation of lactulose and prevent the acidification of colonic contents.
• Do not use other laxatives particularly during the early phase of therapy for portal-systemic encephalopathy.
OVERDOSAGE/ANTIDOTE:
• Overdosage has not been reported. It is expected that diarrhea and abdominal cramps would be the major symptoms.
• Discontinue therapy. Treat supportively as necessary.

Drugs affecting the skin

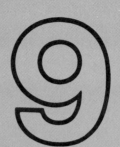

INTRODUCTION

The skin, the largest organ of the body, is exposed to abrasions, infections, and various chemical insults, in addition to the varying and many times adverse atmospheric conditions. The skin varies from a thin, delicate epithelium to a dense, cornified tissue which fortunately is accessible to therapy. The age of the patient and the size of the area to be treated, as well as the extent of the lesion, must be considered in the selection of an appropriate product for treatment. The vehicle in which the active agent is formulated is of utmost importance.

Products for use on specialized epithelial surfaces such as the mucosa of the rectum, mouth, and vagina, are reviewed in Chapter 8, *Drugs Affecting the Gastrointestinal Tract*, Chapter 10, *Drugs Affecting the Teeth and Mouth*, and Chapter 14, *Drugs Affecting the Reproductive Tract*, respectively.

Skin alterations resulting from untoward effects of drugs administered parenterally or orally will be discussed, usually as adverse effects, with the specific drug.

SPECIFIC THERAPEUTIC CLASSIFICATION

Drugs applied topically to treat pathology of the skin may be grouped as follows: anesthetic agents (topical, surface), antiacne agents, anti-infective agents, anti-inflammatory agents, antiseptics/astringents, antipruritic agents/antihistamines, debriding agents, detergents/cleansers, photosensitizers, and sunscreens/sunshades.

Anesthetics, Topical (Surface)

GENERAL CLINICAL USES

The topical (surface) anesthetics are used to control discomfort and pain caused by minor burns, abrasions, scraps, insect bites and stings. In addition, they are used for anesthesia of mucous membranes, endotracheal intubation, and prevention of pain in procedures involving the male and female urethra, in treatment of painful urethritis.

The topical anesthetics are effective when applied to mucous membranes or damaged skin; their effectiveness when applied on intact skin is uncertain, apparently because of poor penetration.

SPECIFIC PRODUCTS AND DOSAGES

GENERIC NAME	TRADE NAME	USE	DOSAGE
benzocaine	HURRICAINE	Mucous membrane anesthesia for dental procedures	Apply liberally as needed
	AMERICAINE Anesthetic Lubricant	On intratracheal catheters, nasogastric and endoscopic tubes, aryngoscopes, proctoscopes	
CII cocaine HCl	(G)*	In ear, nose, throat, rectum, vagina, urethra	Apply as needed

*(G) designates availability as a generic product.

(continued facing page)

GENERIC NAME	TRADE NAME	USE	DOSAGE
cyclomethycaine sulfate	SURFACAINE Jelly	Topical anesthesia in bronchoscopy, cystography, rectal and vaginal examinations, tracheal intubation	Apply as needed
	SURFACAINE Cream, Ointment, Jelly, Suppository	Anorectal conditions	
dibucaine HCl	NUPERCAINAL Ointment, Cream	Skin: cuts, burns, insect bites, sunburn	Apply as needed
	NUPERCAINAL Spray, Suppository	Rectum	
dimethisoquin HCl	QUOTANE Ointment	Skin	bid to qid
dyclonine HCl	DYCLONE Solution	Mouth, pharynx, larynx, trachea, esophagus, urethra prior to endoscopic examination, block gag reflex, relieve pain associated with oral and anogenital lesions	Apply as needed
hexylcaine HCl	CYCLAINE Solution	Intact mucous membranes of the respiratory tract, upper GI tract and urinary tract	Apply as needed
lidocaine HCl	ANESTACON Solution	Male and female urethra; painful urethritis	Apply as needed
	LIDA-MANTLE Cream	Mucous membrane and skin anesthesia	
	XYLOCAINE Solution	Oral and nasal cavity, proximal parts of GI tract	
	XYLOCAINE Viscous	Mouth, pharynx	
	XYLOCAINE Ointment	Oropharynx, for endotracheal intubation	
	XYLOCAINE Jelly	Male and female urethra; painful urethritis	
	XYLOCAINE Suppositories	Rectum	
methyl salicylate	GER-O-FOAM† PANALGESIC†	Skin	bid to tid
pramoxine HCl	TRONOTHANE† Cream, Jelly	Skin	every 3–4 hr.
tetracaine HCl	PONTOCAINE HCl Solution, Cream, Ointment	Nose, throat prior to bronchoscopy, esophagoscopy; skin, rectum	Apply liberally as needed
triethanolamine salicylate	MYOFLEX Creme NEUTROGENA Cream	Skin	bid to tid

†Contains more than one active ingredient.

Benzocaine
Cocaine HCl
Cyclomethycaine Sulfate
Dibucaine HCl
Dimethisoquin HCl
Dyclonine HCl
Hexylcaine HCl
Lidocaine HCl
Methyl Salicylate
Pramoxine HCl
Tetracaine HCl
Triethanolamine Salicylate

PHARMACOLOGY

The surface anesthetics do not readily penetrate the keratinized surface of intact skin. However, they will act on abraded, ulcerated, denuded, or burned skin. They are particularly effective when applied to the mucosa of the mouth, oral and nasal pharynx, larynx, trachea, and urethra.

Application to mucosa of the nasopharynx or respiratory tract may result in blood levels almost as high and as rapidly attained as those occurring after intravenous administration. Therefore, the total dose applied should not exceed one-fourth the maximal recommended dose for injection. Preparation for endoscopy is probably the most common use of surface anesthetics.

The duration of the effect of these anesthetics is quite brief and will persist only if a continuous amount of the drug is in contact with the mucosal surface.

SPECIAL PRECAUTIONS

• Do not use in patients with a history of hypersensitivity to these products or their components.
• Safe use has not been established with respect to adverse fetal development.

• Topical application may produce the same untoward effects as those occurring with parenteral administration.
• In debilitated or elderly patients and children, use dosages commensurate with age and physical condition.
• Use of any of the surface anesthetic agents may interfere with the second stage of swallowing.
• If irritation or sensitivity occurs, discontinue immediately.

ADVERSE EFFECTS

CNS EFFECTS: transient or persistent stimulation followed by depression, twitching, convulsions, tremors, drowsiness
RESPIRATORY EFFECTS: dyspnea, cyanosis, shallow respirations, respiratory arrest
CARDIOVASCULAR EFFECTS: hypotension, quinidinelike changes in cardiac conduction, shock
URINARY TRACT EFFECTS: urethritis rarely
ALLERGIC EFFECTS: urticaria, anaphylactoid reactions, contact dermatitis
OPHTHALMIC EFFECTS: blurred vision
LOCAL EFFECTS: burning, tenderness, swelling, irritation; tissue sloughing and necrosis

CLINICAL GUIDELINES

ADMINISTRATION:
• Since damaged or diseased skin permits penetration of the drug, use of excessive quantities may result in systemic effects.
• Most topical analgesics are ineffective on intact skin.
EFFECTS:
• Redness, swelling, or pain may indicate an allergic reaction; discontinue drug.
DRUG INTERACTIONS:
• Patients with allergic sensitivity to para-aminobenzoic acid derivatives such as procaine, tetracaine, benzocaine have not shown cross sensitivity to lidocaine.

Antiacne Agents (Antiseborrheic and Keratolytic Agents)

GENERAL CLINICAL USES

The antiacne agents contain combinations of antiseborrheic agents, keratolytic agents, and anti-inflammatory agents. The antiseborrheic agents include sulfur, selenium sulfide, zinc pyrethione, pyrithione, parachloromethoxylenol, tar extract, and salicylic acid. The keratolytic agents include salicylic acid, resorcinol, benzoyl peroxide, and tretinoin.

The combinations of antiseborrheic agents and keratolytic agents provide relief from the lesions of acne by providing peeling, drying, and defatting actions.

SPECIFIC PRODUCTS AND DOSAGES

GENERIC NAME	TRADE NAME	USUAL DOSAGE
Antiacne Agents: benzoyl peroxide	BENZAGEL LOROXIDE Acne Lotion PERSADOX Acne Cream, Lotion SULFOXYL Lotion (Regular, Strong)	Apply once to twice daily
resorcinol, resorcinol monoacetate	ACNE-DOME* Cream, Lotion ACNOMEL* Cream, Cake PHISOAC Cream REZAMID* Acne Lotion	Apply bid
salicylic acid	FOSTEX* Cream, Liquid KLARON Acne Lotion KOMED* Acne Lotion	Apply once to twice daily
sulfur, colloidal sulfur	ACNEDERM* Lotion ACNE-DOME* Cream, Lotion BENSULFOID* Lotion FOSTEX* Cream, Liquid LIQUIMAT* Drying Lotion for Acne	Apply once to twice daily

*Contains more than one active ingredient.

(continued overleaf)

GENERIC NAME	TRADE NAME	USUAL DOSAGE
tretinoin	RETIN-A Gel, Cream, Liquid	Apply once or twice daily
Antiseborrheic Agents: benzoyl peroxide	See *ANTIACNE Agents*	Use once or twice weekly
parachlorometaxylenol	METASEP Medicated Shampoo Concentrate	Use once or twice weekly
salicyclic acid	METED* Shampoo FOSTEX* Shampoo Also see *ANTIACNE Agents* and *KERATOLITIC Agents*	Use once or twice weekly
selenium sulfide	EXSEL Lotion SELSUN	Use once or twice weekly
sulfur, colloidal sulfur	See *ANTIACNE Agents*	
tar extract	PENTRAX* Tar Shampoo	Use twice weekly
zinc pyrithione, pyrithione	DANEX Shampoo ZINCON Dandruff Shampoo	Use once or twice weekly

*Contains more than one active ingredient.

Benzoyl Peroxide

PHARMACOLOGY
Benzoyl peroxide provides drying, desquamating, and antiseptic actions. It is a powerful oxidizing agent.

SPECIAL PRECAUTIONS
• Do not use in patients with a history of hypersensitivity to benzoyl peroxide or other components of the formulation.
• Do not use in or near the eyes and mucous membranes; or on highly inflamed or denuded skin.

ADVERSE EFFECTS
LOCAL EFFECTS: stinging, burning, reddening

CLINICAL GUIDELINES
ADMINISTRATION:
• Fair individuals should begin with a single application.
• May bleach colored fabrics.
• Cleanse affected areas prior to administration.
EFFECTS:
• Contact allergy may develop.

Parachlorometoxylenol

PHARMACOLOGY
Parachloromethoxylenol is an antiseborrheic agent. It aids in relief of dandruff and associated conditions.

SPECIAL PRECAUTIONS
• Avoid contact with the eyes.
• Discontinue use if irritation or hyper-

sensitivity occurs.
- Absorption may occur if used over large areas on infants and young children.
- Do not use in acute inflammation, open or infected lesions.

There is no specific antidote; apply bland ointment or cold cream.
- Accidental ingestion generally results in gastrointestinal symptoms. There is no specific antidote; consider emesis or lavage; force fluids.

Resorcinol
Resorcinol Monoacetate

PHARMACOLOGY
Resorcin, resorcinol, and resorcinol monoacetate are keratolytic agents frequently used in combination with sulfur to induce peeling and drying of the skin. In addition, these products have bactericidal and fungicidal activity.

SPECIAL PRECAUTIONS
- Keep away from the eyes and mucous membranes.
- If irritation develops, discontinue use.
- Do not use in patients with a history of hypersensitivity to these or related compounds.
- Persons with sensitive skin may experience mild transitory stinging which disappears on continued use.

ADVERSE EFFECTS
LOCAL EFFECTS: stinging, irritation, itching, scaling

CLINICAL GUIDELINES
OVERDOSAGE/ANTIDOTE:
- Topical overdosage may result in excessive drying and erythema, burning, and itching. Reduce or discontinue medication.

Salicylic Acid

PHARMACOLOGY
Salicylic acid softens keratin and loosens cornified epithelium. The epithelium desquamates easily and makes the underlying viable cells accessible to medication. Viable cells swell and soften, thereby making them more receptive to medication.

SPECIAL PRECAUTIONS
- Avoid contact with the eyes and mucous membranes.
- Do not use in patients with a history of hypersensitivity to salicylic acid or other components of the product.
- If irritation or hypersensitivity occurs, discontinue use.
- Limit use in children under 12 years of age to no more than 1 oz.

ADVERSE EFFECTS
LOCAL EFFECTS: redness, scaling

Selenium Sulfide

PHARMACOLOGY
The mechanism of the antiseborrheic action of selenium sulfide is unknown. Minimal absorption occurs after ap-

plication to the intact skin; with abraded or inflamed skin, absorption occurs to a greater degree.

SPECIAL PRECAUTIONS

• Do not use in patients with a history of hypersensitivity to selenuim sulfide.
• Safe use in infants has not been established.
• Contact with the eyes may result in chemical conjunctivitis.
• Use with caution in the presence of acute inflammation or exudation; increased absorption may occur.

ADVERSE EFFECTS

LOCAL EFFECTS: hair loss, hair discoloration (orange tint), oilness of scalp and hair

CLINICAL GUIDELINES

OVERDOSAGE/ANTIDOTE:
• Accidental oral ingestion usually results in nausea and vomiting. Selenium sulfide is highly toxic.
• There is no specific antidote. Induce vomiting or perform gastric lavage. Administration of a purgative will hasten elimination.

Sulfur/Colloidal Sulfur

PHARMACOLOGY

Sulfur is an antiseborrheic agent which aids in drying the skin and removing excess oil.

SPECIAL PRECAUTIONS

• If undue irritation develops or increases, discontinue use.
• Avoid contact with the eyes.
• Do not use on severely inflamed skin.

ADVERSE EFFECTS

LOCAL EFFECTS: transient warming or smarting sensation, scaling and redness, irritation

Tar Extract

PHARMACOLOGY

Coal tar extract decreases epidermal proliferation and dermal infiltration, thereby helping to correct abnormalities of keratinization.

SPECIAL PRECAUTIONS

• Do not use in patients with a history of hypersensitivity to tar extract or other components of the formulation.
• Staining of the hair and of fabrics may occur.
• Avoid contact with the eyes.

ADVERSE EFFECTS

LOCAL EFFECTS: primary irritation, folliculitis, allergic contact dermatitis, phototoxicity

Tretinoin

PHARMACOLOGY

Tretinoin is an acid derivative of vitamin A, retinoic acid. It affects the follicular epithelium keratinization which causes comedones and is generally considered a strong keratolytic agent.

SPECIAL PRECAUTIONS

• Do not use in patients with a history of hypersensitivity to tretinoin or related compounds.
• If hypersensitivity develops, discontinue use.
• Keep away from the eyes, mouth, an-

gles of the nose, and mucous membranes.
• Concomitant topical medication should be used with caution.

ADVERSE EFFECTS
LOCAL EFFECTS: severe local erythema and peeling, redness, edema, blisters, crusts, temporary hypo- or hyperpigmentation, transitory feeling of warmth, slight stinging.

CLINICAL GUIDELINES
ADMINISTRATION:
• Caution patients to avoid or minimize exposure to tretinoin.
• During early weeks of therapy, an apparent exacerbation of inflammatory lesions may occur.
• Clean skin thoroughly before application.
• Do not apply when the skin is damp or wet.
EFFECTS:
• Therapeutic effects should be noted in 2 to 3 weeks; 6 weeks may be required.

DRUG INTERACTIONS:
• Administer with caution concomitant medications such as peeling agents, sulfur, resorcinol, benzoyl peroxide, or salicylic acid.
• Use with caution with medicated or abrasive soaps and cleansers, soaps and cosmetics that have a drying effect, and products with a high concentration of alcohol, astringents, spices or lime.

Pyrithione
Zinc Pyrithione

PHARMACOLOGY
Zinc pyrithione and pyrithione are antidandruff agents. They aid in removal of sebum without drying the hair.

SPECIAL PRECAUTIONS
• Avoid contact with the eyes; if occurs, wash out with water.
• Discontinue use if irritation or hypersensitivity occurs.

Anti-Infective Agents

GENERAL CLINICAL USES
The anti-infective agents are applied topically to treat infections of the skin caused by susceptible organisms.

Serious and/or extensive infections of the skin may require systemic administration of anti-infective agents. For additional information, see Chapter 2, *Anti-Infective Agents.*

Antifungal agents may be therapeutically successful when applied topically because of the high concentrations attainable in contrast to lower levels usually attained with systemic administration, where toxicity usually limits high serum levels.

At present no topically effective antiviral agents are recognized.

SPECIFIC PRODUCTS AND DOSAGES

GENERIC NAME	TRADE NAME	USUAL DOSAGE
Antibacterial Agents:		
bacitracin/zinc bacitracin	NEOSPORIN* Ointment, Aerosol	tid or qid
chloramphenicol	CHLOROMYCETIN Cream	tid or qid
erythromycin	ILOTYCIN Ointment	tid or qid
gentamicin sulfate	GARAMYCIN Cream, Ointment	tid to qid
gramicidin	CORTISPORIN* Cream MYCOLOG* Cream, Ointment	bid to qid
mafenide	SULFAMYLON Cream	tid or qid
neomycin/neomycin sulfate/ neomycin palmitate	METI-DERM* with Neomycin MYCOLOG* Cream, Ointment NEO-DELTA CORTEF* Ointment NEO-MEDROL* Acetate Topical NEOSPORIN* Ointment, Aerosol NEO-SYNALAR* Cream	bid or tid
nitrofurazone	FURACIN Soluble Dressing FURACIN Soluble Powder FURACIN Solution FURACIN Cream	Daily or weekly Apply to lesion directly from shaker Spray on lesion daily Daily or every few days
oxytetracycline	TERRAMYCIN Ointment TERRA-CORTRIL* Topical Ointment	bid to qid
polymyxin B sulfate	CORTISPORIN* NEOSPORIN* Ointment	tid or qid
sulfacetamide sodium	SEBIZON Lotion	Apply at bedtime and allow to remain overnight
Antifungal Agents:		
acrisorcin	AKRINOL	Apply small quantities bid
amphotericin B	FUNGIZONE Cream, Lotion, Ointment	Apply liberally bid to qid

*Contains more than one active ingredient.

(continued facing page)

GENERIC NAME	TRADE NAME	USUAL DOSAGE
clotrimazole	LOTRIMIN Cream, Solution	bid
haloprogin	HALOTEX Cream, Solution	bid to tid
iodochlorohydroxyquin	HYSONE* VIOFORM	bid or tid; continue 1 week after symptoms abate
miconazole nitrate	MICATIN Lotion, Cream	once or twice daily
nystatin	(G)† MYCOSTATIN Cream, Ointment Topical Powder	bid to qid
sodium thiosulfate	(G) TINVER* Lotion	bid
tolnaftate	TINACTIN* Cream, Lotion, Powder	Apply liberally bid
undecylenic acid	DESENEX	Apply liberally bid
undecylenate calcium	CRUEX Powder	Apply liberally bid
undecylenate zinc	CRUEX Cream	

*Contains more than one active ingredient.
†(G) designates availability as a generic product.

PHARMACOLOGY, SPECIAL PRECAUTIONS, ADVERSE EFFECTS

For detailed information, see Chapter 2, page 10.

CLINICAL GUIDELINES

ADMINISTRATION:
• Wounds should be cleansed and dried prior to application of medication.
• Avoid further contamination of the skin.
• In serious wounds and burns, sterile technique should be used.

EFFECTS:
• Sensitization to many of the topically applied anti-infective agents may occur.
• In fungal infections, if improvement does not occur in 4 weeks, then review diagnosis.

DRUG INTERACTIONS:
• Bacitracin, neomycin, gramicidin, and/or polymyxin B are frequently formulated in combination to provide a wide spectrum of antibacterial activity.
• Local anesthetics related to PABA may antagonize the action of the sulfonamides.

OVERDOSAGE/ANTIDOTE:
• If irritation or sensitization occurs, remove the topical medication by washing with water.
• Treat symptomatically.

Anti-Inflammatory Agents

GENERAL CLINICAL USES

The anti-inflammatory corticosteroids (glucorticoids) applied topically are used to treat corticosteroid-responsive dermatoses such as atopic dermatitis, contact dermatitis, disorders characterized by pruitus such as psoriasis and pruitus ani.

The anti-inflammatory agents administered by intralesional injection are useful in treating keloids; localized hypertrophic lesions of lichen planus, psoriatic plaques, granuloma annulare, and lichen simplex; neurodermatitis, discoid lupus erythematosus, nechrobiosis lipoidica, and alopecia areata.

For additional information about the anti-inflammatory glucocorticoids administered orally, see Chapter 15, page 535.

SPECIFIC PRODUCTS AND DOSAGES

GENERIC NAME	TRADE NAME	USUAL DOSAGE
Corticosteroids: betamethasone	CELESTONE Cream	od to tid

betamethasone acetate
  betamethasone sodium
  phosphate
	CELESTONE SOLUSPAN
	  Injection
		intralesional, intradermal

betamethasone benzoate	BENISONE Lotion, Gel	bid to qid
betamethasone dipropionate	DIPROSONE Cream, Ointment, Lotion, Aerosol	bid
betamethasone sodium phosphate	CELESTONE PHOSPHATE Injection	intralesional
betamethasone valerate	VALISONE Cream, Ointment, Lotion, Aerosol	bid to tid
desonide	TRIDESILON Cream, Ointment	bid to tid

(continued facing page)

GENERIC NAME	TRADE NAME	USUAL DOSAGE
dexamethasone	AEROSEB-DEX* Aerosol	spray as required
	DESABRON Gel	bid to qid
dexamethasone acetate	DECADRON-LA	intradermal, intralesional
dexamethasone sodium phosphate	DECADRON Phosphate	intradermal, intralesional
flumethasone pivalate	LOCORTEN Cream	bid to qid
fluocinolone acetonide	FLUONID Cream Ointment, Solution	bid to qid
	NEO-SYNALAR* Cream	
	SYNALAR Cream, Ointment, Solution	
	SYNEMOL Cream	
fluocinonide	LIDEX Cream, Ointment	bid to qid
	TOPSYN Gel	
fluorometholone	OXYLONE Cream	tid to qid
flurandrenolide	CORDRAN Ointment, Cream, Lotion, Tape	tid to qid
halcinonide	HALOG Cream, Ointment, Solution	bid to tid
hydrocortisone	DERMACORT Cream, Lotion	od to tid
	PRAMOSONE* Cream, Lotion, Ointment	
methylprednisolone acetate	MEDROL Acetate Ointment	bid to tid
	NEO-MEDROL* Acetate Cream	
prednisolone	METI-DERM Cream	bid to qid
prednisolone acetate	METICORTELONE Acetate	intradermal, 1/3-1/2 oral dose up to 0.5 mg/sq in skin
	NEO-DELTA-CORTEF Ointment	od to tid
triamcinolone acetonide	KENALOG Cream, Lotion, Ointment, Spray	bid to qid
	ARISTOCORT Ointment, Cream Lotion	
triamcinolone diacetate	ARISTOCORT Forte	intralesional
triamcinolone hexacetonide	ARISTOSPAN Parenteral	intralesional
Others:		
streptokinase-streptodornase	VARIDASE for Local or Topical use	individualize

*Contains more than one active ingredient.

Corticosteroids (Glucocorticoids)

PHARMACOLOGY

The corticosteroids applied topically provide anti-inflammatory, antipruritic, and vasoconstrictive actions. In severely excoriated skin, systemic absorption may occur. The exact mechanism of action is unclear.

Intralesional or intradermal administration results in a local concentration of active agent and facilitates pharmacologic activities.

SPECIAL PRECAUTIONS

• Do not use in patients with viral diseases of the skin such as varicella and vaccinia; fungal infections; herpes simplex.

• Do not use when circulation is markedly impaired, particularly if stasis dermatitis is present.

• Do not use in patients with a history of hypersensitivity to any of the components.

• Safe use in pregnancy has not been established.

• If infection is present, use appropriate antibiotic therapy; if infection is not controlled, discontinue anti-inflammatory agent until infection is controlled.

• If extensive areas are treated, or if the occlusive technique is used, the possibility of systemic absorption must be considered.

• Do not use in or near the eyes or mucous membranes.

• Avoid inhalation of the aerosol spray.

• Do not use aerosol preparation under occlusive dressings.

• With aerosols avoid freezing tissues by not spraying for more than 3 seconds at distances not less than 6 inches.

• Exposure of aerosol containers to temperatures above 120°F may cause bursting.

ADVERSE EFFECTS

LOCAL EFFECTS: with gel, cream, lotion, ointment, solution—burning sensation, itching, irritation, dryness, folliculitis, secondary infection, skin atrophy, striae, hypertrichosis, acneiform eruptions, hypopigmentation, miliaria, maceration; with spray—transient burning or stinging; with intralesional/intradermal administration—blindness, rarely; hypopigmentation or hyperpigmentation, atrophy, postinjection flare, burning, tingling

• Since systemic absorption is possible, any of the adverse effects associated with any corticosteroid therapy may occur. See Chapter 15, page 535.

CLINICAL GUIDELINES

ADMINISTRATION:

• Wash affected areas thoroughly before topical application.

• Transient discomfort may occur when initially applied.

• For intralesional or intradermal administration, strict aseptic technique is mandatory.

• Topical ethyl chloride spray may be used locally before injection.

EFFECTS:

• Anti-inflammatory action may suppress signs of infection.

DRUG INTERACTIONS:

With intralesional/intradermal administration:

• May be diluted with Dextrose and Sodium Chloride Injection, USP (5% and 10% Dextrose); Sodium Chloride Injection, USP; or Sterile Water for Injection, USP.

• May be mixed with 1% and 2% Lidocaine Hydrochloride using the formulations which do not contain parabens (consult labeling); similar local anesthetics also may be used.

• Diluents containing methylparaben, propylparaben, phenol, etc., should be avoided since these compounds may cause flocculations of the steroid.

• These dilutions will retain full potency

for a week; discard after 7 days.

OVERDOSAGE/ANTIDOTE:

• If sprayed in the eyes, immediately flush with copious amounts of water. Excessive dosage administered intralesionally/intradermally may cause local atrophy.

• There is no known antidote.

Streptokinase-Streptodornase

GENERAL CLINICAL USES

Streptokinase-streptodornase applied topically is useful in dissolution and removal of clotted blood, fibrinous or purulent accumulations, in treatment of acute edema or inflammation in acute and chronic conditions.

PHARMACOLOGY

Streptokinase activates fibrinolytic activity in human serum resulting in dissolution of blood clots and fibrinous exudates. Streptodornase liquifics mucleoprotein of dead cells or pus and has no effect on living cells. It is an anti-inflammatory agent, that is, it relieves pain, swelling, tenderness, and erythema, and aids in resolution of extravasated blood.

SPECIAL PRECAUTIONS

• Do not administer in presence of active hemorrhage.

• Initially, localized leukocytosis and accumulation of tissue fluid occur.

• Streptokinase and streptodornase are antigenic, and antienzymes may develop in patients, particularly following prolonged therapy.

ADVERSE EFFECTS

• Pyogenic and allergic reactions have occurred infrequently.

CLINICAL GUIDELINES

ADMINISTRATION:

• Direct effect must be maintained between enzymes and substrate by use of rubber dam, gauze, or nylon dressings.

• If water was a high calcium content, or if solution contains benzyl alcohol, resultant solution may be cloudy.

EFFECTS:

• Treatment should be on an individual basis.

DRUG INTERACTIONS:

• May be mixed with tetracycline, penicillin, streptomycin, or with dihydrostreptomycin.

Antiseptics/Astringents

GENERAL CLINICAL USES

The antiseptics/astringents applied topically are useful for preoperative washing of the skin to reduce bacterial population, to prevent infections of superficial lacerations and abrasions, and to prevent secondary infections of dermatoses.

SPECIFIC PRODUCTS AND DOSAGES

GENERIC NAME	TRADE NAME	USUAL DOSAGE
Iodine Compounds:		
iodine, tincture of iodine, iodoform	(G)*	1 – 3 times daily and before surgery
povidone-iodine	BETADINE Ointment, Solution, Scrub, Aerosol	1 – 3 times daily and before surgery
Mercury Compounds:		
merbromin	MERCUROCHROME	1 – 3 times daily
thimerosal	MERTHIOLATE	1 – 3 times daily
Others:		
alcohol	(G)	1 – 3 times daily
hexachlorophene	PHISOHEX SOY-DOME Medicated Skin Cleanser	Scrub thoroughly as needed

*(G) designates availability as a generic product.

Iodine Compounds

Iodine
Tincture of Iodine
Iodoform
Povidone-Iodine

PHARMACOLOGY

Solutions of iodine and iodine-releasing compounds are used to disinfect the skin. Iodine tincture or solution is highly germicidal. Povidone-iodine kills gram-negative and gram-positive bacteria, viruses, fungi, protozoa, and yeasts. Microbicidal activity of iodine compounds persists in the presence of blood, serum, or pus.

SPECIAL PRECAUTIONS

• Do not use in patients with a history of hypersensitivity to iodine or related compounds.
• Avoid contact with the eyes.

• Fabrics and skin may be stained golden brown.
• If systemic absorption occurs, results of tests for thyroid function may be affected adversely.

ADVERSE EFFECTS

LOCAL EFFECTS: pain, burning, stinging, hypersensitivity rarely
SYSTEMIC EFFECTS: accidental or intentional ingestion is rarely fatal.

CLINICAL GUIDELINES

OVERDOSAGE/ANTIDOTE:
• Fatalities have occurred when 30 to 250 ml of tincture of iodine has been ingested. Symptoms are chiefly gastrointestinal. Reflex vomiting usually occurs.
• Antidotes include a solution of soluble starch, sodium thiosulfate (5% solution), or protein. Lavage stomach to remove all traces of iodine.

Mercury Compounds

Merbromin
Thimerosal

PHARMACOLOGY

Thimerosal and merbromin, organomercurial antiseptics, provide sustained antimicrobial therapy (bacterial and fungi). They are readily soluble in water and miscible with alcohol and soap. They are not inactivated by soaps, cotton, body lipids, and proteins. Their antibacterial activity is reduced by whole blood.

SPECIAL PRECAUTIONS

• Do not use in patients with a history of hypersensitivity to mercurial compounds.
• Avoid prolonged repeated administration in the mouths of infants.
• Allow surface to dry after administration since bandaging the treated area may result in irritation caused by alcohol and acetone.

ADVERSE EFFECTS

SYSTEMIC EFFECTS: in adults, peripheral neuropathy; in children and infants, anorexia and irritability followed by lethagy, vomiting, and seizures

Alcohol

PHARMACOLOGY

The aliphatic alcohols, namely, ethyl alcohol and isopropyl alcohol, are germicidal in varying degrees. Ethyl alcohol coagulates protein and dissolved sebaceous secretions. Isopropyl alcohol also has bactericidal activity which is due to depression of the surface tension of microorganisms. It has greater fat-solvent properties than ethyl alcohol.

SPECIAL PRECAUTIONS

• Avoid contact with the eyes and mucous membranes

ADVERSE EFFECTS

LOCAL EFFECTS: dry skin, and dermatitis rarely
SYSTEMIC EFFECTS: ingestion results in typical alcoholic intoxication and coma.

Hexachlorophene

PHARMACOLOGY

Hexachlorophene is a bacteriostatic agent effective against gram-positive bacteria, including staphylococci. It is insoluble in water. It is prepared as an emulsion with a detergent which provides an efficient cleansing and antiseptic product. A film remains on the skin after scrubbing, providing an antibacterial residue.

SPECIAL PRECAUTIONS

• Keep out of the eyes.
• Do not apply on burned or denuded skin or any mucous membranes; significant absorption may occur.
• Do not use in premature infants.
• Do not use as an occlusive dressing.

ADVERSE EFFECTS

LOCAL EFFECTS: burning, dermatitis, photosensitivity, sensitivity rare
SYSTEMIC EFFECTS: absorption may result in CNS stimulation, irritation, and sometimes convulsions. Ingestion may result in anorexia, vomiting, abdominal cramps, diarrhea, dehydration, convulsions, hypotension, and shock. Death has occurred. Evacuate stomach by lavage or emesis. There is no specific antidote. If marked hypotension occurs, vasopressor therapy is indicated.

Antipruritic/Antihistaminic Agents

GENERAL CLINICAL USES

The antihistamines, tripelennamine hydrochloride, diphenhydramine hydrochloride, and methapyrilene hydrochloride, are applied topically to alleviate temporarily the itching due to minor skin disorders, ivy and oak poisoning, sunburn, insect bites and stings.

Information concerning orally administered antihistamines which effect skin conditions may be found in Chapter 6, page 302.

SPECIFIC PRODUCTS AND DOSAGES

GENERIC NAME	TRADE NAME	USUAL DOSAGE
diphenhydramine HCl	BENADRYL Cream	prn
methapyrilene HCl	SURFADIL* Cream	prn
tripelennamine HCl	PBZ Hydrochloride Cream, Ointment	prn

*Contains more than one active ingredient.

PHARMACOLOGY

The antihistamines, diphenhydramine hydrochloride, methapyrilene hydrochloride, and tripelennamine hydrochloride, are active histamine antagonists. They also have a modest local anesthetic action when applied topically.

SPECIAL PRECAUTIONS
- Do not use in the eyes.
- If condition persists or irritation develops, discontinue use.
- Do not use in patients with a history of hypersensitivity to this drug or related drugs.

Debriding Agents

Dextranomer

GENERAL CLINICAL USES
Dextranomer is used to cleanse secreting wounds such as venous stasis ulcers, decubitus ulcers, infected, traumatic, and surgical wounds, and infected burns.

SPECIFIC PRODUCTS AND DOSAGES

GENERIC NAME	TRADE NAME	ROUTE OF ADMIN.	DOSAGE
dextranomer	DEBRISAN	topical	Cover wound with 3 mm thickness of beads. Bandage lightly. Change dressing od or bid

PHARMACOLOGY
Dextranomer, hydrophilic unsaturated beads, absorbs exudates and particles impeding tissue repair. Concomitantly, inflammation (edema and pain) is reduced. Bacteria and bacterial toxins may also be removed from the surface of the wound. These effects result in a reduction of wound healing time.

SPECIAL PRECAUTIONS
• Treat any underlying condition concurrently.

ADVERSE EFFECTS
LOCAL EFFECTS: pain when wound dressing is changed

CLINICAL GUIDELINES
ADMINISTRATION:
• Use one container for each patient to minimize cross-contamination.
• Do not pack the wound tightly; allow for expansion.
• Cleanse area with sterile fluid and leave area moist. Bandage lightly after applying dextranomer.

EFFECTS:
- Wounds may appear larger initially because of reduction of edema. When dextranomer becomes grayish-yellow, it is saturated and should be removed.

Detergents/Cleansers

GENERAL CLINICAL USES
Detergents and cleansers are indicated for cleansing skin that is sensitive or irritated, or in dermatitis and eczematous conditions.

SPECIFIC PRODUCTS AND DOSAGES

GENERIC NAME	TRADE NAME	USUAL DOSAGE
entsufon sodium	PHISODERM PHISOHEX*	Apply a small amount; lather thoroughly rinse
sodium lauryl sulfate	CETAPHIL* Lotion	Use daily as needed
sodium lauryl sulfoacetate	LOWILA* Cake	Use daily as needed
sodium tetraborate decahydrate	KOMEX* Scrub	Use daily as needed

*Contains more than one active ingredient.

Entsufon Sodium

PHARMACOLOGY
Entsufon sodium is an effective detergent which acts as an emulsifier of all types of oil.

SPECIAL PRECAUTIONS
- Avoid contact with the eyes.
- Discontinue use if irritation or hypersensitivity occurs.

ADVERSE EFFECTS
- If accidentally swallowed, entsufon sodium may cause gastrointestinal irritation.

Sodium Tetraborate Decahydrate

PHARMACOLOGY
Sodium tetraborate decahydrate provides dissolving particles with abradant action; when combined with surface-active

soapless cleansing agents, the dissolving abradant cleanser is useful in reducing the symptoms of acne.

SPECIAL PRECAUTIONS
• Avoid contact with the eyes; if granules get into the eyes, flush thoroughly with water and avoid rubbing the eyes.
• Do not use on inflamed skin.
• If irritation or excessive dryness develops or increases, discontinue use.

ADVERSE EFFECTS
LOCAL EFFECTS: irritation

Sodium Lauryl Sulfoacetate/Sodium Lauryl Sulfate

PHARMACOLOGY
Sodium lauryl sulfoacetate and sodium lauryl sulfate are defatting agents which remove accumulations of sebum from the skin.

SPECIAL PRECAUTIONS
• Avoid contact with the eyes.
• Discontinue use if irritation or hypersensitivity occurs.

ADVERSE EFFECTS
LOCAL EFFECTS: dryness

Photosensitizers (Melanizing Agents)

GENERAL CLINICAL USES
The photosensitizers or melanizing agents induce pigmentation in vitiliginous skin areas.

SPECIFIC PRODUCTS AND DOSAGES

GENERIC NAME	TRADE NAME	ROUTE OF ADMIN.	USUAL DOSAGE
methoxsalen	OXSORALEN	po	30 mg in one dose taken 2–4 hr. before measured exposure to UV; to increase tolerance to sunlight, 20 mg taken 2 hr. before UV exposure. Do not exceed 280 mg
		topical	Cover affected area; rub in well od or bid
trioxsalen	TRISORALEN	po	**Adults and children over 12 yr.:** 10 mg daily 2–4 hrs. before exposure to ultraviolet rays

Methoxsalen
Trioxsalen

PHARMACOLOGY

Methoxsalen and trioxsalen sensitize the skin to ultraviolet light. The exact mechanism of action is unknown. The increased sensitivity appears within 1 hour after oral ingestion. Topical application may be more effective than systemic. The increased skin sensitivity persists for several days.

SPECIAL PRECAUTIONS

- Caution patients to avoid overexposure to ultraviolet light, which may result in severe burns.
- Patients are hypersensitive to sunlight during the first few days of therapy.
- Do not administer to patients with diseases associated with photosensitivity such as porphyria, lupus erythematosus, and xeroderma pigmentosum.
- Do not administer drugs with photosensitizing properties concurrently.
- Do not administer systemically to patients with hepatic insufficiency.

ADVERSE EFFECTS

LOCAL EFFECTS: acute vesicular cutaneous photosensitization, severe erythema, blistering

SYSTEMIC EFFECTS (ORAL ADMINISTRATION):
CNS EFFECTS: nervousness, insomnia, depressed mood
GASTROINTESTINAL EFFECTS: gastric discomfort, nausea

CLINICAL GUIDELINES
ADMINISTRATIONS:
- To minimize gastric effects, the capsule may be taken with milk or a meal.
- Do not increase dosage.
- Caution patients to wear sunglasses during exposure to ultraviolet light.
- Liver function tests should be performed monthly for the first few months and less frequently thereafter.
EFFECTS:
- Reduction in dosage will produce the same therapeutic effects but more slowly.
OVERDOSAGE/ANTIDOTE:
- Overdosage and/or overexposure to ultraviolet light may result in serious burning and blistering.
- Emesis should be encouraged. In addition, the individual should be kept in a darkened room for 8 hours or until cutaneous reactions subside. The treatment for severe reactions resulting from overdosage or overexposure should follow accepted procedures for treatment of any severe burns.

Sunscreens/Sunshades

GENERAL CLINICAL USES
The sunscreens/sunshades protect the skin from the harmful untraviolet rays of the sun.

SPECIFIC PRODUCTS AND DOSAGES

GENERIC NAME	TRADE NAME	USUAL DOSAGE
cinoxate	SUNDARE Clear Lotion, Creamy Lotion	Apply before exposure to sun
digalloyl trioleate	SUNSTICK Lip Protectant	Apply before exposure to sun; repeat as necessary
2-ethoxyethyl p-methoxycinnamate	RV Paque	Apply before exposure to sun
glyceryl PABA	ECLIPSE* Sunscreen Lotion	Apply every 4–6 hr.
menthyl anthranilate	A-FIL Cream	Repeat every 2 hr.
octyl dimethyl PABA	SUNDOWN Sunscreen Lotion ECLIPSE* Sunscreen Lotion	Apply before exposure to sun
para-aminobenzoic acid	RV PABA* Lipstick PABA PABANOL PRESUN Lotion, Gel	Apply liberally before exposure to sun
pentyl p-(dimethylamino)-benzoate	HERPECIN-L* Cold Sore Lip Balm	Apply bid or prn
red petrolatum	RVP	Apply before exposure to sun
sulisobenzone	UVAL Sunscreen Lotion	Apply before exposure to sun; repeat as necessary

*Contains more than one active ingredient.

Cinoxate

PHARMACOLOGY

Cinoxate effectively screens ultraviolet radiation in the 290 to 320 nanometer range, while permitting tanning rays to reach the skin. Consequently, it prevents sunburn and promotes suntan.

SPECIAL PRECAUTIONS
- Avoid contact with the eyes.
- Do not use the clear lotion near open flames.
- Discontinue use if irritation or hypersensitivity occurs.

- Sun sensitive individuals should use caution by limiting early exposure to the sun.

Digalloyl Trioleate

PHARMACOLOGY

Digalloyl trioleate aids in preventing sun sensitivity skin reactions by screening ultraviolet radiation in the 290 to 320 nanometer range.

SPECIAL PRECAUTIONS
- Discontinue use if irritation or hypersensitivity occurs.

2-Ethoxyethyl p-Methoxycinnamate

PHARMACOLOGY

2-Ethoxyethyl p-methoxycinnamate blocks all actinic rays; it prevents sunburning, tanning, and protects the treated area through the visible light range. It may be used adjunctively with depigmenting agents and bleaching agents.

SPECIAL PRECAUTIONS

- Avoid contact with the eyes.
- Discontinue use if irritation or hypersensitivity occurs.

Glyceryl PABA

PHARMACOLOGY

Glyceryl PABA absorbs those rays of the sun which cause sunburn, wrinkling, dryness, and freckling.

SPECIAL PRECAUTIONS

- Transient stinging may occur.
- Discontinue use if irritation or hypersensitivity occurs.
- Avoid contact with the eyes.
- Staining may occur with some fabrics.

ADVERSE EFFECTS

LOCAL EFFECTS: stinging

Menthyl Anthranilate

PHARMACOLOGY

Menthyl anthranilate provides protection from the sun by absorbing more than 95 percent of the erythema causing spectrum of light between 290 and 320 nanometers; maximum absorption occurs at 340 nanometers.

SPECIAL PRECAUTIONS

- Avoid contact with the eyes.
- Discontinue use if irritation or hypersensitivity occurs.

Octyl Dimethyl PABA

PHARMACOLOGY

Octyl dimethyl PABA, formulated in a moisturing lotion, applied topically prior to sun exposure, aids in preventing harmful effects to the skin, drying, freckling, burning, and tanning.

SPECIAL PRECAUTIONS

- Discontinue use if irritation or hypersensitivity occurs.
- Avoid contact with the eyes.
- Slight staining may occur with some fabrics.
- Excessive or too frequent use may cause a film to form which may peel.

Para-aminobenzoic Acid

PHARMACOLOGY

Para-aminobenzoic acid protects the skin from the sun at 290 to 320 nanometers.

SPECIAL PRECAUTIONS

- Avoid contact with the eyes.
- Discontinue use if irritation or hypersensitivity occurs.
- Avoid contact with light colored clothing or upholstery, especially synthetic materials, as staining may occur.

Pentyl p-(dimethylamino)-Benzoate

PHARMACOLOGY

Pentyl p-(dimethylamino)-benzoate is effective in protecting the skin from light in the range of 290 to 320 nanometers.

SPECIAL PRECAUTIONS
- Do not concurrently administer oral or topical corticosteroid therapy to patients with recurrent cold sores, sun and fever blisters.
- Discontinue use if irritation or hypersensitivity occurs.
- Avoid contact with the eyes.

Red Petrolatum

PHARMACOLOGY
Red petrolatum absorbs erthemal spectrum of light through 340 nanometers but allows the tanning rays to pass.

SPECIAL PRECAUTIONS
- Avoid contact with the eyes.
- Discontinue use if irritation or hypersensitivity occurs.

Sulisobenzone

PHARMACOLOGY
Sulisobenzone absorbs ultraviolet radiation in the wave lengths that are most damaging to human skin.

SPECIAL PRECAUTIONS
- Avoid contact with the eyes.
- Discontinue use if irritation or hypersensitivity occurs.

10

Drugs affecting the mouth and teeth

INTRODUCTION

Drugs specific for treating conditions of the mouth and teeth are limited primarily to those for preventing dental caries, the antiseptic mouthwashes, and preparations for relief of pain and inflammation caused by dentures or dental and/or oral cavity surgical procedures. Drugs to treat infectious conditions are included in Chapter 2, *Anti-Infective Agents*. For specific anesthetic products for use in the oral cavity, see Chapter 9, *Drugs Affecting the Skin—Topical (Surface) Anesthetics*

SPECIFIC THERAPEUTIC CLASSIFICATION

Drugs affecting the mouth and teeth include the fluoride preparations for caries prophylaxis, the antiseptic mouthwashes, and the miscellaneous dental products which contain analgesic, anti-inflammatory, and protective agents for treating trauma, denture irritation, or ulcerative lesions and irritations from nonspecific causes.

Anticaries Preparations

GENERAL CLINICAL USES

The fluoride preparations, acidulated phosphate fluoride and sodium fluoride, are used for prophylaxis against dental caries. These compounds may be applied topically or ingested.

SPECIFIC PRODUCTS AND DOSAGES

GENERIC NAME	TRADE NAME	USUAL DOSAGE
accidulated phosphate fluoride	PHOS-FLUR CHEWABLE Tablets PHOS-FLUR Oral Rinse, Supplement THERA-FLUR Gel, Drops	**Children 3 yrs. and older:** 1 mg daily
sodium fluoride	FLUORITAB Tablets, Liquid PEDIAFLOR Drops FLUORIGARD Mouth Rinse LURIDE Drops, Tablets POLY-VI-FLOR* Vitamins, Fluoride Chewable Tablets, Drops	**Children 3–14 yrs.:** 2.2 mg daily if there is no fluoride in the drinking water **Children 2–3 yrs.:** 1.1 mg daily **Children under 2 yrs.:** 0.5 mg daily

*Contains more than one active ingredient.

Acidulated Phosphate Fluoride Sodium Fluoride

PHARMACOLOGY

Fluoride preparations, applied topically or ingested, prevent caries in children. Once the teeth are formed, fluorides have no effect on them. Drinking water may be fluorinated to provide the necessary amount of fluoride for anticaries effect. The mechanism of action remains obscure.

SPECIAL PRECAUTIONS

• Where water with 0.7 ppm of fluoride is used, dietary fluoride should not be used.

ADVERSE EFFECTS

DENTAL EFFECTS: mottling of teeth with excessive dosage

ALLERGIC EFFECTS: rash, idiosyncratic reactions rarely

CLINICAL GUIDELINES

ADMINISTRATION:

• Can be administered in baby formula or any liquid.

• The mouth rinse should not be swallowed; do not eat or drink or rinse the mouth for at least 15 minutes after using fluoride mouth rinse.

EFFECTS:

• Mottled enamel or dental fluorosis is an

indication of excessive intake of fluoride during childhood.

DRUG INTERACTIONS:

• Do not administer other fluoride-containing drugs concomitantly.

OVERDOSAGE/ANTIDOTE:

• Patients ingesting 263 mg of sodium fluoride have not had any adverse effects. Acute overdosage in children may cause excessive salivation and gastrointestinal disturbances. Excessive ingestion of FLUO-RIGARD Mouth Rinse may cause nausea and/or dental fluorosis.

• For adults the lethal dose of soluble fluoride compounds ranges between 2 and 5 grams. The symptoms of fluoride poisoning are nausea, vomiting, hypersalivation, abdominal pain, diarrhea, myalgia, hyperreflexia, tonic and clonic convulsions, paresthesias, and hypotension. Death may occur from cardiac failure or respiratory arrest.

• Treatment consists of administration of a soluble calcium salt such as calcium chloride solution 5% by lavage, intravenous administration of fluids, and if tetany appears, calcium gluconate injection.

Antiseptic Mouthwashes

GENERAL CLINICAL USES

The antiseptic mouthwashes are useful in maintaining oral hygiene and in relieving local soreness and irritation. In addition to antiseptic properties, some products have anesthetic and deodorizing activities.

SPECIFIC PRODUCTS AND DOSAGES

GENERIC NAME	TRADE NAME	USUAL DAILY DOSAGE
cetylpyridinium chloride	CEPACOL Mouthwash	every 2 to 3 hours
methylbenzethonium chloride	DALIDYNE* Lotion	2 to 3 times daily
phenol, sodium phenolate	CHLORASEPTIC* Mouthwash, Gargle	3 to 5 times daily
povidone-iodine	ISODINE Mouthwash, Gargle	2 to 3 times daily

*Contains more than one active ingredient.

Cetylpyridinium Chloride
Methylbenzethonium Chloride
Phenol/Sodium Phenolate
Povidone-Iodine

PHARMACOLOGY

The antiseptic mouthwashes contain one or more antiseptic or germicidal agents. Phenol, sodium phenolate, methyl-benzethonium chloride, povidone-iodine, and cetylpyridinium chloride are antibacterial agents. They lessen mouth odor by controlling the bacterial population.

Methylbenzethonium chloride, a quarternary ammonium compound, is bactericidal to a wide variety of gram positive and gram-negative bacteria. Povidone-iodine is a complex of iodine and polyvinyl-pyrrolidone with antiseptic properties characteristic of those of iodine.

SPECIAL PRECAUTIONS

• Do not use in patients with a history of hypersensitivity to any of these components.

Miscellaneous Dental Products

GENERAL CLINICAL USES

The miscellaneous dental products include products for relief of denture pain and irritation, protective agents, analgesics, and anti-inflammatory agents. Each product will be identified according to approved clinical use.

SPECIFIC PRODUCTS AND USES

TRADE NAME	COMPOSITION	USES
BUTYN METAPHEN	butacaine, nitromerosol chloride	For temporary relief of denture pain; apply thin layer to denture surface.
GLY-OXIDE Liquid	carbamide peroxide; glycerol	For prophylaxis of oral inflammation caused by canker sores, denture irritation, etc; apply qid; may be expectorated or swallowed.
KENALOG IN ORABASE	triamcinolone acetonide in emollient dental paste	For adjunctive treatment and temporary relief of symptoms associated with oral inflammatory lesions and ulcerative lesions resulting from trauma; apply a small dab (1/4 inch) on lesion until a thin film develops; do not rub in.

(continued overleaf)

TRADE NAME	COMPOSITION	USES
ORABASE	gelatin, pectin, sodium carboxy-methylcellulose	Oral protective paste which provides temporary relief and protection of minor irritations of mouth and gums; press small dab on involved area.
ORABASE with benzocaine	gelatin, pectin, sodium carboxy-methylcellulose, benzocaine	Analgesic oral protective paste which provides temporary relief of pain and covering for minor oral irritations; press small dab on individual area.
ORABASE-HCA	gelatin, pectin, sodium carboxy-methylcellulose, hydrocortisone acetate	Oral paste for adjunctive treatment and temporary relief of symptoms associated with ulcerative lesions resulting from trauma and oral inflammatory lesions; dab on lesions until paste adheres.
PROXIGEL	carbamide peroxide	For relief of minor inflammation of gums and other mucosal surfaces of the mouth and lips; apply a small amount qid on affected area.

PHARMACOLOGY

The products used for adjunctive treatment of oral inflammatory and ulcerative lesions are administered topically only. For detailed information on a specific component, please refer to the appropriate section. Information on the anti-inflammatory agents may be found in Chapter 15, page 535; information on topically active anesthetic agents and antiseptics may be found in Chapter 9, pages 410 and 423, respectively; information on anti-infective agents may be found in Chapter 2, page 10.

SPECIAL PRECAUTIONS

• Do not use in patients with a history of hypersensitivity to the components.

• Do not apply BUTYN METAPHEN to open lesions.

• Do not use corticosteroid-containing products (KENALOG in ORABASE, ORABASE HCA) in the presence of fungal, viral, or bacterial infections of the throat or mouth.

• Do not use corticosteroid-containing products in patients with tuberculosis, peptic ulcer, or diabetes mellitus without the advice of the patient's physician.

• In patients receiving topical corticosteroid therapy, it should be noted that the normal defensive responses of the oral tissues are depressed; virulent strains of oral microorganisms may multiply without producing the usual warning symptoms of oral infections.

• Topical use of the corticosteroid-containing products for a long period of time may result in systemic effects.

• Discontinue treatment if irritation or sensitization develops.

• If significant regeneration or repair of oral tissues has not occurred in 7 days, further investigate etiology of the oral lesion.

ADVERSE EFFECTS

• Not established for local use. For systemic effects which might occur if systemic absorption occurs, see appropriate chapter for each component.

Drugs affecting the eye

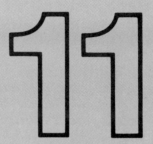

INTRODUCTION

Although many drugs affect the eye, only those products which are used specifically in treating disorders of the eye will be discussed in detail. The majority of drugs, such as the anti-infective agents, because of their broad applicability in therapeutics, have been discussed in other sections and will be appropriately cross-referenced. Because of the specific requirements for ophthalmic use and special formulations that are available, the information about drugs applicable to ophthalmic conditions will be included.

SPECIFIC THERAPEUTIC CLASSIFICATION

Drugs affecting the eye are grouped according to therapeutic or diagnostic activity as follows:
1. Anesthetic agents
2. Anti-infective agents

3. Anti-inflammatory agents
4. Anti-opacity agents
5. Diagnostic agents

6. Miotics/Antiglaucomatous agents
7. Mydriatics/Cycloplegics
8. Zonulytic agents

Local (Surface) Anesthetic Agents

GENERAL CLINICAL USES

Topically applied anesthetic agents for ophthalmic use include benoxinate hydrochloride, proparacaine hydrochloride and tetracaine hydrochloride. These agents are useful for procedures in which a rapid and short-acting anesthetic is indicated such as in tonometry, gonioscopy, removal of corneal foreign bodies, suture removal from the cornea, conjunctival scraping for diagnostic purposes, cataract surgery, and other short corneal and conjunctival procedures.

Lidocaine hydrochloride may be administered by retrobulbar injection for ophthalmic surgery. For information concerning this agent, see Chapter 4, page 164.

SPECIFIC PRODUCTS AND DOSAGES

GENERIC NAME	TRADE NAME	USUAL DOSAGE
Topical Administration: benoxinate HCl	(G)* DORSACAINE	**For deep anesthesia:** 2 drops at 90-second intervals for 3 instillations
proparacaine HCl	(G) ALCAINE 0.5% OPHTHAINE 0.5% OPHTHETIC 0.5%	**For deep anesthesia:** 1–2 drops every 5–10 minutes for 5–7 doses **For removal of sutures and foreign bodies:** 1–2 drops prior to procedure
tetracaine HCl	(G) PONTOCAINE	**For deep anesthesia:** 1–2 drops every 5–10 minutes for 5–7 doses **For removal of sutures and foreign bodies:** 1–2 drops prior to procedure
Retrobulbar Administration: lidocaine HCl	XYLOCAINE HCl 4%	70 kg person—120–200 mg (1.7–3 mg/kg); reduce dosage in children, elderly, and debilitated patients

*(G) designates availability as a generic product.

Topical Anesthetic Agents

Benoxinate HCl
Proparacaine HCl
Tetracaine HCl

PHARMACOLOGY

The local anesthetic agents produce anesthesia by preventing the initiation and transmission of nerve impulses by stabilizing the neural membrane. The local anesthetic agents for ophthalmic use differ primarily in duration of action. Benoxinate produces anesthesia in less than 15 seconds. The duration of action of 1 drop is over 15 minutes. The corneal reflex is fully restored within 1 hour.

Proparacaine produces anesthesia rapidly, in 20 seconds; the duration of this effect is 15 minutes or more. Because its chemical structure differs from the other topical anesthetic agents, cross sensitization is unlikely.

SPECIAL PRECAUTIONS
• Do not use in patients with a history of hypersensitivity to these drugs.
• Prolonged ocular anesthesia may produce permanent corneal opacification with accompanying visual loss.
• Safe use in pregnancy has not been established.
• Repeated use can cause sensitization and local irritation.
• Prolonged ophthalmic use of betacaine sulfate may cause corneal softening.

ADVERSE EFFECTS
LOCAL (OPHTHALMIC) EFFECTS: stinging, burning, conjunctival redness; rare, severe immediate type, apparently hyperallergic corneal reaction with acute, intense, and diffuse epithelial keratitis.

CLINICAL GUIDELINES
ADMINISTRATION:
• Assure that the eye is protected from irritating chemicals, foreign bodies, and rubbing during period of anesthesia.
EFFECTS:
• Blink reflex is temporarily eliminated; protect eye by patching.
DRUG INTERACTIONS:
• Local anesthetics are incompatible with salts of mercury, silver, and other metals.
• Alkalies and antiseptic solutions inactivate most local anesthetics.
OVERDOSAGE/ANTIDOTE:
• With proparacaine hydrochloride, severe systemic reactions from accidental parenteral administration may not occur for approximately 30 minutes after the drug is administered. Hypotension and atrioventricular block which may progress to cardiac and respiratory arrest may occur. Central nervous system effects include tremors, shivering; convulsions may also occur.
• Treat symptomatically and supportively.

Lidocaine Hydrochloride

PHARMACOLOGY
Lidocaine HCl, 4%, administered by retrobulbar injection, exerts its anesthetic activity by preventing the initiation and transmission of nerve impulses. It is metabolized in the liver and excreted by the kidneys. The onset of action is rapid and lasts from 1 to 1.5 hours. For ophthalmic surgery the duration of action may be prolonged by addition of epinephrine.

SPECIAL PRECAUTIONS, ADVERSE EFFECTS, CLINICAL GUIDELINES
For detailed information, see Chapter 4; page 164.

Anti-Infective Agents

GENERAL CLINICAL USES

Anti-infective agents used in ophthalmology may be administered topically, subconjunctively, or systemically. The products for topical administration are formulated to alleviate external bacterial, fungal, protozoan, or viral infections without irritating the eye. The anti-infective agents for subconjunctival and systemic administration are discussed in detail in Chapter 2, page 10.

In selecting an anti-infective agent for ophthalmic use, preference should be given to those drugs that are rarely or never administered systemically to avoid possible sensitization to the more commonly used systemically administered agents.

Subconjunctival administration may be used in combination with topical and/or systemic infections to provide vigorous treatment for serious infections.

Systemic administration of anti-infective agents for ophthalmic infections must be used with the knowledge that most agents do not readily penetrate the eye; large doses must be administered. Chloramphenicol, because of its superior penetration, is frequently the drug of choice in eye infections. Many anti-infective agents not penetrating the normal eye will enter the inflamed eye since the permeability of the blood-aqueous barrier is increased by injury or inflammation.

SPECIFIC PRODUCTS AND DOSAGES

Bacterial sensitivity testing and identification should be performed to determine the causative organism and sensitivity to the appropriate anti-infective agent. For the spectrum of antimicrobial activity see Chapter 2, page 10.

GENERIC NAME	TRADE NAME	ROUTE OF ADMIN.	USUAL DAILY DOSAGE
Bacterial Infections:			
bacitracin	NEOSPORIN*	subconjunct.	**Solution:** 10,000 units in 0.5 ml sodium chloride 1–2 times daily
	NEOSPORIN* Ointment, Solution POLYSPORIN* Ointment	ophth.	**Ointment:** 1–3 times daily
chloramphenicol	(G)† ANTIBIOPTO	ophth.	**Solution:** 2 drops q 3 hr. or more frequently if necessary

*Contains more than one active ingredient.
†(G) designates availability as a generic product.

(continued facing page)

GENERIC NAME	TRADE NAME	ROUTE OF ADMIN.	USUAL DAILY DOSAGE
	Solution, Ointment CHLOROPTIC Solution, Ointment ECONOCHLOR Ointment		**Ointment:** small amount in lower conjunctival sac q 3 hr.
colistin sulfate	COLY-MYCIN S* Ointment, Solution	ophth.	**Ointment:** 1–2 drops q 1–2 hr., a.m. and p.m.
gentamicin sulfate	GARAMYCIN Solution, Ointment	ophth.	**Solution:** 1–2 drops q 4 hr.; in severe infections 2 drops every hr. **Ointment:** a small amount bid or tid
gramicidin	NEOSPORIN* Solution	ophth.	**Solution:** 1–2 drops (0.02–0.04 mg) q 3–4 hr.
lincomycin	LINCOCIN	subconjunct.	**Solution:** 75 mg
neomycin sulfate	NEOSPORIN* Solution, Ointment POLYSPECTRIN* Solution, Ointment STATROL* Solution, Ointment NEO-POLYCIN Solution, Ointment	ophth.	**Solution:** 1–2 drops 4–6 times daily **Ointment:** 1/2 inch tid to qid
oxytetracycline HCl	TERRAMYCIN* with Polymyxin B Sulfate Ointment	ophth.	**Ointment:** 1/2 inch tid or qid
polymyxin B sulfate	AEROSPORIN Solution NEO-POLYCIN* Solution, Ointment NEOSPORIN* Ointment, Solution POLYSPECTRIN* Solution, Ointment STATROL* Solution, Ointment	ophth.	**Solution:** 1 drop (20,000 units/ml) 2–10 times/hr. **Ointment:** small amount in lower conjunctival sac tid to qid
silver nitrate	(G)	ophth.	**Solution:** 2 drops of 1% solution in each eye
sulfacetamide sodium	BLEPHAMIDE S.O.P.* Ointment, Solution CETAMIDE Ointment ISOPTO CETAMIDE Solution METIMYD* Ointment OPTIMYD* Solution SODIUM SULAMYD Solution, Ointment SULFACEL-15* Solution	ophth.	**Solution:** 1–2 drops every 1–2 hr.; increase time intervals as condition responds **Ointment:** apply at night or use during day or before eye is patched

*Contains more than one active ingredient.

(continued overleaf)

GENERIC NAME	TRADE NAME	ROUTE OF ADMIN.	USUAL DAILY DOSAGE
sulfisoxazole	GANTRISIN Solution, Ointment	ophth.	**Solution:** 1–2 drops 3 or more times daily **Ointment:** small amount 1–3 times or more daily
tetracycline HCl	ACHROMYCIN Susp., Ointment	ophth.	**Suspension:** 1–2 drops bid or qid **Ointment:** apply every 2 hr. or more often
Fungal Infections: flucytosine	ANCOBON	po	See Chapter 2, page 67.
natamycin	NATAMYCIN Ophthalmic	ophth.	**Solution:** 1 drop 6–8 times daily
Protozoan Infections: pyrimethamine	DARAPRIM	po	See Chapter 2, pages 81, 84.
Viral Infections: idoxuridine	HERPLEX Solution, S.O.P. Ointment STOXIL Solution, Ointment	ophth.	**Solution:** 1 drop at least every other hour a.m. and p.m. **Ointment:** apply 5 times daily at least
vidarabine monohydrate	VIRA-A Ointment	ophth.	**Ointment:** 1/2 inch 5 times daily at 3-hr. intervals

Drugs for Bacterial Infections

Bacitracin
Chloramphenicol
Colistin Sulfate
Gentamicin Sulfate
Gramicidin
Lincomycin
Neomycin Sulfate
Polymyxin B Sulfate
Sulfacetamide Sodium
Sulfisoxazole
Tetracycline/Oxytetracycline HCl

PHARMACOLOGY, SPECIAL PRECAUTIONS, ADVERSE EFFECTS
For detailed information, see Chapter 2, page 10.

CLINICAL GUIDELINES
ADMINISTRATION:
• Instruct patient to avoid contaminating the applicator tip.
EFFECTS:
• Ointments may retard healing.
• Discontinue use if irritation, hypersensitivity, or bacterial overgrowth occurs; institute appropriate therapy.

Natamycin

PHARMACOLOGY
Natamycin, predominantly a fungicidal compound, produces effective concentrations within the corneal stroma, but not in intraocular fluid. Systemic absorption should not be expected.

SPECIAL PRECAUTIONS
• Do not administer to patients with a history of hypersensitivity to natamycin.

ADVERSE EFFECTS

OPHTHALMIC EFFECTS: conjunctival chemosis and hyperemia (one case)

CLINICAL GUIDELINES

EFFECTS: If improvement does not occur in 7 to 10 days, re-evaluate cause of infection.

Silver Nitrate

PHARMACOLOGY

Silver nitrate ophthalmic solution, used in care of the eyes of newborn babies, prevents ophthalmia neonatorum (gonorrheal conjunctivitis of the newborn). It produces a mild chemical conjunctivitis which should result, when properly performed, in Credé prophylaxis.

SPECIAL PRECAUTIONS

• Do not irrigate eye after instillation of silver nitrate.

ADVERSE EFFECTS

LOCAL EFFECTS: conjunctivitis

Drugs for Viral Infections

Idoxuridine

PHARMACOLOGY

Idoxuridine, applied to the eye, does not penetrate the cornea. It prevents replication of herpes simplex virus. Idoxuridine inhibits enzymes necessary for synthesis of viral DNA.

SPECIAL PRECAUTIONS

• Do not administer to patients with a history of hypersensitivity to idoxuridine.
• Administer with caution to pregnant patients.
• Idoxuridine is not effective in corneal inflammation following herpes simplex keratitis in which the virus is not present.

ADVERSE EFFECTS

OPHTHALMIC EFFECTS: irritation, pain, pruritus, inflammation, edema, photophobia, corneal clouding, stippling, small puncturate effects in the corneal epithelium, rare allergic reactions.

CLINICAL GUIDELINES

ADMINISTRATION:
• If there is no response in 7 or 8 days, consider other therapy.
DRUG INTERACTIONS:
• Do not use boric acid concurrently; irritation may result.
• Antibiotics may be used to control secondary infections.
• Atropine preparations may be used adjunctively.
• Corticosteroids may be used with idoxuridine depending on the judgment of the physician; idoxuridine should be continued for a few days after the steroid has been discontinued.
OVERDOSAGE/ANTIDOTE:
• Although idoxuridine overdosage in the eye is unlikely, if it should occur it may result in small defects in the epithelium of the cornea.
• Accidental ingestion results in no untoward reactions. No treatment is indicated.

Vidarabine Monohydrate

PHARMACOLOGY

Vidarabine has antiviral activity *in vivo* and *in vitro*. It is effective against herpes simplex, types 1 and 2, varicella-zoster, and vaccinia viruses. The mechanism of action has not been established. Vidarabine is rapidly deaminated in the gastrointestinal tract.

SPECIAL PRECAUTIONS

• Do not use in patients with a history of hypersensitivity to vidarabine.

- Do not exceed the recommended frequency and duration of treatment.
- Safe use in pregnancy and lactation has not been established.

ADVERSE EFFECTS

OPHTHALMIC EFFECTS: lacrimation, foreign body sensation, conjunctival injection, burning, irritation, superficial punctate keratitis, pain, photophobia, punctal occlusion, sensitivity

CLINICAL GUIDELINES

ADMINISTRATION:
- May produce a temporary visual haze.

DRUG INTERACTIONS:
- The following drugs have been topically administered concurrently with vidarabine: gentamicin, erythromycin, chloramphenicol, prednisone, and dexamethasone.

OVERDOSAGE/ANTIDOTE:
- Acute massive overdosage by oral ingestion has not occurred. Overdosage by ocular instillation is unlikely because any excess should be quickly expelled from the conjunctival sac.
- No untoward effects should result from ingestion of an entire tube because of the rapid deamination in the gastrointestinal tract.

Anti-Inflammatory Agents

GENERAL CLINICAL USES

The anti-inflammatory corticosteroids (glucocorticoids) are used to treat steroid responsive inflammatory conditions of the palpebral and bulbar conjunctiva, cornea, and anterior segment of the globe, such as allergic conjunctivitis, acne rosacea, superficial punctuate keratitis, herpes zoster keratitis, iritis, cyclitis, selected infective conjunctivitis, and in corneal injuries. The corticosteroids are more effective in acute than in chronic conditions.

Certain products contain, in addition to the corticosteroids, antimicrobial agents such as sulfonamides, polymyxin B sulfate, bacitracin, and/or neomycin. The majority of the combination products have been evaluated by the U.S. Food and Drug Administration as "possibly" effective. This classification requires the manufacturer to conduct further investigations to establish the role of these products in therapeutics.

SPECIFIC PRODUCTS AND DOSAGES

GENERIC NAME	TRADE NAME	USUAL DAILY DOSAGE
dexamethasone	MAXIDEX 0.1% MAXITROL Ophth. Ointment/ Susp.	**Solution:** 1–2 drops every 0.5–1 hr.; reduce to every 2–4 hr. **Ointment:** small amount tid to qid

(continued facing page)

GENERIC NAME	TRADE NAME	USUAL DAILY DOSAGE
dexamethasone sodium phosphate	DECADRON Phosphate	**Solution:** 1–2 drops every hr. during day and every 2 hr. at night **Ointment:** thin coating tid or qid; reduce as condition indicates
fluorometholone	FML LIQUIFILM	**Solution:** 1–2 drops bid to qid
hydrocortisone	CORTISPORIN*	**Ointment:** small amount every 3–4 hr.
medrysone	HMS LIQUIFILM	**Solution:** 1 drop every 4 hr.
prednisolone acetate	CETAPRED* METIMYD* PRED FORTE 1%	**Solution:** 2–3 drops every 1–2 hr.; less often at night **Ointment:** thin film 3–4 times a day and at night
prednisolone sodium phosphate	HYDELTRASOL INFLAMASE METRETON* OPTIMYD*	**Solution:** 1–2 drops every hr. during day and every 2 hr. at night; reduce dosage as condition indicates **Ointment:** thin coating tid to qid

*Contains more than one active ingredient.

Dexamethasone
Dexamethasone Sodium Phosphate
Fluorometholone
Hydrocortisone
Medrysone
Prednisolone Acetate
Prednisolone Sodium Phosphate

PHARMACOLOGY

The anti-inflammatory corticosteroids (glucocorticoids) inhibit the inflammatory response to mechanical, chemical, or immunological stimuli. The exact mechanism of action is unknown. For additional information, in particular pertaining to systemic administration, see Chapter 15, page 535.

SPECIAL PRECAUTIONS

• The corticosteroids are contraindicated in acute superficial herpes simplex keratitis, fungal diseases of ocular structures, vaccinia, varicella, and most other viral diseases of the cornea and conjunctiva, and in tuberculosis of the eye.

• Do not use in patients with a history of hypersensitivity to these agents.

• When treating stromal herpes simplex, use extreme caution; frequent use of slit-lamp microscopy is manditory.

• Prolonged use may result in glaucoma, damage to the optic nerve, defects in visual acuity and fields of vision, or posterior subcapsular cataract formation, or may aid in the establishment of secondary ocular infections from pathogens liberated from ocular tissues.

• Use of topical steroids in these conditions may cause thinning of the cornea or sclera which may result in perforation.

• Acute purulent infections of the eye may be masked or activity enhanced by the presence of steroid medications.

• Safety of intensive or protracted use of topical steroids during pregnancy has not been substantiated.

• Fungal infections of the cornea are prone to develop coincidentally with long-term local steroid use.

ADVERSE EFFECTS

LOCAL (OPHTHALMIC) EFFECTS: with topical use, glaucoma with optic nerve damage, visual acuity and field defects, posterior subcapsular cataract formation, secondary ocular infection from pathogens including herpes simplex liberated from ocular tissues, perforation of the globe, exacerbation of viral and fungal infections of the cornea,

stinging or buring rarely, lacrimation, mydriasis, loss of accommodation, ptosis; with subconjunctival administration, pain, ulceration, granulomatous formation.

CLINICAL GUIDELINES

ADMINISTRATION:

• Caution and instruct patients to avoid contaminating applicator and/or medication.

EFFECTS:

• Check intraocular pressure frequently since prolonged use may result in glaucoma.

• Watch for signs of fungal infection such as persistent ulceration.

Antiopacity Agents

GENERAL CLINICAL USES

Abortion or suppression of the formation of opacities of the lens has been accomplished by local application of a lymphagogue. Opacities well advanced as characteristic in senility have responded less favorably to treatment than those in the eye with metabolic functions less impaired.

SPECIFIC PRODUCTS AND DOSAGES

GENERIC NAME	TRADE NAME	USUAL DAILY DOSAGE
senecio cineraria compound solution	SUCCUS CINERARIA MARITIMA (SCM-WALKER)	Instill in the affected eye, 2 drops morning and evening

Senecio Cineraria Compound

PHARMACOLOGY

Senecio cineraria compound solution, a senecio alkaloid, is formulated as an ophthalmic solution which stimulates circulation in and around the eye. Opacities have been checked or aborted, particularly in patients with minimally deteriorated metabolic functions.

SPECIAL PRECAUTIONS

• Do not use in patients with a history of hypersensitivity to any of the senecio alkaloids or to hamamelis vulgaris (witch hazel).

• Patients with a history of allergy are more likely to experience sensitivity reactions than other patients.
• If excessive irritation occurs, discontinue treatment.
• Do not use in patients with glaucoma.

ADVERSE EFFECTS
LOCAL (OPHTHALMIC) EFFECTS: irritation

CLINICAL GUIDELINES
ADMINISTRATION:
• Caution patients not to contaminate solution by touching tip of dropper to any surface.

Diagnostic Agents

GENERAL CLINICAL USES
Fluorescein sodium is administered intravenously in retinal angiography to distinguish between viable and nonviable tissue, malignant and nonmalignant tissue, and to determine the vascular circulatory relationship. The fluorescein strips are used for staining the anterior segment of the eye when fitting contact lenses, in disclosing corneal injury, and in applanation tonometry.

SPECIFIC PRODUCTS AND DOSAGES

GENERIC NAME	TRADE NAME	ROUTE OF ADMIN.	USUAL DOSAGE
fluorescein sodium	FLUORESCITE Inj. 10% FLURESS* Solution FUL-GLO Strips	iv topical	**Adults:** 500 mg (3–5 ml) **Children:** 35 mg/10 lb body wt **Solution:** 1–3 drops placed in the conjunctival sac **Strips:** moisten with sterile water. Touch conjunctiva or fornix with moistened tip. Closing the eyelid distributes the stain.

*Contains more than one active ingredient.

Fluorescein Sodium

PHARMACOLOGY

Fluorescein sodium has a yellowish-green fluorescence which demarcates the vascular area under observation, distinguishing it from adjacent area. It is administered intravenously and also topically in combination with a local anesthetic or as sodium fluorescein strips. When administered intravenously, the fluorescein sodium should appear in the central retinal artery in 11 to 13 seconds.

SPECIAL PRECAUTIONS

• Do not use in patients with a history of hypersensitivity to fluorescein sodium or related compounds.
• Use cautiously in patients with a history of allergies, asthma, or hypersensitivity.

ADVERSE EFFECTS

CNS EFFECTS: headache, syncope, pyrexia
RESPIRATORY EFFECTS: transient dyspnea
CARDIOVASCULAR EFFECTS: cardiac arrest, basilary artery ischemia, thrombophlebitis at injection site, severe
URINARY TRACT EFFECTS: urine is bright yellow and fluoresces for 24 to 36 hours after administration.
GASTROINTESTINAL EFFECTS: with intravenous administration, nausea, vomiting, strong taste, gastrointestinal distress
ALLERGIC EFFECTS: urticaria, pruritus, angioneurotic edema
DERMATOLOGIC EFFECTS: temporary yellowish skin discoloration

CLINICAL GUIDELINES

ADMINISTRATION:
• Administer a small test dose prior to the diagnostic injection.
• Warn patient that skin will be discolored yellowish and urine will be bright yellow and fluoresce for 24 to 36 hours.
EFFECTS:
• In 9 to 14 seconds, luminescence appears in the retinal and choroidal vessels.
• Fluorescein is an intense fluorescent green in a more alkaline medium such as the aqueous humor.
DRUG INTERACTIONS:
• Fluorescein detoxifies the aniline dye in indelible pencil when accidently placed in the eye. The aniline dye may cause edema and necrosis of ocular tissue which may result in loss of vision.
• The usual preservatives used in ophthalmic preparations may be inactivated by fluorescein.
OVERDOSAGE/ANTIDOTE:
• Up to 1250 mg have been well tolerated in adults.
• For emergency use, intravenous epinephrine 1:1000 should be available at the time of administration. An antihistamine should also be available. There is no specific antidote.

Miotics/Antiglaucomatous Agents

GENERAL CLINCIAL USES

The miotics and other antiglaucomatous agents are used primarily to treat glaucoma but are used also in accomocative estropia or convergent strabismus. The miotics may be used to prevent the iris from moving into the surgical incision after intraocular surgery.

SPECIFIC PRODUCTS AND DOSAGES

GENERIC NAME	TRADE NAME	USUAL DOSAGE
Parasympathomimetic Agents: acetylcholine chloride	MIOCHOL*	**Intraocular:** 0.5–1 ml into anterior chamber **Topical:** 1–2 drops bid to tid
carbachol	CARBACEL ISOPTO CARBACHOL	**Intraocular:** 0.5 ml into anterior chamber **Topical:** 1–2 drops bid to tid
demecarium bromide	HUMORSOL	**Topical:** 1–2 drops weekly to bid as needed
echothiophate iodide	PHOSPHOLINE	**Topical:** 1–2 drops bid
isoflurophate	FLOROPRYL	**Topical:** 1/4 inch ointment tid to bid
physostigmine	ESERINE ISOPTO ESERINE MIOCEL*	**Topical:** apply small quantity of ointment in lower lid **Topical:** 1–2 drops bid to tid
pilocarpine hydrochloride	(G)† ADSORBOCARPINE MI-PILO MISTURA P	**Topical:** 1—2 drops bid or tid; may be increased up to 6 times daily **Topical:** Apply small quantity of ointment in lower lid
pilocarpine nitrate	P-V CARPINE PILOFRIN	**Topical:** 1–2 drops bid to qid
pilocarpine ocular therapeutic system	OCUSERT PILO-20 OCUSERT PILO-40	20 mcg/hr. for 1 week—one application 40 mcg/hr. for 1 week—one application
Carbonic Anhydrase inhibitors: acetazolamide	(G) DIAMOX HYDRAZOL	250 mg to 1 gm po daily in divided doses; **Maximum:** 1 gm/day
dichlorphenamide	DARANIDE	100–200 mg po; then 100 mg bid; maintenance dose 25–50 mg od to tid
ethoxzolamide	ETHAMIDE	62.5–250 mg po bid to qid
methazolamide	NEPTAZANE*	50–100 mg po bid or tid
Sympathomimetic Agents: epinephrine HCl	(G) EPIFRIN	1 drop od to qid

*Contains more than one active ingredient.
†(G) designates availability as a generic product.

(continued overleaf)

GENERIC NAME	TRADE NAME	USUAL DOSAGE
epinephrine bitartrate	E-CARPINE* EPITRATE MYTRATE	1–2 drops bid; more frequently if necessary
epinephrine HCl	(G) GLAUCON	1 drop od at bedtime or bid
epinephryl borate	EPINAL	1 drop od to bid
hydroxyamphetamine hydrobromide	PAREDRINE	1–2 drops into conjunctival sac
Osmotic Agents: glycerin 50%	OSMOGLYN 50%	1–1.5 gm/kg po 1–1.5 hr. prior to surgery
mannitol	(G)	1.5–2.0 gm/kg as 20% solution or 25% solution administered iv over 30 min. or less; administer 1–1.5 hr. before surgery
urea	UREAPHIL	Slow iv infusion, 60 drops/min; do not exceed 120 gm/day; **adult:** 1–1.5 gm/kg; **children:** 0.5–1.5 gm/kg; **young children:** less
Beta Blocking Agent: timolol maleate	TIMOPTIC	1 drop in each eye bid; increase if necessary

*Contains more than one active ingredient.

Parasympathomimetic Agents

Acetylcholine Chloride
Carbachol
Demecarium Bromide
Echothiophate Iodide
Isoflurophate
Physostigmine
Pilocarpine

PHARMACOLOGY

Acetylcholine chloride, carbachol, and pilocarpine, parasympathomimetic agents, produce miosis by activating the neuron and affecting the iris spincter.

The duration of action of acetylcoholine is short. Carbachol produces rapid and prolonged miosis. In contrast to acetylcholine chloride, it is not destroyed by cholinesterase. Carbachol stimulates the motor end plate of the muscle cell and partially inhibits the action of cholinesterase. When administered intraocularly, maximal miosis usually occurs within 2 to 5 minutes. Administered topically, it is slightly more potent than pilocarpine but does not penetrate the eye as well.

Pilocarpine, the most important miotic agent is use, produces miosis by affecting the ciliary muscle. It acts directly on parasympathetic end organs, improving the outflow facility in patients with open-angle glaucoma. After topical application of pilocarpine, miosis begins in 15 to 30 minutes and lasts 4 to 8 hours. Maximal reduction of intraocular pressure occurs in 75 minutes. The rate of production of aqueous humor is not affected.

Demecarium bromide, echothiophate iodide, isoflurophate, and physostigmine, cholinesterase inhibitors with sustained activity, act mainly on erythrocytic cholinesterase. Ethothiophate iodide also depresses plasma cholinesterase.

Topical application of demecarium bromide to the eye produces intense miosis and ciliary muscle contraction accompanied by increased permeability of the ciliary body and iris, increased permeability of the blood-aqueous barrier, and vasodilation. Maximal reduction of intraocular pressure occurs in 2 to 4 hours and the effect lasts for 9 or more days.

Echothiophate iodide also enhances the effect of endogenously liberate acetylcholine on the iris, ciliary muscle, and other parasympathetically innervated structures of the eye, causing miosis, increasing the outflow of aqueous humor and decreasing the intraocular pressure and potentiating accommodation. After a single application, the intraocular pressure is reduced maximally in 24 hours and the effect may persist for as long as 4 days.

Isoflurophate, a long-acting miotic agent, reduces the intraocular pressure maximally within 24 hours; reduction persists for as long as 1 week.

Physostigmine provides rapid and intense miosis which occurs in about 3 to 4 minutes. A maximal effect is noted within 30 minutes. The duration of action may range from 12 to 36 hours.

SPECIAL PRECAUTIONS
• Do not use in patients with corneal injury, with a history of hypersensitivity of any of these compounds, or with active uveal inflammation.

• Administer cautiously after any procedure that reduces the epithelial barrier of the cornea and conjunctiva, such as instrumental tonometry or topical anesthesia.
• Administer with caution to patients with bronchial asthma since these drugs have bronchoconstrictor activity.
• Administer with extreme caution to patients with myasthenia gravis who are receiving systemic anticholinesterase therapy.
• Use cholinesterase inhibitors with great caution, if at all, in patients with a history of retinal detachment.
• Safe use in pregnancy has not been established.
• Warn patients who are receiving cholinesterase inhibitors that exposure to organophosphate-type insecticides and pesticides may cause added systemic effects.
• Use with extreme caution in patients with marked vagotonia, bronchial asthma, spastic gastrointestinal disturbances, peptic ulcer, pronounced bradycardia and hypotension, recent myocardial infarction, epilepsy, parkinsonism, and other disorders that may respond adversely to vagotonic effects.
• Use extreme caution prior to intraocular surgery because of the possibility of hyphema.

ADVERSE EFFECTS
LOCAL (OPHTHALMIC) EFFECTS: stinging, burning, lacrimation, lid muscle twitching, conjunctival and ciliary redness, brow ache, headache, induced myopia with visual blurring; activation of latent iritis or uveitis; retinal detachment; iris cysts occurring more frequently in children than adults; conjunctival thickening and obstruction of nasolacrimal canals, lens opacites; with physostigmine, hyperreactivity of pupil and accommodative reflexes

SYSTEMIC EFFECTS: salivation, nausea, abdominal cramps, vomiting, diarrhea, incontinence (urinary), dyspnea, bradycardia, cardiac irregularities

CLINICAL GUIDELINES

ADMINISTRATION:
- Gonioscopy should be performed prior to administration.
- Do not allow tip of applicator to become contaminated by touching the eyelid or other moist surfaces since isoflurophate is rapidly hydrolyzed by water.
- Keep tube tightly closed.
- Apply at night before retiring to lessen visual blurring.
- Wash hands immediately after administration.
- Keep frequency of use at a minimum in all patients, particularly children, to reduce the chance of iris cysts developing.
- Compress lacrimal sac during and following instillation for 1 to 2 minutes to minimize drainage into the nasal chambers, which have extensive absorptive surfaces.

DRUG INTERACTIONS:
- Administer succinylcholine with extreme caution before or during general anesthesia to patients receiving cholinesterase inhibitors because of possible respiratory and cardiovascular collapse.
- See Special Precautions for concurrent use of organophosphate insecticides and pesticides.

OVERDOSAGE/ANTIDOTE:
- If accidentally ingested or if topical overdosage occurs, atropine sufate, 0.4 to 0.6 ng, for adults, should be administered parenterally (intravenously if necessary); reduce dosage for children. Pralidoxime chloride (PROTOPAM Chloride) has been used in addition to (not as a substitute for) atropine sulfate in treating the systemic effects due to cholinesterase inhibitors.

Carbonic Anhydrase Inhibitors

Acetazolamide
Dichlorphenamide
Ethoxzolamide
Methazolamide

PHARMACOLOGY

Acetazolamide is a potent carbonic anhydrase inhibitor which, administered orally in ophthalmologic use, is effective in controlling fluid secretion of aqueous humor and results in a decrease in intraocular pressure. It is a nonbactericidal sulfonamide which is distinctly different pharmacologically from the bacteriostatic sulfonamides. Also, its use as a diuretic agent is discussed in Chapter 5, page 253.

Dichlorphenamide is a carbonic anhydrase inhibitor which reduces intraocular pressure by partially suppressing the secretion of aqueous humor (inflow); the mechanism of action if not fully understood. After oral administration, dichlorphenamide acts within 1 hour and has a maximal effect in 2 to 4 hours. The intraocular tension may be lowered for approximately 6 to 12 hours.

Ethoxzolamide, a carbonic anhydrase inhibitor, reduces intraocular pressure by partially suppressing the secretion of aqueous humor. It is absorbed rapidly following oral administration, and the effects last about 8 hours.

Methazolamide, a sulfonamide derivative and a potent carbonic anhydrase inhibitor, is absorbed somewhat slowly from the intestinal tract and disappears more slowly from the plasma than does acetazolamide. The onset of action and duration of activity are delayed in comparison with acetazolamide.

SPECIAL PRECAUTIONS
- Do not use in patients with severe or absolute glaucoma and chronic noncon-

gestive angle-closure glaucoma, adrenocortical insufficiency, hepatic insufficiency, renal insufficiency, or an electrolyte imbalance state such as hyperchloremic acidosis or sodium and potassium depletion states, or with a history of hypersensitivity to these drugs.
• Safe use in pregnancy has not been established.
• Use with caution in patients with hepatic cirrhosis and in those in whom advanced pulmonary disease may have impaired respiratory capacities and also elevated pCO_2 values.

ADVERSE EFFECTS
CNS EFFECTS: headache, weakness, nervousness, globus hystericus, sedation, lassitude, depression, confusion, disorientation, dizziness, ataxia, tremor, paresthesias of the hands, feet, and tongue
URINARY TRACT EFFECTS: frequency, colic, calculi
GASTROINTESTINAL EFFECTS: anorexia, nausea, vomiting, constipation
METABOLIC AND ENDOCRINE EFFECTS: loss of weight
HEMATOLOGIC EFFECTS: leukopenia, agranulocytosis, thrombocytopenia
DERMATOLOGIC EFFECTS: eruptions, and pruritus
OTIC EFFECTS: tinnitus

CLINICAL GUIDELINES
ADMINISTRATION:
• Supplement diet with foods high in potassium to avoid hypokalemia.
• Adverse reactions common to all sulfonamide derivatives may occur with acetazolamide and methazolamide. See Chapter 5 for detailed information.
EFFECTS:
• Acidotic state may be corrected by administration of bicarbonate.
• Signs of hypokalemia may be noted.

DRUG INTERACTIONS:
• When administered with miotics such as carbachol, demecarium bromide, isoflurophate, physostigmine, or pilocarpine, best results may be obtained.
• May be used with other miotics and osmotic agents to reduce intraocular tension rapidly.
OVERDOSAGE/ANTIDOTE:
• Overdosage is characterized by an exaggeration of the adverse effects.
• There is no specific antidote. Treat supportively.

Sympathomimetic Agents

Epinephrine
Epinephrine Bitartrate
Epinephrine HCl
Epinephryl Borate

PHARMACOLOGY
Epinephrine and related compounds are sympathomimetic drugs which act on both alpha and beta receptors to produce dilation of pupils and enhance outflow of aqueous humor, thereby reducing intraocular pressure. The formation of aqueous humor is decreased and vasoconstriction is also produced. For additional information, see Chapter 6, page 321.

SPECIAL PRECAUTIONS
• Do not use in patients with a history of hypersensitivity to epinephrine and related compounds; with narrow-angle (congestive) glaucoma, shock, during anesthesia with halogenated hydrocarbons or cyclopropane, and also in individuals with organic brain damage.
• Safe use in pregnancy has not been established.

- Administer cautiously to elderly patients, those with cardiovascular disease, in psychoneurotic individuals, to pregnant patients, and to patients with long-standing bronchial asthma and emphysema who may also have developed cardiovascular damage.

ADVERSE EFFECTS

CNS EFFECTS: anxiety, headache, fear, trembling
CARDIOVASCULAR EFFECTS: palpitations, tachycardia, extrasystoles
AUTONOMIC EFFECTS: perspiration
LOCAL EFFECTS: necrosis at injection site; conjunctival pigmentation, blurred vision, eye ache or pain, lacrimation
ALLERGIC EFFECTS: contact dermatitis, allergic lid reaction, conjunctivitis

CLINICAL GUIDELINES

ADMINISTRATION:
- Protect from exposure to light.
- Discard solution if it is brown or contains a precipitate.
- Advise patient to avoid contamination of applicator tip.

EFFECTS:
- "Epinephrine-fastness" can occur with prolonged use.

DRUG INTERACTIONS:
- Epinephrine has been used in combination with pilocarpine and other miotics.
- Administration during anesthesia with halogenated hydrocarbons or cyclopropane is contraindicated.
- Do not administer concurrently with excessive doses of digitalis, mercurial diuretics or other drugs that sensitize the heart to arrhythmias.
- Epinephrine is destroyed readily by alkalies and oxidizing agents such as oxygen, chlorine, bromine, iodine, permanganates, chromates, nitrates, and salts of easily reducible metals, especially iron.

- The effects may be potentiated by tricyclic antidepressants and by certain antihistamines, e.g., diphenhydramine, tripelennamine, d-chlorpheniramine, and sodium l-thyroxine.

OVERDOSAGE/ANTIDOTE:
- Overdosage or inadvertent intravenous administration may cause cardiovascular hemorrhage resulting in hypertension. Fatalities may result from pulmonary edema because of the cardiovascular effects.
- Rapidly acting vasodilators such as nitrites, or alpha blocking agents, may counteract the marked pressor effects of epinephrine and related compounds.

Hydroxyamphetamine Hydrobromide

PHARMACOLOGY

Hydroxyamphetamine hydrobromide dilates the pupil, probably by stimulation of the dilator muscles of the iris. The maximal effect is produced in 45 to 60 minutes; recovery is complete in about 6 hours.

SPECIAL PRECAUTIONS

- Do not use in patients with narrow-angle glaucoma.
- Use with caution in patients with hypertension, hyperthyroidism, and diabetes.

ADVERSE EFFECTS

LOCAL (OPHTHALMIC) EFFECTS: increased intraocular pressure, photophobia, blurred vision.

CLINICAL GUIDELINES

ADMINISTRATION:
- Avoid contamination of applicator tip.

DRUG INTERACTIONS:
- Hydroxyamphetamine hydrobromine has been administered concomitantly with homatropine.

OVERDOSAGE/ANTIDOTE:
- Topical overdosage is characterized by dilation of the pupils. Accidental ingestion may cause hypertension, palpitation, cardiac arrhythmias, substernal discomfort, headache, sweating, nausea, vomiting, and gastrointestinal irritation.
- There is no specific antidote. Topical overdosage may be treated with pilocarpine 1%.

Osmotic Agents

Glycerin

PHARMACOLOGY
Glycerin 50%, a hypertonic solution for oral administration, is useful in reducing intraocular pressure. An immediate decrease in intraocular pressure is measured, with the maximal reduction occurring in 1 hour. It is often used in patients who do not respond to miotics and carbonic anhydrase inhibitors.

SPECIAL PRECAUTIONS
- Do not use in patients with a history of hypersensitivity to glycerin or related compounds.
- Administer cautiously in senile, diabetic, or severely dehydrated patients.

ADVERSE EFFECTS
CNS EFFECTS: headache
GASTROINTESTINAL EFFECTS: nausea, vomiting, diarrhea
METABOLIC AND ENDOCRINE EFFECTS: hyperglycemia, glycosuria

CLINICAL GUIDELINES
ADMINISTRATION:
- Administer orally to avoid the hazards of intravenous administration.

- May be used prior to surgery performed under local anesthesia.

DRUG INTERACTIONS:
- Has been used with miotics and carbonic anhydrase inhibitors.

Mannitol
Urea

PHARMACOLOGY, SPECIAL PRECAUTIONS, ADVERSE EFFECTS, CLINICAL GUIDELINES
For detailed information, see the discussion of diuretic agents in Chapter 5, page 249.

Beta Blocking Agent

Timolol Maleate

PHARMACOLOGY
Timolol maleate is a general beta adrenergic receptor blocking agent. When applied topically to the eye it acts to reduce elevated as well as normal intraocular pressure with little or no effect on pupil size or visual acuity due to increased accommodation.

Reduction in intraocular pressure can usually be detected within 30 minutes after administration.

SPECIAL PRECAUTIONS
- Do not use in patients hypersensitive to timolol maleate.
- Use with caution in patients with bronchial asthma; sinus bradycardia and greater than first degree block; cardiogenic shock; heart failure; and in patients concomitantly receiving adrenergic-augmenting psychotropic drugs.
- Efficacy in patients with narrow-angle

or angle-closure glaucoma has not been established.

• Safe use in pregnancy and in children has not been established.

ADVERSE EFFECTS
CARDIOVASCULAR EFFECTS: slight reduction in resting heart rate
LOCAL EFFECTS: irritation, hypersensitivity

CLINICAL GUIDELINES
ADMINISTRATION:
• Monitor pulse rates in patients with history of severe cardiac disease.
DRUG INTERACTIONS:
• Patients who are receiving beta adrenergic blocking agents orally along with timolol maleate should be observed for additive effects.

Mydriatic and Cycloplegic Agents

GENERAL CLINICAL USES
The anticholinergic and adrenergic agents applied topically to the eye produce mydriasis and cycloplegia for refraction, or for iris dilation and relaxation of the ciliary muscle in acute inflammatory conditions of the anterior uveal tract.

SPECIFIC PRODUCTS AND DOSAGES

GENERIC NAME	TRADE NAME	USUAL DOSAGE
atropine sulfate	(G)* BUF OPTO ISOPTO ATROPINE	**Solution:** 1–2 drops up to tid **Ointment:** small amount od to bid
cyclopentolate HCl	(G) CYCLOGYL	**Solution:** adults—1 drop; 2nd drop in 5 min.; children—1 drop; 2nd drop in 10 min.
homatropine hydrobromide	HOMATROCEL ISOPTO HOMATROPINE	**Solution:** 1–2 drops; repeat as necessary
scopolamine hydrobromide	(G) ISOPTO HYOSCINE	**Solution:** 1–2 drops
tropicamide	MYDRIACYL	**Solution:** 1–2 drops; repeat in 5 min.

*(G) designates availability as a generic product.

Anticholinergic Agents

Atropine Sulfate
Cyclopentolate HCl
Homatropine Hydrobromide
Scopolamine Hydrobromide
Tropicamide

PHARMACOLOGY

Atropine sulfate, cyclopentolate hydrochloride, homatropine hydrobromide, scopolamine hydrobromide, and tropicamide produce mydriasis and cycloplegia by blocking cholinergic stimulation of the sphincter muscle of the iris and the ciliary muscle of the lens.

Atropine sulfate has a slow onset of action but the action may persist for 6 days.

Homatropine hydrobromide also has a slow onset of action but a maximal effect is reached in approximately 60 minutes and the effects last for 36 to 48 hours.

Cyclopentolate hydrochloride acts rapidly but has a shorter duration of action than atropine. Cycloplegia continues for 25 to 75 minutes; recovery is complete in 6 to 24 hours.

Scopolamine hydrobromide has cycloplegic effects comparable to those of atropine but its duration of action is shorter.

Tropicamide acts rapidly and the duration of activity is relatively short, 20 to 35 minutes.

SPECIAL PRECAUTIONS

• Do not use in patients with glaucoma or predisposition to narrow-angle glaucoma, or with a history of hypersensitivity to these compounds.

• Safe use in pregnancy has not been established.
• Use cautiously in the elderly and others who have increased intraocular pressure.

ADVERSE EFFECTS

LOCAL (OPHTHALMIC) EFFECTS: irritation, congestion, hyperemia, edema, follicular conjunctivitis, dermatitis; with cyclopentolate HCl and tropicamide, increased intraocular pressure, transient stinging, blurred vision, photophobia

SYSTEMIC EFFECTS: dry mouth and skin, flushing, fever, rash, thirst, tachycardia, confusion, somnolence, hallucinations, delirium; with cyclopentolate HCl and tropicamide, psychotic reactions and behavioral disturbances may occur in children especially with 2% solution; ataxia, incoherent speech, restlessness, hallucinations, disorientation as to time and place, failure to recognize people, tachycardia

CLINICAL GUIDELINES

ADMINISTRATION:
• Tonometric examination is advised prior to treatment.
• Minimize systemic absorption by gentle compression of the lacrimal sac for a minute or two after instillation.

EFFECTS:
• Discontinue if irritation or sensitization occurs.
• Systemic effects may occur, particularly in children and elderly patients.

OVERDOSAGE/ANTIDOTE:
• Overdosage may produce peripheral symptoms of atropine poisoning. Exaggeration of the adverse effects is noted.
• Treat symptomatically and supportively.

Zonulytic Agents

GENERAL CLINICAL USES
Zonulytic agents are useful in intracapsular lens extraction. Chymotrypsin is the only enzymed marketed for this purpose.

SPECIFIC PRODUCTS AND DOSAGES

GENERIC NAME	TRADE NAME	USUAL DOSAGE
chymotrypsin	ALPHA CHYMAR CATARASE ZOLYSE	Irrigate posterior chamber using 2 ml or more, approximately one half at 3 o'clock and the remainder at 9 o'clock positions.

Chymotrypsin

PHARMACOLOGY
Chymotrypsin is a proteolytic enzyme obtained from the pancreas. Its enzymatic action causes dissolution of zonular fibers attached to the lens.

SPECIAL PRECAUTIONS
• Do not use in patients with high vitreous pressure and a gaping incisional wound.
• Do not use in patients with congenital cataracts.
• Do not use in patients under 20 years of age.
• Do not use in patients with a history of hypersensitivity to chymotrypsin or related compounds.
• Note that the enzyme is extremely toxic to the retina and should not be allowed to penetrate into the vitreous, as posterior diffusion could occur.

ADVERSE EFFECTS
LOCAL (OPHTHALMIC) EFFECTS: transient increase in intraocular pressure, moderate uveitis, corneal edema, striation, delay of healing of incisions

CLINICAL GUIDELINES
ADMINISTRATION:
• Do not use the reconstituted solution if it is cloudy or contains a precipitate.
• Do not autoclave the powder or the reconstituted solution.
• After use discard any unused portion, including the diluent.
• All instruments and syringes used must be free of enzyme-inactivation alcohol and other chemicals.
EFFECTS:
• The transient glaucoma which frequently occurs lasts about 1 week.
• Pilocarpine may be useful in reducing the intraocular pressure.

Drugs affecting the ear

12

INTRODUCTION

The various pathologic conditions of the external and middle ear may be treated by medications administered topically or systemically. Only topically administered medications will be included herein; systemically administered medications, such as the anti-infective agents, are discussed in the appropriate chapter, e.g., Chapter 2, *Anti-infective Agents*, page 10.

SPECIFIC THERAPEUTIC
CLASSIFICATION

Drugs affecting the ear are grouped into five categories: analgesics and anesthetics, anti-infective agents, anti-inflammatory agents, ceruminolytic agents, and irrigating solutions. Since the anti-infective agents are discussed in detail in Chapter 2, the specific products formulated for treating otic infections topically will be listed here, and only information related to this use will be included. Similarly, the anti-inflammatory agents, discussed in detail in Chapter 15, *Endocrine and Other Drugs Affecting Metabolism*, page 535, will be listed and discussed only in relation to topical treatment of pathology of the ear.

Analgesics/Anesthetics for Otic Use

GENERAL CLINICAL USES
Various local (surface) anesthetic agents, namely, benzocaine, dibucaine hydrochloride, and lidocaine, are used alone or, frequently, in combination with anti-infective and/or anti-inflammatory agents for relief of pain and pruritus in acute congestive and serous otitis media, otitis externa, and acute swimmer's ear.

SPECIFIC PRODUCTS AND DOSAGES

GENERIC NAME	TRADE NAME	USUAL DOSAGE
benzocaine	AMERICAINE* AURALGAN OTIC* MYRINGACAINE* TYMPAGESIC*	**Adults and children:** fill ear canal and plug with cotton, qid
dibucaine hydrochloride	OTOCORT*	**Adults and children:** 3–5 drops tid or qid
lidocaine hydrochloride	LIDOSPORIN*	**Adults:** 3–4 drops tid or qid **Infants and children:** 2–3 drops tid or qid

*Contains more than one active ingredient.

Benzocaine

PHARMACOLOGY
Benzocaine is a local anesthetic agent which is poorly soluble in water and therefore is absorbed slowly.

For additional information see *Chapter 9*, page 410.

SPECIAL PRECAUTIONS
• Do not use in patients with a history of hypersensitivity to benzocaine or related compounds.
• Do not use in infants under one year of age.
• Discontinue if sensitivity or irritation occurs.
• Indiscriminate use of anesthetic ear-

drops may mask symptoms of fulminating infections of the middle ear.
• Do not use in patients with a perforated eardrum.

ADVERSE EFFECTS
• Although adverse effects have not been established for the otic formulation of benzocaine, those effects occurring with other formulations, namely, dermatitis and sensitivity reactions, might also occur with the otic formulation.

CLINICAL GUIDELINES
ADMINISTRATION:
• Avoid touching the ear with the dropper; do not rinse dropper after use.
• Cleanse the ear prior to administration.

Dibucaine Hydrochloride

PHARMACOLOGY
Dibucaine hydrochloride produces local anesthesia when applied topically. It is a quinoline derivative and the most potent and longest acting of the commonly employed local anesthetics.

For additional information, see Chapter 9, *Drugs Affecting the Skin*, page 410.

SPECIAL PRECAUTIONS
• Avoid prolonged use.
• Do not use in patients with a history of hypersensitivity to dibucaine hydrochloride and related compounds.
• If irritation develops, discontinue use immediately.
• Indiscriminate use of anesthetic eardrops may mask the symptoms of fulminating infections of the middle ear.

• Do not use in patients with a perforated eardrum.

CLINICAL GUIDELINES
ADMINISTRATION:
• Avoid touching the ear with the dropper; do not rinse dropper after use.
• Cleanse the ear prior to administration.
DRUG INTERACTIONS:
• Formulated in combination with polymyxin B, neomycin sulfate, and hydrocortisone.

Lidocaine Hydrochloride

PHARMACOLOGY
Lidocaine, a topically effective analgesic agent, relieves the pain often associated with otitis externa by preventing the initiation and transmission of nerve impulses. It stabilizes the neural membrane.

For additional information, see Chapter 9, *Drugs Affecting the Skin*, page 410.

SPECIAL PRECAUTIONS
• Do not use in patients with a history of hypersensitivity to lidocaine or related compounds.
• Indiscriminate use of anesthetic eardrops may mask symptoms of fulminating infections of the middle ear.
• Do not use in patients with a perforated eardrum.

ADVERSE EFFECTS
• Not established.

CLINICAL GUIDELINES
ADMINISTRATION:
• Warm solution to body temperature; avoid overheating.
• Avoid touching the ear with the dropper; do not rinse the dropper after use.
• Cleanse the ear prior to administration.

EFFECTS:
• In combination with antibiotics, prolonged use may result in overgrowth of nonsusceptible organisms.

DRUG INTERACTIONS:
• Lidocaine is used in combination with polymyxin B and other topically applied antibiotics.

Anti-Infective Agents

GENERAL CLINICAL USES
Infections of the external ear caused by bacteria and/or fungi are treated with anti-infective agents applied topically. Since these infections are frequently caused by more than one organism, products are available containing more than one anti-infective agent. The organisms causing otic infections most commonly are *Pseudomonas, Proteus, Staphylococcus aureus*, and *Candida* species.

The antibacterial and antifungal agents usually used include acetic acid, chloramphenicol, colistin, neomycin, nystatin, and polymyxin B.

SPECIFIC PRODUCTS AND DOSAGES

GENERIC NAME	TRADE NAME	USUAL DOSAGE
acetic acid	(G)† VOSOL* VOLSOL* HCl	**Adults and children:** 5 drops tid or qid
chloramphenicol	CHLOROMYCETIN	**Adults and children:** 2–3 drops tid
colistin sulfate	COLY-MYCIN S* with neomycin and hydrocortisone	**Adults:** 4 drops tid or qid **Infants and children:** 3 drops tid or qid
neomycin sulfate	COLY-MYCIN S* NEO-CORTEF* NEO-MEDROL* OTOBIONE*	**Adults and children:** 3–4 drops tid or qid
nystatin	FLOROTIC*	2–3 drops tid or qid
polymyxin B sulfate	AEROSPORIN* CORTISPORIN* LIDOSPORIN*	**Adults and children:** 3–4 drops tid or qid

*Contains more than one active ingredient.
†(G) designates availability as a generic product.

Acetic Acid
Chloramphenicol
Colistin
Neomycin
Nystatin
Polymixin B

PHARMACOLOGY

The anti-infective agents used in local treatment of infections of the ear are those commonly applied topically for dermatologic infections. Frequently the anti-infective agents are combined with local anesthetic and/or anti-inflammatory agents.

The antibacterial agents, polymyxin B sulfate, colistin sulfate, neomycin, and chloramphenicol are effective when applied topically against a wide range of gram-negative and gram-positive bacteria. These agents are administered systemically infrequently, therefore if sensitization or resistance develops, it does not jeopardize therapy in life-threatening infections.

The antifungal agents, nystatin and acetic acid, are usually used in combination with antibacterial and/or anti-inflammatory agents for *Candida* infections.

For additional information, see Chapter 2, page 10.

SPECIAL PRECAUTIONS

• Prolonged or repeated use may result in overgrowth of nonsusceptible organisms.
• Do not use in patients with a history of hypersensitivity to any of the components.
• Use with care in patients with perforated eardrum because of possible systemic absorption and ototoxicity (neomycin).

ADVERSE EFFECTS

LOCAL EFFECTS: not established
SYSTEMIC EFFECTS: see Chapter 2, *Anti-Infective Agents*, for specific information concerning each drug.

CLINICAL GUIDELINES

ADMINISTRATION:
• Warm before administering; avoid overheating; if overheated, antibiotic potency may be lost.
• Ear should be cleansed thoroughly and dried prior to administration of medication.
• Avoid contamination of dropper or solution.
• Instill when affected ear is turned upwards; maintain this position for a few minutes after instillation.
EFFECTS:
• Watch for signs of overgrowth of nonsusceptible organisms, including fungi.

Anti-Inflammatory Agents

GENERAL CLINICAL USES

Inflammation and pruritus usually accompany infections and other disorders of the external and middle ear. The corticosteroids applied topically have been used to alleviate these symptoms.

SPECIFIC PRODUCTS AND DOSAGES

GENERIC NAME	TRADE NAME	USUAL DOSAGE
dexamethasone	DECADRON	3 or 4 drops bid or tid
hydrocortisone	AURAL ACUTE* CORTISPORIN* OTOCORT*	**Adults:** 4 drops tid or qid **Infants and children:** 3 drops tid or qid
hydrocortisone acetate	COLY-MYCIN S* NEO-CORTEF*	**Adults:** 4 drops tid or qid
prednisolone acetate	NEO-DELTA-CORTEF*	**Adults:** 4 drops tid or qid

*Contains more than one active ingredient.

PHARMACOLOGY, SPECIAL
PRECAUTIONS, ADVERSE EFFECTS,
CLINICAL GUIDELINES
For detailed information see Chapter 15, *Endocrine and Other Drugs Affecting Metabolism*, page 535, and Chapter 9, *Drugs Affecting the Skin*, page 420.

Ceruminolytic Agents

GENERAL CLINICAL USES
Glands in the outer third of the ear produce cerumen which is hydroscopic and bacteriostatic. Accumulation of large amounts of cerumen may interfere with hearing and visualization of the eardrum. The ceruminolytic agents aid in removal of cerumen. There are no drugs marketed which either retard or stimulate production of cerumen.

SPECIFIC PRODUCTS AND DOSAGES

GENERIC NAME	TRADE NAME	USUAL DOSAGE
carbamide peroxide	DEBROX	Administer 5 to 10 drops twice daily for 3 to 4 days; remove wax by irrigating with warm water.
triethanolamine polypeptide oleate-condensate	CERUMENEX	Fill ear canal with medication with patients head held at 45° angle. Insert cotton plug and wait 15 to 20 minutes. Then gently flush ear with lukewarm water. Repeat if necessary.

Carbamide Peroxide

PHARMACOLOGY

Carbamide peroxide, formulated in anhydrous glycerol for application to the ear canal, penetrates and softens cerumen, thereby facilitating its removal.

SPECIAL PRECAUTIONS

• Do not use in patients with a history of hypersensitivity to carbamide peroxide or related compounds.
• Do not use in patients with knowledge or suspicion of a perforated eardrum.

ADVERSE EFFECTS

LOCAL EFFECTS: redness, irritation

CLINICAL GUIDELINES

ADMINISTRATION:
• Residual cerumen may be removed by gentle irrigation with warm water.
EFFECTS:
• Carbamide peroxide may be used prophylactically.

Triethanolamine Polypeptide Oleate-Condensate

PHARMACOLOGY

Triethanolamine polypeptide oleate-condensate emulsifies and disperses excess or impacted ear wax, facilitating its removal. It is an aqueous miscible solution with low surface tension; the solution is slightly acidic, which is similar to the surface of the normal ear canal.

SPECIAL PRECAUTIONS

• Do not use in patients with a history of hypersensitivity to this product or in patients with a positive patch test to it.
• Do not use in patients with knowledge or suspicion of a perforated eardrum.
• Use with extreme caution if at all in patients with otitis media.
• Use with extreme caution in patients with demonstrable dermatologic idiosyncrasies or with a history of allergic reactions in general.
• Do not expose the ear canal to this medication for over 15 to 30 minutes.

ADVERSE EFFECTS

LOCAL EFFECTS: dermatitis ranging from a very mild erythema and pruritus to a severe eczematoid reaction.

CLINICAL GUIDELINES

ADMINISTRATION:

• Instruct patients not to exceed the time of exposure, nor to use the medication more frequently than directed by the physician.

• Avoid undue exposure to the periaural skin during instillation and the flushing out of the medication.

• Advise patients to discontinue medication if an adverse reaction occurs.

EFFECTS:

• If medication comes in contact with the skin, wash area with soap and water to avoid irritation or possible dermatitis.

Irrigating Solutions

GENERAL CLINICAL USES

For topical therapy to be effective, it is necessary to maintain a clean, dry ear canal. Desquamated material, cerumen, purulent material, or residual medications should be removed prior to application of a specific medication. The irrigating solutions aid in cleansing the ear canal and aid in acidification; acidification of the canal aids in restoring normal flora.

SPECIFIC PRODUCTS AND DOSAGES

GENERIC NAME	TRADE NAME	USUAL DOSAGE
acetic acid 2%	(G)* DOMEBORO otic	4 to 6 drops every 2 to 3 hrs.
aluminum acetate solution (Burow's solution)	BURO-SOL BUROWETS	2 to 4 drops every 2 to 3 hrs.
hydrogen peroxide	(G)	4 to 6 drops every 2 to 3 hrs.

*(G) designates availability as a generic product.

Acetic Acid Solution 2%
Aluminum Acetate Solution

PHARMACOLOGY

Acetic acid solution and aluminum acetate solution (modified Burow's) restore the normal acidic pH to the ear canal. These solutions also suppress bacterial growth and multiplication.

SPECIAL PRECAUTIONS

• If undue irritation or sensitivity develops, discontinue treatment.
• Store at room temperature (59°–86°F).
• Do not use in patients with a perforated eardrum.

CLINICAL GUIDELINES
ADMINISTRATION:
• Warm solution prior to use.

Hydrogen Peroxide

PHARMACOLOGY

Hydrogen peroxide, a very unstable compound, rapidly breaks down, releasing nascent oxygen, which has germicidal action and also aids in removal of tissue debris from inaccessible regions.

SPECIAL PRECAUTIONS

• Do not use in patients with a perforated eardrum.

Drugs affecting the musculoskeletal system

INTRODUCTION

Disorders of the musculoskeletal system amenable to drug therapy include acute and chronic rheumatic conditions, spastic disorders, infections, inflammations resulting from trauma or degenerative processes, parkinsonism, and drug-induced extrapyramidal disorders. Although few of the drugs available have a "curative" effect, they usually reduce the inflammation and pain, and may slow the progress of the condition.

SPECIFIC THERAPEUTIC CLASSIFICATION

Drugs affecting the musculoskeletal system are classified as follows:
1. Antiarthritic agents: gold compounds and nonsteroidal anti-inflammatory agents
2. Antigout/uricosuric agents

3. Anti-inflammatory agents: steroid and salicylates (nonsteroids)
4. Skeletal muscle relaxants: curarelike preparations, centrally acting muscle relaxants, dantrolene sodium
5. Skeletal muscle stimulants

Analgesic agents frequently used in orthopedic conditions are reviewed in Chapter 4, *Drugs Affecting the Brain and Spinal Cord,* page 127.

Anti-infective agents used for treating infections of the musculoskeletal system are reviewed in Chapter 2, *Anti-Infective Agents,* page 10.

Information concerning products for treating metabolic conditions which have a direct effect on the musculoskeletal system such as paget's disease (osteitis deformans) can be found in Chapter 15, *Endocrine and Other Drugs Affecting Metabolism,* page 532.

Antiarthritic Agents

GENERAL CLINICAL USES

In general, the antiarthritic agents are used to relieve the symptoms of arthritis; there is no known drug to cure the disease. Aurothioglucose and other gold compounds are indicated for use in treating active rheumatoid arthritis in adults and children. Fenoprofen sodium, ibuprofen, indomethacin, naproxyn, sulindac and tolmetin sodium are useful in the relief of the signs and symptoms of rheumatoid arthritis and osteoarthritis, including treatment of acute flares and in the long-term management of the diseases.

Phenylbutazone and oxyphenbutazone afford relief in rheumatoid arthritis, rheumatoid spondylitis, gout, osteoarthritis, psoriatic arthritis, acute superficial thrombophlebitis, painful shoulder (peritendinitis, capsulitis, bursitis, and acute arthritis of that joint).

Sulindac is also indicated for acute or long term use for the relief of signs and symptoms of osteoarthritis, rheumatoid arthritis, ankylosing spondylitis, acute painful shoulder, and acute gouty arthritis.

Hydroxychloroquine sulfate is indicated for the treatment of rheumatoid arthritis and of discoid and systemic lupus erythematosus. It is also indicated for suppressive treatment of acute attacks of malaria.

Penicillamine is indicated in the treatment of patients with severe, active rheumatoid arthritis who have failed to respond to an adequate trial of conventional therapy.

SPECIFIC PRODUCTS AND DOSAGES

GENERIC NAME	TRADE NAME	ROUTE OF ADMIN.	USUAL DOSAGE	
			ADULTS	CHILDREN
Gold Preparations: aurothioglucose	SOLGANAL	im	10–50 mg/week maximum: 0.8–1 gm (total dose)	1/4 adult dose
gold sodium thiomalate	MYOCHRYSINE	im	10–50 mg/week	**Under 12 yrs.:** 25 mg single dose
gold thiosulfate with sodium thiosulfate	(G)†	im	25 mg/week, maximal total dose 1000 mg	Not established
Antiarthritic Preparations: fenoprofen calcium	NALFON	po	300–600 mg qid; maximum 3200 mg/day	Not established
ibuprofen	MOTRIN	po	300–600 mg tid or qid; maximum 2400 mg/day	Not established
indomethacin	INDOCIN	po	25–50 mg bid or tid; maximum 200 mg/day	Not established
naproxen	NAPROSYN	po	250 mg od to bid; maximum 750 mg/day	Not established
oxyphenbutazone	OXALID TANDEARIL	po	100–600 mg/day divided in 3–4 equal doses	Not established
phenylbutazone	AZOLID BUTAZOLIDIN STERAZOLIDIN*	po	100–600 mg/day divided in 3–4 equal doses	Not established
sulindac	CLINORIL	po	150–200 mg bid	Not established
tolmetin sodium	TOLECTIN	po	400 mg tid; maximum 2000 mg/day	**2 yrs. and over:** 20 mg/kg/day divided in 3–4 doses; maximum 30 mg/kg/day
Others: hydroxychloroquine sulfate	PLAQUENIL Sulfate	po	**Initial:** 400–600 mg/day in divided doses **Maintenance:** 200–400 mg/ day in divided doses	Not established
penicillamine	CUPRIMINE DEPEN	po	**Initial:** 125–250 mg increased by 125–250 mg/day at 1–3-month intervals; maximum: 1500 mg/day **Maintenance:** individualize; 500–750 mg/day may be adequate	Not established

*Contains more than one active ingredient.
†(G) designates availability as a generic product.

Gold Preparations

Aurothioglucose
Gold Sodium Thiomalate
Gold Thiosulfate with Sodium
   Thiosulfate

PHARMACOLOGY

Gold preparations, when administered intramuscularly, are gradually absorbed and produce prolonged therapeutic effects. The exact mechanism of action is unknown. They are excreted primarily by the kidney. These preparations appear to have a suppressive effect on the synovitis of rheumatoid arthritis.

SPECIAL PRECAUTIONS

• Do not use in patients with severe diabetes, renal disease, hepatitis, marked hypertension, heart failure, a history of agranulocytosis and hemorrhagic diathesis, or in pregnant patients.
• Patients with blood dyscrasias or those who have recently had radiation should not receive aurothioglucose.
• Do not use in patients with urticaria, eczema, or colitis.
• Use with extreme caution in patients with allergy or hypersensitivity, skin rash, previous kidney or liver disease, compromised cerebral or cardiovascular circulation.

ADVERSE EFFECTS

CNS EFFECTS: headache
RESPIRATORY EFFECTS: inflammation of the upper respiratory tract
GASTROINTESTINAL EFFECTS: diarrhea, and colic
HEPATIC EFFECTS: toxic hepatitis, acute yellow atrophy, jaundice
HEMATOLOGIC EFFECTS: rarely aplastic anemia, hemorrhagic diathesis, thrombocytopenia, agranulocytosis, eosinophilia, leukopenia
DERMATOLOGIC EFFECTS: dermatitis, pruritus, erythema, stomatitis, vaginitis

CLINICAL GUIDELINES
ADMINISTRATION:
• Perform urine examination and complete blood count every 2 weeks throughout treatment period.
• Inquire about occurrence of pruritus, sore mouth, or indigestion each time before treatment.
• Never administer intravenously.
• Protect from light.
• Needle and syringe must be dry.
• Shake thoroughly and warm to body temperature before administration.
EFFECTS:
• Gold is poorly tolerated by aged patients.
• If toxic effects occur, interrupt treatment immediately.
DRUG INTERACTIONS:
• Do not administer concomitantly with antimalarials, immune suppressants, phenylbutazone or oxyphenbutazone because of their potential for causing blood dyscrasias.
OVERDOSAGE/ANTIDOTE:
• Overdosage or toxicity is characterized by severe dermatitis (papular, vesicular, and exfoliative), stomatitis, and jaundice.
• Glucocorticoids (systemic) may be used to treat severe dermatitis or stomatitis, or for renal, hematologic, or most other adverse effects. Treatment may be required for many months. Severe reactions to gold may be treated with dimercaprol. Start therapy at first signs of severe untoward reaction. Dimercaprol promotes the excretion of gold. For detailed information see Chapter 20, page 692.

Fenoprofen Calcium

PHARMACOLOGY

Fenoprofen calcium is a nonsteroidal anti-inflammatory antiarthritic agent. The mode of action is unknown. It is rapidly absorbed following oral administration and is excreted in the urine as the glucuronide.

SPECIAL PRECAUTIONS

• Do not use in Functional Class IV (incapacitated, largely or wholly bedridden or confined to a wheelchair; little or no self-help) rheumatoid arthritis patients.
• Safety and effectiveness for children has not been established.
• Do not use in patients with a history of hypersensitivity to fenoprofen calcium.
• Because the potential exists for cross sensitivity to aspirin and other nonsteroidal anti-inflammatory drugs, fenoprofen calcium should not be given to patients in whom such drugs induce the symptoms of asthma, rhinitis, or urticaria.
• Give under close supervision to patients with a history of upper gastrointestinal tract disease; gastrointestinal bleeding, sometimes severe, has occurred.
• Do not use in patients with active peptic ulcer.
• Do not use in patients with significantly impaired renal function.
• Safe use in pregnancy and lactation has not been established.
• Use with caution in patients with compromised cardiac function.

ADVERSE EFFECTS

CNS EFFECTS: somnolence, dizziness, tremor, confusion, insomnia, headache, nervousness, fatigue, malaise
RESPIRATORY EFFECTS: dyspnea
CARDIOVASCULAR EFFECTS: palpitations, tachycardia
URINARY TRACT EFFECTS: dysuria
AUTONOMIC EFFECTS: increased sweating
GASTROINTESTINAL EFFECTS: dyspepsia, constipation, nausea, vomiting, abdominal pain, anorexia, occult blood in stool, diarrhea, flatulence, dry mouth, peptic ulcer and/or gastrointestinal hemorrhage (3 cases)

METABOLIC AND ENDOCRINE EFFECTS: peripheral edema
HEPATIC EFFECTS: increased alkaline phosphatase, LDH, and SGOT
HEMATOLOGIC EFFECTS: anemia
DERMATOLOGIC EFFECTS: pruritus, rash, urticaria
OPHTHALMIC EFFECTS blurred vision
OTIC EFFECTS: tinnitus, decreased hearing

CLINICAL GUIDELINES

ADMINISTRATION:
• Monitor hemoglobin level periodically.
• Since food decreases blood levels of fenoprofen, the drug should be given 30 minutes before or 2 hours after meals.
• During prolonged treatment, monitor hearing by auditory tests.
• Periodic liver function tests should be performed.
EFFECTS:
• With single doses of fenoprofen there is less suppression of collagen-induced platelet aggregation than with aspirin.
• Fenoprofen decreases platelet aggregation and prolongs bleeding time.
• Caution should be exercised by patients whose activities require alertness if they experience central nervous system side effects with fenoprofen.
DRUG INTERACTIONS:
• The potential exists for cross sensitivity between aspirin and other nonsteroidal anti-inflammatory agents, and fenoprofen.
• Coadministration of aspirin decreases the biologic half-life of fenoprofen because of an increase in metabolic clearance which results in a greater amount of hydroxylated fenoprofen in the urine; the clinical significance is unknown.
• Chronic administration of phenobarbital may be associated with a decrease in plasma half-life of fenoprofen; clinical significance is unknown.
• When phenobarbital is added or with-

drawn, dosage adjustment of fenoprofen may be required.

• Concomitant administration of antacids (aluminum and magnesium hydroxide) does not interfere with absorption of fenoprofen.

• Food ingestion decreases the rate and extent of absorption of fenoprofen.

• In patients receiving coumarin-type anticoagulants, the addition of fenoprofen to therapy could prolong the prothrombin time.

• In patients receiving fenoprofen and steroids concomitantly, any reduction in steroid dosage should be gradual to avoid the possible complications of sudden steroid withdrawal.

OVERDOSAGE/ANTIDOTE:

• Overdosage is characterized by an exaggeration of the adverse effects.

• There is no specific antidote. Empty stomach by vomiting or lavage. Supportive therapy should be used as needed. Since fenoprofen is acidic and is excreted in the urine, it may be beneficial to administer an alkali and induce diuresis.

• Furosemide (LASIX) does not lower blood levels.

Ibuprofen

PHARMACOLOGY

Ibuprofen, a nonsteroidal anti-inflammatory agent, possesses analgesic and antipyretic activities. Its mode of action is unknown. It does not alter the course of the underlying disease. Following oral administration it is absorbed rapidly; peak blood levels are reached in 1 hour; maximal clinical benefits may not occur until 1 to 2 weeks after initiation of therapy. Ibuprofen is excreted primarily in the urine. It has not been detected in the milk of lactating mothers.

SPECIAL PRECAUTIONS

• Do not use in Functional Class IV (incapacitated, largely or wholly bedridden or confined to a wheelchair; little or no self-care) rheumatoid arthritis patients.

• Do not use in children, in patients with a history of hypersensitivity to ibuprofen, or in individuals with the syndrome of nasal polyps, angioedema, and bronchospastic reactivity to aspirin or other nonsteroidal anti-inflammatory agents.

• Anaphylactoid reactions have occurred in patients with known aspirin hypersensitivity.

• Give under close supervision to patients with a history of upper gastrointestinal tract disease.

• Use with caution in patients with a history of cardiac decompensation because of fluid retention and edema.

• Use with caution in patients with intrinsic coagulation defects and those on anticoagulant therapy because ibuprofen has been shown to prolong bleeding time.

• Safe use in pregnancy and in nursing mothers has not been established.

ADVERSE EFFECTS

CNS EFFECTS: dizziness, headache, nervousness, depression, insomnia

CARDIOVASCULAR EFFECTS: congestive heart failure in patients with marginal cardiac function, elevated blood pressure

GASTROINTESTINAL EFFECTS: nausea, epigastric pain, heartburn, diarrhea, abdominal distress, nausea, vomiting, indigestion, constipation, abdominal cramps or pain, bloating, flatulence, gastric or duodenal ulcer with bleeding and/or perforation, gastric hemorrhage, melena

METABOLIC AND ENDOCRINE EFFECTS: decreased appetite, edema, fluid retention

HEMATOLOGIC EFFECTS: leukopenia, decreased hemoglobin and hematocrit

DERMATOLOGIC EFFECTS: rash (including

maculopapular type), pruritus, vesicul-obullous eruptions, urticaria, erythema multiforme

OPHTHALMIC EFFECTS: amblyopia, blurred and/or diminished vision, scotomata and/or changes in color vision

OTIC EFFECTS: tinnitus

CLINICAL GUIDELINES

ADMINISTRATION:
• Administer with meals or milk to minimize gastrointestinal complaints.
• Advise patient to report signs and symptoms of gastrointestinal ulceration or bleeding, blurred vision or other eye symptoms, skin rash, weight gain or edema.
• Patients with rheumatoid arthritis seem to require higher doses than patients with osteoarthritis.

EFFECTS:
• A therapeutic response is sometimes seen in a few days to a week but most often is observed by 2 weeks.
• If the patient develops blurred and/or diminished vision, scotomata, and/or changes in color vision, discontinue drug; patient should have complete ophthalmologic examination.

DRUG INTERACTIONS:
• May be used in combination with gold salts and/or corticosteroids.
• When ibuprofen and other nonsteroidal anti-inflammatory agents are administered to patients on coumarin-type anticoagulants, bleeding has been reported.
• When administered concurrently with aspirin, the effectiveness of aspirin is nullified.

OVERDOSAGE/ANTIDOTE:
• Overdosage (8000 mg) of ibuprofen in an adult has caused dizziness or nystagmus. After hospitalization, parenteral hydration, and bed rest, the patient recovered with no reported sequelae. In a child, apnea and cyanosis occurred.

• The stomach should be emptied by lavage or vomiting; little or no drug will likely be recovered if more than 1 hour has elapsed since ingestion. Because the drug is acidic and is excreted in the urine, it is theoretically beneficial to administer an alkali and induce diuresis.

Indomethacin

PHARMACOLOGY

Indomethacin is a potent, nonsteroidal drug with anti-inflammatory, antipyretic, and analgesic properties. The mode of action is unknown. After oral administration, indomethacin is promptly absorbed. Peak plasma levels are reached within 2 hours and excretion is primarily by way of the kidneys. Indomethacin crosses the placental barrier.

SPECIAL PRECAUTIONS

• Do not use in Functional Class IV (incapacitated, largely or wholly bedridden or confined to a wheelchair; little or no self-care) rheumatoid arthritis patients.
• Do not use in children 14 years of age and younger.
• Do not use in pregnant women and nursing mothers.
• Do not use in patients with active gastrointestinal lesions or a history of recurrent lesions.
• Do not use in patients allergic to aspirin or indomethacin.
• Gastrointestinal reactions, at times severe, may occur; be alert for any sign or symptom signaling possible gastrointestinal reaction.
• Use with great caution in elderly patients; adverse reactions appear to increase with age.
• With prolonged therapy watch for possible ocular effects: corneal deposits and reti-

nal disturbances including those of the macula.

• Use with caution since indomethacin may aggravate psychiatric disturbances, epilepsy, and parkinsonism; if severe central nervous system effects develop, discontinue drug.

ADVERSE EFFECTS

CNS EFFECTS: psychotic episodes, depersonalization, depression, mental confusion, coma, convulsions, peripheral neuropathy, drowsiness, light headedness, dizziness, syncope, headache

CARDIOVASCULAR EFFECTS: hypotension, epistaxis

URINARY TRACT EFFECTS: hematuria

GASTROINTESTINAL EFFECTS: ulcerations including perforation and hemorrhage of esophagus, stomach, duodenum or small intestines; gastrointestinal bleeding, perforation of pre-existing sigmoid lesions, increased abdominal pain in ulcerative colitis; ulcerative colitis, regional ileitis rarely; gastritis, nausea, vomiting, anorexia, epigastric distress, abdominal pain, diarrhea, ulcerative stomatitis

METABOLIC AND ENDOCRINE EFFECTS: edema, vaginal bleeding, hyperglycemia, glyosuria

HEPATIC EFFECTS: toxic hepatitis, jaundice rarely

HEMATOLOGIC EFFECTS: aplastic anemia, hemolytic anemia, bone marrow depression, agranulocytosis, leukopenia, thrombocytopenic purpura rarely

ALLERGIC EFFECTS: acute respiratory distress including dyspnea and asthma, angiitis, urticaria, angioedema, skin rash, and purpura

DERMATOLOGIC EFFECTS: alopecia, erythema nodosum

OPHTHALMIC EFFECTS: corneal deposits, retinal disturbances including those of the macula, blurred vision

OTIC EFFECTS: deafness rarely; hearing disturbances; tinnitus

CLINICAL GUIDELINES

ADMINISTRATION:

• The gastrointestinal effects may be reduced by giving the drug immediately after meals, with food, or with antacids.

EFFECTS:

• Adverse effects appear to correlate with the size of the dose.

• Existing psychiatric disturbances may be aggravated.

• Maximal benefits usually occur within 3 to 4 weeks.

DRUG INTERACTIONS:

• When given to patients receiving probenecid, the plasma levels of indomethacin are likely to be increased.

• Aspirin may interfere with the absorption of indomethacin if administered simultaneously.

• Effects of coumarin-type anticoagulants may be increased.

• Concomitant administration of cortisone-related drugs may result in the enhancement of gastrointestinal disturbances; dosage adjustment may be required.

• Concurrent administration of thyroid preparations may increase the risk of adverse effects on the cardiovascular system.

OVERDOSAGE/ANTIDOTE:

• Overdosage is characterized by an exaggeration of the adverse effects, namely, nausea, vomiting, diarrhea, confusion, and agitation. Symptoms may progress with larger doses to convulsions, coma, hemorrhage from the stomach and intestines.

• There is no specific antidote. Empty the stomach by inducing vomiting or gastric lavage. Treat symptomatically and supportively as indicated by patient's condition.

Naproxen

PHARMACOLOGY

Naproxen, a nonsteroidal anti-inflammatory agent, also has analgesic and antipyretic properties. Following oral administration it is absorbed rapidly and also completely. Peak plasma levels are attained in 2 to 4 hours. Naproxen is excreted in the urine; it readily crosses the placental barrier and has been found in the milk of lactating women.

SPECIAL PRECAUTIONS

- Do not use in Functional Class IV (incapacitated, largely or wholly bedridden or confined to a wheelchair; little or no self-care) rheumatoid arthritis patients.
- Safety and effectiveness in children has not been established.
- Do not use in patients with a history of hypersensitivity to naproxen.
- Because the potential exists for cross sensitivity reactions, naproxen should not be given to patients in whom aspirin or other nonsteroidal anti-inflammatory drugs induce the syndrome of asthma, rhinitis, or urticaria.
- Give under close supervision to patients prone to upper gastrointestinal tract disease; gastrointestinal bleeding, sometimes severe, has occurred.
- Safe use in pregnancy and lactation has not been established.
- Use with caution in patients with significantly impaired renal function.
- Use with caution in patients with questionable or compromised cardiac function.

ADVERSE EFFECTS

CNS EFFECTS: headache, drowsiness, dizziness, light-headedness, vertigo, inability to concentrate, depression

RESPIRATORY EFFECTS: dyspnea

CARDIOVASCULAR EFFECTS: palpitations

GASTROINTESTINAL EFFECTS: heartburn, nausea, dyspepsia, adominal pain, constipation, stomatitis, diarrhea, vomiting, melena, gastrointestinal bleeding, peptic ulceration, thirst

METABOLIC AND ENDOCRINE EFFECTS: edema

HEPATIC EFFECTS: jaundice

HEMATOLOGIC EFFECTS: thrombocytopenia, agranulocytosis

DERMATOLOGIC EFFECTS: pruritus, eruptions, sweating, ecchymoses, rash, urticaria, purpura, angioneurotic edema

OPHTHALMIC EFFECTS: visual disturbances

OTIC EFFECTS: tinnitus, hearing disturbances

CLINICAL GUIDELINES

ADMINISTRATION:
- Monitor serum creatinine and/or creatinine clearance because of possible renal effects.
- Caution patients about engaging in activities requiring alertness, particularly if they experience drowsiness, vertigo, or depression.
- Monitor hemoglobin value frequently.

EFFECTS:
- Symptomatic improvement usually begins within 2 weeks.

DRUG INTERACTIONS:
- May be used in combination with gold salts and/or corticosteroids.
- Aspirin administered concurrently increases the rate of excretion of naproxen.
- The potential for cross sensitivity reactions exists for aspirin, other anti-inflammatory steroids and naproxen.
- Patients receiving bishydroxycoumarin, hydantoin, sulfonamides, or sulfonylurea concurrently with naproxen should be observed carefully for drug interaction.

Naproxen may displace certain drugs from their binding sites because of its affinity for protein.

• Naproxen decreases platelet aggregation and prolongs bleeding time.

• Increased 17-ketosteroid levels may occur because of an interaction between the drug and/or its metabolites with m-dinitrobenzene used in this assay.

OVERDOSAGE/ANTIDOTE:

• Overdosage (1900 to 3000 mg for 3 to 7 days in 4 patients) resulted in drowsiness, heartburn, and a single episode of vomiting. There was no evidence of toxicity or late sequelae 5 to 15 months later.

• There is no specific antidote. The stomach should be emptied by inducing vomiting or gastric lavage. Supportive measures should be employed as necessary. Administration of activated charcoal (5 grams) would reduce markedly the absorption of naproxen.

Sulindac

PHARMACOLOGY

Sulindac is a nonsteroidal anti-inflammatory drug which also has analgesic and antipyretic activities. The mode of action is unknown. Inhibition of prostaglandin synthesis may be involved.

Following oral administration, approximately 90 percent of sulindac is absorbed. The peak plasma concentration is reached in 2 to 3 hours. The mean half-life of sulindac is 7.8 hours and that of the sulindac metabolite is 6.4 hours. Sulindac is excreted in the urine as unchanged drug and as the glucuronide.

SPECIAL PRECAUTIONS

• Do not use in patients who are hypersensitive to sulindac.

• Do not use in patients in whom acute asthmatic attacks, urticaria, or rhinitis is precipitated by aspirin or other nonsteroidal anti-inflammatory agents.

• Since peptic ulceration and gastrointestinal bleeding have been reported with sulindac, use with caution in patients with active gastrointestinal bleeding or an active peptic ulcer.

• Patients with impaired renal funtion should be monitored closely and may require a reduction in sulindac dosage to avoid excessive drug accummulation.

• Use with caution in patients with compromised cardiac function, hypertension, or other conditions predisposing to fluid retention. Peripheral edema has been observed in some patients taking sulindac.

• Do not use in pregnant women or nursing mothers; safety has not been established.

• Safe use in children has not been established.

• Use with caution in patients receiving oral anticoagulants or oral hypoglycemic agents.

ADVERSE EFFECTS

CNS EFFECTS: dizziness, headache, nervousness, vertigo, paresthesias, neuritis, depression

CARDIOVASCULAR EFFECTS: hypertension, epistaxis

GASTROINTESTINAL EFFECTS: gastrointestinal pain, dyspepsia, nausea, vomiting, diarrhea, constipation, flatulence, anorexia, cramps, gastritis, gastroenteritis, gastrointestinal bleeding

METABOLIC AND ENDOCRINE EFFECTS: edema

DERMATOLOGIC EFFECTS: rash, pruritus, stomatitis, sore or dry mucous membranes

ALLERGIC EFFECTS: hypersensitivity

OPHTHALMIC EFFECTS: transient visual disturbances

OTIC EFFECTS: tinnitus, decreased hearing

CLINICAL GUIDELINES

ADMINISTRATION:

• Institute an appropriate ulcer regimen in patients with an active peptic ulcer or with active gastrointestinal bleeding.

• Monitor patient's progress carefully if peptic ulcer or gastrointestinal bleeding is present.

EFFECTS:

• Sulindac inhibits platelet function; therefore carefully observe patients who may be adversely affected.

• Abnormalities of liver function tests, particularly elevation of alkaline phosphatase, may occur. Monitor until it returns to normal, or if a significant abnormality persists, discontinue sulindac.

• Since adverse eye findings have been reported with nonsteroidal anti-inflammatory agents, any patient developing eye complaints with sulindac should have appropriate ophthalmologic studies.

DRUG INTERACTIONS:

• Concomitant administration of aspirin with sulindac significantly depressed the plasma levels of the active sulfide metabolite.

• Concomitant administration of probenecid had only a slight effect on plasma sulfide levels, while plasma levels of sulindac and sulfone were increased. Sulindac produced a modest reduction in the uricosuric action of probenecid, which probably is not significant.

• Neither propoxyphene hydrochloride nor acetaminophen had any effect on the plasma levels of sulindac or its sulfide metabolites.

OVERDOSAGE/ANTIDOTE:

• Overdosage is characterized by an exaggeration of the adverse effects.

• Empty stomach by inducing vomiting or by gastric lavage. Treat symptomatically and supportively as necessary.

Tolmetin Sodium

PHARMACOLOGY

Tolmetin sodium is a nonsteroidal anti-inflammatory agent which also possesses analgesic and antipyretic activity. The mode of action is unknown. Following oral administration it is rapidly absorbed; peak plasma levels are reached within 30 to 60 minutes. The drug is eliminated in the urine. Clinical effects may not occur for 1 to 2 weeks.

SPECIAL PRECAUTIONS

• Do not use in Functional Class IV (incapacitated, largely or wholly bedridden or confined to a wheelchair; little or no self-care) rheumatoid arthritis patients.

• Safe use in children has not been established.

• Do not use in patients who have previously exhibited intolerance to tolmetin.

• Because the potential exists for cross sensitivity to aspirin and other nonsteroidal anti-inflammatory drugs, tolmetin should not be given to patients in whom such drugs induce the symptoms of asthma, rhinitis or urticaria.

• Give only under close supervision to patients with a history of upper gastrointestinal tract disease; peptic ulceration and gastrointestinal bleeding, sometimes severe, have been reported.

• Use with caution in patients with impaired renal function.

• Bleeding time may be prolonged.

• Use with caution in patients with compromised cardiac function since some retention of salt and water and mild peripheral edema has occurred.

• Safe use in pregnancy and lactation has not been established.

ADVERSE EFFECTS

CNS EFFECTS: headache, dizziness, light-headedness, tension, nervousness, and drowsiness

GASTROINTESTINAL EFFECTS: abdominal pain, nausea, vomiting, indigestion, heart-burn, constipation, dyspepsia, peptic ulcer, gastrointestinal bleeding

METABOLIC AND ENDOCRINE EFFECTS: mild edema

HEMATOLOGIC EFFECTS: small and transient decrease in hemoglobin and hematocrit, granulocytopenia

DERMATOLOGIC EFFECTS: maculopapular rash, urticaria, pruritus

OTIC EFFECTS: tinnitus

CLINICAL GUIDELINES

ADMINISTRATION:
- Ophthalmologic examination should be conducted at periodic intervals during therapy.
- Monitor renal function, particularly in patients with impaired renal function.
- Administer with meals, milk, or antacids other than sodium bicarbonate.

EFFECTS:
- A therapeutic response can be expected in a few days up to a week; progressive improvement can be anticipated during succeeding weeks of therapy.

DRUG INTERACTIONS:
- Does not interfere with the clinical assessment of the tuberculin skin test or the immediate-type hypersensitivity skin test or the immune mechanism as measured by skin testing.
- Concurrent administration of gold salts or corticosteroids has produced additional therapeutic benefit.
- Concurrent administration of salicylates is not recommended; there is no additional benefit, and potential for adverse reactions is increased.

- Urinary metabolites of tolmetin may give false positive tests for proteinuria when tests which rely on acid precipitation as the endpoint are used; no interference is seen with the reagent test strips (ALBUSTIX or URISTIX).
- Although tolmetin binds extensively to protein (*in vitro*), it does not alter the dosage of warfarin required to maintain a uniform prothrombin time.
- In adult diabetic patients under treatment with either sulfonylureas or insulin, there is no change in the clinical effects of either tolmetin or the hypoglycemic agent.

OVERDOSAGE/ANTIDOTE:
- Overdosage is characterized by an exaggeration of the adverse effects, particularly those on the gastrointestinal tract.
- There is no specific antidote. Empty the stomach by inducing vomiting or by gastric lavage followed by administration of activated charcoal. Use supportive therapy as indicated.
- Animal studies indicate that urinary excretion of tolmetin is enhanced when the urine is made alkaline by administering sodium bicarbonate.

Oxyphenbutazone
Phenylbutazone

PHARMACOLOGY

Oxyphenbutazone and phenylbutazone are nonhormonal antiarthritic anti-inflammatory agents; they also have antipyretic, analgesic, and mild uricosuric properties. Both phenylbutazone and oxyphenbutazone are absorbed rapidly and completely from the gastrointestinal tract following oral administration. Peak plasma levels are reached in 2 hours. Both compounds are metabolized in the liver and excreted slowly in the urine. The mechanism of action is unknown.

SPECIAL PRECAUTIONS
• Do not use in children 14 years of age or less or in senile patients.
• Do not use in patients with a history or symptoms of gastrointestinal inflammation or ulceration, including severe or recurrent or persistent dyspepsia.
• Do not use in patients with a history of hypersensitivity to phenylbutazone or oxyphenbutazone; with blood dyscrasias; renal, hepatic, or cardiac dysfunction; hypertension; thyroid disease, systemic edema; salivary gland enlargement due to the drug; polymyalgia rheumatica; temporal arteritis.
• Do not use in patients receiving other potent chemotherapeutic agents or on long-term anticoagulant therapy.
• In patients 60 years of age and older, treatment should be restricted to 1 week. The appearance of clinical edema is an indication to discontinue treatment with the drug.
• Patients 40 years of age or older have an increased susceptibility to the toxicity of the drug.
• Since serious, and even fatal, blood dyscrasias have occured, monitor hemogram and discontinue drug if significant changes occur.
• Observe careful detailed history for disease and the detection of the earliest signs of adverse reactions.

ADVERSE EFFECTS
CNS EFFECTS: agitation, confusional state, lethargy
CARDIOVASCULAR EFFECTS: cardiac decompensation, hypertension, pericarditis, diffuse interstitial myocarditis with muscle necrosis, perivascular granulomata, aggravation of thyroid arteritis in patients with polymyalgia rheumatica
URINARY TRACT EFFECTS: proteinuria, hematuria, oliguria, anuria, renal failure with azotemia, glomerulonephritis, acute tubular necrosis, nephrotic syndrome, bilateral renal cortical necrosis, renal stones, ureteral obstruction with uric acid crystals, impaired renal function
GASTROINTESTINAL EFFECTS: ulcerative esophagitis, acute and reactivated gastric and duodenal ulcer with perforation and hemorrhage, ulceration and perforation of large bowel, occult gastrointestinal bleeding with anemia, gastritis, epigastric pain, hematemesis, dyspepsia, nausea, vomiting, diarrhea, abdominal distention, ulcerative stomatitis, salivary gland enlargement
METABOLIC AND ENDOCRINE EFFECTS: sodium and chloride retention and edema, plasma dilution, toxic and nontoxic goiter, myxedema, hypoglycemia, respiratory alkalosis, metabolic alkalosis
HEPATIC EFFECTS: fatal and nonfatal hepatitis (cholestasis may or may not be prominent)
HEMATOLOGIC EFFECTS: agranulocytosis, aplastic anemia, hemolytic anemia, anemia due to blood loss, thrombocytopenia, pancytopenia, leukopenia, bone marrow depression
ALLERGIC EFFECTS: erythema multiforme; Stevens-Johnson syndrome, Lyell's syndrome, toxic necrotizing epidermolysis; exfoliative dermatitis; serum sickness, hypersensitivity angiitis (polyarteritis); anaphylactic shock, urticaria, arthralgia, fever, rash
DERMATOLOGIC EFFECTS: petechiae, purpura without thrombocytopenia, toxic pruritus, erythema nodosum
OPHTHALMIC EFFECTS: blurred vision, optic neuritis, retinal hemorrhage, toxic ambylopia, retinal detachment
OTIC EFFECTS: hearing loss

CLINICAL GUIDELINES

ADMINISTRATION:

• Administer before or after meals or with a glass of milk to minimize any gastric upset.

• Check patients weekly or every 2 weeks for weight gain.

• Obtain complete hemogram weekly or every 2 weeks, particularly in elderly patients.

EFFECTS:

• Caution patient to report to physician the occurrence of fever, sore throat, oral lesions, salivary gland enlargement, black or tarry stools, weight gain, edema.

• Caution patient not to engage in activities requiring alertness such as driving a car or operating machinery.

DRUG INTERACTIONS:

• Effects of insulin, sulfonylurea, and sulfonamide-type agents may be potentiated.

• Reduces iodine uptake by thyroid.

OVERDOSAGE/ANTIDOTE:

• Overdosage is characterized by convulsions, euphoria, psychosis, depression, headache, hallucinations, giddiness, vertigo, coma, hyperventilation and insomnia.

• There is no specific antidote. Empty stomach by inducing vomiting or gastric lavage. Supportive therapy is indicated.

Hydroxychloroquine Sulfate

PHARMACOLOGY, SPECIAL PRECAUTIONS, ADVERSE REACTIONS, CLINICAL GUIDELINES

For detailed information, see Chapter 2, page 80.

Penicillamine

PHARMACOLOGY

The mechanism of action of penicillamine in rheumatoid arthritis is unknown. It appears to suppress disease activity. Unlike cytotoxic immunosuppressants, penicillamine markedly lowers IgM rheumatoid factor but produces no significant depression in absolute levels or serum immunoglobulins.

SPECIAL PRECAUTIONS

• Do not administer to patients who are pregnant, or who have a history of penicillamine-related aplastic anemia or agranulocytosis.

• Do not administer to patients with a history or other evidence of renal insufficiency.

• Penicillamine has been associated with fatalities due to certain diseases such as aplastic anemia, agranulocytosis, thrombocytopenia, Goodpasture's syndrome, and myasthenic syndrome.

• If drug fever occurs, then discontinue therapy.

ADVERSE EFFECTS

CNS EFFECTS: hyperpyrexia

RESPIRATORY EFFECTS: allergic alveolitis, obliterative bronchiolitis

CARDIOVASCULAR EFFECTS: thrombophlebitis

GASTROINTESTINAL EFFECTS: anorexia, epigastric pain, nausea, vomiting, diarrhea, reactivation of peptic ulcer, pancreatitis

HEPATIC EFFECTS: hepatic dysfunction, cholestatic jaundice

ENDOCRINE AND METABOLIC EFFECTS: thyroiditis, mammary hyperplasia

MUSCULOSKELETAL EFFECTS: polyarthralgia, migratory; synovitis, polymyositis

URINARY TRACT EFFECTS: proteinuria, hematuria, nephrotic syndrome, Goodpasture's syndrome

DERMATOLOGIC EFFECTS: alopecia, anetoderma

ALLERGIC EFFECTS: pruritus, rashes, phemphigoid reactions, lupuslike syn-

drome, urticaria, exfoliative dermatitis
HEMATOLOGIC EFFECTS: thrombocytopenia, agranulocytosis, aplastic anemia, thrombotic thrombocytopenic purpura, hemolytic anemia, red cell aplasia, monocytosis, leukocytosis, eosinophilia, and thrombocytosis
OPHTHALMIC EFFECTS: optic neuritis
OTIC EFFECTS: tinnitus

CLINICAL GUIDELINES
ADMINISTRATION:
- Give on an empty stomach at least 1 hour before meals and at least 1 hour apart from any other drug, food, or milk. This permits maximal absorption and reduces the likelihood of inactivation by metal binding.
- Monitor hematoligic parameters routinely including RBC, WBC, platelets (direct count), urinalysis, and hepatic parameters.
- Instruct patients to report immediately symptoms such as fever, sore throat, chills, bleeding or bruising.
EFFECTS:
- Two or 3 months may be required before the first evidence of a clinical response is noted.
- The first evidence of supression is relief of pain, tenderness, and swelling.

- If remissions occur, they may last from months to years, but usually require continued treatment.
- Increases in serum alkaline phosphatase, lactic dehydrogenase, positive cephalin flocculation, and thymol turbidity tests have occurred.
DRUG INTERACTIONS:
- Do not use in patients who are receiving gold therapy, antimalarial or cytotoxic drugs, oxyphenbutazone, or phenylbutazone because they have similar serious hematologic and renal adverse effects.
- Salicylates, other nonsteroidal anti-inflammatory drugs, or systemic corticosteroids may be continued when penicillamine is initiated.
- Mineral supplements should not be administered since they may block the response to penicillamine.
- Penicillamine reduces serum digoxin levels.
- Concomitant administration of iron reduces absorption and anticupruretic activity of penicillamine.
OVERDOSAGE/ANTIDOTE:
- In one patient overdosage (16 capsules) resulted in hemolytic anemia and thrombocytopenia. This patient responded well to penicillamine withdrawal and prednisone 20 mg tid.

Antigout/Uricosuric Agents

GENERAL CLINICAL USES
The antigout/uricosuric agents either terminate the attack, decrease uric acid content of the body, or relieve the discomfort caused by urate deposits.

Allopurinol reduces the serum uric acid level in patients with gout per se and in that associated with blood dyscrasias and their therapy. It is also useful in treating patients with recurrent uric acid stone formation.

Colchicine, specific for treating gout, is also useful in treating primary or secondary uric acid nephropathy by preventing tissue and urate deposits. When colchicine and probenecid are administered together, the incidence of acute attacks of gout appears to be reduced. The residual pain and mild discomfort accompanying gout are also relieved.

Indomethacin, a nonsteroidal anti-inflammatory agent, has been found effective in relieving pain and reducing fever, swelling and tenderness in acute gouty arthritis. See *Antiarthritic Agents*, page 471, for detailed information.

Phenylbutazone and oxyphenbutazone depress the formation of uric acid by inhibiting secretion. See *Antiarthritic Agents*, page 471, for detailed information.

Probenecid, also administered orally, is used to treat hyperuricemia associated with gout and gouty arthritis. It is also used adjunctively with penicillin for elevation and prolongation of plasma levels by whatever route the antibiotic is given.

Sulfinpyrazone, an orally administered uricosuric agent, is useful for maintenance therapy in chronic gout. It is not intended for relief of an acute attack.

SPECIFIC PRODUCTS AND DOSAGES

GENERIC NAME	TRADE NAME	ROUTE OF ADMIN.	USUAL DAILY DOSAGE
allopurinol	ZYLOPRIM	po	**Adults:** 200–300 mg/day to 400–600 mg/day for severe conditions; administer in divided doses **Children 6–10 yrs.:** 300 mg/day **Under 6 yrs.:** 150 mg/day
colchicine	(G)†	po iv	0.6–1.2 mg every 2 hr. as necessary 0.5–1.0 mg od or bid
	COLBENEMID*	po	0.5–1.0 mg od or bid
indomethacin	INDOCIN	po	50 mg tid; then decrease
oxyphenbutazone	OXALID TANDEARIL	po	400 mg initially; then 100 mg q 4 hr. See *Antiarthritic Agents*
phenylbutazone	AZOLID AZOLID-A* BUTAZOLIDIN	po	400 mg initially; 100 mg q 4 hr. usually for 4 days. Discontinue therapy after 7 days in patients 60 yrs. or older
probenecid	(G) BENEMID COLBENEMID*	po	250–500 mg bid
sulfinpyrazone	ANTURANE	po	**Initial:** 100–200 mg od to bid **Maintenance:** 200–400 mg bid

*Contains more than one active ingredient.
†(G) designates availability as a generic product.

Allopurinol

PHARMACOLOGY

Allopurinol reduces the production of uric acid by inhibiting the biochemical reactions immediately preceding its formation. Its action differs from that of uricosuric agents which lower the serum uric acid level by increasing urinary excretion of uric acid. Allopurinol reduces both the serum and urinary uric acid levels thereby avoiding hyperuricosuria in patients with gouty nephropathy or with a predisposition to formation or uric acid stones.

SPECIAL PRECAUTIONS

• Do not use in children except those with hyperuricemia that is secondary to malignancy.
• Do not use in nursing mothers.
• Do not restart therapy in patients who have had a severe reaction to allopurinol.
• Periodic liver function tests should be performed since hepatotoxicity has occurred; increases in serum alkaline phosphatase or serum transaminase have been measured.
• Do not administer to immediate relative of patients with idiopathic hemochromatosis.
• Safe use in pregnancy has not been established.
• Use with caution in patients with pre-existing renal disease since both a rise and a decrease in BUN have been reported; patients with renal impairment may require less drug.
• In patients with severely impaired renal function, the half-life may be greatly prolonged; adjust dosage accordingly.
• Evaluate kidney function periodically, particularly during the first few months of therapy.
• Administer with great caution, if at all, to patients with renal failure.

• May precipitate gouty attack with mobilization of uric acid pool before excretion takes place. Concomitant administration of colchicine may prevent this.

ADVERSE EFFECTS

CNS EFFECTS: peripheral neutitis, and drowsiness
AUTONOMIC EFFECTS: fever, chills
GASTROINTESTINAL EFFECTS: nausea, vomiting, diarrhea, intermittent abdominal pain
HEMATOLOGIC EFFECTS: mild reticulocytosis, erythema multiforme, leukopenia, leukocytosis, eosinophilia
ALLERGIC EFFECTS: exfoliative, urticarial, and purpuric lesions
DERMATOLOGIC EFFECTS: maculopapular rash, dermatitis, alopecia, pruritus
MUSCULOSKELETAL EFFECTS: arthralgia
OPHTHALMIC EFFECTS: cataracts

CLINICAL GUIDELINES

ADMINISTRATION:
• Caution patients that drowsiness may occur and to use caution in engaging in actitivies where alertness is mandatory.
• Assure adequate fluid intake to produce daily urine output of at least 2 liters; a slightly alkaline urine is desirable to avoid formation of xanthine calculi and to prevent renal precipitation of urates in patients receiving uricosuric agents concomitantly.
• Advise patients to take drug with meals to minimize gastrointestinal complaints.
EFFECTS:
• Several months of therapy may be necessary to deplete the uric acid pool sufficiently to achieve control of acute attacts of gout.
• Normal serum urate levels are achieved in 1 to 3 weeks.
• Discontinue drug if rash appears; in some instances, rashes have been followed by severe hypersensitivity reactions.

DRUG INTERACTIONS:
• Do not administer iron salts concomitantly.
• In patients receiving mercaptopurine or azathioprine, the concomitant administration of allopurinol, 300 to 600 mg daily, will require reduction in dose 1/3 or 1/4 of the usual dose of mercaptopurine or azathioprine; subsequent adjustments in dosage should be made on the basis of therapeutic response and any toxic effects.
• Concomitant administration of a uricosuric agent with allopurinol may result in a decrease in urinary excretion of oxypurines as compared with their excretion with allopurinol alone.
• Allopurinol prolongs the half-life of the anticoagulant dicumarol; reassess coagulation time.
• Alkaline phosphatase and transaminase levels may increase.

OVERDOSAGE/ANTIDOTE:
• Overdosage is characterized by an exaggeration of the adverse effects.
• There is no specific antidote. Treat supportively.

Colchicine

PHARMACOLOGY
Colchicine, although effective in relieving the pain of acute attacts of gout, has no uricosuric activity. The mechanism of action is unknown. It is not an analgesic.

SPECIAL PRECAUTIONS
• Administer with caution in patients who are aged and debilitated, especially those with renal, gastrointestinal, or heart disease.
• Do not use in patients with a history of hypersensitivity to colchicine or related compounds.
• Use with caution in patients with hepatic dysfunction since colchicine toxicity may be increased.

ADVERSE EFFECTS
CNS EFFECTS: peripheral neuritis, and weakness
GASTROINTESTINAL EFFECTS: nausea, vomiting, diarrhea, anorexia abdominal pain
HEMATOLOGIC EFFECTS: bone marrow depression, agranulocytosis, thrombocytopenia; aplastic anemia may occur with prolonged administration
DERMATOLOGIC EFFECTS: depilation

CLINICAL GUIDELINES
ADMINISTRATION:
• It is generally necessary to reach dose levels which produce nausea, vomiting, and diarrhea for a clinical effect. Paregoric may be given either concurrently or when diarrhea develops.
• Therapy should be initiated at the first warning of an acute attack of gout.
EFFECTS:
• If weakness, anorexia, nausea, vomiting, or diarrhea occurs dosage should be reduced.
• Pain, redness, and swelling may abate within 12 hours.
OVERDOSAGE/ANTIDOTE:
• The first symptoms to appear are gastrointestinal—nausea, vomiting, abdominal pain, and diarrhea. The diarrhea may be severe and bloody due to hemorrhagic gastroenteritis. Burning sensations in the throat, stomach, and skin may also occur. Extensive vascular damage may result in shock. Hematuria and oliguria, and marked muscular weakness, ascending paralysis, delirium, and convulsions may occur. Death is usually the result of respiratory depression.
• Death has occurred with as little as 8 mg. There is usually a latent period between overdosage and onset of symptoms, regardless of route of administration.

• There is no specific antidote. Empty stomach by gastric lavage. Hemodialysis or peritoneal dialysis have been used. Combat shock. Atropine and morphine may relieve the abdominal pain. Respiratory assistance may be required.

Indomethacin

See *Antiarthritic Agents*, page 476.

Oxyphenbutazone
Phenylbutazone

See *Antiarthritic Agents*, page 471, in this chapter for detailed information.

Probenecid

PHARMACOLOGY
Probenecid, a uricosuric agent, acts by inhibiting tubular reabsorption or urates; urinary excretion of uric acid is increased and serum uric acid level decreased.

The tubular secretion of penicillin is inhibited, thereby increasing the plasma level.

SPECIAL PRECAUTIONS
• Do not administer to patients with a history of hypersensitivity to probenecid or related compounds.
• Do not use in patients with blood dyscrasias or uric acid kidney stones.
• Do not initiate therapy until an acute gouty attack has subsided.
• Do not administer salicylates concomitantly because of the antagonism of the uricosuric acid by probenecid.
• If urine is alkalinized, monitor patient's acid-base balance.

• Use cautiously in patients with a history of peptic ulcer.
• In patients with renal impairment, dosage increase may be required.

ADVERSE EFFECTS
CNS EFFECTS: headache, dizziness
URINARY TRACT EFFECTS: frequency; nephrotic syndrome rarely
AUTONOMIC EFFECTS: flushing
GASTROINTESTINAL   EFFECTS: anorexia, nausea, vomiting, sore gums
METABOLIC AND ENDOCRINE EFFECTS: exacerbation of gout and uric acid stones with or without renal colic, hematuria, and pain
HEPATIC EFFECTS: hepatic necrosis rarely
HEMATOLOGIC EFFECTS: anemia, hemolytic, anemia; aplastic anemia rarely
ALLERGIC EFFECTS: anaphylaxis, dermatitis, pruritus, fever

CLINICAL GUIDELINES
ADMINISTRATION:
• Advise patients to consume liberal amounts of fluids.
• Administer with food, milk, or antacids to relieve gastric disturbances.
EFFECTS:
• Prevent hematuria, renal colic, costovertebral pain, and formation of urate stones by alkalinization of urine and liberal fluid intake.
• Urine may be alkalinized by ingestion of sodium bicarbonate 3 to 7.5 gm daily or potassium citrate 7.5 gm daily.
• Exacerbation of gout may follow probenecid therapy.
• Decreases both renal and hepatic excretion of BSP.
• Tubular reabsorption of phosphorus is inhibited in hypoparathyroid but not in euparathyroid individuals.
• Insignificant increases in free sulfa plasma concentration, but significant increase in total sulfa plasma level; excretion of con-

jugated sulfa drugs decreased.

DRUG INTERACTIONS:
- Decreases urinary excretion of amino-salicylic acid, aminohippuric acid, phenol-sulfonphthalein, pantothenic acid, 17-keto-steroids, and sodium idomethamate.
- Increase in indomethacin plasma levels occurs.
- Excretion of salicylates, streptomycin, chloramphenicol, chlortetracycline, oxyte-tracycline, or neomycin *not* influenced.
- A reducing substance may appear in the urine which will give a false positive Benedicts' test (for reducing substances, e.g., glucose).

OVERDOSAGE/ANTIDOTE:
- Gastric intolerance may be indicative of overdosage. Huge overdosage may result in central nervous stimulation and death from respiratory failure.
- There is no specific antidote. Treat supportively.

Sulfinpyrazone

PHARMACOLOGY
Sulfinpyrazone, a potent uricosuric agent, controls serum urate levels by po-tentiating the urinary excretion of uric acid. In addition, it has a minimal anti-in-flammatory effect. Sulfinpyrazone prevents or reduces tophi and the joint changes in chronic gouty arthritis.

SPECIAL PRECAUTIONS
- Do not use in patients with active pep-tic ulcer; peptic ulcer may be aggravated or reactivated.
- Use with caution in pregnant women; weigh potential risks against possible bene-fits.
- Do not administer salicylates to patients receiving sulfinpyrazone.
- Use with caution in patients with known sensitivity to phenylbutazone and other pyrazoles.
- Do not administer to patients with pre-existing stones.
- Dosage may require adjustment in pa-tients with renal impairment.
- Assess renal function periodically in pa-tients with significant renal impairment.

ADVERSE EFFECTS
GASTROINTESTINAL EFFECTS: nausea, vom-iting, diarrhea, epigastric pain
HEMATOLOGIC EFFECTS: anemia; leukope-nia, agranulocytosis, and thrombocytopenia rarely
ALLERGIC EFFECTS: hypersensitivity reac-tions
DERMATOLOGIC EFFECTS: rash

CLINICAL GUIDELINES
ADMINISTRATION:
- To minimize gastrointestinal distur-bances, administer with food, milk or ant-acids.
- Periodic blood counts are recom-mended.
- Alkalinization of the urine is desirable.
EFFECTS:
- May precipitate or exacerbate attacks of gout initially.
- Urolithiasis and renal colic may be pre-cipitated, particularly in initial stage of therapy.
DRUG INTERACTIONS:
- When sulfinpyrazone and sulfonamides are administered concomitantly, the effect of the sulfonamides may be potentiated.
- Some other pyrazoles potentiate hypo-glycemic sulfonylurea agents as well as in-sulin.
- Salicylates antagonize the action of sul-finpyrazone.

• May accentuate the action of coumarin-type anticoagulants and further depress prothrombin time when administered concurrently.

OVERDOSAGE/ANTIDOTE:

• Signs of overdosage are nausea, vomiting, diarrhea, epigastric pain, ataxia, labored respiration, convulsions, and coma. Possible symptoms after overdosage with other pyrazolone derivatives include anemia and ulceration.

• No specific antidote is known. Empty stomach by inducing vomiting or gastric lavage. Treat supportively with intravenous glucose infusion and analeptics as needed.

Anti-Inflammatory Agents

Glucocorticoids

GENERAL CLINICAL USES

The glucocorticoids may be administered orally or intramuscularly for control of serious inflammation seen in rheumatic conditions of the muscles and joints. Rheumatic conditions which may be treated include psoriatic arthritis, rheumatoid arthritis, ankylosing spondylitis, acute and subacute bursitis, acute nonspecific tenosynovitis, acute gouty arthritis, juvenile rheumatoid arthritis.

Intra-articular or periarticular administration of glucocorticoids is useful as adjunctive short-term therapy in synovitis of osteoarthritis, acute and subacute bursitis, epicondylitis, post-traumatic osteoarthritis, rheumatoid arthritis, acute nonspecific tenosynovitis.

Intrabursal administration of glucocorticoids is useful as adjunctive short-term therapy in bursitis and associated inflammatory disorders of the tendons such as tenosynovitis, and inflammatory disorders of the muscles such as fibrositis and myositis.

SPECIFIC PRODUCTS AND DOSAGES

Information for products used for oral and intramuscular administration is presented in Chapter 15, *Endocrine and Other Drugs Affecting Metabolism,* page 532.

GENERIC NAME	TRADE NAME	ROUTE OF ADMIN.	USUAL DOSAGE
betamethasone acetate and betamethasone sodium phosphate	CELESTONE SOLUSPAN Suspension	intrabursal, intra-articular, peri-articular	0.5–2 ml
dexamethasone acetate	DECADRON-LA	intra-articular	4–16 mg
dexamethasone sodium phosphate	DECADRON Phosphate	intra-articular	0.8–4 mg
methylprednisolone acetate	DEPO-MEDROL	intra-articular	4–80 mg
prednisolone acetate	(G)* STERANE	intra-articular	5–100 mg
triamcinolone acetonide	KENALOG-40	intra-articular, intra-bursal	2.5–15 mg
triamcinolone hexacetonide	ARISTOSPAN	intra-articular	2–20 mg

*(G) designates availability as a generic product.

PHARMACOLOGY

The glucocorticoids have anti-inflammatory, antipruritis, and vasoconstrictive actions. They also have salt-retaining properties and can cause profound and varied metabolic effects. These drugs modify the body's immune response to diverse stimuli.

SPECIAL PRECAUTIONS

• For systemic effects, see Chapter 15, page 534.
• Intra-articular injections may produce systemic as well as local effects.
• Appropriate examination of any joint fluid present is necessary to exclude a septic process.
• A marked increase in pain accompanied by local swelling, further restriction of joint motion, fever, and malaise are suggestive of septic arthritis. If this complication occurs and the diagnosis of sepsis is confirmed, appropriate antimicrobial therapy should be instituted.
• Local injection of a steroid into a previously infected joint is to be avoided.
• Corticosteroids should not be injected into unstable joints.
• Do not inject in infected areas or to alleviate joint pain arising from infectious states such as gonococcal or tuberculous arthritis.

ADVERSE EFFECTS

LOCAL EFFECTS: transient pain at injection site, postinjection flare, Charcot-like arthropathy, hypopigmentation, hyperpigmentation, sterile abscess
SYSTEMIC EFFECTS: see Chapter 15, *Endocrine and Other Drugs Affecting Metabolism*, page 534.

CLINICAL GUIDELINES

ADMINISTRATION:

• Sterile administrative technique is mandatory.

• Caution patient to avoid overuse of joint in which symptomatic benefit has been obtained.

• When the amount of synovial fluid is increased, aspiration may be performed before administration.

• Attention should be paid to avoid deposition of drug along the needle path, which might produce atrophy.

EFFECTS:

• To avoid possible joint destruction from repeated doses of intra-articular corticosteroid, injection should be as infrequent as possible.

Salicylates

Acetylsalicylic Acid (Aspirin)
Choline Salicylate
Magnesium Salicylate
Potassium Salicylate
Sodium Salicylate

GENERAL CLINICAL USES

The salicylates are nonsteroidal, anti-inflammatory, antipyretic, and analgesic agents useful in treating rheumatoid arthritis, rheumatic fever, osteoarthritis, and other conditions for which an anti-inflammatory–analgesic agent is desired.

PHARMACOLOGY, SPECIAL PRECAUTIONS, ADVERSE EFFECTS, CLINICAL GUIDELINES
See Chapter 4, *Drugs Affecting the Brain and Spinal Cord*, page 130.

SPECIFIC PRODUCTS AND DOSAGES

GENERIC NAME	TRADE NAME	ROUTE OF ADMIN.	USUAL DOSAGE
acetylsalicylic acid (aspirin)	(G)† ASCRIPTIN* BUFFERIN*	po	**Adult:** 4.5–7.5 gm/day in divided doses **Children:** 60–110 mg/kg/day in divided doses
choline salicylate	ARTHROPAN Liquid	po	0.87–1.74 gm up to qid
magnesium salicylate	HYALEX* MOBIDIN	po	3.6–9.6 gm/day in divided doses
potassium salicylate	PABALATE-SF*	po	1.3–1.9 gm/day in divided doses
sodium salicylate	(G) PABALATE*	po	1.3–1.9 gm/day in divided doses

*Contains more than one active ingredient.
†(G) designates availability as a generic product.

Skeletal Muscle Relaxants

GENERAL CLINICAL USES

It is desirable to induce skeletal muscle relaxation in a variety of conditions such as during anesthesia; in spastic conditions as in spinal cord injury, stroke, cerebral palsy, or muscle sclerosis; and also when muscle spasms are present due to local pathology such as inflammation of the muscles or joints, or secondary to trauma. The skeletal muscle relaxants are divided into three groups:

The *centrally or directly acting products* are useful for the relief of skeletal muscle spasms due to reflex spasm caused by local pathology such as inflammation of the muscles or joints, or secondary to trauma; spasticity caused by upper motor neuron disorders such as cerebral palsy and paraplegia; athetosis, stiff-arm syndrome, and tetanus.

When it is necessary to control the manifestations of clinical spasticity resulting from spinal cord injury, cerebral palsy, or muscular sclerosis, *dantrolene sodium* is indicated. It is not indicated for rheumatic disorders.

The *curarelike preparations*, classified as neuromuscular blocking agents, are useful when it is desirable to induce skeletal muscle relaxation in combination with anesthesia and also during pharmacologically or electrically induced convulsions.

SPECIFIC PRODUCTS AND DOSAGES

GENERIC NAME	TRADE NAME	ROUTE OF ADMIN.	SUGGESTED DAILY DOSAGE		
			ADULTS	MRDD†	CHILDREN
Central-acting Skeletal Muscle Relaxants:					
baclofen	LIORESAL	po	5–20 mg tid	80 mg	Not established
carisoprodol	RELA SOMA SOMA* Compound	po	350 mg qid	1400 mg	**Under 12 yrs.:** not recommended **Over 12 yrs.:** 25 mg/kg/day divided in 4 equal doses

*Contains more than one active ingredient.
†MRDD = maximum recommended daily dose.

(continued overleaf)

GENERIC NAME	TRADE NAME	ROUTE OF ADMIN.	SUGGESTED DAILY DOSAGE		
			ADULTS	MRDD†	CHILDREN
chlorphenesin carbamate	MAOLATE	po	**Initial:** 800 mg tid **Maintenance:** 400 mg qid or less	2400 mg	Not recommended
chlorzoxazone	PARAFLEX PARAFON* Forte	po	250–750 mg tid or qid	3000 mg	125–500 mg tid or qid
cyclobenzaprine HCl	FLEXERIL	po	20–40 mg/day in divided doses	60 mg	Not established
diazepam	VALIUM Injection	im/iv	5–10 mg; repeat in 3–4 hr. if necessary; larger doses may be used	Not established	**5 yrs. and over:** 5–10 mg every 3–4 hr. **Infants over 30 days:** 1–2 mg
		po	2–10 mg bid to qid	40 mg	1–2.5 mg tid to qid
meprobamate	MILTOWN Intramuscular	im	400 mg every 3–4 hr.	———	**Children:** 200 mg every 3–4 hr. **Infants:** 125 mg every 6 hr.
metaxalone	SKELAXIN	po	800 mg tid or qid	———	**Over 12 yrs.:** 800 mg tid or qid
methocarbamol	(G)†† ROBAXIN Injection	im/iv	1–3 gm	3 gm	15 mg/kg qid (in tetanus)
	ROBAXIN	po	1.5 gm tid to qid	8 gm	Not established
orphenadrine citrate	(G)	po	100 mg bid	200 mg	Not established
	NORFLEX	im/iv	60 mg bid	120 mg	Not recommended
Peripherally Acting Skeletal Muscle Relaxant: dantrolene sodium	DANTRIUM	po	25–100 mg bid to qid	400 mg	1–3 mg/kg od to qid
		iv	**Initial:** 1 mg/kg; may repeat up to cumulative dose 10 mg/kg		Not recommended
Curarelike Skeletal Muscle Relaxants: decamethonium bromide	SYNCURINE	iv	0.5–3 mg at rate of 1 mg/min at 10- to 30-min. intervals	———	Not recommended
gallamine triethiodide	FLAXEDIL IV	iv	0.5–1 mg/kg	———	0.5–1 mg/kg

*Contains more than one active ingredient.
†MRDD = maximum recommended daily dose.
††(G) designates availability as a generic product.

(continued facing page)

GENERIC NAME	TRADE NAME	ROUTE OF ADMIN.	SUGGESTED DAILY DOSAGE		
			ADULTS	MRDD†	CHILDREN
hexafluorenium bromide	MYLAXEN	iv	0.2–0.4 mg/kg	36 mg	Consult labeling
metocurine iodide	METUBINE Iodide	iv	1.5–5 mg depending on type of anesthesia	————	Not recommended
pancuronium bromide	PAVULON	iv	0.04–0.1 mg/kg	————	Same as for adults; test with 0.02 mg/kg in neonates
succinylcholine chloride	(G) ANECTINE QUELICIN SUCOSTRIN	iv im	25–75 mg 25–75 mg	150 mg	2 mg/kg 2.5 mg/kg
tubocurarine chloride	(G)	iv	40–60 U; then 20–30 U (0.1–0.3 mg/kg)	————	0.15–0.3 mg/kg

†MRDD = maximum recommended daily dose.

Centrally Acting Skeletal Muscle Relaxants

Baclofen

PHARMACOLOGY

Baclofen is capable of inhibiting both monosynaptic and polysynaptic reflexes at the spinal level. The precise mechanism of action is not fully known.

Baclofen is rapidly and extensively absorbed after oral administration. It is excreted primarily unchanged by the kidneys.

SPECIAL PRECAUTIONS

- Do not use in patients hypersensitive to baclofen.
- Do not withdraw drug abruptly; hallucinations have occurred.
- In patients with impaired renal function, dosage reduction may be necessary.
- Safe use in pregnancy, children, or nursing mothers has not been established.

ADVERSE EFFECTS

CNS EFFECTS: drowsiness, dizziness, weakness, fatigue, confusion, headache, insomnia, euphoria, excitement, depression, hallucinations, paresthesia, slurred speech, coordination disorder, tremor, rigidity, dystonia, ataxia, dysarthria, epileptic seizure

CARDIOVASCULAR EFFECTS: hypotension

RESPIRATORY EFFECTS: dyspnea, chest pain, syncope, nasal congestion

GASTROINTESTINAL EFFECTS: nausea, constipation, anorexia, taste disorder, abdominal pain, vomiting, diarrhea, occult blood in stool

AUTONOMIC EFFECTS: dry mouth, excessive perspiration

URINARY TRACT EFFECTS: frequency, enuresis, urinary retention, dysuria, nocturia, hematuria

METABOLIC AND ENDOCRINE EFFECTS: impotence, inability to ejaculate, ankle edema, weight gain

DERMATOLOGIC EFFECTS: rash, pruritus

OPHTHALMIC EFFECTS: blurred vision, nystagmus, strabismus, miosis, mydriasis, and diplopia

OTIC EFFECTS: tinnitus

CLINICAL GUIDELINES

ADMINISTRATION:
- Avoid abrupt withdrawal of drug.
- Caution patients that since drowsiness and sedation may occur, it may be hazardous to drive a motor vehicle or operate dangerous machinery.

EFFECTS:
- In patients with epilepsy, monitor clinical state and EEG since seizure control has deteriorated in some cases.
- SGOT increases, alkaline phosphatase elevations, and blood sugar elevations have been reported.

DRUG INTERACTIONS:
- Effects may be additive to those of alcohol and other CNS depressants.

OVERDOSAGE/ANTIDOTE:
- Overdosage is characterized by vomiting, muscle hypotonia, drowsiness, accommodation disorders, coma, respiratory depression, and seizures.
- In the conscious patient, empty stomach by inducing vomiting followed by lavage. In the obtunded patient, secure the airway with a cuffed endotracheal tube before beginning lavage. Maintain adequate respiratory exchange; do not use respiratory stimulants.

Carisoprodol
Meprobamate

PHARMACOLOGY

The mode of action of carisoprodol and meprobamate has not been clearly identified but may be related to their sedative properties. These drugs do not directly relax skeletal muscle in man. Following oral administration of carisoprodol, relief of symptoms usually begins within 30 minutes and lasts for 4 to 6 hours. Meprobamate administered intramuscularly relaxes skeletal muscle by way of the CNS; the action is obvious within 30 minutes.

Carisoprodol and meprobamate are metabolized in the liver and excreted by the kidneys. They are present in breast milk at a concentration higher than that of maternal plasma.

SPECIAL PRECAUTIONS

- Do not use in patients with acute intermittent prophyria or with a history of allergic or idosyncratic reactions to carisoprodol, meprobamate or related compounds, such as mebutamate or tybamate.
- On very rare occasions, the first dose has been followed by idiosyncratic reactions appearing within minutes or hours. These reactions have included extreme weakness, transient quadriplegia, dizziness, ataxia, temporary loss of vision, diplopia, mydriasis, dysarthria, agitation, euphoria, confusion, and disorientation. The symptoms usually subside over the course of the next several hours. Supportive and symptomatic therapy, including hospitalization, may be necessary.
- Safe use in pregnancy, lactation, or children under 12 years has not been established.
- Use with caution in addiction-prone patients.
- Abrupt withdrawal has resulted in mild withdrawal effects such as abdominal cramps, insomnia, chilliness, headache, and nausea.
- Use with caution in patients with compromised liver or kidney function.
- Do not use meprobamate intramuscular in patients with pre-existing renal damage;

polyethylene glycol, the vehicle in meprobamate im, may cause further damage.
• Meprobamate im controls the spasms of tetanus evoked by somatic stimuli but not those evoked by proprioceptive stimuli. If ineffective in relieving spasms of tetanus, search for a visceral trigger point.

ADVERSE EFFECTS
CNS EFFECTS: drowsiness, dizziness, vertigo, ataxia, tremor, agitation, irritability, headache, depressive reactions, syncope, insomnia
CARDIOVASCULAR EFFECTS: tachycardia, postural hypotension, facial flushing
GASTROINTESTINAL EFFECTS: nausea, vomiting, hiccups, epigastric distress
ALLERGIC EFFECTS: rash, erythema multiforme, pruritus, eosinophilia, fixed drug eruption with cross reaction to meprobamate/carisoprodol, asthmatic episodes, fever, weakness, dizziness, angioneurotic edema, smarting eyes, hypotension, anaphylactoid shock
LOCAL EFFECTS: with meprobamate im, induration, nodules, asceptic abscess

CLINICAL GUIDELINES
ADMINISTRATION:
• Warn patients that these drugs may impair the mental and/or physical abilities required to perform potentially hazardous tasks such as driving a car or operating machinery.
• Do not administer meprobamate im, intravenously; thrombosis or hemolysis may occur.
EFFECTS:
• If drowsiness occurs, reduction of dosage may alleviate it.
• Meprobamate im may precipitate seizures in epileptic patients.
DRUG INTERACTIONS:
• The effects of carisoprodol/meprobamate and alcohol and other central nervous system depressants or psychotropic drugs may be additive.
OVERDOSAGE/ANTIDOTE:
• Overdosage has produced stupor, coma, shock, respiratory depression, and, very rarely, death. The effects of an overdosage of carisoprodol and alcohol or other CNS depressants can be additive even when one of the drugs has been taken in the usual recommended dosage.
• Remove any remaining drug from the stomach. Use supportive therapy including respiratory assistance, CNS stimulants, and/or pressor agents. Diuresis, osmotic (mannitol) diuresis, peritoneal dialysis, and hemodialysis have been used. Carisoprodol and meprobamate are dialyzable. Monitor urinary output to avoid overhydration. Observe patient for possible relapse due to incomplete gastric emptying and delayed absorption.

Chlorphenesin Carbamate
Chlorzoxazone

PHARMACOLOGY
Chlorphenesin carbamate and chlorzoxazone are centrally acting skeletal muscle relaxants which act primarily at the level of the spinal cord and subcortical areas of the brain. These drugs are absorbed rapidly following oral administration, metabolized rapidly, and excreted in the urine as glucuronides. An effect is noted in 1 to 3 hours.

SPECIAL PRECAUTIONS
• Do not use in patients with a history of hypersensitivity to either of these drugs.
• Use with caution in patients with a history of allergic reactions to drugs.
• If signs or symptoms of liver dysfunction are noted, discontinue drug immediately.

- Safe use in pregnancy has not been established.

ADVERSE EFFECTS
CNS EFFECTS: drowsiness, dizziness, light-headedness, malaise, overstimulation occasionally, confusion; paradoxical stimulation, insomnia, nervousness and headache with chlorophenesin carbamate
URINARY TRACT EFFECTS: discoloration of urine rarely
GASTROINTESTINAL EFFECTS: bleeding, nausea, epigastric distress
HEPATIC EFFECTS: hepatic necrosis after prolonged therapy (1 year with chlorzoxazone); jaundice
HEMATOLOGIC EFFECTS: with chlorphenesin carbamate, leukopenia, thrombocytopenia, agranulocytosis, pancytopenia
ALLERGIC EFFECTS: rash, petechiae, ecchymoses; angioneurotic edema, anaphylactoid reactions extremely rare; drug fever

CLINICAL GUIDELINES
ADMINISTRATION:
- Caution patients to avoid engaging in hazardous activities such as driving a car or operating machinery.
DRUG INTERACTIONS:
- Do not administer concurrently with other potentially hepatotoxic drugs, central nervous system depressants, and other skeletal muscle relaxants; the effects may be additive.
OVERDOSAGE/ANTIDOTE:
- Overdosage is characterized by an exaggeration of the adverse effects, particularly the CNS effects. One case of overdosage with 12 grams of chlorphenesin carbamate resulted in slight nausea and drowsiness for about 6 hours.
- There is no known antidote. Induce vomiting or use gastric lavage and/or saline catharsis. Use supportive therapy as indicated.

Cyclobenzaprine Hydrochloride

PHARMACOLOGY
Cyclobenzaprine relieves skeletal muscle spasm without interfering with muscle function. It appears to act within the central nervous system at the brain stem. It is well absorbed after oral administration, metabolized to glucuronidelike conjugates, and eliminated quite slowly by the kidneys.

The drug is excreted in the milk of nursing mothers.

This drug is structurally and pharmacologically similar to the tricyclic antidepressants.

SPECIAL PRECAUTIONS
- Do not use in patients with a history of hypersensitivity to this drug.
- Do not administer during the acute recovery phase of myocardial infarction or to patients with arrhythmias, heart block or conduction disturbances, congestive heart failure or hyperthyroidism.
- CNS reactions noted with tricyclic antidepressants have occurred with large doses of cyclobenzaprine.
- May impair mental or physical abilities required for performance of hazardous tasks.
- Use with caution in patients with a history of urinary retention, angle-closure glaucoma, and increased intraocular pressure.
- Safe use in pregnancy, lactation, and children less than 15 years old has not been established.

ADVERSE EFFECTS
CNS EFFECTS: drowsiness, dizziness, weakness, paresthesia, insomnia, tremor, euphoria, nervousness, disorientation, confusion, headache, ataxia
RESPIRATORY EFFECTS: dyspnea

CARDIOVASCULAR EFFECTS: increased heart rate, tachycardia

URINARY TRACT EFFECTS: retention, decreased bladder tone

AUTONOMIC EFFECTS: dry mouth, and sweating

GASTROINTESTINAL EFFECTS: dyspepsia, unpleasant taste, abdominal pain, constipation, coated tongue

OPHTHALMIC EFFECTS: blurred vision

MUSCULOSKELETAL EFFECTS: myalgia, dysarthria

CLINICAL GUIDELINES

ADMINISTRATION:

• Administration for longer than 2 to 3 months is not recommended.

DRUG INTERACTIONS:

• Do not use concomitantly with MAO-inhibitors or within 14 days after their discontinuation; hyperpyretic crises, severe convulsions and deaths have occurred.

• Concurrent administration with alcohol, barbiturates, and other CNS depressants has resulted in enhanced effects.

• Use with caution in patients taking anticholinergic medication; cyclobenzaprine has atropinelike action.

• Tricyclic antidepressants may block the antihypertensive action of guanethidine and similarly acting compounds.

OVERDOSAGE/ANTIDOTE:

• Overdosage is characterized by drowsiness, hypothermia, tachycardia, and other cardiac rhythm abnormalities such as bundle branch block, impaired conduction, and congestive heart failure. Pupils may be dilated. Severe hypotension, convulsions, and coma may occur.

• No specific antidote is known. Empty stomach. Monitor cardiac function for arrhythmias; treat as necessary. Digitalis will control cardiac failure. Anticonvulsants may be given to control seizures. Dialysis is probably of no value because of low drug plasma concentrations.

Diazepam

PHARMACOLOGY, SPECIAL PRECAUTIONS, ADVERSE EFFECTS, CLINICAL GUIDELINES
See Chapter 3, page 102.

Metaxalone

PHARMACOLOGY

The mechanism of action of metaxalone has not been established, but may be due to general central nervous system depression. It is not known if this drug is found in mother's milk.

SPECIAL PRECAUTIONS

• Do not use in patients with a history of hypersensitivity to metaxalone, with a known tendency to drug-induced hematolytic or other anemias, or in patients with significantly impaired renal or hepatic function.

• Safe use in pregnancy and lactation and in children 12 years of age or less has not been established.

ADVERSE EFFECTS

CNS EFFECTS: drowsiness, dizziness, headache, nervousness, irritability

GASTROINTESTINAL EFFECTS: nausea, vomiting, gastrointestinal upset

HEPATIC EFFECTS: jaundice

HEMATOLOGIC EFFECTS: leukopenia, hemolytic anemia

ALLERGIC EFFECTS: light rash with or without pruritus

CLINICAL GUIDELINES

ADMINISTRATION:

• Monitor liver function during treatment.

DRUG INTERACTIONS:
• Elevations in cephalin flocculation tests without concurrent changes in other liver function parameters have been noted.
• False positive Benedicts' test, due to an unknown reducing substance, has been noted; a glucose-specific test will differentiate findings.

OVERDOSAGE/ANTIDOTE:
• Overdosage is characterized by an exaggeration of the adverse effects. No documented case of major toxicity has been reported.
• Empty stomach by gastric lavage. Use supportive therapy as indicated.

Methocarbamol

PHARMACOLOGY
Methocarbamol has no direct action on skeletal muscle or nerve fiber; the action may be due to general central nervous system depression. The exact mechanism of action has not been established. It is effective following oral, intravenous, or intramuscular administration.

SPECIAL PRECAUTIONS
• Do not use in patients with a history of hypersensitivity to methocarbamol.
• Safe use in pregnancy, nursing mothers, women of childbearing potential, or children less than 12 years of age has not been established.
• Methocarbamol injection should not be used in patients with known or suspected renal pathology; this is because of the polyethylene glycol 300 present.
• Use caution when administering the injectable form in patients with known or suspected epilepsy.
• Do not exceed a dose of 30 ml/day for 3 consecutive days except in the treatment of tetanus.

ADVERSE EFFECTS
CNS EFFECTS: light-headedness, dizziness, drowsiness; with the injection, vertigo, fainting, syncope
CARDIOVASCULAR EFFECTS: with injection, hypotension, thrombophlebitis, bradycardia
GASTROINTESTINAL EFFECTS: nausea, metallic taste
ALLERGIC EFFECTS: urticaria, pruritus, rash, conjunctivitis with nasal congestion, blurred vision; with injection, anaphylactoid reaction
OPHTHALMIC EFFECTS: with injection, nystagmus, diplopia, blurred vision
MUSCULOSKELETAL EFFECTS: with injection, mild muscle incoordination
LOCAL EFFECTS: with injection, pain at site of injection

CLINICAL GUIDELINES
ADMINISTRATION:
• The rate of intravenous administration should not exceed 3 ml/min or one vial in approximately 3 minutes.
• Avoid extravasation; this is a hypertonic solution.
• Blood aspirated into the syringe does not mix with the methocarbamol solution.
• The patient should be in recumbent position to reduce the incidence of adverse effects.

DRUG INTERACTIONS:
• May cause a color interference in certain screening tests for 5-hydroxy-indolacetic acid (5-HIAA) and vanilmandelic acid (VMA).
• For intravenous use, may be added to Sodium Chloride Injection or 5% Dextrose Injection.

OVERDOSAGE/ANTIDOTE:
• Overdosage with the injectable formulation is usually due to rapid intravenous administration. It may result in syncope. Convulsive seizures have been reported during intravenous administration, includ-

ing instances in known epileptics.
• In most cases, recovery has been spontaneous. In others, epinephrine, injectable steroids, and/or injectable antihistamines were employed to hasten recovery.
• Overdosage with the oral form has resulted in an exaggeration of the adverse effects.
• There is no specific antidote. Empty the stomach and use supportive therapy as indicated.

Orphenadrine Citrate

PHARMACOLOGY
Orphenadrine citrate has muscle-relaxing activity which may be related to the analgesic properties. It does not directly relax skeletal muscles which are tense or spastic. This agent has anticholinergic actions. When administered intravenously it relieves spasms for brief periods. Orphenadrine citrate is an analogue of the antihistamine, diphenhydramine.

SPECIAL PRECAUTIONS
• Do not use in patients with glaucoma, duodenal or pyloric obstruction, stenosing peptic ulcers, prostatic hypertrophy, obstruction of the bladder neck, cardiospasm, or myasthenia gravis.
• Do not use in patients with a history of hypersensitivity to orphenadrine citrate.
• Safe use in pregnancy or in children has not been established.
• Patients may experience light-headedness, dizziness, or syncope; these effects are usually transient.
• Use with caution in patients with cardiac decompensation, coronary insufficiency, cardiac arrhythmias, or tachycardia.

ADVERSE EFFECTS
CNS EFFECTS: weakness, headache, dizziness, drowsiness, hallucinations, agitation, tremor; mental confusion in elderly patients rarely
CARDIOVASCULAR EFFECTS: tachycardia
AUTONOMIC EFFECTS: dry mouth
GASTROINTESTINAL EFFECTS: nausea, vomiting, constipation, gastric irritation
HEMATOLOGIC EFFECTS: aplastic anemia very rarely
ALLERGIC EFFECTS: hypersensitivity reactions; urticaria rarely; anaphylactic reactions
DERMATOLOGIC EFFECTS: pruritus, dermatoses
OPHTHALMIC EFFECTS: blurred vision, dilatation of pupils, increased ocular tension

CLINICAL GUIDELINES
ADMINISTRATION:
• Caution patients that drowsiness may occur which may interfere with driving a motor vehicle or operating machinery.
OVERDOSAGE/ANTIDOTE:
• Overdosage with the oral form may result in an exaggeration of the adverse effects.
• The gastric irritation produced may result in evacuation of the stomach. If not, empty stomach by gastric lavage. Treat supportively.

Peripherally Acting Skeletal Muscle Relaxant

Dantrolene Sodium

PHARMACOLOGY
Dantrolene sodium is a direct acting muscle relaxant. After oral administration absorption is slow but consistent, producing skeletal muscle relaxation by interfering with muscle contraction. Central nervous system effects may also occur. Dantrolene sodium is absorbed incompletely and slow-

ly following oral administration and is probably metabolized in the liver.

SPECIAL PRECAUTIONS

• Hepatotoxicity, including fatal hepatitis, has occurred in patients receiving dantrolene sodium for 60 days or longer; fatal and nonfatal liver disorders have been reported.
• If benefits are not evident within 45 days, discontinue therapy.
• Do not use in patients with active hepatic disease such as acute hepatitis and active cirrhosis, or with a history of previous liver disease or dysfunction.
• Do not use in patients where spasticity is utilized to sustain upright posture and balance in locomotion or whenever spasticity is localized to obtain or maintain increased function.
• Use with particular caution in females and in patients over 35 years of age in view of apparent greater likelihood of drug-induced, potentially fatal hepatocellular disease in these groups.
• Safe use in pregnancy, in women of childbearing potential, or in nursing mothers, or in children under 5 years of age, has not been established.
• Use with caution in patients with impaired pulmonary function, particularly in those with obstructive pulmonary diseases, and in patients with severely impaired cardiac function due to myocardial disease.
• Caution patients to avoid exposure to sunlight because of possible photosensitivity reaction.

ADVERSE EFFECTS

CNS EFFECTS: drowsiness, dizziness, weakness, general malaise, fatigue, speech disturbance, seizure, headache, light-headedness, insomnia, mental depression; also mental confusion, increased nervousness
RESPIRATORY EFFECTS: feeling of suffocation

CARDIOVASCULAR EFFECTS: tachycardia, erratic blood pressure, phlebitis
URINARY TRACT EFFECTS: frequency, crystalluria, incontinence/nocturia, difficult urination and/or retention
AUTONOMIC EFFECTS: sweating, chills, and fever
GASTROINTESTINAL EFFECTS: diarrhea may be severe, necessitating withdrawal; constipation, gastrointestinal bleeding, anorexia, swallowing difficulty, gastric irritation, abdominal cramps, alteration of taste
METABOLIC AND ENDOCRINE EFFECTS: difficult erection
HEPATIC EFFECTS: hepatitis
DERMATOLOGIC EFFECTS: abnormal hair growth, acnelike rash, pruritus, urticaria, eczematoid eruption
OPHTHALMIC EFFECTS: visual disturbances, diplopia, excessive tearing
MUSCULOSKELETAL EFFECTS: myalgia and backache

CLINICAL GUIDELINES

ADMINISTRATION:
• Monitor hepatic function including frequent determinations of SGOT or SGPT; if abnormalities occur, discontinue therapy.
• Caution patients against driving a car and particularly those engaged in hazardous occupations while taking dantrolene sodium.
• CNS adverse effects may be minimized by beginning therapy with a low dose and increasing gradually until an optimal regimen is established.
EFFECTS:
• Photosensitivity reactions may be evoked.
DRUG INTERACTIONS:
• Interaction with estrogen therapy has not been established but hepatotoxicity has occurred more often in women over 35 years of age receiving concomitant estrogen therapy.

• Concurrent administration of tranquilizing agents may result in excessive drowsiness.

• Neither phenobarbital nor diazepam appears to effect dantrolene sodium metabolism.

OVERDOSAGE/ANTIDOTE:

• Overdosage is characterized by flaccid muscle paralysis.

• For acute overdosage, general supportive measures should be employed along with immediate gastric lavage. Administer intravenous fluids in fairly large quantities to avert the possibility of crystalluria. Maintain adequate airway and use artificial respiration. Monitor electrocardiogram.

• No experience has been reported with dialysis.

Curarelike Agents

Decamethonium Bromide
Succinylcholine Chloride

PHARMACOLOGY

The curarelike agents, decamethonium bromide and suscinylcholine chloride, ultra-short-acting muscle relaxants, block neural transmission at the myoneural junction by depolarization. A flaccid paralysis of skeletal muscle is produced within a few minutes after intravenous administration. The effects of a single paralyzing dose generally disappear within 10 minutes. Although succinylcholine chloride may be administered intramuscularly or intravenously, intravenous administration is more predictable. These agents have no known effect on consciousness, the pain threshold, or cerebration; they should only be used during adequate anesthesia.

SPECIAL PRECAUTIONS

• These drugs should be used only by physicians familiar with their actions, characteristics, and hazards, and those skilled in the management of artificial respiration. Facilities for endotracheal intubation and for providing adequate ventilation of the patient must be instantly available. It may be necessary to control or assist respiration.

• Do not use in patients with a history of hypersensitivity to succinylcholine chloride or decamethonium bromide.

• Safe use in pregnancy has not been established with respect to the possible adverse effects upon fetal development.

• Prolonged respiratory depression or apnea because of low or abnormal variants of plasma cholinesterase may follow use of succinylchloine.

• Administer with extreme caution and at minimal dosages to patients with severe liver disease, severe anemia, malnutrition, severe dehydration, changes in body temperature, exposure to neurotoxic insecticides or those receiving antimalarial drugs because of low level of plasma cholinesterase.

• Administer with great caution to patients with severe burns, those recovering from severe trauma, those suffering from electrolyte imbalance, those receiving quinine, those who have been digitalized recently or who may have digitalis toxicity, as serious cardiac arrhythmias or cardiac arrest may occur.

• Use great caution in patients with pre-existing hyperkalemia or who are paraplegic, have suffered spinal neuraxis injury, or who have dystrophic neuromuscular disease, as such patients tend to become severely hyperkalemic when decamethonium or succinylcholine are given.

• Use with caution in patients undergoing ocular surgery and in patients with glaucoma, fractures, or muscle spasms; the muscle fasciculations may cause additional trauma.

ADVERSE EFFECTS

CNS EFFECTS: hyperthermia

RESPIRATORY EFFECTS: depression, apnea

CARDIOVASCULAR EFFECTS: tachycardia, hypertension, hypotension, arrhythmias, bradycardia, cardiac arrest

AUTONOMIC EFFECTS: excessive salivation

HEMATOLOGIC EFFECTS: myoglobinemia

ALLERGIC EFFECTS: hypersensitivity rarely

OPHTHALMIC EFFECTS: increased intraocular pressure

MUSCULOSKELETAL EFFECTS: profound and prolonged muscle relaxation, muscle fasciculation, postoperative muscle pain

CLINICAL GUIDELINES

ADMINISTRATION:
- Monitor patient's temperature continuously since malignant hyperthermia may be triggered by these drugs.

EFFECTS:
- Tachyphylaxis may occur after repeated doses.
- If other muscle relaxants are used concurrently, the possibility of a synergistic or antagonistic effect should be considered.
- In patients with severely impaired renal function or hypotension, the effects may be prolonged.

DRUG INTERACTIONS:
- Do not mix with short-acting barbiturates in the same syringe or administer simultaneously during intravenous infusion through the same needle. Free barbituric acid may be precipitated or succinylcholine hydrolyzed.
- Do not administer concurrently drugs such as neostigmine or echothiophate iodide, which inhibit plasma cholinesterase or compete with succinylcholine for the enzyme, such as procaine administered intravenously.
- Compatible with procaine or thiopental sodium; may be mixed without precipitate formation.

OVERDOSAGE/ANTIDOTE:
- Overdosage is characterized by apnea or prolonged muscle paralysis.
- Treat with controlled respiration. Edro-phonium or neostigmine preceded by atropine may be used if the primary depolarizing block has become a nondepolarizing block. Small repeated doses of neostigmine may shorten the action of succinylcholine or decamethonium. Use supportive therapy as indicated.

Gallamine Triethiodide
Metocurine Iodide
Pancuronium Bromide
Tubocurarine Chloride

PHARMACOLOGY

The curarelike preparations which are nondepolarizing neuromuscular blocking agents include metocurine iodide, gallamine triethiodide, tubocurarine chloride, and pancuronium bromide. They block impulses to skeletal muscles at the myoneural junction. Following intravenous administration, flaccid paralysis occurs within a few minutes and may last for as long as 90 minutes. Repeated doses may result in a cumulative effect. These drugs are excreted by the kidneys. Cerebration and consciousness are not affected.

SPECIAL PRECAUTIONS

- Do not use in patients with a history of hypersensitivity to these drugs.
- Do not use in patients in whom histamine release is a definite hazard.
- These drugs should be used only by physicians experienced in the technique of artificial respiration and the administration of oxygen under positive pressure.
- Use with extreme caution in patients with known myasthenia gravis.
- Safe use in pregnancy has not been established.
- Use with caution in patients with respiratory depression or with renal, hepatic, or pulmonary disease.

• Severe renal disease or hypotension may result in a prolonged action.

ADVERSE EFFECTS
RESPIRATORY EFFECTS: depression, apnea
CARDIOVASCULAR EFFECTS: depression, hypotension
GASTROINTESTINAL EFFECTS: salivation
ALLERGIC EFFECTS: hypersensitivity reactions rarely
DERMATOLOGIC EFFECTS: with pancuronium bromide, a transient rash occasionally
MUSCULOSKELETAL EFFECTS: profound and prolonged muscle relaxation

CLINICAL GUIDELINES
ADMINISTRATION:
• Rapid intravenous administration may produce increased release of histamine with decreased respiratory capacity due to bronchospasm and paralysis of respiratory muscles.
EFFECTS:
• Hypotension due to ganglionic blockage may occur following administration of large doses.
• Neonates are especially sensitive to nondepolarizing neuromuscular blocking agents during the first month of life.
DRUG INTERACTIONS:
• Concurrent administration of general anesthetics (halothane, ether, enflurance, methoxyflurane) and certain antibiotics (neomycin, streptomycin, kanamycin, gentamicin), as well as abnormal states such as acidosis, electrolyte imbalance, and neuromuscular disease, has caused potentiation.
• When administering concurrently with a barbiturate solution (with a high pH such as methohexital sodium of thiopental sodium), precipitation may occur. Administer each component from a separate syringe.
OVERDOSAGE/ANTIDOTE:
• Overdosage usually results in prolonged apnea with its attendant hazards due to hypoxia; hypotension, skeletal muscle weakness, decreased respiratory reserve, low tidal volume, or apnea also may occur.
• Edrophonium or neostigmine may antagonize the skeletal muscle relaxant action of metacurine iodide. Neostigmine should be accompanied or preceded by an injection of atropine sulfate or its equivalent. Ventilate manually or mechanically; maintain airway until recovery of normal respiration is complete.

Hexafluorenium Bromide

PHARMACOLOGY
Hexafluoronium bromide, a plasma cholinesterase inhibitor, is used as an adjunct to succinylcholine to prolong its effect. It prolongs the neuromuscular blockage of succinylcholine and obviates the muscular fasciculations which may occur when succinylcholine is administered alone. It has no effect on consciousness, cerebration, or pain threshold. The duration of effect is from 20 to 30 minutes.

SPECIAL PRECAUTIONS
• Do not use in patients with a history of hypersensitivity to it or to bromides.
• Do not administer unless adequate facilities are available for intubation, artificial respiration, and oxygen therapy.
• Safe use in pregnancy has not been established.

ADVERSE EFFECTS
CNS EFFECTS: hypothermia
RESPIRATORY EFFECTS: depression, apnea, bronchospasm
CARDIOVASCULAR EFFECTS: bradycardia, tachycardia, hypertension, hypotension, cardiac arrest, arrthythmia
GASTROINTESTINAL EFFECTS: salivation
OPHTHALMIC EFFECTS: increased intraocular pressure

CLINICAL GUIDELINES

ADMINISTRATION:
• Administer only after unconsciousness has been induced.

DRUG INTERACTIONS:
• If other muscle relaxants are adminis-

tered concurrently, the possibility of synergistic or antagonistic actions should be considered.

OVERDOSAGE/ANTIDOTE:
   See *Succinylcholine*, page 503.

Skeletal Muscle Stimulants (Anticholinesterase Muscle Stimulants)

GENERAL CLINICAL USES

The anticholinesterase or parasympathomimetic muscle stimulants are used primarily for diagnosis and treatment of myasthenia gravis. Edrophonium chloride is useful whenever a curare antagonist is needed to reverse neuromuscular block by curare, tubocurarine, gallamine triethiodide, or dimethyl tubocurarine. It is not effective against decamethonium bromide or succinylcholine chloride. It also may be used for differential diagnosis of myasthenia gravis and as an adjunct in the evaluation of treatment requirements in this disease.

SPECIFIC PRODUCTS AND DOSAGES

GENERIC NAME	TRADE NAME	ROUTE OF ADMIN.	USUAL DOSAGE	
			ADULTS	CHILDREN
ambenonium chloride	MYTELASE	po	Individualize; 5–75 mg tid or qid; maximum dose 200 mg/day	Not established
edrophonium chloride	TENSILON	iv/im	2–10 mg; maximum dose 40 mg	**Infants up to 75 lb:** initial 1 mg may increase to 5 mg; **over 75 lb:** initial 2 mg may increase to 10 mg
guanidine hydrochloride	(G)*	po	10–35 mg/kg/day divided in 3–4 doses	Not established

*(G) designates availability as a generic product.

(continued facing page)

GENERIC NAME	TRADE NAME	ROUTE OF ADMIN.	USUAL DOSAGE	
			ADULTS	**CHILDREN**
neostigmine bromide	(G) PROSTIGMIN Bromide	po	15–375 mg/day in divided doses; average dose 150 mg/day	Not established
neostigmine methylsulfate	(G) PROSTIGMIN Methylsulfate	sc/im iv	0.5–2.5 mg 0.5–2.0 mg	Not established Not established
pyridostigmine bromide	MESTINON	po	600–1500 mg/day spaced to provide maximum strength as needed	Not established
		iv/im	1/30 oral dose	**Neonates:** 0.05–0.15 mg/kg

Ambenonium Chloride
Edrophonium Chloride
Guanidine Hydrochloride
Neostigmine Bromide
Neostigmine Methylsulfate
Pyridostigmine Bromide

PHARMACOLOGY

These drugs inhibit the destruction of acetylcholine by cholinesterase, thereby facilitating transmission of impulses across the myoneuronal junction. The drugs differ primarily in their duration of action and adverse effects.

Pyridostigmine bromide and ambenonium chloride have a longer duration of action than neostigmine, and they produce fewer side effects. Edrophonium has a rapid onset of action and shorter duration of action. Orally administered products act more slowly than those administered parenterally.

SPECIAL PRECAUTIONS

• Do not use in patients with a history of hypersensitivity to anticholinesterase agents.

• Do not use compounds containing bromide in patients with a previous history of reaction to bromides.
• Do not use in patients with intestinal or urinary obstruction of the mechanical type.
• Use with caution in patients with bronchial asthma or cardiac dysrhythmias.
• Safe use in pregnancy and lactation has not been established.
• Patients may develop "anti-cholinesterase insensitivity" for brief or prolonged periods.

ADVERSE EFFECTS

CNS EFFECTS: convulsions, dysphonia
RESPIRATORY EFFECTS: increased tracheobronchial secretions, laryngospasm, bronchiolar constriction, paralysis of muscles of respiration, central respiratory paralysis
CARDIOVASCULAR EFFECTS: bradycardia, cardiac standstill, arrhythmia, fall in cardiac output leading to hypotension
URINARY TRACT EFFECTS: frequency, incontinence
AUTONOMIC EFFECTS: diaphoresis
GASTROINTESTINAL EFFECTS: increased salivary, gastric, and intestinal secretion; nau-

sea, vomiting, increased peristalsis, diarrhea, abdominal cramps, dysphagia

OPHTHALMIC EFFECTS: increased lacrimation, pupillary constriction, spasms of accommodation, dyplopia, conjunctival hyperemia

MUSCULOSKELETAL EFFECTS: dysarthria, weakness, fasciculations

CLINICAL GUIDELINES

DRUG INTERACTIONS:
- Certain antibiotics, especially neomycin, streptomycin, and kanamycin, have a mild but definite nondepolarizing blocking action which may accentuate neuromuscular block; dosage adjustment may be required.
- In patients with symptoms of myasthenia gravis who are receiving other anticholinergic drugs, symptoms of anticholinesterase overdose (cholinergic crisis) may mimic underdosage (muscular weakness); the patient's condition may worsen.

- Administer cautiously with anticholinergic drugs which may slow down intestinal motility.
- Concurrent administration of atropine and ambenonium chloride results in excessive gastrointestinal stimulation.
- Do not administer to patients receiving mecamylamine, a ganglionic blocking agent.

OVERDOSAGE/ANTIDOTE:
- Overdosage is characterized by severe cholinergic reactions, namely, muscle weakness, including muscles of respiration, which may result in death. Muscarinic symptoms, namely, nausea, vomiting, diarrhea, sweating, increased bronchial and salivary secretions, may occur. The airway may be obstructed by bronchial secretions.
- Atropine sulfate is the antidote; doses may reach 1.2 mg intravenously initially. Pralidoxime chloride, a cholinesterase reactivator, may be given intravenously.

Drugs affecting the reproductive tract in the male and female

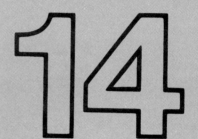

INTRODUCTION

The drugs affecting the reproductive tract in both the male and female include anti-infective agents specific for infections of the reproductive tract and the hormone preparations, both natural and synthetic, which control, prevent, or enhance fertility.

SPECIFIC THERAPEUTIC CLASSIFICATION

Drugs affecting the reproductive tract will be separated into the following groups:

1. Abortifacients: dinoprostone, dinoprost tromethamine
2. Androgens: synthetic and natural hormones commercially available
3. Anti-infective agents products used topically in vaginal douches, gels, and inserts, and in urethral inserts
4. Contraceptives: locally applied prod-

ucts—creams, foams, jellies, and suppositories; also the orally administered contraceptive agents consisting of a combination of an estrogen and a progestogen

5. Estrogens and progestogens: synthetic and natural hormones commercially available

6. Fertility agents: clomiphene citrate and menotropins which induce ovulation; also chorionic gonadotropin

7. Uterine muscle stimulants (oxytocic agents): oxytocin, a synthetic posterior pituitary hormone, and the ergot derivatives which stimulate uterine contractions

Abortifacients

GENERAL CLINICAL USES
The abortifacients are used for aborting pregnancy. Dinoprost trimethamine, administered intra-amniotically, is used for aborting second trimester pregnancy. Dinoprostone, administered as a vaginal suppository, is used for termination of pregnancy from the twelfth gestational week through the second trimester; for evacuation of the uterine contents in the management of missed abortion or intrauterine fetal deaths up to 28 weeks of gestational age; and in the management of nonmetastatic gestational trophoblastic disease.

SPECIFIC PRODUCTS AND DOSAGES

GENERIC NAME	TRADE NAME	ROUTE OF ADMIN.	USUAL DOSAGE
dinoprostone	PROSTIN E$_2$	intravaginal (suppository)	20 mg; repeat every 3–5 hr. until abortion occurs
dinoprost tromethamine	PROSTIN F$_2$ alpha	intra-amniotic	40 mg

Dinoprostone

PHARMACOLOGY
Dinoprostone, administered intravaginally, stimulates contraction of the myometrium similar to that seen during labor. It is not established with certainty that action results from a direct effect of the drug on the myometrium. The smooth muscle of the gastrointestinal tract is also stimulated.

SPECIAL PRECAUTIONS
• Do not use in patients with a history of hypersensitivity to dinoprostone or in pa-

tients with acute pelvic inflammatory disease.
- For use only by medically trained personnel in the hospital.
- May result in birth of a live-born fetus, particularly as gestation approaches the end of the second trimester.
- Any failed pregnancy termination should be completed by some other means.
- Dinoprostone-induced abortion sometimes may be incomplete; take measures to assure complete abortion.
- Use with caution in patients with a history of asthma, hypo- or hypertension, cardiovascular disease, renal disease, hepatic disease, anemia, jaundice, diabetes, or epilepsy.
- Use with caution in presence of cervicitis, infected endocervical lesions, or acute vaginitis.
- When a pregnancy is diagnosed as a missed abortion and is electively interrupted with dinoprostone, uterine death should be confirmed with a negative pregnancy test for chorionic gonadotropin activity. When a pregnancy involving late fetal intrauterine death is interrupted with dinoprostone, fetal death should be confirmed prior to treatment.

ADVERSE EFFECTS

CNS EFFECTS: transient pyrexia, headache, chills, shivering, dizziness, tension, tremor
RESPIRATORY EFFECTS: tightness in chest, coughing, wheezing
CARDIOVASCULAR EFFECTS: transient diastolic blood pressure decrease, chest pain, cardiac arrhythmia
AUTONOMIC EFFECTS: flushing, hot flashes, diaphoresis
GASTROINTESTINAL EFFECTS: vomiting, diarrhea, nausea
METABOLIC AND ENDOCRINE EFFECTS: vaginal pain, breast tenderness, dehydration, vaginismus

DERMATOLOGIC EFFECTS: rash, and skin discoloration
MUSCULOSKELETAL EFFECTS: backache, point inflammation or pain, arthralgia, muscle cramp or pain, nocturnal leg cramps, myalgia, stiff neck
OPTHALMIC EFFECTS: blurred vision, eye pain

CLINICAL GUIDELINES

ADMINISTRATION:
- Insert suppository high into the vagina.
- Patient should remain supine for 10 minutes after insertion.
- Additional intravaginal administration of each subsequent suppository should be at 3 to 5-hour intervals until abortion occurs.

Dinoprost Tromethamine

PHARMACOLOGY

When administered intra-amniotically, dinoprost stimulates the myometrium of the gravid uterus to contract. These contractions are sufficient to produce evacuation of the uterus in the majority of cases.

SPECIAL PRECAUTIONS

- Do not use in patients with a history of hypersensitivity to dinoprost or to patients with pelvic inflammatory disease.
- Use should be limited to medically trained personnel in a hospital.
- Failed pregnancy termination should be completed with other means.
- There exists the possibility that a live-born fetus may occur, particularly as gestational age approaches the end of the second trimester.
- Induced abortion sometimes may be incomplete; assure complete abortion. If treatment is not successful, delay use of hypertonic saline until uterus is no longer contracting.

• Use with caution in patients with a history of asthma, glaucoma, hypertension, cardiovascular disease, or epilepsy.

ADVERSE EFFECTS

CNS EFFECTS: pain, headache, backache, dizziness, epileptiform convulsion, paresthesia, anxiety, drowsiness, malaise

RESPIRATORY EFFECTS: dyspnea, hyperventilation, chest constriction, bronchospasm, rales, hiccups

CARDIOVASCULAR EFFECTS: bradycardia, hypertension, vasomotor symptoms, vasovagal symptoms, second degree heart block

URINARY TRACT EFFECTS: retention, dysuria, hematuria

AUTONOMIC EFFECTS: flushing, chills

GASTROINTESTINAL EFFECTS: vomiting, nausea, and diarrhea

METABOLIC AND ENDOCRINE EFFECTS: posterior cervical perforation, endometritis, breast tenderness, burning sensation in breast, uterine rupture, polydipsia

OPHTHALMIC EFFECTS: burning sensation in eye, diplopia

CLINICAL GUIDELINES

ADMINISTRATION:

• Withdraw at least 1 ml of amniotic fluid before administering drug.

• Inject slowly; do not inject medication in case of a bloody tap.

• If abortion has not been established in 24 hours, an additional 10–40 mg may be administered.

EFFECTS:

• Dinoprost stimulates the gastrointestinal tract, causing vomiting and/or diarrhea.

DRUG INTERACTIONS:

• Concomitant administration of intravenous oxytocin should be used with caution in the absence of adequate cervical dilation; cervical perforation has occurred in a few primigravidas.

Androgens

GENERAL CLINICAL USES

Androgens are used in the male to treat impotence due to androgenic deficiency, eunuchoidism and eunuchism, male climacteric, symptoms when due to androgen deficiency, postpubertal cryptorchidism with evidence of hypogonadism.

In the female, the androgens are used in the prevention of postpartum breast engorgement and pain, palliation of advancing inoperable breast cancer, and in androgen-responsive tumors proven to be hormone dependent.

The androgens also have anabolic activity. For detailed information concerning this use, see Chapter 15, page 540.

SPECIFIC PRODUCTS AND DOSAGES

GENERIC NAME	TRADE NAME	ROUTE OF ADMIN.	USUAL DOSAGE
fluoxymesterone	HALOTESTIN ORA-TESTRYL	po	2–10 mg daily; individualize therapy
methyltestosterone	(G)* ANDROID-5 METANDREN Linguet	buccal	5–40 mg daily
	(G) ORETON Methyl	po	10–80 mg daily
testosterone	(G) ORETON Pellets	sc implant	150–450 mg for 3–4 months; individualize dosage
		im	10–50 mg 2–3x/week
testosterone cypionate	DEPO-TESTOSTERONE MALOGEN CYP	im	100–400 mg every 4–6 weeks
testosterone enanthate	(G) DELATESTRYL	im	100–400 mg every 4 weeks
testosterone propionate	ORETON Propionate Buccal Tabs	buccal	5–40 mg daily
	(G) NEO-HOMBREOL	im	20–100 mg 2–4 times/week

*(G) designates availability as a generic product.

PHARMACOLOGY

The androgens, including naturally occurring testosterone, stimulate and maintain the secondary sexual characteristics associated with the adult male. In addition, the androgens influence closure of epiphyseal lines and reduce urinary excretion of nitrogen, sodium, potassium, chloride, phosphorus, and water in males and some females.

Testosterone propionate is an active androgen which may be administered buccally, thereby permitting the testosterone to be absorbed directly into the venous circulation. Methyltestosterone is a short-acting androgen for oral administration, as is fluoxymesterone. Testosterone enanthate and testosterone cypionate are long-acting androgens (2–4 weeks); they are absorbed slowly and the sustained effect resembles closely the endogenous production of testosterone.

SPECIAL PRECAUTIONS
• Do not use in patients with known or suspected carcinoma of the prostate or carcinoma of the male breast, severe liver disease, or prostatic hypertrophy with obstructive symptoms.
• Do not use in pregnancy or in breast-feeding mothers.
• Watch female patients for signs of

virulization such as hoarseness or deepening of the voice, oily skin, acne, hirsutism, enlarged clitoris, stimulation of libido, and menstrual irregularities.
• If SGOT increases or BSP retention increases, or if cholestatic hepatitis with jaundice occurs, discontinue therapy.
• Prolonged administration may result in sodium and fluid retention, especially in patients with compromised cardiac reserve or renal disease.
• In treating males for climacteric symptoms, avoid stimulation to point of increasing nervous, mental, and physical activities that are beyond the patient's cardiovascular capacity.
• If priapism or other signs of excessive sexual stimulation develop, discontinue therapy.
• In the male, prolonged administration or excessive dosage may cause inhibition of testicular function.
• Hypersensitivity and gynecomastia may occur rarely.
• Concomitant administration of ACTH or adrenal steroids may add to the edema.
• Use cautiously in patients with a history of myocardial infarction or coronary artery disease since serum cholesterol levels may increase.

ADVERSE EFFECTS

CNS EFFECTS: sleeplessness, chills
URINARY TRACT EFFECTS: irritability of urinary bladder
GASTROINTESTINAL EFFECTS: with oral preparations, nausea, vomiting, diarrhea
METABOLIC AND ENDOCRINE EFFECTS: oligospermia, decreased ejaculatory volume, hypercalcemia, gynecomastia, sodium and water retention, priapism, virilization; serum cholesterol may increase or decrease
HEPATIC EFFECTS: cholestatic hepatitis with jaundice
HEMATOLOGIC EFFECTS: leukopenia

ALLERGIC EFFECTS: dermatitis, anaphylactoid reactions
DERMATOLOGIC EFFECTS: flushing of skin, acne, rash
LOCAL EFFECTS: with intramuscular preparations—urticaria at injection site, postinjection induration, furunculosis; with pellets—slough following implantation.

CLINICAL GUIDELINES

ADMINISTRATION:
• Buccal tablets should be placed under the tongue or in the upper or lower buccal pouch between the gum and cheek. Advise patients to avoid eating, drinking, chewing, or smoking while tablet is in place.
EFFECTS:
• Hypercalcemia may occur, particularly during any therapy for metastatic breast cancer.
• Testicular function may be inhibited and ejaculatory volume decreased with high androgen doses.
• Monitor serum cholesterol levels during therapy.
DRUG INTERACTIONS:
• Methandrostenolone decreases metabolism of oxyphenbutazone; a longer and more unpredictable response is obtained; avoid concurrent administration.
• Increases occur in BSP retention and SGOT level.
• PBI may decrease.
• May increase sensitivity to anticoagulants; dosage of anticoagulant may have to be decreased to maintain prothrombin time and the desired therapeutic level.
• Concomitant administration of corticosteroids may enhance edema resulting from androgen use.
• May alter glucose tolerance test; insulin or oral hypoglycemic agent dosage may be adjusted accordingly.
• Metapyrone test results may be altered.
• Decrease in protein bound iodine, de-

crease in thyroid binding capacity and radi-oactive iodine uptake, increase in T_3 up-take.

• Increase clotting factors II, V, VII, and X

• Decreased creatinine and creatine ex-cretion lasting up to 2 weeks.

• Increased 17-ketosteroid excretion.

OVERDOSAGE/ANTIDOTE:

• Overdosage is characterized by an exag-geration of the masculinizing adverse ef-fects.

• There is no specific antidote; discontinue or reduce dosage.

Anti-Infective Agents

GENERAL CLINICAL USES

Infections of the male and female genital tracts may be treated by systemic or local anti-infective agents. The anti-infective agents administered systemi-cally to treat infections of the reproductive tract are reviewed in Chapter 2, *Anti-Infective Agents.*

Topically administered products which have specific formulations for use in this area are included and are arranged by active ingredient.

SPECIFIC PRODUCTS AND USES

GENERIC NAME	TRADE NAME	USES
candicidin	CANDEPTIN Vaginal Capsules, Vaginal Ointment, Vaginal Tablets VANOBID Vaginal Tablets, Vaginal Ointment	Vulvovaginal candidiasis (moniliasis)
clotrimazole	GYNE-LOTRIMIN Vaginal Tablets	Vulvovaginal candidiasis (moniliasis)
furazolidone	FUROXONE TRICOFURAN*	Vaginitis
gentian violet	GVS Vaginal Insert HYVA Vaginal Tablets	Vulvovaginal candidiasis
metronidazole	FLAGYL Tablets	Oral administration for trichomoniasis in the male and female

*Contains more than one active ingredient.

(continued overleaf)

GENERIC NAME	TRADE NAME	USES
miconazole nitrate	MONISTAT 7 Vaginal Cream	Vulvovaginal candidiasis (moniliasis)
nystatin	KOROSTATIN Vaginal Tablets MYCOSTATIN Vaginal Tablets NILSTAT Vaginal Tablets	Vulvovaginal candidiasis (moniliasis)
oxytetracycline hydrochloride	TERRAMYCIN* with Polymyxin B Vaginal Tablets	Chronic vaginitis due to susceptible bacteria (gram-negative or gram-positive)
polymyxin B sulfate	TERRAMYCIN* with Polymyxin B Vaginal Tablets	Chronic vaginitis due to susceptible bacteria (gram-negative), including *Pseudomonas aeruginosa*
povidone-iodine	BETADINE Vaginal Gel, Douche	Vaginitis, vaginal moniliasis, *Trichomonas vaginalis* vaginitis
sulfanilamide	AVC Cream, Suppositories BENEGYN* Vaginal Cream SULFAMAL* VAGITROL Cream, Suppositories	Vulvovaginitis due to *Trichomonas vaginalis, Candida albicans, Hemophilus vaginalis*
sulfathiazole, sulfacetamide, sulfabenzamide	SULTRIN* Triple Sulfa Vaginal Tablets	*Hemophilus vaginalis* vaginitis
sulfisoxazole	VAGILIA* Vaginal Cream	Vaginitis due to trichomonads, *C. albicans,* and bacteria

*Contains more than one active ingredient.

PHARMACOLOGY

Effective concentrations (bactericidal or bacteriostatic, fungicidal or fungistatic) of the anti-infective agents formulated for use in the male and female reproductive tracts are attainable without producing undesirable effects. Absorption of these agents through intact mucous membranes is minimal. However, because of the irregular structure of the vagina, even and complete distribution may be difficult to achieve and thereby limit the effectiveness of the product.

Detailed information about each anti-infective product may be found in the following locations:

Candicidin

See Chapter 2, page 74.

Clotrimazole

See Chapter 2, page 69.

Furazolidone

See Chapter 2, page 46.

Gentian Violet

See Chapter 2, page 75.

Metronidazole

See Chapter 2, page 97.

Miconazole Nitrate/Nystatin

See Chapter 2, page 72.

Oxytetracycline Hydrochloride

See Chapter 2, page 61.

Polymyxin B Sulfate

See Chapter 2, page 52.

Povidone Iodine

See Chapter 9, page 424.

Sulfabenzamide
Sulfacetamide Sodium
Sulfanilamide
Sulfathiazole
Sulfisoxazole

See Chapter 2, page 56.

SPECIAL PRECAUTIONS
• Do not use in patients with a history of hypersensitivity to each agent.
• Discontinue use of gentian violet if acute chemical vulvovaginitis develops.
• Intractable candidiasis may be a pre-

senting symptom of unrecognized diabetes mellitus.
• Safe use of sulfonamides in pregnancy has not been established.
• Use sulfonamides with caution in patients with impaired hepatic or renal disease, severe allergy, or bronchial asthma.
• Do not use metronidazole in patients with a history of blood dyscrasias, organic disease of the central nervous system, or during the first trimester of pregnancy.
• Discontinue if irritation develops.

ADVERSE EFFECTS
For systemic effects which might occur with absorption of these compounds, refer to Chapter 2, page 10.
LOCAL EFFECTS:
• gentian violet—purple staining on clothing and/or skin
• sulfonamides—mild, transient stinging or burning
• miconazole nitrate—burning, itching, irritation, pelvic cramps, hives, skin rash, headache
• candicidin—irritation rarely
• clotrimazole—mild burning, rash, lower abdominal cramps, slight urinary frequency, burning or irritation in sexual partner rarely

Contraceptives, Oral and Local

GENERAL CLINICAL USES
Contraceptives prevent impregnation of the ovum. They may be products applied topically, preventing the entrance of sperm into the fallopian tubes and uterus, or products administered systemically, the oral contraceptives, which prevent impregnation or nidation.

SPECIFIC PRODUCTS AND DOSAGES: ORAL CONTRACEPTIVES

GENERIC NAME	TRADE NAME
norethindrone 0.35 mg	MICRONOR NOR-QD
norethindrone 0.5 mg/ethinyl estradiol 0.035 mg	BREVICON
norethindrone 0.5 mg/ethinyl estradiol 0.035 mg/inert	BREVICON 28 days
norethindrone 1 mg/mestranol 0.05 mg	NORINYL 1 50 21 days
norethindrone 1 mg/mestranol 0.05 mg/inert	NORINYL 1 50 28 days
norethindrone 1 mg/mestranol 0.08 mg	NORINYL 1 80 21 days
norethindrone 1 mg/mestranol 0.08 mg/inert	NORINYL 1 80 28 days
norethindrone 2 mg/mestranol 0.1 mg	NORINYL 2 mg
norethindrone 2 mg/mestranol 0.10 mg	ORTHO-NOVUM 2 mg 21
norethindrone 10 mg/mestranol 0.06 mg	ORTHO-NOVUM 10 mg
norethindrone 1 mg/mestranol 0.05 mg	ORTHO-NOVUM 1/50 21
norethindrone 1 mg/mestranol 0.05 mg/inert	ORTHO-NOVUM 1/50 28
norethindrone 1 mg/mestranol 0.08 mg	ORTHO-NOVUM 1/80 21
norethindrone 1 mg/mestranol 0.08 mg/inert	ORTHO-NOVUM 1/80 28
norethindrone acetate 1 mg/ethinyl estradiol 20 mcg	LOESTRIN 1/20
norethindrone acetate 1 mg/ethinyl estradiol 20 mcg/ferrous fumerate 75 mg	LOESTRIN Fe 1/20
norethindrone acetate 1 mg/ethinyl estradiol 30 mcg	LOESTRIN 21 1.5/30
norethindrone acetate 1.5 mg/ethinyl estradiol 30 mcg/ferrous fumerate 75 mg	LOESTRIN 1.5/30
norethindrone acetate 1 mg/ethinyl estradiol 50 mcg	NORLESTRIN 21 1/50
norethindrone acetate 2.5 mg/ethinyl estradiol 50 mcg	NORLESTRIN 21 2.5/50
norethindrone acetate 2.5 mg/ethinyl estradiol 50 mcg/ferrous fumerate 75 mg	NORLESTRIN Fe 2.5/50
norethindrone acetate 1 mg/ethinyl estradiol 50 mcg/ferrous fumerate 75 mg	NORLESTRIN Fe 1/50
norgestrel 0.075 mg	OVRETTE
norgestrel 0.5 mg/ethinyl estradiol 0.05 mg	OVRAL
norgestrel 0.5 mg/ethinyl estradiol 0.05 mg/inert	ORVAL 28
norgestrel 0.3 mg/ethinyl estradiol 0.03 mg	LO/OVRAL
norgestrel 0.3 mg/ethinyl estradiol 0.03 mg/inert	LO/ORVAL 28

(continued facing page)

GENERIC NAME	TRADE NAME
norethynodrel 5 mg/mestranol 75 mcg	ENOVID 5 mg
norethynodrel 2.5 mg/mestranol 100 mcg	ENOVID-E
norethynodrel 5 mg/mestranol 100 mcg	ENOVID 5 mg
ethynodiol diacetate 1 mg/ethinyl estradiol 50 mcg	DEMULEN
ethynodiol diacetate 1 mg/ethinyl estradiol 50 mcg/placebo	DEMULEN-28
ethynodiol diacetate 1 mg/mestranol 0.1 mg	OVULEN
ethynodiol diacetate 1 mg/mestranol 0.1 mg	OVULEN-21
ethynodiol diacetate 1 mg/mestranol 0.1 mg/placebo	OVULEN-28

PHARMACOLOGY

The oral contraceptive agents consist of a combination of an estrogen and a progestogen. The estrogens, ethinyl estradiol and mestranol, and the progestogens, norethindrone, norethindrone acetate, norgestrel, and ethynodiol diacetate, act by suppressing gonadotropins. Alterations in the cervical mucus and endometrium occur which impede conception.

SPECIAL PRECAUTIONS

• All Special Precautions involving estrogens and progesterone/progestogens are applicable to the combination products.

• The use of hormonal contraceptives has been shown to subject users to an increased risk of thromboembolic disease.

• Other risks include elevated blood pressure and reduced tolerance to carbohydrates; liver disease has also occurred.

• Discontinue oral contraceptives if there is gradual or sudden, partial or complete loss of vision.

• Pregnancy should be ruled out before initiating or continuing the contraceptive regime; fetal abnormalities have occurred in offspring of women who have taken progestogens and/or estrogens during pregnancy.

ADVERSE EFFECTS

CNS EFFECTS: mental depression, chorea, headache, nervousness, dizziness, fatigue

CARDIOVASCULAR EFFECTS: thrombophlebitis, pulmonary embolism, myocardial infarction, cerebral thrombosis, cerebral hemorrhage, hypertension

URINARY TRACT EFFECTS: cystitislike syndrome

GASTROINTESTINAL EFFECTS: nausea, vomiting, abdominal cramps and bloating, changes in appetite

METABOLIC AND ENDOCRINE EFFECTS: changes in libido, breakthrough bleeding, spotting, changes in menstrual flow, amenorrhea, changes in cervical erosion and cervical secretion, increase in size of uterine fibromyomata, temporary infertility after discontinuance, vaginitis, edema; breast enlargement, tenderness, secretion; changes in body weight, diminution in lactation pospartum, reduced tolerance to carbohydrates, porphyria

HEPATIC EFFECTS: gallbladder disease, cholestatic jaundice

ALLERGIC EFFECTS: rash

DERMATOLOGIC EFFECTS: cholasma or melasma, hirsutism, loss of scalp hair, erythema multiforme, erythema nodosum, hemorrhagic eruption, itching

OPTHALMIC EFFECTS: intolerance to contact lenses, changes in corneal curvature (steepening), cataracts

MUSCULOSKELETAL EFFECTS: backache

CLINICAL GUIDELINES

ADMINISTRATION:
- Caution patients that nonadherence to dosage schedule increases the risk of pregnancy.

EFFECTS:
- Fetal abnormalities have occurred in offspring of women who have taken these products during pregnancy.
- Increased sulfobromophthalein retention; alteration of other hepatic function tests.
- Increase in prothrombin time, factors VII, VIII, IX, and X.
- Decrease in anti-thrombin III.
- Increase in norepinephrine-induced platelet aggregability.
- Increase PBI and butanol extractable protein bound iodine.
- Decrease in T_3 uptake
- Reduced response to metyrapone test.
- Decreased pregnanediol.
- Decreased glucose tolerance.
- Decreased serum folate.

OVERDOSAGE/ANTIDOTE:
- Overdosage may cause nausea; withdrawal bleeding may occur.
- There is no specific antidote. Treat supportively.

SPECIFIC PRODUCTS AND DOSAGES: LOCAL CONTRACEPTIVES

GENERIC NAME	TRADE NAME
nonoxynol 9 2%	ORTHO Creme
nonoxynol 9 5%	CONCEPTROL Birth Control Cream DELFEN Contraceptive Cream
nonoxynol 9 10%	SEMICID Contraceptive Suppositories
nonoxynol 9 12.5%	DELFEN Contraceptive Foam ENCARE Oval Vaginal Suppositories KOROMEX Contraceptive Foam
nonyl phenoxy polyethylene ethanol 8.0%	EMKO Pre-Fil EMKO Vaginal Foam
nonyl phenoxy polyoxyethylene ethanol 8.0%	BECAUSE Birth Control Foam
octoxynol 1.0%	KOROMEX II* Jelly
octoxynol 3.0%	KOROMEX II Cream
phenylmercuric acetate 0.4 mg	LOROPHYN Suppositories
phenylmercuric acetate 0.05%	LOROPHYN Jelly

*Contains more than one active ingredient.

(continued facing page)

GENERIC NAME	TRADE NAME
p-diisobutylphenoxy-polyethoxyethanol	PRECEPTIN Contraceptive Gel ORTHO-GYNOL Contraceptive Jelly
dodecaethyleneglycol monolaurate 5%	RAMSES "10-Hour" Vaginal Jelly

PHARMACOLOGY

The local contraceptives, nonoxynol 9, nonyl phenoxy polyoxyethylene ethanol, nonyl phenoxy polyethylene ethanol, octoxynol, phenylmercuric acetate, p-diiso-butylphenoxypolyethoxyethanol, and dode-caethyleneglycol monolaurate, are spermicidal agents. Also, the physical properties of the formulations provide a physical barrier preventing the sperm from entering the fallopian tubes.

SPECIAL PRECAUTIONS

• When pregnancy is contraindicated, the contraceptive program should be prescribed by the physician.
• Do not use in patients with a history of hypersensitivity to the ingredients.
• Discontinue use if burning and/or irritation of the vagina or penis occur.

ADVERSE EFFECTS

LOCAL EFFECTS: burning, irritation, itching, redness

Estrogens/Progestogens

GENERAL CLINICAL USES

Natural and synthetic ovarian hormones, estrogen and progesterone, administered systemically, are used to replace deficient hormones. They may be used to treat menopausal and premenopausal states, dysfunctions of the reproductive system, and postpartum breast engorgement, and to control fertility. Administered topically, estrogens have been used to relieve the symptoms of senile and atrophic vaginitis. Certain estrogens have been used to treat malignancies in the male and female; these products are reviewed in Chapter 17, *Antineoplastic/Anticancer Agents.*

Progesterone and the progestogens are indicated for treating habitual and threatened abortion, premature labor, functional uterine bleeding, functional dysmenorrhea, primary and secondary amenorrhea, female hypogonadism, and other progesterone deficiency states.

Combinations of estrogens and progestogens, and certain progestogens alone, are used for contraception. See the discussion of contraceptives, in the preceding section.

Estrogens

SPECIFIC PRODUCTS AND DOSAGES

GENERIC NAME	TRADE NAME	ROUTE OF ADMIN.	USUAL DOSAGE
chlorotrianisene	TACE	po	12–25 mg od to qid
dienestrol	(G)†	topical (intravaginal)	od to bid
diethylstilbestrol	(G)	intravaginal po	up to 1 mg daily 0.2–0.5 mg daily cyclically
diethylstilbestrol diphosphate	STILPHOSTROL	po iv	50–200 mg tid 0.5–1 gm 1–2 x/week
estrogens, conjugated	PREMARIN FEMEST	po intravaginal	0.3–1.25 mg daily and cyclically or as needed od or bid od or bid
estrogens, esterified	(G) AMNESTROGEN MENEST	po	0.3–7.5 mg daily, cyclically, or as needed
estradiol	(G) ESTRACE (G)	po im	1–2 mg daily 1.0 mg 1–3 x/week
estradiol cypionate	DEPO-ESTRADIOL Cypionate	im	1–5 mg/2–3 weeks
estradiol valerate	(G) DELADUMONE* DELESTROGEN*	im	5–30 mg every 2–4 weeks
estrone	THEELIN	im	0.1–2 mg 2–3 x/week
ethinyl estradiol	(G) ESTINYL FEMINONE Estinyl	po	0.02–1 mg daily
piperazine estrone sulfate	OGEN	po	0.625–5 mg/day
polyestradiol phosphate	ESTRADURIN	im	40 mg every 2–4 weeks

*Contains more than one active ingredient.
†(G) designates availability as a generic product.

PHARMACOLOGY

Estrogens are responsible for the development and maintenance of the female reproductive tract and secondary sex characteristics. The estrogens also inhibit the secretion of pituitary gonadotropins. Exogenously administered estrogens are excreted in mother's milk.

Ethinyl estradiol, one of the most active estrogens known, is a naturally occurring estrogen altered chemically to render it effective when administered orally. Estradiol is also one of the more potent of the naturally occurring estrogens. Estrogen valerate is a long-acting estrogen which after intramuscular administration produces an estrogenic effect which lasts for 2 to 3 weeks.

Estrone is claimed to have a more prompt effect than insoluble estrone suspensions. The piperazine sulfate salt is slightly less potent than estrone sodium or potassium sulfate.

The nonsteroidal estrogens include diethylstilbestrol and the related compounds, dienestrol and chlorotrianisone; these compounds are effective when administered orally.

Conjugated estrogens are made up of a mixture of estrogens from pregnant mares' urine. It is effective when administered orally.

Esterified estrogens are a water-soluble mixture of estrogenic substances for oral administration.

Polyestradiol phosphate for intramuscular administration leaves the bloodstream within 24 hours. It is stored passively in the reticuloendothelial system.

Piperazine estrone sulfate, soluble in water, acts similarly to estrone. Gastrointestinal absorption is usually prompt and complete.

SPECIAL PRECAUTIONS

• Estrogens are contraindicated in patients with thrombophlebitis, thromboembolic disorders, cerebral apoplexy or a past history of these conditions.
• Do not administer to women with a personal or family history of mammary or genital malignancy or with precancerous mammary lesions.
• Do not use in women with recurrent mastitis, markedly impaired liver function or undiagnosed abnormal genital bleeding.
• Be alert to the early manifestations of thrombolic disorders such as thrombophlebitis or pulmonary emboli; if they occur, discontinue immediately.
• In cyclic therapy, withdrawal bleeding may occur during the 1 week off medication.
• Use judiciously in young patients because of a retarding effect on epiphyseal closure.
• If unexplained or excessive vaginal bleeding occurs, be sure to check for organic pathology.
• Do not use in patients with hypertrichosis or with blood dyscrasias.
• Do not use in patients with a history of hypersensitivity to estrogens.
• Use with caution in patients with cardiac or renal disease, asthma, or epilepsy.
• Diabetic patients may require regulation of insulin during mediction with estrogens.
• Discontinue use if there is a sudden, partial or complete loss of vision, or a sudden onset of proptosis, diplopia, migraine, papilledema or retinal vascular lesions.
• Safe use in pregnancy has not been established.

ADVERSE EFFECTS

CNS EFFECTS: headache, vertigo, mental depression, increased or decreased libido, malaise, irritability, fatigue, dizziness, nervousness, aggravation of migraine headache
RESPIRATORY EFFECTS: pulmonary embolism
CARDIOVASCULAR EFFECTS: thromboembolism, hypertension, cerebrovascular accident
URINARY TRACT EFFECTS: stress incontinence with large doses, cystitislike syndrome
GASTROINTESTINAL EFFECTS: anorexia, nausea, vomiting, mild diarrhea, abdominal cramps or bloating, changes in appetite

METABOLIC AND ENDOCRINE EFFECTS: in females, edema, hypercalcemia, sodium retention, soreness and enlargement of breast, gynecomastia, amenorrhea, breakthrough bleeding and spotting, increased cervical mucus, decreased glucose tolerance, increased blood glucose, melasma, cholasma, increase or decrease in body weight, reactivation of endometriosis; in males, loss of libido, gynecomastia, interference with spermatogenesis, and testicular atrophy

HEPATIC EFFECTS: cholestatic jaundice, hepatic cutaneous prophyria

ALLERGIC EFFECTS: rash, pruritus

DERMATOLOGIC EFFECTS: hemorrhagic eruption, hair loss, erythema nodosum, erythema multiforme

LOCAL EFFECTS: pain at injection site, localized dermatitis, sterile abscess; with creams, burning sensation

MUSCULOSKELETAL EFFECTS: backache

CLINICAL GUIDELINES

ADMINISTRATION:
- Inject deeply into upper, outer quadrant of the gluteal muscle.
- Administer tablets after meals to reduce nausea and vomiting.

EFFECTS:
- Clinical laboratory tests should not be considered definitive unless estrogen therapy has been discontinued for at least 60 days.
- Pre-existing fibromyomata may increase in size during estrogen therapy.
- Treatment may mask signs of the climacteric.

DRUG INTERACTIONS:
- A decrease in glucose tolerance has been measured; antidiabetic medication may require adjustment accordingly.
- Estrogens may cause an elevation of the PBI and BEI, and decrease in T_3 uptake.
- Alterations in the metapyrone test and pregnanediol determinations have been reported.
- Increases in BSP and in prothrombin and factors VII, VIII, IX, and X have occurred.

OVERDOSAGE/ANTIDOTE:
- Overdosage of estrogenic vaginal creams and suppositories may stimulate uterine bleeding in menopausal women.
- With large doses of estrogens, nausea, anorexia, vomiting, and mild diarrhea are the most common signs.
- There is no specific antidote. Terminate therapy; withdrawal bleeding may occur.

Progesterone
Progestogens

SPECIFIC PRODUCTS AND DOSAGES

GENERIC NAME	TRADE NAME	ROUTE OF ADMIN.	USUAL DAILY DOSAGE
dydrogesterone	DUPHASTON GYNOREST	po	10–20 mg daily in divided doses

(continued facing page)

GENERIC NAME	TRADE NAME	ROUTE OF ADMIN.	USUAL DAILY DOSAGE
ethisterone	(G)*	po	25–100 mg daily
hydroxyprogesterone caproate	DELALUTIN	im	250–375 mg as needed
medroxyprogesterone acetate	AMEN PROVERA	im po	50 mg weekly 2.5–50 mg daily
megestrol acetate	MEGACE	po	40–320 mg daily in divided doses; also see Chapter 17, *Antineoplastic/Anticancer Agents,* page 617.
norethindrone	NORLUTIN	po	Usually 5–20 mg daily
norethindrone acetate	NORLUTATE	po	Usually 2.5–10 mg daily
norethynodrel	See *Contraceptives, Oral and Local,* page 518		
norgestrel	See *Contraceptives, Oral and Local,* page 518		
progesterone	(G) GESTEROL LIPO-LUTIN	im	10–50 mg daily or every other day

*(G) designates availability as a generic product.

PHARMACOLOGY

Progesterone and the progestogens cause the secretory phase of the endometrium to develop and establish all of the effects of the corpus luteum hormone. Progesterone is the natural progestational substance and is administered intramuscularly. Synthetic forms such as dehydroprogesterone, which is structurally related to naturally occurring progesterone, have been developed for oral administration. Detectable amounts of progestogens have been identified in mother's milk.

Hydroxyprogesterone caproate, a derivative of progesterone, is a long-acting progestational agent for intramuscular administration. It is approximately 7 times more potent than progesterone and its action lasts about 9 to 17 days.

Medroxyprogesterone acetate, a progesterone derivative, may be administered orally or intramuscularly.

Norethindrone, norethindrone acetate, and ethisterone, derivatives of testosterone, are potent progestational agents. The acetate is approximately twice as potent as norethindrone. Ethisterone is not as active as the other testosterone derivatives.

Megestrol acetate is a progestational agent used in treating carcinoma. See Chapter 17, page 616 for detailed information.

SPECIAL PRECAUTIONS

- Do not use in patients with missed or incomplete abortion, carcinoma of the breast, and undiagnosed genital bleeding.
- Do not use in patients with a history of hypersensitivity to these compounds or related compounds.
- Do not use in patients with a history of or presence of thrombophlebitis, thromboembolic disorders, cerebrovascular accident, or pulmonary embolism.
- Discontinue if there is a sudden, partial, or complete loss of vision, or if there is sudden onset of proptosis, diplopia, or migraine.
- Administer with caution to patients who have had periodic attacks of asthma, migraine, or epilepsy.
- Observe carefully patients with psychic depression; depression may recur.
- Use with caution in patients with cardiac or renal dysfunction, or markedly impaired hepatic function.

ADVERSE EFFECTS

CNS EFFECTS: headache, insomnia, somnolence, fatigue, dizziness, nervousness
RESPIRATORY EFFECTS: coughing, dyspnea
CARDIOVASCULAR EFFECTS: thromboembolism
AUTONOMIC EFFECTS: hyperpyrexia rarely
GASTROINTESTINAL EFFECTS: nausea, vomiting, diarrhea, ulcerative stomatitis
METABOLIC AND ENDOCRINE EFFECTS: edema, weight gain, changes in libido, masculinization with certain progestogens but not dehydroprogesterone, breakthrough bleeding, galactorrhea, melasma, cholasma
HEPATIC EFFECTS: jaundice, including neonatal jaundice
ALLERGIC EFFECTS: urticaria, pruritus, pruritus vulvae, angioneurotic edema, rash, and anaphylaxis with medroxyprogesterone acetate
LOCAL EFFECTS: irritation

CLINICAL GUIDELINES

ADMINISTRATION:
- Immerse vial of injectable preparation in warm water to facilitate filling syringe.
- Using a wet needle or syringe may cause solution to become cloudy; the potency is not affected.

EFFECTS:
- Masculinization of the female fetus has occurred when progestogens have been used in pregnant women.

DRUG INTERACTIONS:
- Endocrine and liver (BSP) function tests may be affected; also metapyrone and pregnanediol determinations.
- Coagulation tests including increases in prothrombin time and factors VII, VIII, IX, and X have occurred.
- Effect may be decreased by phenylbutazone.
- Effect may be increased by phenothiazines.

Fertility Agents/Ovulation Stimulants

The fertility agents, clomiphene citrate, menotropins, and chorionic gonadotropin, are used to induce ovulation in the anovulatory infertile patient.

SPECIFIC PRODUCTS AND DOSAGES

GENERIC NAME	TRADE NAME	ROUTE OF ADMIN.	USUAL DOSAGE
chorionic gonadotropin	(G)* A.P.L. Secules FOLLUTIN	im	500–5000 units every second day to daily
clomiphene citrate	CLOMID	po	Individualize; usually 25–100 mg daily. Do not increase dosage or duration of therapy beyond 100 mg/day for 5 days
menotropins	PERGONAL	im	Individualize dosage. Usually 75–150 IU

*(G) designates availability as a generic product.

Chorionic Gonadotropin

GENERAL CLINICAL USES

Chorionic gonadotropin is used in treating cryptorchidism not due to anatomic obstruction; male hypogonadism secondary to pituitary failure; and in the induction of ovulation and pregnancy in the anovulatory, fertile woman.

PHARMACOLOGY

Chorionic gonadotropin is a gonad-stimulating substance obtained from the urine of pregnant women. It is a polypeptide hormone produced by the human placenta. It stimulates production of gonadal steroid hormones.

SPECIAL PRECAUTIONS

• Do not use in patients with precocious puberty, prostatic carcinoma or other androgen-dependent neoplasia.
• Do not use in patients with a history of hypersensitivity to chorionic gonadotropin.
• Use with caution in patients with epilepsy, migraine, asthma, cardiac or renal disease because of possible fluid retention.

ADVERSE EFFECTS

CNS EFFECTS: headache, irritability, restlessness, depression, tiredness
RESPIRATORY EFFECTS: pleural effusion
CARDIOVASCULAR EFFECTS: arterial thromboembolism
METABOLIC AND ENDOCRINE EFFECTS: ovarian enlargement, ascites with or without pain, multiple births, rupture of ovarian cysts, precocious puberty, edema, gynecomastia
LOCAL EFFECTS: pain at site of injection

CLINICAL GUIDELINES
ADMINISTRATION:
• Administer by intramuscular route only.
EFFECTS:
• Chorionic gonadotropin has no known effect on appetite, hunger, fat mobilization, or body fat distribution.

Clomiphene Citrate

PHARMACOLOGY

Clomiphene citrate, a nonsteroidal agent, may stimulate ovulation in anovulatory women with functional hypothalmic-pituitary-ovarian systems and adequate endogenous estrogen. The mechanism of action remains unclear; clomiphene may stimulate pituitary gonadotropin release. Clomiphene is an antiestrogen.

SPECIAL PRECAUTIONS
• Do not use in patients with a history of hypersensitivity to clomiphene citrate.
• Do not administer to pregnant women or those with liver disease, history of liver dysfunction, or bleeding of undetermined origin.
• Discontinue if any visual abnormalities occur.
• Do not administer to women with ovarian cysts.

ADVERSE EFFECTS
CNS EFFECTS: headache, vertigo, lightheadedness, insominia
AUTONOMIC EFFECTS: hot flushes
GASTROINTESTINAL EFFECTS: nausea, bloating, and vomiting
METABOLIC AND ENDOCRINE EFFECTS: cystic enlargement of ovaries, cyclic ovarian pain, abnormal uterine bleeding, breast engorgement
DERMATOLOGIC EFFECTS: rash, hair loss
OPHTHALMIC EFFECTS: blurred vision, scintillating scotomata, loss of visual acuity, photophobia

CLINICAL GUIDELINES
ADMINISTRATION:
• Caution patients that visual symptoms may interfere with driving a motor vehicle or operating machinery.
• Advise patient of the possibility of multiple pregnancy and the potential hazards of multiple pregnancy.
EFFECTS:
• Multiple pregnancies have occurred;

the incidence is approximately eight times the normal.
• Ovarian cysts may occur; they appear to be dose related.
• BSP retention may be increased.
OVERDOSAGE/ANTIDOTE:
• Overstimulation of the ovary may produce pelvic pain, enlarged ovaries, and cyst formation.
• No antidote is known. Treat symptomatically.

Menotropins

PHARMACOLOGY
Menotropins, a combination of follicle stimulating hormone (FSH) and luteinizing hormone (LH) activity obtained from urine of postmenopausal women, is used to stimulate ovarian follicular growth in women who do not have primary ovarian failure. Ovulation is not produced by menotropins; human chorionic gonadotropin must be given to effect ovulation.

SPECIAL PRECAUTIONS
• Do not use in patients with primary ovarian failure as indicated by a high level of urinary gonadotropins, in patients with overt thyroid and adrenal dysfunction, or in those with organic intracranial lesions such as a pituitary tumor.
• Avoid use in patients with abnormal bleeding of undetermined origin.
• Do not use in patients with ovarian cysts or enlargement not due to polycystic ovary syndrome, or in pregnant patients.
• Occasionally (approximately 20% of patients treated) abnormal ovarian enlargement may occur accompanied by abdominal distention and/or abdominal pain.
• Hyperstimulation syndrome characterized by sudden ovarian enlargement accompanied by ascites with or without pain

and/or pleural effusion may occur in approximately 0.4 percent of patients treated.
• Caution patients that multiple births, usually twins, have occurred in approximately 20 percent of patients treated.

ADVERSE EFFECTS
RESPIRATORY EFFECTS: pleural effusion
CARDIOVASCULAR EFFECTS: arterial thromboembolism, hypotension
URINARY TRACT EFFECTS: oliguria
HEMATOLIGIC EFFECTS: hemoperitoneum, hypercoagulability
ALLERGIC EFFECTS: sensitivity
GASTROINTESTINAL EFFECTS: flatulence, and discomfort

METABOLIC AND ENDOCRINE EFFECTS: ovarian enlargement, hyperstimulation syndrome, birth defects, ascites

CLINICAL GUIDELINES
ADMINISTRATION:
• Pregnancy or primary ovarian failure should be ruled out prior to initiation of therapy.
• Any unused reconstituted drug should be discarded.
EFFECTS:
• Multiple pregnancies have occurred in a remarkable number of patients.
• Birth defects have occurred.

Uterine Muscle Stimulants (Oxytocic Agents)

GENERAL CLINICAL USES
The uterine muscle stimulants (oxytocic agents)—ergonovine maleate, methyl ergonovine maleate, and oxytocin—are used for induction, management, or stimulation of labor; to control postpartum hemorrhage or atony; and for initial milk letdown in postpartum patients.

SPECIFIC PRODUCTS AND DOSAGES

GENERIC NAME	TRADE NAME	ROUTE OF ADMIN.	USUAL DOSAGE
ergonovine maleate	(G)*	im/iv	0.2 mg; may be repeated in 2 to 4 hrs.
	ERGOTRATE Maleate	po	0.2–0.4 mg bid to qid

*(G) designates availability as a generic product.

(continued overleaf)

GENERIC NAME	TRADE NAME	ROUTE OF ADMIN.	USUAL DOSAGE
methylergonovine maleate	METHERGINE	im po	0.2 mg; may be repeated in 2 to 6 hrs. 0.2 mg tid or qid
oxytocin	(G)* PITOCIN	iv iv infusion	0.025–1.0 ml; repeat in 20 min. if necessary 1 ml in 1,000 ml 5% dextrose injection; 14 drops/min.
	SYNTOCINON PITOCIN CITRATE SYNTOCINON	im buccal nasal spray	3–10 units (0.3–1 ml) 200 units; repeat in 30 min. One spray into one or both nostrils 2–3 min. before nursing

*(G) designates availability as a generic product.

Ergonovine Maleate
Methylergonovine Maleate
Oxytocin

PHARMACOLOGY

Ergonovine maleate and methylergonovine induce rapid and sustained uterine contractions. Following intravenous administration, the onset of action is immediate; after intramuscular administration, the onset of action is 2 to 5 minutes; after oral administration, 5 to 10 minutes.

Oxytocin, a synthetic posterior pituitary product, stimulates uterine contractions and induces milk ejection in lactating females. The sensitivity of the uterus to oxytocin increases gradually during gestation and sharply before parturition.

SPECIAL PRECAUTIONS

• Do not administer when the following conditions are present: cephalopelvic disproportion, unfavorable fetal position, presentations which are undeliverable without conversion, in obstetrical emergencies when the benefit-to-risk rates for either the fetus or mother favor surgical intervention, fetal distress when delivery is not imminent, hypertonic uterine patterns.

• Do not use in patients with a history of hypersensitivity to the drug.

• Improper administration resulting in overstimulation of the uterus can be hazardous to both mother and fetus.

• Do not administer if the following conditions are present: prematurity, placenta previa, abruptio placentae, previous major surgery on cervix or uterus including cesarian section, overdistention of the uterus, grand multiparity, past history of uterine sepsis or of traumatic delivery.

• If tetany should occur, discontinue immediately.

• Use with caution in patients with puerperal infection, obliterative vascular disease, and hepatic, cardiac, or renal disease.

ADVERSE EFFECTS

CNS EFFECTS: dizziness, headache
RESPIRATORY EFFECTS: temporary chest pain, dyspnea
CARDIOVASCULAR EFFECTS: fetal bradycardia, cardiac arrhythmias, pelvic hematoma, premature ventricular contractions, transient hypertension, palpitation
AUTONOMIC EFFECTS: diaphoresis
GASTROINTESTINAL EFFECTS: nausea, vomiting

METABOLIC AND ENDOCRINE EFFECTS: severe water intoxication with convulsions and coma

HEMATOLOGIC EFFECTS: afibrinogenemia (one fatality)

ALLERGIC EFFECTS: anaphylactic reaction

OTIC EFFECTS: tinnitus

CLINICAL GUIDELINES

ADMINISTRATION:

• Intravenous administration produces a greater incidence of adverse effects than other routes of administration.

• Intravenous administration gives more predictable contraction patterns and more concise control than other routes of administration.

• Do not administer simultaneously by more than one route.

EFFECTS:

• Hypertensive episodes, subarachnoid hemorrhage, rupture of the uterus, and fetal deaths have occurred with oxytocin therapy.

• Oxytocin has an intrinsic antidiuretic effect, acting to increase water reabsorption from the glomerular filtrate.

DRUG INTERACTIONS:

• Oxytocin may not be effective in patients anesthetized with potent uterine relaxants such as halothane and chloroform until anesthetic is completely eliminated.

• Concomitant administration of oxytocic and vasopressors during surgical anesthesia may cause severe hypertension and result in cerebral hemorrhage.

• Calcium gluconate administered intravenously may restore uterine sensitivity in hypocalcemic patients; do not administer calcium gluconate to digitalized patients.

OVERDOSAGE/ANTIDOTE:

• Overdosage is characterized by an exaggeration of the adverse effects.

• Hypertension may be controlled promptly by intravenous administration of chlorpromazine 15 mg. Severe cramping may be controlled by terminating use of oxytocic agent. There is no specific antidote.

15

Endocrine and other drugs affecting metabolism

INTRODUCTION

The majority of drugs affect metabolism to some extent or in some manner. However, the endocrine products, both natural and synthetic, have a profound effect on metabolism. These products are used for replacement therapy or for their supplemental therapeutic effects on metabolism.

SPECIFIC THERAPEUTIC CLASSIFICATION

The endocrine products affecting metabolism include the following:

1. Adrenocortical hormones
   a. Mineralocorticoids
   b. Glucocorticoids
2. Anabolic steroids
3. Anterior pituitary hormones
   a. Corticotropin
   b. Somatotropin
   c. Thyrotropin

4. Antialcohol drug—disulfiram
5. Cholesterol/lipid-reducing agents
6. Gonadotropin
7. Hyperglycemic/hypoglycemic (anti-diabetic) agents
8. Parathyroid and calcium regulators
9. Posterior pituitary hormones
10. Potassium replacements and supplements
11. Sex hormones
    a. Androgens
    b. Estrogens
12. Thyroid/antithyroid preparations

Adrenocortical Hormones

Mineralocorticoids

GENERAL CLINICAL USES

The mineralocorticoids, desoxycorticosterone acetate, desoxycorticosterone pivalate, and fludrocortisone acetate, are used as partial replacement therapy for primary and secondary adrenocortical insufficiency in Addison's disease and for the treatment of salt-losing adrenogenital syndrome.

SPECIFIC PRODUCTS AND DOSAGES

GENERIC NAME	TRADE NAME	ROUTE OF ADMIN.	USUAL DOSAGE
desoxycorticosterone acetate (DOCA)	(G)* PERCORTEN Acetate in Oil	im	1–5 mg daily; maximum 10 mg/day
	PERCORTEN Acetate Pellets	sc	Use twice the number of mg of solution in oil for 8–12 months plus an extra pellet
desoxycorticosterone pivalate	PERCORTEN Pivalate Intramuscular Repository	im	25 mg for each mg of oil preparation; administer every 4 wks
fludrocortisone acetate	FLORINEF Acetate	po	0.05–0.2 mg daily

*(G) designates availability as a generic product.

Desoxycorticosterone Acetate
Desoxycorticosterone Pivalate
Fludrocortisone Acetate

PHARMACOLOGY

The effects of these drugs are dose-related; small doses produce marked sodium retention and increased urinary potassium excretion, rise in blood pressure; larger doses inhibit endogenous adrenal cortical secretion, thymic activity, and pituitary corticotropin excretion, promote deposition of liver glycogen, and induce negative nitrogen balance. Desoxycorticosterone has pure mineralocorticoid activity in contrast to fludrocortisone acetate, which has both mineralocorticoid and glucocorticoid activities.

SPECIAL PRECAUTIONS
• Do not use in patients with systemic fungal infections.
• Some signs of infection may be masked; new infections may appear during use.
• Do not vaccinate patients against smallpox or use other immunization procedures during therapy.
• In patients with active tuberculosis restrict use to those cases of fulminating or disseminated tuberculosis in which the corticosteroid is used for management of the disease in conjunction with an appropriate antituberculous regimen.
• If used in patients with latent tuberculosis or tuberculin reactivity, watch for signs of reactivation of the disease.
• Safe use in pregnancy, nursing mothers, and women of childbearing potential has not been established.
• Adverse effects may be produced by too rapid withdrawal or by continued use of large doses.
• To avoid drug-induced adrenal insufficiency, supportive dosage may be required in times of stress (such as trauma, surgery,

or severe illness) both during treatment and for a year afterward.
• Use with caution in patients with diverticulitis, fresh intestinal anastomoses, active or latent peptic ulcer, renal insufficiency, hypertension, osteoporosis, acute glomerulonephritis, vaccinia, varicella, exanthema, Cushing's syndrome, antibiotic-resistant infections, diabetes mellitus, congestive heart failure, chronic nephritis, thromboembolic tendencies, thrombophlebitis, convulsive disorders, metastatic carcinoma, and myasthenia gravis.

ADVERSE EFFECTS
CNS EFFECTS: convulsions, increased intracranial pressure with papilledema usually after treatment, vertigo, headache, severe mental disturbances, insomnia, syncopal episodes

CARDIOVASCULAR EFFECTS: hypertension, necrotizing angiitis, thrombophlebitis, congestive heart failure

GASTROINTESTINAL EFFECTS: peptic ulcer with possible perforation and hemorrhage, pancreatitis, abdominal distention, ulcerative esophagitis

METABOLIC AND ENDOCRINE EFFECTS: sodium and fluid retention, potassium loss, hypokalemic alkalosis, menstrual irregularities, development of Cushing state, suppression of growth in children, secondary adrenocortical and pituitary unresponsiveness, manifestations of diabetes mellitus, increased requirement for insulin or oral hypoglycemic agents in diabetics, hyperglycemia, glucosuria, negative nitrogen balance due to protein catabolism

ALLERGIC EFFECTS: anaphylactoid reactions

DERMATOLOGIC EFFECTS: impaired wound healing, thin fragile skin, bruising, petechiae, ecchymoses, facial erythema, increased sweating, subcutaneous fat atrophy, purpura, striae, hyperpigmentation of skin and

nails, hirsutism, acneiform eruptions; reactions of skin tests may be suppressed
OPHTHALMIC EFFECTS: posterior subcapsular cataracts, increased intraocular pressure, glaucoma, exophthalmos
MUSCULOSKELETAL EFFECTS: muscle weakness, steroid myopathy, loss of muscle mass, osteoporosis, vertebral compression fractures, aseptic necrosis of femoral and humeral heads, pathologic fractures of long bones, spontaneous fractures

CLINICAL GUIDELINES

ADMINISTRATION:
• Monitor dosage and salt intake carefully to avoid development of hypertension, edema, and weight gain.
EFFECTS:
• If an infection occurs during therapy, it should be promptly controlled by suitable antimicrobial therapy.

• Dietary salt restriction and potassium supplementation may be necessary; therefore monitor serum electrolyte levels.
• Calcium excretion is increased.
• There is an enhanced corticosteroid effect in patients with hypothyroidism and in those with cirrhosis.
DRUG INTERACTIONS:
• Use aspirin with caution in conjunction with corticosteroids in patients with hypoprothrombinemia; bleeding may occur.
OVERDOSAGE/ANTIDOTE:
• Overdosage is characterized by changes in the CNS (anxiety, depression, stimulation), gastrointestinal bleeding, elevated blood sugar, hypertension and edema.
• The signs of overdosage or underdosage can be corrected by varying the salt intake or giving the steroid intramuscularly if necessary. There is no specific antidote. Treat supportively.

Glucocorticoids

GENERAL CLINICAL USES
The glucocorticoids, consisting of the basic compound and/or the salts of beclomethasone, betamethasone, cortisone, dexamethasone, fludrocortisone, hydrocortisone, meprednisone, methylprednisolone, paramethasone, prednisolone, prednisone, and triamcinolone, are indicated for serious or life-threatening conditions such as:

1. *Endocrine disorders:* primary or secondary adrenocortical insufficiency, congenital adrenal hyperplasia, nonsuppurative thyroiditis; hypercalcemia associated with cancer.
2. *Rheumatic disorders:* as adjunctive therapy for short-term administration in psoriatic arthritis; rheumatoid arthritis, ankylosing spondylitis; acute and subacute bursitis; acute nonspecific tenosynovitis; acute gouty arthritis, juvenile rheumatoid arthritis.
3. *Collagen diseases:* during an exacerbation or as maintenance therapy in selected cases of systemic lupus erythematosus, acute rheumatic carditis.
4. *Dermatologic diseases:* bullous dermatitis herpetiformis, severe exfoliative dermatitis, mycosis fungoides, severe psoriasis.
5. *Allergic states:* control of severe or incapacitating allergic conditions intractable to adequate trials of conventional treatment, such as sea-

sonal or perennial allergic rhinitis, bronchial asthma, contact dermatitis, atopic dermatitis, serum sickness.

6. *Ophthalmic diseases:* severe acute and chronic allergic and inflammatory processes involving the eye and its adnexa such as allergic conjunctivitis, keratitis, allergic corneal marginal ulcers, herpes zoster ophthalmicus, iritis and iridocyclitis, chorioretinitis, anterior segment inflammation, diffuse posterior uveitis, choroiditis, optic neuritis, sympathetic ophthalmia.

7. *Respiratory diseases:* symptomatic sarcoidosis, Loffler's syndrome not manageable by other means, berylliosis, fulminating or disseminated pulmonary tuberculosis when accompanied by appropriate antituberculous chemotherapy.

8. *Hematologic disorders:* idiopathic and secondary thrombocytopenia in adults, acquired (autoimmune) hemolytic anemia, erythroblastopenia (RBC anemia), congenital (erythroid) hypoplastic anemia.

9. *Neoplastic diseases:* for palliative management of leukemias and lymphomas in adults, acute leukemia of childhood.

10. *Edematous states:* to induce diuresis or remission of proteinuria in the nephrotic syndrome, without uremia, of the idiopathic type or that due to lupus erythematosus.

11. *Gastrointestinal disease:* to tide the patient over a critical period of disease as ulcerative colitis (systemic therapy), regional enteritis (systemic therapy).

12. *Miscellaneous disorders:* tuberculous meningitis with subarachnoid block or impending block when concurrently accompanied by appropriate antituberculous chemotherapy; systemic dermatomycositis (polymyositis).

For clinical uses of glucocorticoids administered topically, intralesionally or intradermally, see Chapter 9, *Drugs Affecting the Skin.* For clinical uses of formulations for intrabursal, intra-articular or periarticular administration, see Chapter 13, *Drugs Affecting the Musculoskeletal System.* Ophthalmic uses and preparations are included in Chapter 11, *Drugs Affecting the Eye.*

SPECIFIC PRODUCTS AND DOSAGES

GENERIC NAME	TRADE NAME	ROUTE OF ADMIN.	USUAL DOSAGE
beclomethasone dipropionate	VANCERIL Inhaler	inhalation	100 mcg tid or qid; maximal daily intake should not exceed 20 inhalations (1000 mcg) in adults

(continued facing page)

GENERIC NAME	TRADE NAME	ROUTE OF ADMIN.	USUAL DOSAGE
			Children 6–12 yrs.: 50–100 mcg tid or qid; maximal daily dose 500 mcg
betamethasone	CELESTONE Tablet, Syrup, Cream	po topical	0.6–7.2 mg daily Small amount bid to tid
betamethasone acetate and betamethasone sodium phosphate	CELESTONE SOLUSPAN Suspension	intradermal intralesional periarticular intra-articular intrabursal intramuscular	0.2 ml/sq cm; maximum 1 ml/wk 0.2 ml/sq cm 1.0 ml 0.5–2.0 ml 0.25–1.0 ml 1.0–2.0 ml weekly
betamethasone dipropionate	DIPROSONE Cream, Ointment, Lotion, Aerosol	topical	Thin film bid
betamethasone valerate	VALISONE Aerosol, Cream, Lotion, Ointment	topical	Thin film 1–3 times daily
cortisone acetate	(G)† CORTONE Sterile Aqueous Suspension Tablet	im po	20–300 mg daily 25–300 mg daily
dexamethasone	(G) DERONIL Tablet DECADRON Elixir, Tablet DEXONE HEXADROL AEROSEB-D Topical Spray DECADERM Gel	po topical	0.5–9 mg daily Thin film bid to tid
dexamethasone acetate	DECADRON-LA	im intralesional intradermal intra-articular	8–16 mg 0.8–1.6 mg 0.8–1.6 mg 4–16 mg
dexamethasone sodium phosphate	(G) DECADRON Phosphate DECADRON Phosphate Respihaler DECADRON Phosphate Turbinaire	iv im intra-articular intradermal intralesional inhalation intranasal	2–40 mg 4–20 mg 0.8–4 mg 0.4–6 mg 0.4–6 mg **Adults:** 3 inhalations tid or qid; maximum: 12 inhalations/day **Children:** 2 inhalations tid or qid; maximum: 8 inhalations/day **Adults:** 2 sprays bid or tid **Children 6–12 yrs:** 1–2 sprays bid

†(G) designates availability as a generic product.

(continued overleaf)

GENERIC NAME	TRADE NAME	ROUTE OF ADMIN.	USUAL DOSAGE
	HEXADROL Phosphate	im	0.5–9.0 mg daily
		iv	0.5–9.0 mg daily
	DECADRON Sterile Ophth. Oint.	ophth.	Thin coating tid to qid
	DECADRON Sterile Ophth. Sol.	ophth.	1–2 drops hourly then every 2 hr.
fludrocortisone acetate	FLORINEF Acetate	po	0.05–0.2 mg daily
hydrocortisone	(G)† CORTEF Tablet	po	20–240 mg daily in divided doses
hydrocortisone sodium succinate	SOLU-CORTEF Plain, MIX-O-VIAL	im	100–250 mg
meprednisone	BETAPAR	po	8–60 mg daily
methylprednisolone	(G) MEDROL	po	4–48 mg daily
methylprednisolone acetate	(G) DEPO-MEDROL	im	40–120 mg wkly
		intra-articular	4–80 mg
		intralesional	20–60 mg
	MEDROL Acetate	topical	Thin film 1–3 times daily
	MEDROL Enpak	rectal	20–40 mg as retention enema
methylprednisolone sodium succinate	SOLU-MEDROL	iv	10–250 mg
		im	40–120 mg
paramethasone acetate	HALDRONE Tablet	po	2–24 mg daily
prednisone	(G) DELTASONE Tablet METICORTEN Tablet ORASONE SK-PREDNISONE	po	5–60 mg daily
prednisolone	(G) ATARAXOID*	po	5–60 mg daily
	DELTA-CORTEF METI-DERM Aerosol, Cream METI-DERM* with Neomycin Aerosol	topical	Thin film tid to qid
prednisolone acetate	(G) STERANE Aqueous Suspension	im	4–60 mg
		intra-articular	5–50 mg

*Contains more than one active ingredient.
†(G) designates availability as a generic product.

(continued facing page)

GENERIC NAME	TRADE NAME	ROUTE OF ADMIN.	USUAL DOSAGE
	METICORTELONE Acetate	intralesional	5–50 mg
	METIMYD* Ophth. Oint., Suspension	ophth. oint.	Thin film tid to qid
	NEO-DELTA CORTEF* Oint., Ophth. Oint., Suspension	ophth. susp. topical	2–3 drops hourly or every 2 hr. Thin film tid or qid
prednisolone sodium phosphate	METRETON Ophth. Soln. OPTIMYD* Ophth. Soln.	ophth.	2–3 drops hourly or every 2 hr.
triamcinolone	(G) ARISTOCORT Tablet KENACORT Tablet SK-TRIAMCINO-LONE	po	4–48 mg daily
triamcinolone acetonide	ARISTOCORT Cream, Oint.	topical	Thin film bid to qid
	ARISTOCORT-A Cream, Oint.	topical	Thin film tid to qid
	KENALOG-10	intrabursal Intralesional	2.5–5.0 mg 1 mg
	KENALOG-40	im intra-articular intrabursal	40–60 mg 10–40 mg 10–40 mg
	MYCOLOG* Cream	topical	Thin film daily
	MYCOLOG OINT.*	topical	Thin film tid or bid
	KENALOG	topical	Thin film daily
	KENALOG Oint., Spray	topical	Thin film bid or tid
	KENALOG in Orabase	topical (dental)	Small dab bid or tid
triamcinolone diacetate	(G) ARISTOCORT Forte ARISTOCORT Syrup KENACORT Syrup	intradermal im po	5–48 mg 3–48 mg/day 4–48 mg/day
triamcinolone hexacetonide	ARISTOSPAN	intralesional intra-articular	Up to 0.5 mg per sq in 2–20 mg

*Contains more than one active ingredient.

PHARMACOLOGY

The glucocorticoids have anti-inflammatory, antipruritic, and vasoconstrictive actions. They also have salt-retaining properties. The glucocorticoids cause profound and varied metabolic effects and also modify the body's immune responses to diverse stimuli. They are clinically effective by all routes of administration.

SPECIAL PRECAUTIONS

For detailed information, see the discussion of mineralocorticoids, page 534.

ADVERSE EFFECTS

LOCAL EFFECTS: with intramuscular administration, severe pain, abscess formation, tissue atrophy, local depigmentation

SYSTEMIC EFFECTS: see *Mineralocorticoids.*

CLINICAL GUIDELINES

See, *Mineralocorticoids,* page 535.

Anabolic Steroids

GENERAL CLINICAL USES

The anabolic steroids are used primarily as adjunctive therapy in senile and postmenopausal osteoporosis and also in pituitary dwarfism. They promote weight gain in convalescence and in patients in the catabolic state. In addition they may be useful in increasing hemoglobin levels in some patients with aplastic (congenital and idiopathic) anemia.

Anabolic steroids do not enhance athletic ability.

SPECIFIC PRODUCTS AND DOSAGES

GENERIC NAME	TRADE NAME	ROUTE OF ADMIN.	USUAL DOSAGE	
			ADULTS	**CHILDREN**
ethylestrenol	MAXIBOLIN	po	4–8 mg daily	1–3 mg daily
methandriol dipropionate	ANABOLIN IM ANABOLIN LA-100	im	10–40 mg daily or 50–100 mg once or twice weekly	5–10 mg daily
methandrostenolone	DIANABOL	po	2.5–5 mg daily	Not established
nandrolone decanoate	DECA-DURABOLIN	im	50–100 mg every 3–4 weeks	**2–13 yrs.:** 25–50 mg every 3–4 weeks
nandrolone phenpropionate	DURABOLIN	im	25–50 mg weekly	**2–13 yrs.:** 12.5–25 mg every 2–4 weeks
				(continued facing page)

GENERIC NAME	TRADE NAME	ROUTE OF ADMIN.	USUAL DOSAGE	
			ADULTS	**CHILDREN**
oxandrolone	ANAVAR	po	5–10 mg daily in divided doses	0.25 mg/kg/day
oxymetholone	ADROYD ANADROL-50	po	1–5 mg/kg/day	1–5 mg/kg/day
stanozolol	WINSTROL	po	6 mg daily in divided	**6–12 yrs.:** 2 mg tid **Under 6 yrs.:** 1 mg bid

Ethylestrenol
Methandriol Dipropionate
Methandrostenolone
Nandrolone Decanoate
Nandrolone Phenpropionate
Oxandrolone
Oxymetholone
Stanozolol

PHARMACOLOGY

The anabolic steroids, weak androgens, are derivatives of testosterone. They promote or restore body tissues without clinical signs of virilism in patients who are receiving an appropriate diet. Complete dissociation of the anabolic and androgenic effects of the anabolic steroids has not been achieved.

SPECIAL PRECAUTIONS

• Use with extreme caution, if at all, in patients with carcinoma of the prostate, benign prostatic hypertrophy, carcinoma of the breast in the male patient; in pregnancy, infancy; in patients with nephrosis or the nephrotic phase of nephritis; hypersensitivity or hepatic dysfunction.

• Virilization may occur in the female patient; amenorrhea usually occurs even in the presence of thrombocytopenia.

• Since iron deficiency anemias manifested by a low serum iron and decreased percent saturation of transferrin have occurred, periodic determination of the serum iron and iron-binding capacity is recommended.

• In patients with aplastic anemia treated with anabolic steroids, leukemia has occurred; the role of the anabolic steroids is unclear.

• Administer with caution to patients with cardiac or hepatic disease.

• Since hepatotoxic effects have occurred, periodic liver function tests are recommended.

• Use with caution in patients with or without congestive heart failure since edema has occurred occasionally.

• Since serum cholesterol levels may increase or decrease during therapy, use cautiously in patients with coronary artery disease or a history of myocardial infarction; serial determinations of serum cholesterol levels are suggested.

• In women with disseminated breast carcinoma, hypercalcemia may then develop spontaneously and as a result of hormonal therapy.

ADVERSE EFFECTS

CNS EFFECTS: excitation, sleepiness, chills

URINARY EFFECTS: bladder irritability

GASTROINTESTINAL EFFECTS: nausea, vomiting, diarrhea

METABOLIC AND ENDROCRINE EFFECTS: in prepubertal males—phallic enlargement, increased frequency of erections; in postpubertal males—inhibition of testicular function, oligospermia, gynecomastia; in females—hirsutism, male pattern baldness, deepening of voice, clitoral enlargement, increase or decrease in libido

HEMATOLOGIC EFFECTS: bleeding

DERMATOLOGIC EFFECTS: acne

CLINICAL GUIDELINES

ADMINISTRATION:

• Administer just before or with meals to minimize gastrointestinal irritation.

• Therapy should be intermittent.

EFFECTS:

• Clinical laboratory test alterations may persist for 2 to 3 weeks after stopping anabolic steroid therapy.

• Alterations may occur in the metyrapone test, glucose tolerance test; decrease in protein bound iodine, decrease in thyroxine-binding capacity and radioactive iodine uptake; retention of sodium, chloride, water, potassium, phosphates, calcium; decrease in BSP, serum cholesterol, serum glutamic oxalotransaminase, serum bilirubin, alkaline phosphatase, suppression of clotting factors II, V, VII, and X; decrease in 17-ketosteroid excretion.

• A well balanced diet should accompany the administration of anabolic steroids.

DRUG INTERACTIONS

• The anabolic steroids may increase the sensitivity to anticoagulants; the anticoagulant dosage may have to be decreased to maintain the prothrombin time at the desired level.

• Anabolic steroids enhance antidiabetic activity of insulin or oral hypoglycemic agents; the dosage of insulin or oral hypoglycemic agent should be adjusted accordingly.

• Concomitant administration of adrenal steroids or ACTH may add to edema.

• Serum cholesterol may increase during therapy.

• Gonadotropin secretion is inhibited.

• Methandrostenolone decreases the metabolism of oxyphenbutazone; a longer, more intense, and unpredictable response to oxyphenbutazone is obtained.

OVERDOSAGE/ANTIDOTE:

• Overdosage is characterized by an exaggeration of the adverse effects.

• There is no specific antidote; discontinue therapy. Treat supportively.

Anterior Pituitary Hormones

GENERAL CLINICAL USES

Of the anterior pituitary hormones, corticotropin, somatropin, and thyrotropin are available commercially. Corticotropin is useful for diagnostic testing for adrenocortical function.

Somatropin is used to stimulate linear growth in patients with pituitary growth hormone deficiency.

Thryotropin is used in the management of certain types of thyroid carcinoma and resulting metastases. It is also used to determine subclinical hypothyroidism or low thyroid reserve, to differentiate between primary and secondary hypothyroidism, to evaluate the need for thyroid medication in patients already receiving thyroid therapy, and to aid in the detection of remnants and metastases of thyroid carcinoma.

SPECIFIC PRODUCTS AND DOSAGES

GENERIC NAME	TRADE NAME	ROUTE OF ADMIN.	USUAL DOSAGE
corticotropin injection (ACTH)	(G)* ACTHAR	iv im/sc	**Diagnosis:** 10–25 units dissolved in 500 ml of 5% glucose infused over 8 hr. **Therapy:** 20 units qid
corticotropin injection, repository	(G) HP ACTHAR GEL	im/sc	40–80 units every 24–72 hr.
somatropin	ASELLACRIN	im	1 ml (2 IU) 3 times/week with a minimum of 48 hr between injections
thyrotropin injection (thyroid stimulating hormone)	THYTROPAR	im/sc	**Diagnosis:** 10 IU for 1–7 days **Therapy:** 10 IU for 3–8 days

*(G) designates availability as a generic product.

Corticotropin (ACTH)

PHARMACOLOGY
Corticotropin and repository corticotropin are anterior pituitary hormones which stimulate the functioning adrenal cortex to produce and secrete the adrenocortical hormones which have both glucocorticoid (anti-inflammatory) and mineralocorticoid (salt-retaining) properties. The corticotropin is of porcine origin.

SPECIAL PRECAUTIONS, ADVERSE EFFECTS
For detailed information, see the discussion of mineralocorticoids in this chapter, page 534.

CLINICAL GUIDELINES
ADMINISTRATION:
• Do not administer intravenously.
• Dietary salt restriction and potassium supplementation may be necessary.
EFFECTS:
• Corticotropin may only suppress symptoms and signs of chronic disease without altering the natural course of the disease.
• Corticotropin increases calcium excretion.
• There is an enhanced effect of corticotropin in patients with hypothyroidism and in those with cirrhosis.
DRUG INTERACTIONS
• Aspirin should be used cautiously in conjunction with corticotropin in patients with hypoprothrombinemia; bleeding may occur.

- Increased dosages of insulin or oral hypoglycemia agents may be necessary in patients taking corticotropin.

Somatotropin

GENERAL CLINICAL USES
Somatotropin is useful when growth failure due to a deficiency of pituitary growth hormone exists.

PHARMACOLOGY
Somatotropin does stimulate linear growth in patients with pituitary growth hormone deficiency. Somatotropin also is an anabolic agent that stimulates intracellular transport of amino acids. Retention of nitrogen, phosphorus, and potassium occurs. Other metabolic parameters are stimulated which result in body growth.

SPECIAL PRECAUTIONS
- Do not use in patients with closed epiphyses; somatotropin is ineffective.
- Do not use in patients with any progression of an underlying intracranial lesion.
- Use with caution in patients with diabetes mellitus or with a family history of diabetes mellitus because of its diabetogenic actions.

ADVERSE EFFECTS
ALLERGIC EFFECTS: antibodies to somatotropin are formed in 30 to 40 percent of patients treated.

CLINICAL GUIDELINES
ADMINISTRATION:
- Subcutaneous administration may lead to lipoatrophy or lipodystrophy at site of administration.

- Test patients for glycosuria frequently.
- Monitor bone age annually, especially in pubertal patients, or those receiving thyroid hormone concomitantly.

EFFECTS:
- Treatment should be continued until the patient reaches adult height.

DRUG INTERACTIONS:
- Concomitant administration of glucocorticoids may inhibit response to somatotropin.

Thyrotropin

PHARMACOLOGY
Thyrotropin, thyroid stimulating hormone, increases iodine uptake by the thyroid, increases formation of thyroid hormone, and causes hyperplasia of thyroid cells. Thyrotropin is isolated from bovine anterior pituitary gland.

SPECIAL PRECAUTIONS
- Do not use in patients hypersensitive to thyrotropin, with coronary thrombosis, and with untreated Addison's disease.
- Use with caution in patients with angina pectoris or cardiac failure.
- Use with care in presence of hypopituitarism since varying degrees of adrenal cortical atrophy are generally present with this condition.
- Adrenal cortical suppression as may be seen with corticosteroid therapy should not be overlooked.

ADVERSE EFFECTS
CNS EFFECTS: fever, headache
CARDIOVASCULAR EFFECTS: transitory hypotension, tachycardia, auricular fibrillation
GASTROINTESTINAL EFFECTS: nausea and vomiting

METABOLIC AND ENDOCRINE EFFECTS: menstrual irregularities, thyroid swelling

ALLERGIC EFFECTS: urticaria, anaphylactic reactions, hypotension

LOCAL EFFECTS: postinjection flare

CLINICAL GUIDELINES

ADMINISTRATION:

• Thyrotropin will retain its potency for approximately two weeks after reconstitution if refrigerated.

OVERDOSAGE/ANTIDOTE:

• Overdosage is characterized by headache, irritability, nervousness, sweating, tachycardia, increased bowl motility, and menstrual irregularities. Angina pectoris or congestive heart failure may be induced or aggravated. Shock may develop. Excessive doses may result in symptoms resembling "thyroid storm." Chronic excessive dosage will produce the signs and symptoms of hyperthyroidism.

• There is no specific antidote. Discontinue thyrotropin administration. If shock occurs, use supportive measures; treatment of unrecognized adrenal insufficiency should be considered.

Antialcohol Agent

Disulfiram

GENERAL CLINICAL USES

Disulfiram is an aid in the management of selected chronic alcoholic patients.

SPECIFIC PRODUCTS AND DOSAGES

GENERIC NAME	TRADE NAME	ROUTE OF ADMIN.	USUAL DOSAGE
disulfiram	ANTABUSE	po	250–500 mg/day

PHARMACOLOGY

Disulfiram interferes with the oxidation of alcohol resulting in disagreeable sensations which, it is hoped, discourage ingestion of alcohol. After disulfiram therapy, the ingestion of alcohol, even in small amounts, may produce the following reactions: flushing, throbbing in the head and neck, throbbing headache, respiratory difficulty, nausea, copious vomiting, dyspnea, hyperventilation, tachycardia, hypotension, syncope, marked uneasiness, weakness, vertigo, blurred vision, and confusion. The reaction may last from 30 to 60 minutes to several hours, as long as there is alcohol in the blood.

SPECIAL PRECAUTIONS
- Do not use in patients with severe myocardial disease or coronary occlusion, psychoses, or hypersensitivity.
- Severe reactions, including respiratory depression, cardiovascular collapse, arrhythmias, myocardial infarction, acute congestive heart failure, unconsciousness, convulsions, and death, have occurred.
- Use with extreme caution in patients with diabetes mellitus, hypothyroidism, epilepsy, cerebral damage, chronic and acute nephritis, hepatic cirrhosis, or hepatic insufficiency because of possible accidental disulfiram-alcohol reaction.
- Safe use in pregnancy has not been established.

ADVERSE EFFECTS
CNS EFFECTS: drowsiness, fatigability, headache; psychotic reactions with high doses or with concomitant administration of metronidazole or isoniazid

METABOLIC AND ENDOCRINE EFFECTS: impotence, metallic or garliclike aftertaste.

HEPATIC EFFECTS: cholestatic hepatitis (unconfirmed)

ALLERGIC EFFECTS: dermatitis

DERMATOLOGIC EFFECTS: acneiform eruptions

CLINICAL GUIDELINES
ADMINISTRATION:
- Monitor hepatic function (transaminase tests at 10 to 14 days); also CBC, SMA-12 (every 6 months).
- Patient must abstain from alcohol for at least 12 hours before administration.
- Warn patient of disulfiram-alcohol reaction; caution to avoid alcohol in any form including sauces, vinegars, cough medications, aftershave lotion, etc.
- Advise patient to carry identification indicating that he is receiving disulfiram and physician or institution to contact.

EFFECTS:
- The disulfiram reaction may occur with alcohol up to 14 days after the patient has ingested disulfiram.
- Disulfiram appears to decrease the rate at which certain drugs are metabolized and may increase the blood levels and possibility of clinical toxicity of drugs given concomitantly.

DRUG INTERACTIONS:
- Barbiturates have been administered concurrently without untoward effects; the possibility of initiating a new abuse should be considered.
- Do not administer to patients who have recently received metronidazole, paraldehyde, alcohol, or alcohol-containing preparations such as cough syrups, tonics; do not administer these produced concurrently with disulfiram.
- With diphenylhydantoin and its congeners, toxic levels may be produced.
- Adjustment of dosage of oral anticoagulants may be necessary, particularly at the beginning and end of therapy; disulfiram may prolong the prothrombin time.
- Disulfiram and isoniazid may produce unsteady gait or marked changes in mental status.

Cholesterol- and Lipid-Reducing Agents (Antihyperlipidemic Agents)

GENERAL CLINICAL USES

The cholesterol- and lipid-reducing agents are indicated for adjunctive therapy to diet and other measures for the reduction of elevated serum cholesterol and/or triglycerides.

SPECIFIC PRODUCTS AND DOSAGES

GENERIC NAME	TRADE NAME	ROUTE OF ADMIN.	USUAL DAILY DOSAGE	
			ADULTS	CHILDREN
cholestyramine	QUESTRAN	po	4 gm tid to qid before meals	Not established
clofibrate	ATROMID-S	po	2 gm daily in divided doses	Not established
colestipol hydrochloride	COLESTID	po	15–30 gm daily in divided doses 2–4 times daily	Not established
dextrothyroxine sodium	CHOLOXIN	po	**Initial:** 1–2 mg daily; **Maintenance:** 4–8 mg daily	**Initial:** 0.05 mg/kg/day **Maintenance:** 0.1 mg/kg/day
niacin (nicotinic acid)	(G)* NICO-SPAN NICOLAR	po	0.5–3 gm daily divided in 3 doses	Not established
probucol	LORELCO	po	500 mg bid	Not established
sitosterols	CYTELLIN	po	3–6 gm before meals; **Maximum:** 24–36 gm daily	Not established

*(G) designates availability as a generic product.

Cholestyramine
Colestipol Hydrochloride

PHARMACOLOGY

Colestipol HCl and cholestyramine are anion exchange resins. The chloride anion can be replaced by other anions with greater affinity for the resin, such as the bile salts. These drugs are not hydrolyzed by digestive enzymes and are not absorbed from the gastrointestinal tract. The increased fecal loss of bile acids leads to an increased oxidation of cholesterol to bile acids, with a decrease in beta lipoprotein and in serum cholesterol levels.

SPECIAL PRECAUTIONS

- Do not use in patients with a history of hypersensitivity to colestipol HCl and cholestyramine.
- Do not use in patients with complete biliary obstruction where bile is not secreted into the intestines.
- Safe use in pregnancy and lactation has not been established.
- Absorption of fat-soluble vitamins A, D, and K may be prevented; supplemental vitamin administration may be necessary with long-term treatment.
- May interfere with normal fat digestion.
- Measure serum triglycerides to insure that significant changes have not occurred.

ADVERSE EFFECTS

GASTROINTESTINAL EFFECTS: constipation, fecal impaction, hemorrhoids, steatorrhea, abdominal gas, distention, flatulence, nausea, vomiting, diarrhea, heartburn, indigestion

METABOLIC AND ENDOCRINE EFFECTS: hyperchloremic acidosis, osteoporosis

HEPATIC EFFECTS: biliary colic

HEMATOLOGIC EFFECTS: with cholestyramine—bleeding tendency

DERMATOLOGIC EFFECTS: rash; irritation of skin, tongue, and perianal area

CLINICAL GUIDELINES

ADMINISTRATION:
- Advise patients to take other medications at least 1 hour before or 4 to 6 hours after cholestyramine to avoid impeding absorption; cholestyramine may bind other drugs.
- Advise patients always to mix with water or other fluids before ingesting.
- Evaluate gastrointestinal function prior

to administration so that severe constipation may be averted, especially in patients with coronary artery disease.
- Monitor cholesterol levels.

EFFECTS:
- Hypoprothrombinemia may occur because of vitamin K deficiency.
- May produce or severely worsen pre-existing constipation; in patients with constipation, impaction may occur.

DRUG INTERACTIONS:
- Cholestyramine and colestipol hydrochloride may have a strong affinity for acidic materials and may also absorb neutral, or, less likely, basic materials to some extent; consequently, absorption of the following drugs may be delayed or reduced: phenylbutazone, warfarin, chlorothiazide, tetracycline, phenobarbital, thyroid and thyroxine preparations, digitalis
- Discontinuance could potentiate digitalis effects to a toxic level.

OVERDOSAGE/ANTIDOTE:
- Prolonged use or overdosage may result in severe constipation leading to impaction. Large dosages may interfere with normal fat digestion.
- To avoid constipation related to prolonged or large doses, use of laxatives may be required.

Clofibrate

PHARMACOLOGY

Clofibrate, administered orally, reduces elevated serum lipids, especially the beta lipoprotein fraction, and/or triglyceride levels. It reduces cholesterol formation early in the synthetic process.

SPECIAL PRECAUTIONS

- Do not use in pregnant or lactating patients or in those with clinically significant

renal or hepatic dysfunction, including primary biliary cirrhosis.
• Use caution when administering concomitantly with anticoagulants.
• Women of childbearing potential undergoing clofibrate therapy should practice strict birth control procedures; clofibrate should be withdrawn several months before conception.
• Attempts should be made to control serum lipids with appropriate dietary regimens, weight loss in obese patients, and control of diabetes mellitus, prior to initiating therapy with clofibrate.
• If the drug is discontinued, the patient should be placed on an appropriate hypolipidemic diet.
• Use with caution in patients with peptic ulcer; the reactivation of ulcers has been reported.

ADVERSE EFFECTS

CNS EFFECTS: headache, dizziness, fatigue, weakness
CARDIOVASCULAR EFFECTS: increase or decrease in angina; arrhythmias, phlebitis, increase phosphokinase
URINARY TRACT EFFECTS: dysuria, hematuria, proteinuria, decreased output
GASTROINTESTINAL EFFECTS: nausea, vomiting, stomatitis, gastritis, loose stools, dyspepsia, flatulence, abdominal distress
METABOLIC AND ENDOCRINE EFFECTS: impotence, decreased libido, weight gain, polyphagia
HEPATIC EFFECTS: hematomegaly, increased SGOT and SGPT, BSP retention, increased thymol turbidity
HEMATOLOGIC EFFECTS: leukopenia, potentiation of anticoagulant effect, anemia, eosinophilia
ALLERGIC EFFECTS: urticaria
DERMATOLOGIC EFFECTS: rash, pruritus, dry brittle hair, alopecia
MUSCULOSKELETAL EFFECTS: muscle cramping, aching, weakness; arthralgia

CLINICAL GUIDELINES

ADMINISTRATION:
• Measure serum lipids prior to and periodically after initiation of therapy.
• Frequently monitor serum transaminase and other liver function tests and hematologic parameters.
EFFECTS:
• Flulike symptoms (muscle aching, soreness, cramping) may be produced.
DRUG INTERACTIONS:
• When anticoagulants are administered concomitantly, the anticoagulant dosage should be reduced, usually by one half, to maintain the prothrombin time at the desired level.
OVERDOSAGE/ANTIDOTE:
• There has been no reported case of overdosage. Should it occur, symptomatic supportive measures are suggested.

Dextrothyroxine Sodium

PHARMACOLOGY

Dextrothyroxine sodium reduces serum cholesterol levels; elevated levels of beta lipoprotein and triglyceride fractions may also be reduced. The mechanism of action is by stimulation of the liver to increase catabolism and excretion of cholesterol and its degradation products; cholesterol synthesis is increased.

SPECIAL PRECAUTIONS

• Do not use in patients with known organic heart disease, hypertension, advanced liver or kidney disease; pregnancy, nursing mothers, or patients with a history of iodism.
• Withdrawal of the drug 2 weeks prior to surgery is suggested if anticoagulants may be used.

- Use with caution in patients with coronary artery disease since the cardiac condition may be aggravated.
- If used in women of childbearing potential, those patients should exercise strict birth control procedures.
- Discontinue therapy if signs of iodism develop.
- Use with caution in children with familial hypercholesterolemia; continue use only if significant reduction in serum cholesterol occurs.
- Use with caution in patients receiving anticoagulants and insulin or oral hypoglycemic agents.

ADVERSE EFFECTS

CNS EFFECTS: insomnia, nervousness, tremors, headache, dizziness, tiredness, psychic changes, paresthesia

RESPIRATORY EFFECTS: hoarseness

CARDIOVASCULAR EFFECTS: angina pectoris, arrhythmias, ECG evidence of ischemic myocardial changes, increased heart size, palpitations

URINARY TRACT EFFECTS: diuresis

AUTONOMIC EFFECTS: sweating, flushing, hyperthermia

GASTROINTESTINAL EFFECTS: dyspepsia, nausea, vomiting, constipation, diarrhea, decreased appetite

METABOLIC AND ENDOCRINE EFFECTS: loss of weight, menstrual irregularities, changes in libido, peripheral edema

HEPATIC EFFECTS: cholestatic jaundice (1 patient)

DERMATOLOGIC EFFECTS: hair loss, rash, pruritus

OPHTHALMIC EFFECTS: lid lag, visual disturbances

OTIC EFFECTS: tinnitus

MUSCULOSKELETAL EFFECTS: muscle pain

CLINICAL GUIDELINES

EFFECTS:
- In diabetic patients, the blood sugar level may increase with a resultant increase in insulin or oral hypoglycemic agent requirement.
- Hypothyroid patients are more sensitive to dextrothyroxine than euthyroid patients.

DRUG INTERACTIONS:
- Concomitant use of epinephrine may precipitate an episode of coronary insufficiency which may be enhanced in patients receiving thyroid analogs. Keep in mind when catecholamine injections are required in patients with coronary artery disease.
- Serum protein bound iodine levels will be greatly increased.
- Concomitant administration of digitalis may result in an additive effect.
- May potentiate effects of coumarin anticoagulants such as dicumarol and warfarin.

Niacin (Nicotinic Acid)

PHARMACOLOGY, SPECIAL PRECAUTIONS, ADVERSE EFFECTS

For detailed information, see Chapter 16, page 595.

CLINICAL GUIDELINES

ADMINISTRATION:
- Administration of a sustained-release formulation minimizes undesirable side effects, namely, flushing, pruritus, and gastrointestinal irritation.

EFFECTS:
- Diabetic or potential diabetic patients may have a decreased glucose tolerance; diet or hypoglycemic therapy may require adjustment.
- Elevated uric acid levels have occurred and may cause problems in patients predisposed to gout.

DRUG INTERACTIONS:
- Niacin may potentiate hypotensive drugs and phenothiazine derivatives, and may inactivate fibrinolysin.
- Liver function tests may be abnormal;

glucose tolerance may be decreased.
• Antihypertensive drugs of the adrenergic blocking type may have an additive vasodilating effect and produce postural hypotension.

OVERDOSAGE/ANTIDOTE:
• Overdosage is characterized by an exaggeration of the adverse effects.
• There is no specific antidote; discontinue use of niacin.

Probucol

PHARMACOLOGY
The mechanism of action of probucol in lowering serum lipids is unknown. It does not appear to affect the later stages of cholesterol biosynthesis.

SPECIAL PRECAUTIONS
• Do not use in patients with a history of hypersensitivity.
• Safe use in pregnancy, lactation, or in children has not been established.

ADVERSE EFFECTS
CNS EFFECTS: dizziness, syncope, headache, paresthesias
CARDIOVASCULAR EFFECTS: palpitations, chest pain
AUTONOMIC EFFECTS: hyperhidrosis, fetid sweat
GASTROINTESTINAL EFFECTS: diarrhea, flatulence, abdominal pain, nausea, vomiting, heartburn, anorexia
URINARY TRACT EFFECTS: nocturia
ENDOCRINE AND METABOLIC EFFECTS: angioneurotic edema; increased uric acid, BUN, blood glucose
HEPATIC EFFECTS: elevated SGOT, SGPT, bilirubin, alkaline phosphatase, creatine phosphokinase
HEMATOLOGIC EFFECTS: eosinophilia, thrombocytopenia

DERMATOLOGIC EFFECTS: rash
OPHTHALMIC EFFECTS: tearing, conjunctivitis, blurred vision
OTIC EFFECTS: tinnitus

CLINICAL GUIDELINES
ADMINISTRATION:
• Absorption from the gastrointestinal tract is limited and variable. When administered with food, peak blood levels are higher and less variable than when administered on an empty stomach.

Sitosterols

PHARMACOLOGY
Sitosterols may lower elevated serum cholesterol by interfering with intestinal absorption. The exact mechanism of action is unknown.

SPECIAL PRECAUTIONS
• Safe use during pregnancy and lactation has not been established.
• May interfere with the absorption of other substances and drugs.

ADVERSE EFFECTS
GASTROINTESTINAL EFFECTS: loose stools

CLINICAL GUIDELINES
ADMINISTRATION:
• Warn patients that bulky light-colored stools may be produced.
• Administer mixed with coffee, tea, fruit juices, or milk to increase palatability; administer immediately before meals.
EFFECTS:
• A slight laxative effect may occur.
DRUG INTERACTIONS:
• Other drugs administered orally may not be absorbed, since sitosterols interfere with intestinal absorption of cholesterol and may also interfere with absorption of other materials.

Gonadotropin

GENERAL CLINICAL USES

Chorionic gonadotropin is useful in treating cryptorchidism not due to anatomic obstruction; selected cases of male hypogonadism secondary to pituitary failure; and in induction of ovulation and pregnancy in the anovulatory, infertile female. It has no effect in the treatment of obesity.

SPECIFIC PRODUCTS AND DOSAGES

GENERIC NAME	TRADE NAME	ROUTE OF ADMIN.	USUAL DOSE
chorionic gonadotropin	(G)* A.P.L. Secules ANTUITRIN-S FOLLUTEIN	im	**Cryptorchidism:** 4000 USP units three times weekly, then gradually reduced **Male hypogonadism:** 500–1000 USP units 3 times weekly, increase gradually to 2000–4000 USP units 3 times weekly **Induction of ovulation:** 5000–10000 USP units 1 day after last dose of menotropins

*(G) designates availability as a generic product.

PHARMACOLOGY

Chorionic gonadotropin, a polypeptide produced by the placenta, is a gonad-stimulating hormone. Chorionic gonadotropin promotes production of gonadal steroid hormones by stimulating the interstitial cells of the testis to produce androgens and the corpus luteum of the ovary to produce progesterone.

Human chorionic gonadotropin has no known effect on fat mobilization, appetite, sense of hunger, or body fat distribution.

SPECIAL PRECAUTIONS

• Do not use in precocious puberty, prostatic carcinoma, or other androgen-dependent neoplasia.

• Do not use in patients with a history of hypersensitivity to human chorionic gonadotropin.

• Human chorionic gonadotropin should be used in conjunction with human menopausal gonadotropins only by physicians experienced with infertility problems and familiar with patient selection, contraindications, warnings, precautions, and adverse effects described for menotropins.

• Use with caution for induction of androgen secretion, since chorionic gonadotropin may induce precocious puberty in patients treated for cryptorchidism; if signs of precocious puberty occur, therapy should be discontinued.

• Since androgens may cause fluid retention, chorionic gonadotropin should be used with caution in patients with epilepsy, migraine, asthma, or cardiac or renal disease.

ADVERSE EFFECTS

CNS EFFECTS: headache, irritability, restlessness, depression, tiredness

METABOLIC AND ENDOCRINE EFFECTS: edema, precocious puberty, gynecomastia

LOCAL EFFECTS: pain at site of injection

Hyperglycemic/Hypoglycemic Agents

Antidiabetic Agents

Insulins

GENERAL CLINICAL USES

Insulin is used to control the blood sugar level in patients with diabetes mellitus.

SPECIFIC PRODUCTS AND DOSAGES

GENERIC NAME	TRADE NAME	AVAILABLE CONC. (units/cc)	CLINICAL EFFECT (in hrs)		
			onset	peak	duration
Prompt-acting: insulin injection	(G)* REGULAR ILETIN	U-40, U-80, U-100	1/2–1	2–3	approx 8
	REGULAR (CONCENTRATED) ILETIN	U-500			

*(G) designates availability as a generic product.

(continued overleaf)

GENERIC NAME	TRADE NAME	AVAILABLE CONC. (units/cc)	CLINICAL EFFECT (in hrs)		
			onset	peak	duration
prompt insulin zinc suspension	(G)* SEMILENTE INSULIN SEMILENTE ILETIN	U-40, U-80, U-100	1/2 –1	5–7	approx 12–18
Intermediate-acting: insulin zinc suspension	(G) LENTE ILETIN LENTE INSULIN	U-40, U-80, U-100	1–1 1/2	8–12	approx 24
globin zinc insulin injection	(G)	U-40, U-80, U-100	2	8–16	approx 24
isophane insulin suspension	(G) NPH ILETIN	U-40, U-80, U-100	1–1 1/2	8–12	approx 24
Long-acting: extended insulin zinc suspension	(G) ULTRALENTE ILETIN ULTRALENTE INSULIN	U-40, U-80, U-100	4–8	16–18	approx 36
protamine zinc insulin suspension	(G) PROTAMINE ZINC ILETIN	U-40, U-80, U-100	4–8	14–20	approx 36

*(G) designates availability as a generic product.

PHARMACOLOGY

The insulins are divided into three groups based on the type of action: fast, intermediate, or long. The fast-acting forms consist of insulin injection (regular, unmodified) which has a short duration of action, and prompt insulin zinc suspension, which has a prolonged duration of action without the addition of a modifying protein. Both products are obtained from beef, pork, or a mixture of beef and pork pancreas. The prompt insulin zinc suspension is not to be adapted for use in place of regular (unmodified) insulin in dealing with acidosis and emergencies.

The intermediate-acting insulins consist of globin zinc insulin injection, which contains globin, a beef protein, to delay absorption; insulin zinc suspension, a mixture of extended insulin zinc suspension 70% and prompt insulin zinc suspension 30%; and isophane insulin suspension, a form conjugated with protamine to delay absorption. These products are obtained from beef, pork, or a mixture of beef and pork pancreas. Globin zinc insulin injection may be used in patients who exhibit sensitivity to protamine.

The long-acting insulins, protamine zinc insulin suspension and extended insulin zinc suspension, are not to be adapted for use in place of regular (unmodified) insulin in dealing with acidosis and emergencies. The extended insulin zinc suspension is derived from beef pancreas, whereas the protamine zinc insulin suspension is derived from pork, beef, or a mixture of beef and pork pancreas. With these products a decrease in blood sugar may come about so slowly that marked hypoglycemia without apparent symptoms is produced.

ADVERSE EFFECTS

Adverse effects occurring with the insulin preparations are primarily pharmacological actions and are due to overdosage. See *Overdosage/Antidote*, below, for detailed information. Additionally, hypersensitivity reactions, characterized by generalized urticaria, angioneurotic edema, and anaphylaxis, have occurred; these reactions are due primarily to the proteins present.

SPECIAL PRECAUTIONS

• The patient should be cautioned to follow carefully a course of diet and exercise prescribed by the physician.
• Caution patient that if he finds it necessary to omit a meal because of nausea or vomiting, the physician should be notified and the urine should be tested every 3 or 4 hours.
• Caution patient to notify physician if any illness occurs from any cause.
• Do not use in patients with a history of hypersensitivity to that product.

CLINICAL GUIDELINES

ADMINISTRATION:
• Instruct patient fully in administration techniques, personal hygiene, diet, exercise, testing of urine for sugar and ketones.
• Advise patient to carry candy or lump sugar to counteract hypoglycemia.
• Administer insulin before breakfast.
• Advise patient to rotate sites of injection.
• Prepare card for patient to identify him as a diabetic.
• Advise patient to refrigerate insulin.

EFFECTS:
• Hypoglycemia may occur following increased work or exercise; when food is not being absorbed in the usual manner; because of postponement or omission of a meal or in illness with vomiting, diarrhea, or delayed digestion; when insulin is administered too long before a meal; when the patient's requirement for insulin declines; or when large doses of insulin are given at insufficient or irregular intervals.
• An early symptom of hypoglycemia is fatigue; it is of utmost importance for the patient to understand clearly that the presence of vague symptoms of fatigue, headache, drowsiness, lassitude, tremulousness or nausea demands immediate attention.
• The presence of sugar in the urine means unsuitable dosage of insulin or dietary imbalance.

DRUG INTERACTIONS:
• Prompt insulin zinc suspension may be mixed with insulin zinc suspension and extended insulin zinc suspension.
• Insulin injection may be mixed with all other insulin products.
• Insulin zinc suspension may be mixed with regular crystalline insulin and prompt insulin zinc suspension.
• Extended insulin zinc suspension may be mixed with regular crystalline insulin and prompt insulin zinc suspension.
• Protamine zinc insulin suspension may be mixed with regular crystalline insulin.
• Isophane insulin suspension may be mixed with regular crystalline insulin.

OVERDOSAGE/ANTIDOTE:
• An excessive dose of insulin causes hypoglycemia. The initial symptoms are vague and consist of fatigue, headache, drowsiness, lassitude, tremulousness, or nausea. More marked symptoms include weakness, sweating, tremor, or nervousness.
• Treatment consists of candy or a lump of sugar, which should always be carried by the patient. If the patient becomes delirious or mentally confused, dilute corn syrup or orange juice with sugar should be ad-

ministered by mouth. In severe hypoglycemic reactions, dextrose in water, 5%, 10%, or 20%, sterile solution may be administered intravenously.

Oral Hypoglycemic Agents

Acetohexamide   Tolazamide
Chlorpropamide Tolbutamide

GENERAL CLINICAL USES
The orally administered hypoglycemic agents, the sulfonylureas, may be effective in controlling stable adult diabetes mellitus of the maturity onset or nonketotic type.

SPECIFIC PRODUCTS AND DOSAGES

GENERIC NAME	TRADE NAME	USUAL DAILY DOSAGE
acetohexamide	DYMELOR	250–1500 mg daily
chlorpropamide	DIABINESE	**Adults:** 250–500 mg daily **Geriatric:** 100–125 mg daily **Maximum:** 750 mg daily
tolazamide	TOLINASE	100–250 mg daily
tolbutamide	(G)* ORINASE	250–3000 mg daily

*(G) designates availability as a generic product.

PHARMACOLOGY
The sulfonylureas, sulfonamide derivatives, are devoid of antibacterial activity. They lower blood glucose following oral administration in both diabetics and nondiabetics. They are absorbed from the gastrointestinal tract and exert a hypoglycemic effect. The hypoglycemic effect of chlorpropamide is noted within 1 hour; this effect is maximal at 3 to 6 hours and persists for 24 hours. Acetohexamide has a rapid onset of action and the effects last 12 to 24 hours. Tolazamide produces a peak hypoglycemic effect in 4 to 6 hours; the effect lasts about 10 hours. Tolbutamide is rapidly absorbed from the gastrointestinal tract and the effect may last 6 to 12 hours.

The mode of action of the sulfonylureas appears to be stimulation and release of endogenous insulin.

SPECIAL PRECAUTIONS
• Do not use in patients with juvenile or growth-onset diabetes mellitus, with severe or unstable "brittle" diabetes, with diabetes complicated by ketosis or acidosis, diabetic coma, major surgery, severe infection, severe trauma.
• Safe use in pregnancy or in women who may become pregnant has not been established.
• Do not use in patients with serious impairment of hepatic, renal, or thyroid function.

- Dosage adjustment may be required to prevent the occurrence of hypoglycemia in patients with impaired hepatic and/or renal function and in debilitated or malnourished patients.

ADVERSE EFFECTS

CNS EFFECTS: fever, weakness, paresthesias, vertigo, malaise, headache

GASTROINTESTINAL EFFECTS: diarrhea, rarely severe, sometimes accompanied by bleeding into the lower bowel; anorexia, nausea, vomiting, epigastric discomfort.

METABOLIC AND ENDOCRINE EFFECTS: edema associated with hyponatremia infrequently

HEPATIC EFFECTS: eosinophilia, leukopenia, thrombocytopenia, mild anemia, aplastic anemia, agranulocytosis, pancytopenia

ALLERGIC EFFECTS: urticaria, pruritus, erythema; urticarial, morbilliform, or maculopapular eruptions

DERMATOLOGIC EFFECTS: rash, exfoliative dermatitis, phototoxicity rarely

CLINICAL GUIDELINES

ADMINISTRATION:

- Administer before breakfast.
- Contact patient weekly; observe for evidence of occasional drug reactions.
- Patient should be advised to contact physician if pruritus, rash, jaundice, dark urine, light-colored stools, low-grade fever, sore throat or diarrhea occurs.
- Administering the drug in divided doses may reduce gastrointestinal adverse effects.

EFFECTS:

- Pseudodiabetes with azotemia due to chronic renal disease has been misdiagnosed as diabetes mellitus.
- Elderly patients may be hyperresponsive.

DRUG INTERACTIONS:

- Use barbiturates cautiously in patients receiving chlorpropamide; in animals the action of barbiturates has been prolonged.
- A disulfiramlike reaction may be produced by the ingestion of alcohol.
- Caution should be exercised when antibacterial sulfonamides, oxyphenbutazone/phenylbutazone, salicylates, insulin, probenecid, dicumarol, bishydroxycoumarin, phenyramidol, or MAO-inhibitors are administered concurrently; hypoglycemia may result from either potentiation or accumulation of sulfonylureas.
- Tolbutamide may cause reduction in I^{131} uptake.
- Alcohol and decreased diet may lead to hypoglycemia, ketosis, coma, and death.
- Thiazides suppress insulin secretion and contribute to hyperglycemia; dosage adjustment may be required.
- Alkaline phosphatase increase is indicative of cholangiolitic jaundice; withdraw drug.
- A false positive reaction for urine albumin may occur because of sulfonylurea metabolites; this does not occur with tolazamide.

OVERDOSAGE/ANTIDOTE:

- In accidental ingestion by children, note that 3 to 5 days are required for complete elimination of these drugs. Hypoglycemia may occur.
- Treat hypoglycemia. Dextrose, 10 to 50% in water, may be used if patient has protracted hypoglycemia.

Hyperglycemic Agents

GENERAL CLINICAL USES

The hyperglycemic agents, glucagon and diazoxide, increase blood glucose concentration.

Diazoxide administered orally is useful in the management in adults of hypoglycemia due to hyperinsulinism associated with inoperable islet cell adenoma or carcinoma; extrahepatic malignancy; in children in leucine sensitivity, islet cell hyperplasia, nesidioblastosis, extrahepatic malignancy, islet cell adenoma or adenomatosis.

Glucagon is used to counteract severe hypoglycemic reactions in diabetic patients or during insulin shock therapy in psychiatric patients.

SPECIFIC PRODUCTS AND DOSAGES

GENERIC NAME	TRADE NAME	ROUTE OF ADMIN.	USUAL DOSAGE
diazoxide	PROGLYCEM Capsules, Suspension	po	**Adults:** 3–8 mg/kg/day divided in 2 or 3 equal doses **Infants and newborns:** 8–15 mg/kg/day divided in 2 or 3 equal doses
glucagon for injection	(G)*	sc/im/iv	0.5 to 1 unit; may be repeated one or two additional times

*(G) designates availability as a generic product.

Diazoxide

PHARMACOLOGY

Diazoxide, a benzothiadiazine derivative, when administered orally, causes a prompt dose-related increase in blood glucose concentration. This effect is due primarily to an inhibition of insulin release from the pancreas. The hyperglycemic effect usually begins within 1 hour and lasts no more than 8 hours in the presence of normal renal function. Diazoxide is excreted by the kidneys; it crosses the placental barrier in animals.

SPECIAL PRECAUTIONS

• Do not use in patients with functional hypoglycemia and in patients who are hypersensitive to diazoxide or other thiazides.

• Safe use in pregnancy has not been established.

• The antidiuretic property of diazoxide may result in significant fluid retention, which may precipitate congestive heart failure in patients with compromised cardiac reserve.

• Ketoacidosis and nonketotic hyperosmolar coma have been reported in patients with diazoxide, usually during other illnesses.

• Use with caution in patients with impaired renal function.

ADVERSE EFFECTS

CNS EFFECTS: headache, weakness, malaise, anxiety, dizziness, insomnia, fever, polyneuritis, paresthesia, extrapyramidal signs

CARDIOVASCULAR EFFECTS: hypotension

occasionally; transient hypertension in few cases; chest pain rarely; congestive heart failure, tachycardia, palpitations

URINARY TRACT EFFECTS: glycosuria, decreased creatinine clearance, reversible nephrotic syndrome, decreased urinary output, hematuria, albuminuria

GASTROINTESTINAL EFFECTS: anorexia, nausea, vomiting, abdominal pain, ileus, diarrhea, transient loss of taste

METABOLIC AND ENDOCRINE EFFECTS: sodium and fluid retention, diabetic ketoacidosis, hyperosmolar nonketotic coma, hyperglycemia, gout, increased uric acid level, pancreatitis, pancreatic necrosis, galactorrhea, enlargement of lump in breast

HEPATIC EFFECTS: increased SGOT, alkaline phosphatase; azotemia

HEMATOLOGIC EFFECTS: eosinophilia, decreased hemoglobin/hematocrit, excessive bleeding, decreased IgG, lymphadenopathy

DERMATOLOGIC EFFECTS: hirsutism of lanugo type, reversible; rash, alopecia, pruritus, monilial dermatitis, herpes

OPHTHALMIC EFFECTS: cataracts, transient; subconjunctival hemorrhage, ring scotoma, blurred vision, diplopia, and lacrimation

MUSCULOSKELETAL EFFECTS: advance in bone age

CLINICAL GUIDELINES

ADMINISTRATION:
- Monitor blood glucose levels closely until patient's condition has stabilized; this usually requires several days.
- Regular monitoring of blood glucose and urine glucose and ketones is required during prolonged treatment.

EFFECTS:
- The presence of hypokalemia potentiates the effects of diazoxide.
- In some patients, higher blood levels have been obtained with the liquid (suspension) than with the capsules; dosage may require adjustment if patient is changed from one formulation to another.

DRUG INTERACTIONS:
- Concomitant administration of thiazide diuretics or other potent diuretics may intensify the hyperglycemic and hyperuricemic effects of diazoxide.
- Alpha adrenergic blocking agents antagonize the inhibition of insulin release by diazoxide.
- The effects of antihypertensive drugs may be enhanced by diazoxide.
- Since diazoxide binds to protein (over 90 percent), administration with coumarin or its derivatives may require reduction in the dosage of the anticoagulant.
- Diazoxide may possibly displace bilirubin from albumin; this should be kept in mind, particularly when treating newborns with increased bilirubinemia.

OVERDOSAGE/ANTIDOTE:
- Overdosage induces hyperglycemia which may be associated with ketoacidosis.
- Hyperglycemia may be reversed by the administration of insulin or tolbutamide; restore fluid and electrolyte balance. Because of the long half-life of diazoxide, patient must be observed for about 7 days.
- Both peritoneal dialysis and hemodialysis have been used successfully, each in one patient.

Glucagon

PHARMACOLOGY

Glucagon, a polypeptide hormone produced by the pancreas, causes an increase in blood glucose concentration by converting hepatic glycogen to glucose. When administered parenterally, the effect is rapid but is only useful when hepatic glycogen is available.

SPECIAL PRECAUTIONS
- Since glucagon is a protein, hypersensitivity is a possibility.
- In the treatment of hyperglycemic shock, liver glycogen must be available; glucose administered intravenously or by gavage should be considered in the hypoglycemic patient.

ADVERSE EFFECTS

GASTROINTESTINAL EFFECTS: nausea, vomiting

CLINICAL GUIDELINES

ADMINISTRATION:
- Reconstitute glucagon using sterile conditions; the solution will remain potent for as long as 3 months if kept refrigerated.

EFFECTS:
- If unconscious, the patient usually will awaken in 5 to 20 minutes.
- Give patient supplemental carbohydrates to restore liver glycogen and prevent secondary hypoglycemia.

DRUG INTERACTIONS:
- Glucagon and glucose may be used together without precipitating or decreasing the efficacy of glucose administration.
- Glucagon precipitates when mixed with solutions containing sodium chloride, potassium chloride, or calcium chloride.

OVERDOSAGE/ANTIDOTE:
- Overdosage of glucagon results in hyperglycemia.
- Hyperglycemia may be reversed by the administration of insulin.

Parathyroid/Calcium Regulators

Parathyroid Regulators

GENERAL CLINICAL USES

Calcitonin-salmon is indicated for the treatment of moderate to severe symptomatic Paget's disease of the bone. Effectiveness has been demonstrated principally in patients with moderate to severe disease characterized by polyosteotic involvement with elevated serum alkaline phosphatase and urinary hydroxyproline excretion.

Dihydrotachysterol is used to treat hypocalcemia associated with idiopathic and postoperative hypoparathyroidism and pseudohypoparathyroidism.

Etidronate disodium is indicated for treatment of symptomatic Paget's disease of bone (osteitis deformans).

Parathyroid hormone may be used in the treatment of acute hypoparathyroidism with tetany. Long-continued use is not recommended since patients soon become refractory to injections of this substance.

SPECIFIC PRODUCTS AND DOSAGES

GENERIC NAME	TRADE NAME	ROUTE OF ADMIN.	USUAL DOSAGE
calcitonin-salmon	CALCIMAR	sc/im	50–100 MRC units/day
dihydrotachysterol	(G)* HYTAKEROL	po	**Initial:** 0.8–2.4 mg/day **Maintenance:** 0.2–1.0 mg/day
etidronate disodium	DIDRONEL	po	5–10 mg/kg/day **Maximum:** 20 mg/kg/day
parathyroid injection	(G)	sc/im/iv	20–40 units q 12 hr.

*(G) designates availability as a generic product.

Calcitonin-Salmon

PHARMACOLOGY

Calcitonin-salmon, a semisynthetic compound of salmon origin, acts primarily on bone but also has direct renal and gastrointestinal effects. The potency of the compound is greater than calcitonin from other sources. Calcitonin causes a marked transient inhibition of ongoing bone resorptive processes. With prolonged use, there is a persistent, small decrease in the rate of bone absorption. Bone formation may be augmented by calcitonin.

SPECIAL PRECAUTIONS
• Do not use in patients hypersensitive to synthetic calcitonin-salmon or its gelatin diluent.
• Safe use in pregnancy has not been established.
• Do not administer to nursing mothers.
• Because calcitonin and gelatin (diluent) are proteins, systemic allergic reactions may occur.
• Consider skin testing prior to treatment with calcitonin-salmon.
• The administration of calcitonin could possibly lead to hypocalcemic tetany under special circumstances; no cases have been reported. Provide for administration of parenteral calcium if needed.

ADVERSE EFFECTS
GASTROINTESTINAL EFFECTS: nausea, and vomiting
AUTONOMIC EFFECTS: facial flushing
LOCAL EFFECTS: after subcutaneous or intramuscular injection, inflammation

CLINICAL GUIDELINES
ADMINISTRATION:
• Monitor serum alkaline phosphatase and 24-hour urinary hydroxyproline and evaluate symptoms.
EFFECTS:
• A decrease of serum calcium and serum alkaline phosphatase toward normal values usually occurs with the first few months of therapy.

Dihydrotachysterol

PHARMACOLOGY

Dihydrotachysterol elevates serum calcium by stimulation of calcium absorption and metabolism of bone calcium in the absence of parathyroid hormone. After oral administration, it is well absorbed and has a prolonged effect. It is faster acting than vitamin D and less persistent after cessation of treatment.

SPECIAL PRECAUTIONS

• Do not use in patients with hypercalcemia, hypocalcemia associated with renal insufficiency and hyperphosphatemia.

• Do not administer to patients with abnormal sensitivity to the effects of vitamin D and hypervitaminosis D.

• Safe use in pregnancy has not been established.

• Administer with caution to patients with renal stones because of the effect on serum calcium.

• Maintain a normal serum phosphorus level in patients with renal osteodystrophy accompanied by hyperphosphatemia.

ADVERSE EFFECTS

CNS EFFECTS: languor, convulsions, vertigo, headache

GASTROINTESTINAL EFFECTS: anorexia, nausea, vomiting, diarrhea, abdominal cramps

METABOLIC AND ENDOCRINE EFFECTS: osteoporosis, weight loss, metastatic calcifications, thirst

URINARY TRACT EFFECTS: renal damage, polyurea, albuminuria

HEMATOLOGIC EFFECTS: anemia

DERMATOLOGIC EFFECTS: band keratitis, xanthemia

MUSCULOSKELETAL EFFECTS: ataxia of lower extremities

OTIC EFFECTS: tinnitus

CLINICAL GUIDELINES

ADMINISTRATION:

• Monitor serum calcium levels during therapy; maintain level between 9 and 10 mg/100 ml.

DRUG INTERACTIONS:

• Concurrent administration of thiazide diuretics may cause hypercalcemia.

OVERDOSAGE/ANTIDOTE:

• Overdosage is characterized by the symptoms of hypercalcemia: weakness, headache, anorexia, nausea, vomiting, abdominal cramps, vertigo, tinnitus, ataxia, exanthema; renal impairment and metastatic calcifications may also occur.

• Withdraw drug; administer low-calcium diet and a laxative. Hydrate patient. Dialysis may be used, also administration of citrates, sulfates, phosphates, corticosteroids, EDTA, and mithramycin.

Etidronate Disodium

PHARMACOLOGY

Etidronate disodium acts primarily on bone by inhibiting either calcium crystal resorption or crystal growth. It slows the rate of bone turnover in Pagetic bone lesions and in the normal remodeling process.

Patients absorb about 1 percent of an oral dose of 5 mg/kg/day. Absorption increases with increase in dosage. Etidronate disodium is not metabolized. The majority of the drug is cleared from the blood within 6 hours. Absorbed drug is excreted in the urine and unabsorbed drug in the feces.

SPECIAL PRECAUTIONS

• Avoid overtreatment; adhere to recommended dosage regimen.

- Use with caution in patients with impaired renal function since etidronate disodium is excreted in the urine.
- Since increased frequency of bowel movements and diarrhea has occurred with etidronate disodium, it may be advisable to withhold the drug from patients with enterocolitis.
- Use only when clearly needed in women who are or may become pregnant.
- Advise nursing mothers to stop nursing if they are taking etidronate disodium.
- Safe use in children has not been established.

ADVERSE EFFECTS
GASTROINTESTINAL EFFECTS: diarrhea, loose bowel movements, nausea
MUSCULOSKELETAL EFFECTS: bone pain

CLINICAL GUIDELINES
ADMINISTRATION:
- Assure that patient maintains an adequate nutritional status, particularly, an adequate intake of calcium and vitamin D.
OVERDOSAGE/ANTIDOTE:
- There is no experience with acute overdosage. Theoretically, overdosage may result in hypocalcemia.
- Treat symptomatically and supportively.

Parathyroid Injection

PHARMACOLOGY
Parathyroid injection, prepared from beef glands, is standardized by its capacity to increase the total serum calcium in normal dogs. One USP parathyroid unit is defined as one one-hundredth of the amount required to raise the calcium content of 100 ml of blood serum of normal dogs 1 mg within 16 to 18 hours after administration.

SPECIAL PRECAUTIONS
- Do not give to patients whose blood calcium levels are already above normal.
- Use with caution in the presence of renal or cardiac disease.
- Use caution when administering intravenously because parathyroid extracts have some of the properties of proteins.
- Do not use in patients with a history of hypersensitivity to the product.

ADVERSE EFFECTS
LOCAL EFFECTS: after subcutaneous injection, moderate inflammatory reaction
SYSTEMIC EFFECTS: physiologic effects of hormone, hyperphosphaturia, hypophosphatemia, hypercalcemia, hypocalcuria

CLINICAL GUIDELINES
ADMINISTRATION:
- Control dosage to maintain the serum calcium level at not more than 12 mg per 100 ml.
EFFECTS:
- In postoperative patients or those with idiopathic hypoparathyroidism, a twofold or greater increase in phosphorus excretion may occur.
- Patients with pseudohypoparathyroidism have a twofold or less increase in phosphorus levels.
DRUG INTERACTIONS:
- If parathyroid injection is to added to other intravenous solutions, dextrose 2.5 to 5% should be used; saline solutions often cause formation of a precipitate.
OVERDOSAGE/ANTIDOTE:
- Overdosage is characterized by anorexia, vomiting, diarrhea, and weakness.
- There is no specific antidote. Discontinue therapy. Treat supportively.

Calcium Regulators

GENERAL CLINICAL USES

The calcium regulators include products to treat both hypocalcemia and hypercalcemia.

The calcium supplements are useful in increasing the serum calcium levels in conditions associated with hypocalcemia, tetany (nocturnal leg cramps), and hypoparathyroidism (postoperative and idiopathic). Hypocalcemia is defined as a serum calcium below 8 mg/100 ml or 4 mEq/liter. The calcium supplements are usually administered orally, but intravenous administration of calcium solutions may be necessary for prompt relief of symptoms.

Calcium is necessary for normal cardiac and skeletal muscle functions and for the coagulation of blood. Calcium solutions may be administered in cardiac resuscitation when epinephrine fails to improve weak or ineffective myocardial contractions.

The antihypercalcemic agents are useful in treating hypercalcemia occurring with neoplasms with or without osseous metasteses, hyperparathyroidism, thiazide therapy, multiple myeloma, sarcoidosis, hypervitaminosis D, milk-alkali syndrome, and overdosage of calcium supplements.

The Recommended Dietary Allowances of calcium are:
1. Adults—800 mg
2. Pregnant and lactating women—1200 mg
3. Children
   a. 1/2–1 yr.—540 mg
   b. 1–10 yrs.—800 mg
   c. 11–18 yrs.—1200 mg

Calcitriol is indicated in the management of hypocalcemia in patients undergoing chronic renal dialysis. Calcitriol has been shown to reduce elevated parathyroid hormone levels in some of these patients.

Calcium Supplements

SPECIFIC PRODUCTS AND DOSAGES

GENERIC NAME	TRADE NAME	ROUTE OF ADMIN.	USUAL DAILY DOSAGE	
			ADULTS	**CHILDREN**
calcitriol	ROCALTROL	po	0.25 mcg/day; may increase by 0.25 mcg/day at 2- to 4-week intervals *Hemodialysis patients:* 0.5–1 mcg/day	Not established

(continued facing page)

GENERIC NAME	TRADE NAME	ROUTE OF ADMIN.	USUAL DAILY DOSAGE	
			ADULTS	CHILDREN
calcium carbonate	(G)† FOSFREE*	po	1–2 gm tid	Not established
calcium chloride	(G)	iv po	0.5–1.0 gm/day 6–8 gm/day in divided doses	Not established Not established
calcium glubionate	NEO-CALGLUCON	po	15 ml tid **Pregnant or lactating Patients:** 15 ml qid	**4 yrs. and older:** 15 ml tid **Under 4 yrs.:** 10 ml tid **Infants:** 5 ml 5x/day
calcium gluceptate	(G)	im/iv	2–5 ml	Not established
calcium gluconate	(G) FOSFREE* KALCINATE	po iv	1–2 gm bid to tid 0.5–2.0 gm	Not established Not established
calcium glycerophosphate	CALPHOSAN* CALORA FORTE*	im po	10 ml 1–2 times/wk 40–120 mg daily	Not established Not established
calcium lactate	(G) FOSFREE*	po	0.32–1.3 gm tid	Not established
calcium levulinate	(G)	im/iv/sc	1 gm daily	0.2–0.5 mg daily
calcium orotate	CALORA FORTE*	po	40–120 mg daily	Not established
calcium phosphate dibasic	(G) DISAL-D*	po	0.5–1.5 mg tid or bid	Not established
calcium phosphate tribasic	(G) CA-PLUS ELECAL	po	1–2 gm tid	Not established

*Contains more than one active ingredient.
†(G) designates availability as a generic product.

Calcitriol

PHARMACOLOGY
Calcitriol, a product naturally occurring in humans, is also known as 1,25-dihydroxycholecalciferol, the active form of vitamin D_3. The two known sites of action are intestine and bone. Calcitriol stimulates intestinal calcium transport.

Calcitriol, after oral administration, is rapidly absorbed from the intestines. The pharmacologic activity of calcitriol is about 3 to 5 days.

SPECIAL PRECAUTIONS
• Withhold all vitamin D. Calcitriol is the most potent metabolite of vitamin D available.
• Do not administer to patients with hypercalcemia or evidence of vitamin D toxicity.

• Aluminum carbonate or hydroxide gel should be used to control serum phosphate levels in patients undergoing dialysis.

• The serum calcium times phosphate (Ca × P) product should not be allowed to exceed 70.

• Use with caution in patients on digitalis because hypercalcemia in such patients may precipitate cardiac arrhythmias.

• Safe use in pregnancy, nursing mothers, or children has not been established.

ADVERSE EFFECTS

CNS EFFECTS: weakness, headache, somnolence, psychosis (overt)

CARDIOVASCULAR EFFECTS: hypertension, cardiac arrhythmias

RESPIRATORY EFFECTS: rhinorrhea

AUTONOMIC EFFECTS: dry mouth

GASTROINTESTINAL EFFECTS: nausea, vomiting, constipation, metallic taste, polydipsia, anorexia, pancreatitis

METABOLIC AND ENDOCRINE EFFECTS: loss of weight, hyperthermia, decreased libido, hypercholesterolemia

URINARY TRACT EFFECTS: polyuria, albuminuria, elevated BUN

HEPATIC EFFECTS: elevated SGOT and SGPT

ALLERGIC EFFECTS: pruritus

OPHTHALMIC EFFECTS: photophobia

CLINICAL GUIDELINES

ADMINISTRATION:

• Early in treatment, determine serum calcium twice weekly to avoid overdosage. A fall in serum alkaline phosphatase antedates the appearance of hypercalcemia and may be an indication of impending hypercalcemia.

• Determine serum calcium, phosphorus, magnesium, and alkaline phosphatase and 24 hour urinary calcium and phosphorus periodically.

• Inform patient/spouse about compliance with dosage instructions.

DRUG INTERACTIONS:

• Magnesium-containing antacid and calcitriol should not be used concomitantly, because such use may lead to the development of hypermagnesemia.

• Overdosage of any form of vitamin D is dangerous.

• Avoid use of nonprescription drugs.

• Cholestyramine may impair intestinal absorption of calcitriol.

OVERDOSAGE/ANTIDOTE:

• Excessive dosage of calcitriol induces hypercalcemia and in some instances hypercalciuria.

• Discontinue drug immediately. Institute low calcium diet and withdraw calcium supplements. Determine calcium levels daily. Persistant or markedly elevated serum calcium levels may be corrected by dialysis against a calcium free dialysate.

Calcium Salts

PHARMACOLOGY

Calcium salts available for oral administration include calcium chloride, calcium carbonate, calcium glubionate, calcium gluconate, calcium lactate, calcium orotate, dibasic calcium phosphate, and tribasic calcium phosphate; for intramuscular and/or intravenous administration, calcium chloride, calcium gluceptate, calcium gluconate, calcium levulinate, calcium lactate, and calcium glycerophosphate. All calcium preparations are used to preserve or restore the functional integrity of the nervous and muscular systems, normal cardiac function, and blood coagulation.

Dibasic calcium phosphate supplies both calcium and phosphorus and is useful in those individuals who must restrict their intake of dairy products.

SPECIAL PRECAUTIONS

- Patients with achlorhydria may not absorb orally administered calcium salts.
- Administer with caution to patients who are digitalized because of a possible additive effect.
- Calcium gluceptate should be administered intramuscularly only in emergencies in young patients when technical difficulty makes intravenous injection impossible.
- Do not administer to patients with renal calculi.
- Do not administer calcium lactate or calcium glycerophosphate intramuscularly in infants and young children.
- Use of calcium is contraindicated in the presence of ventricular fibrillation in patients undergoing cardiac resuscitation.
- Periodically measure calcium levels to avoid hypercalcemia.

ADVERSE EFFECTS

CNS EFFECTS: with calcium glubionate—polyuria tingling sensation, sense of oppression, "heat waves"

URINARY TRACT EFFECTS: with calcium glubionate—polyuria

GASTROINTESTINAL EFFECTS: with calcium gluceptate—chalklike taste; with calcium glubionate—anorexia, nausea, vomiting, constipation, abdominal pain, dry mouth, thirst

LOCAL EFFECTS: irritation with parenteral administration

CLINICAL GUIDELINES

ADMINISTRATION:

- Administer with meals to minimize gastrointestinal side effects.
- When administering calcium gluceptate parenterally, the solution should be warmed to body temperature and administered slowly; discontinue administration if patient complains of any discomfort; resume when symptoms disappear.
- Patient should remain recumbent for a short time after receiving a calcium injection.
- Administer calcium glubionate before meals to enhance absorption.
- Milk is a good vehicle for administration of calcium gluconate.

EFFECTS:

- When calcium glubionate is administered in therapeutic amounts for prolonged periods, hypercalcemia and hypercalciuria may occur.
- Administration of calcium gluconate in large doses intramuscularly may cause abscess formation.

DRUG INTERACTIONS:

- Administration of corticosteroids may interfere with calcium absorption.
- Certain dietary substances interfere with the absorption of calcium; these substances include oxalic acid (found in large quantities in rhubarb and spinach), phytic acid (in bran and whole cereals), and phosphorus (milk and other dairy products).

OVERDOSAGE/ANTIDOTE:

- Overdosage is characterized by all the signs and symptoms of hypercalcemia.
- The products listed in the following section on *Antihypercalcemic Agents* may be used; hemodialysis or peritoneal dialysis may be considered.

Antihypercalcemic Agents

SPECIFIC PRODUCTS AND DOSAGES

GENERIC NAME	TRADE NAME	ROUTE OF ADMIN.	USUAL DOSAGE
disodium edetate	ENDRATE SODIUM VERSENATE	iv infusion	**Adults:** 50 mg/kg; maximum: 3 gm/day **Children:** 40 mg/kg (1 gm/55 lb) Maximum: 70 mg/kg/day
mithramycin	MITHRACIN	iv	25 mcg/kg/day; dilute in 1 liter of 5% glucose in water

Disodium Edetate

PHARMACOLOGY

Disodium edetate is a chelating agent which increases the urinary excretion of calcium by forming soluble complexes with it and other divalent and trivalent metals. These complexes are not reabsorbed to any great extent by the renal tubules. Chelation occurs in the blood, decreasing the ionized calcium concentration in serum before calcium is excreted.

SPECIAL PRECAUTIONS

• Do not use in anuric patients or in patients with generalized arteriosclerosis associated with advancing age.
• Use is limited to emergency treatment of calcium intoxication since prolonged use and doses exceeding 3 grams has caused acute tubular necrosis of the kidney.
• Treatment should not exceed 48 hours.
• Do not administer rapidly or insufficiently diluted.

• Safe use in pregnancy has not been established.

ADVERSE EFFECTS

CNS EFFECTS: circumoral paresthesia, numbness, headache
CARDIOVASCULAR EFFECTS: hypotension
URINARY TRACT EFFECTS: albuminuria, urinary casts, oliguria, RBC and WBC in urine
GASTROINTESTINAL EFFECTS: nausea, vomiting, diarrhea
METABOLIC AND ENDOCRINE EFFECTS: hypocalcemia, hyperuricemia
HEMATOLOGIC EFFECTS: anemia, hemorrhagic tendencies
DERMATOLOGIC EFFECTS: exfoliative dermatitis
LOCAL EFFECTS: pain at site of infusion, thrombophlebitis

CLINICAL GUIDELINES

ADMINISTRATION:
• It is a tissue irritant; serious side effects

may occur with administration in the undiluted form.

- Assess renal excretory function prior to treatment.
- Patient should remain in bed for a short time after infusion because of possible postural hypotension.

EFFECTS:
- Electrolyte imbalance may be induced during treatment; evaluate by appropriate laboratory determinations and status of cardiac function periodically.
- Hypomagnesemia and/or hypokalemia may occur, particularly during prolonged therapy.

DRUG INTERACTIONS:
- Treatment lowers blood sugar and insulin requirements in diabetic patients receiving insulin.

OVERDOSAGE/ANTIDOTE:
- Overdosage is characterized by a precipitous drop in serum calcium level.

- A calcium replacement suitable for intravenous administration (e.g., calcium gluconate) should be available for use. However, in digitalized patients the replacement of calcium ions may produce a reversal of the desired digitalis effect.

Mithramycin

PHARMACOLOGY

Mithramycin, a potent antineoplastic agent, may be considered in the treatment of certain symptomatic patients with hypercalcemia and hypercalcemia associated with a variety of advanced neoplasms. The mechanism of action is unknown.

SPECIAL PRECAUTIONS, ADVERSE EFFECTS, CLINICAL GUIDELINES
See Chapter 17, page 609.

Posterior Pituitary Hormones

GENERAL CLINICAL USES
The posterior pituitary hormones, lypressin, vasopressin, and vasopressin tannate, are vasopressors. They are used to control or prevent the diuresis of diabetes insipidus due to a deficiency of posterior pituitary antidiuretic hormone.

The other posterior pituitary hormone, oxytocin, acts similarly to ergonovine and methylergonovine; these drugs are discussed in Chapter 14, *Drugs Affecting the Reproductive Tract.*

Desmopressin acetate is indicated as antidiuretic replacement therapy in the management of cranial diabetes insipidus and for temporary polyuria and polydipsia associated with trauma to, or surgery in, the pituitary region.

SPECIFIC PRODUCTS AND DOSAGES

GENERIC NAME	TRADE NAME	ROUTE OF ADMIN.	USUAL DAILY DOSAGE
desmopressin acetate	DDAVP	intranasal	**Adults:** 0.1–0.4 ml daily **Children 3 mos–12 yrs.:** 0.05–0.3 ml daily
lypressin	DIAPID Nasal Spray	intranasal	1–2 sprays in one or both nostrils whenever the frequency of urination becomes increased or significant thirst develops, usually qid
vasopressin	PITRESSIN	im/sc	0.25–0.5 ml bid or tid
vasopressin tannate	PITRESSIN Tannate	im	0.3–1 ml; repeat as required

Desmopressin Acetate

PHARMACOLOGY

Desmopressin acetate is a synthetic analogue of the natural hormone, argininevasporessin. It has an antidiuretic activity of about 400 IU as compared with arginine vasopressin.

Desmopressin acetate provides a prompt onset of antidiuretic action with a long duration of action. This product also has decreased actions on the visceral smooth muscle and decreased vasopressor action in relation to the enhanced antidiuretic activity.

SPECIAL PRECAUTIONS
• Do not use in patients hypersensitive to desmopressin acetate.
• In very young and elderly patients in particular, fluid intake should be adjusted in order to decrease the potential occurrence of water intoxication and also hyponatremia.

• Use with caution in patients with coronary artery insufficiency and/or hypertensive cardiovascular disease.
• Safe use in pregnancy has not been established.

ADVERSE EFFECTS
CNS EFFECTS: headache
RESPIRATORY EFFECTS: nasal congestion, rhinitis
GASTROINTESTINAL EFFECTS: nausea, abdominal cramps
AUTONOMIC EFFECTS: flushing
METABOLIC AND ENDOCRINE EFFECTS: vulvar pain

CLINICAL GUIDELINES
EFFECTS:
• At high doses, a slight elevation of blood pressure has been produced. It disappears with a reduction in dosage.
OVERDOSAGE/ANTIDOTE:
• Overdosage is characterized by elevation of blood pressure, headache, and exaggeration of the other adverse effects.
• There is no known specific antidote.

Discontinue drug immediately. If considerable fluid retention is causing concern, a saluretic such as furosemide may induce a diuresis.

Lypressin
Vasopressin
Vasopressin Tannate

PHARMACOLOGY

The antidiuretic agents, lypressin and vasopressin tannate, are similar to the posterior pituitary antidiuretic hormone. They act by increasing the rate of reabsorption of water from the distal renal tubules. Other actions produced with high doses include contraction of smooth muscle of the gastrointestinal tract and contraction of all parts of the vascular bed.

The action of lypressin nasal spray begins rapidly with a peak occurring within 1 hour. The usual duration of action is 3 to 8 hours. The action of vasopressin tannate may last as long as 48 to 96 hours.

SPECIAL PRECAUTIONS

• Administer with extreme caution to patients with vascular disease, particularly disease of the coronary arteries; anginal pain may be precipitated.

• Do not administer vasopressin to patients with chronic nephritis with nitrogen retention until reasonable nitrogen levels have been attained.

• Use vasopressin cautiously in patients with epilepsy, migraine, asthma, and heart failure.

• Do not administer to patients known to be hypersensitive to vasopressin or lypressin or related drugs.

• Safe use in pregnancy has not been established.

ADVERSE EFFECTS

CNS EFFECTS: tremor, vertigo, circumoral pallor, pounding in head, headache

RESPIRATORY EFFECTS: bronchial constriction; inadvertent inhalation of lypressin nasal spray has caused substernal tightness, coughing, transient dyspnea

CARDIOVASCULAR EFFECTS: cardiac arrest

AUTONOMIC EFFECTS: sweating

GASTROINTESTINAL EFFECTS: abdominal cramps, flatus, nausea, vomiting, heartburn

ALLERGIC EFFECTS: vasopressin—urticaria, anaphylaxis

LOCAL EFFECTS: lypressin nasal spray—rhinorrhea, nasal congestion, irritation, pruritus of nasal passages, nasal ulceration

OCULAR EFFECTS: lypressin nasal spray—conjunctivitis

CLINICAL GUIDELINES

ADMINISTRATION:

• Caution patients to avoid inhalation of lypressin nasal spray.

• Local irritation may result from lypressin nasal spray.

• NEVER administer vasopressin tannate intravenously.

EFFECTS:

• Vasopressin tannate may produce water intoxication characterized by drowsiness, listlessness, or headache.

OVERDOSAGE/ANTIDOTE:

• Symptoms of overdosage of the antidiuretic agents are exaggerations of their pharmacologic effects.

• There is no known antidote.

Potassium Replacements and Supplements

GENERAL CLINICAL USES

Potassium supplements are useful in treating and preventing hypokalemia which may occur secondary to treatment with diuretics or corticosteroids, after severe vomiting and diarrhea, or with low dietary uptake of potassium. The potassium supplements may also be useful in the treatment of cardiac arrhythmias due to digitalis intoxication.

If the basic disturbance produces metabolic acidosis, as in some renal tubular disorders, an organic salt such as potassium gluconate or an alkalinizing potassium salt mixture may be administered.

Sugar-free preparations are available and are identified by "(SF)" after the trade name.

Preparations are available for both oral and parenteral administration. Parenteral administration is indicated when oral replacement is not feasible such as in severe vomiting and diarrhea, gastrointestinal intubation or fistulas, prolonged diuresis, and in the treatment of cardiac arrhythmias, particularly those due to digitalis glycosides.

SPECIFIC PRODUCTS AND DOSAGES

GENERIC NAME	TRADE NAME	ROUTE OF ADMIN.	USUAL DAILY DOSAGE
For Oral Administration: potassium acetate, potassium bicarbonate, potasssium citrate	POTASSIUM TRIPLEX	po	15 mEq tid to qid
potassium bicarbonate, potassium citrate	K-LYTE Effervescent Tablets	po	25–50 mEq/day
potassium and chloride	KAOCHLOR-EFF (SF) KLORVESS Effervescent Tablets (SF)	po	20 mEq bid to tid
potassium chloride	(G)* KAOCHLOR 10% Liquid, 20% Liquid (SF) KAON-CL Tabs KAY CIEL Elixir 10% K-LYTE/CL Powder SLOW-K*	po	20–80 mEq/day

*(G) designates availability as a generic product.

(continued facing page)

GENERIC NAME	TRADE NAME	ROUTE OF ADMIN.	USUAL DAILY DOSAGE
potassium chloride, potassium bicarbonate	PFIKLOR* Effervessent Tablets (SF)	po	20 mEq bid to qid
potassium chloride supplement	KATO Powder K-LOR	po	20–40 mEq/day
potassium gluconate	KAON Elixir (SF) Tablets KOLYUM Liquid (SF), Powder (SF)	po	40–80 mEq/day
For Parenteral Administration: potassium acetate	(G)	iv	If serum level exceeds 2.5 mEq/l, administer K at rate not exceeding 10 mEq/hr. in a conc. less than 30 mEq/min. Maximum: 200 mEq/day
potassium chloride	(G)	iv	Individualize

PHARMACOLOGY

Potassium salts correct or reverse potassium depletion states. Potassium chloride supplement is a spray-dried tomato powder product which when reconstituted provides a low sodium tomato juice drink which supplies 20 mEq potassium per dose. Potassium gluconate or the combination of potassium bicarbonate, potassium citrate, or potassium acetate may be particularly useful in treating hypokalemic hypochloremic alkalosis; these are alkalinizing products.

Potassium intoxication may result from either therapeutic doses or overdoses. Usually intoxication is caused by administering the drug too rapidly or by acute or chronic renal insufficiency.

SPECIAL PRECAUTIONS

• Do not use in patients with hyperkalemia since further increase in serum potassium may lead to cardiac arrest.
• Use with caution in patients with heart disease.
• In cardiac patients with esophageal compression due to an enlarged left atrium, wax matrix potassium chloride preparations (SLO-K Tablets) have produced esophageal ulceration.
• All solid dosage forms are contraindicated in patients in whom a delay or arrest in tablet passage through the gastrointestinal tract may occur.
• In patients with impaired mechanism for excreting potassium, hyperkalemia may develop rapidly and asymptomatically; cardiac arrest may occur.
• Do not administer to patients with severe renal impairment, with oliguria or azotemia, untreated Addison's disease, adynamia episodica hereditaria, acute dehydration, heat cramps, or hyperkalemia.
• Carefully monitor serum potassium concentrations in patients with chronic renal disease or any other condition which impairs potassium excretion.
• Hypokalemia should not be treated with concomitant administration of potassium salts and a potassium-sparing diuretic such as spironolactone or triamterene.
• Potassium chloride tablets have produced stenosis and/or ulcerative lesions of the small bowel and death.
• Hypokalemia in patients with metabolic acidosis should be treated with an alkalinizing potassium salt such as potassium bi-

carbonate, potassium citrate, or potassium acetate.

ADVERSE EFFECTS

Effects in ( ) are characteristic of potassium intoxication.

CNS EFFECTS: (paresthesias of the extremities, flaccid paralysis, listlessness, mental confusion, weakness, heaviness of the legs)

CARDIOVASCULAR EFFECTS: (decrease in blood pressure, cardiac arrhythmias, heart block, disappearance of P wave, widening and slurring of QRS complex, changes in S-T segment, tall peaked T waves)

GASTROINTESTINAL EFFECTS: nausea, vomiting, abdominal discomfort, diarrhea, gastrointestinal tract obstruction, bleeding, perforation

METABOLIC AND ENDOCRINE EFFECTS: (hyperkalemia)

CLINICAL GUIDELINES

ADMINISTRATION:
- Minimize gastrointestinal irritation by diluting preparation, administering the dose with meals, or reducing the dose. Administer in full glass of water or fruit juice.
- Do not administer potassium salts to patient with an empty stomach.

EFFECTS:
- Hyperkalemia may complicate chronic renal failure, systemic acidosis such as diabetic acidosis, acute dehydration, extensive tissue breakdown such as in severe burns, adrenal insufficiency, or the administration of a potassium-sparing diuretic such as spironolactone or triamterene.

DRUG INTERACTIONS:
- Do not use concomitantly with potassium-sparing diuretics such as spironolactone and triamterene.

OVERDOSAGE/ANTIDOTE:
- Overdosage is usually asymptomatic and may be manifested only by increasing serum potassium concentration and characteristic electrocardiographic changes, namely, peaking of T waves, loss of P wave, depression of S-T segment, and prolongation (widening and slurring) of the QT interval. Late manifestations include muscle paralysis and cardiovascular collapse from cardiac arrest.
- Treat hyperkalemia with dextrose solution, 10 or 25%, containing 10 units of crystalline insulin per 20 gm of dextrose, given iv in a dose of 300 to 500 ml/hr. Intravenous infusion of sodium bicarbonate 7.5% reduces the serum potassium level by causing potassium to shift into cells. The ECG should be monitored constantly. Intravenous administration of dextrose solution containing insulin also causes potassium to shift into the cells but less rapidly than sodium bicarbonate. Correction of acidosis, use of ion exchange resins, hemodialysis and peritoneal dialysis may be considered.

Sex Hormones

Androgens

GENERAL CLINICAL USES

Of the androgens, the anabolic steroids, which are weak androgens and derivatives of testosterone, are used primarily as adjunctive therapy in senile and postmenopausal osteoporosis and for stimulation of some forms of hematopoiesis.

For products and detailed information, please refer to Chapter 14, *Drugs Affecting the Reproductive Tract*, page 521.

Estrogens

GENERAL CLINICAL USES
The estrogens, both natural and synthetic, are administered systemically to replace deficient hormones. Conditions which may be treated include menopausal and premenopausal states, dysfunction of the reproductive system, postpartum breast engorgement, and control of fertility.

See Chapter 14, *Drugs Affecting the Reproductive Tract* for specific products and information.

Thyroid Preparations

GENERAL CLINICAL USES
The thyroid preparations, levothyroxine sodium, liothyronine sodium, liotrix, thyroglobulin, and thyroid hormone provide thyroid replacement therapy for conditions involving inadequate endogenous thyroid production.

Thyrotropic hormone, thyrotropin, is used to diagnose hypothyroidism and in the management of certain types of thyroid carcinoma and resulting metastases.

SPECIFIC PRODUCTS AND DOSAGES

GENERIC NAME	TRADE NAME	ROUTE OF ADMIN.	USUAL DOSE	
			ADULTS	CHILDREN
levothyroxine sodium (T$_4$)	(G)* SYNTHROID	im/iv	0.2–0.5 mg daily	Not established
	(G)	po	0.1–0.2 mg/day	0.3–0.4 mg/day

*(G) designates availability as a generic product.

(continued overleaf)

GENERIC NAME	TRADE NAME	ROUTE OF ADMIN.	USUAL DOSE	
			ADULTS	CHILDREN
liothyronine sodium (T₃)	(G)* CYTOMEL Tablets RO-THYRONINE	po	**Initial:** 5–25 mcg/day followed by 5-mcg increments depending on clinical response **Maintenance:** 25–75 mcg/day	**Infants and children less than 3 yrs.:** 5–50 mcg **Children over 3 yrs.:** adult dose
liotrix	EUTHROID	po	15–60 mg daily	Not established
thyroglobulin	(G) PROLOID Tablets	po	**Initial:** 0.5 gr, increase gradually **Maintenance:** 0.5–3.0 gr (32–190 mg) daily	Not established
thyroid hormone	(G) THYROCRINE THYRO-TERIC	po	**Initial:** 7.5–30 mg/day followed by increments of 30–60 mg **Maintenance:** 120–180 mg/day	Same as adults
thyrotropin (TSH)	THYTROPAR	im/sc	10 IU for 3–5 days; see *Anterior Pituitary Hormones*, page 544, for detailed information	

*(G) designates availability as a generic product.

Levothyroxine Sodium
Liothyronine Sodium
Liotrix
Thyroglobulin
Thyroid Hormone
Thyrotropin

PHARMACOLOGY

Levothyroxine sodium (T_4) a synthetic form of thyroid hormone, is readily absorbed from the gastrointestinal tract and is effective by any parenteral route of administration. It has a relatively slow onset of action. Administration of sodium levothyroxine alone will result in complete physiologic thyroid replacement.

Liothyronine sodium (T_3) a synthetic form of natural thyroid hormone, has all of the pharmacologic activities of the natural hormone. It is not firmly bound to serum protein and consequently is readily available to body tissues. After oral administration, about 85 percent is absorbed from the gastrointestinal tract. The onset of activity is noted within a few hours and the maximal pharmacologic effect occurs within 2 to 3 days.

Liotrix is a mixture of synthetic salts of levothyroxine sodium (T_4) and liothyronine sodium (T_3) combined in a constant 4:1 ratio. In contrast to the individual metabolically active hormones, liotrix will usually produce normal results for PBI, T, and other thyroid function tests when thyroid deficiencies are made euthyroid.

Thyroglobulin, obtained from frozen hog thyroid, maintains the normal metabolism of the organs throughout the body. The potency is equal to that of thyroid hormone.

The thyroid hormones increase the

metabolic rate. The effect develops slowly but may be prolonged. Thyroid hormone prepared from fresh, dessicated animal thyroid glands also increases the metabolic rate of body tissues. The effect develops slowly, beginning within 48 hours, and reaches a maximum in 8 to 10 days. The effect continues for several weeks.

Thyrotropin, thyroid-stimulating hormone, is a secretion of the anterior pituitary gland. It regulates the activity of the thyroid gland. Thyrotropin is isolated from bovine anterior pituitary gland.

SPECIAL PRECAUTIONS

- Do not use in patients with thyrotoxicosis or acute myocardial infarction uncomplicated by hypothyroidism.
- Do not use in patients with concurrent hypothyroidism and hypoadrenalism unless treatment of hypoadrenalism with adrenocortical steroids precedes the initiation of thyroid therapy.
- Use with extreme caution in patients with cardiovascular disease, including hypertension.
- If chest pain or other aggravation of cardiovascular disease occurs, then decrease dosage.
- Patients receiving thyroid hormone should be observed carefully if catecholamines are administered.
- Patients with coronary artery disease receiving thyroid hormone may experience cardiac arrhythmias when undergoing surgery.
- Rule out morphologic hypogonadism and nephrosis before treating with sodium liothyronine.
- Diabetic patients receiving thyroid hormone may require an increased dosage of insulin or oral hypoglycemic agents.

ADVERSE EFFECTS

The adverse effects are due primarily to overdosage and are characteristic of the symptoms of hyperthyroidism.

CNS EFFECTS: tremors, headache, nervousness, insomnia

CARDIOVASCULAR EFFECTS: palpitations, tachycardia, cardiac arrhythmias, angina pectoris

AUTONOMIC EFFECTS: sweating, intolerance to heat, fever

GASTROINTESTINAL EFFECTS: diarrhea

METABOLIC AND ENDOCRINE EFFECTS: weight loss

CLINICAL GUIDELINES

ADMINISTRATION:
- Monitor patients carefully for signs of hyperthyroidism.

EFFECTS:
- All thyroid preparations alter the results of thyroid function tests.
- The PBI usually remains at levels below normal during sodium liothyronine therapy because of the less firm binding to serum protein than is noted with thyroxine.
- Patients with hypothyroidism and especially myxedema are particularly sensitive to thyroid preparations; initiate therapy with small doses and increase gradually.

DRUG INTERACTIONS:
- I^{131} thyroid uptake may be depressed, particularly if dosage exceeds 75 mcg sodium liothyronine daily; useful I^{131} thyroid uptake studies may be conducted within 2 weeks following discontinuance of the drug.
- Concomitant administration of thyroid hormone and epinephrine in patients with coronary artery disease may precipitate coronary insufficiency.
- Possible alterations in the prothrombin time must be considered and closely monitored in patients on anticoagulant therapy.
- In diabetic patients (diabetes mellitus), an increased dosage of insulin or oral hypoglycemic agents may be required.
- Possible alterations in the prothrombin time must be considered and closely moni-

tored in patients on anticoagulant therapy (warfarin, bishydroxycoumarin); dosage reduction may be necessary.
• Maximum dosage of liotrix in patients receiving digitalis is 4 mg.

OVERDOSAGE/ANTIDOTE:
• Overdosage is characterized by the signs of hyperthyroidism, namely, palpitations, tachycardia, cardiac arrhythmia, weight loss, angina pectoris, tremors, headache, diarrhea, nervousness, insomnia, sweating, and intolerance to heat. Shock may develop.
• There is no known antidote. Discontinue therapy or reduce dosage. In shock, supportive measures and treatment of unrecognized adrenal insufficiency should be considered.

Antithyroid Preparations

GENERAL CLINICAL USES
The antithyroid preparations, methimazole and propylthiouracil, are useful in treating hyperthyroidism or ameliorating hyperthyroidism prior to thyroid surgery. Sodium iodide I^{131} may also be used.

SPECIFIC PRODUCTS AND DOSAGES

GENERIC NAME	TRADE NAME	ROUTE OF ADMIN.	USUAL DOSAGE ADULTS	CHILDREN
methimazole	TAPAZOLE	po	**Initial:** 15–60 mg/day divided in equal doses **Maintenance:** 5–15 mg/day divided in 3 equal doses	**6–10 yrs.:** 5–10 mg/day divided in 3 equal doses
propylthiouracil	(G)*	po	**Initial:** 200–400 mg/day divided in 3 equal doses **Maintenance:** 50–150 mg/day divided in 3 equal doses	**10 yrs. and over:** 150–300 mg/day divided in 3 equal doses **6–10 yrs.:** 50–150 mg/day divided in 3 equal doses
sodium iodide I^{131}	(G) ORIODIDE-131 IODOTOPE-131 THERIODIDE-131	po	4–10 millicuries	

*(G) designates availability as a generic product.

Methimazole
Propylthiouracil

PHARMACOLOGY

Methimazole and propylthiouracil inhibit the synthesis of thyroid hormone but do not inactivate existing thyroid hormone or interfere with its activity.

Methimazole and propylthiouracil cross the placental membrance and can induce goiter and cretinism in the developing fetus.

SPECIAL PRECAUTIONS

• Use judiciously in pregnant patients since these drugs cross the placental membranes.
• Postpartum patients should not breast-feed their babies.
• Caution patients to report any evidence of illness such as sore throat, skin eruptions, fever, headache, or general malaise.
• Do not use in patients with a history of hypersensitivity to either drug.
• Use with care when given to patients receiving drugs known to cause agranulocytosis.
• Since these drugs may cause hypoprothrombinemia, bleeding may occur.

ADVERSE EFFECTS

CNS EFFECTS: paresthesias, headache, drowsiness, neuritis, vertigo
CARDIOVASCULAR EFFECTS: lymphenadenopathy, periarteritis
GASTROINTESTINAL EFFECTS: nausea, vomiting, epigastric distress, loss of taste
METABOLIC AND ENDOCRINE EFFECTS: edema
HEPATIC EFFECTS: jaundice, hepatitis
HEMATOLOGIC EFFECTS: agranulocytosis, granulocytopenia, thrombocytopenia, hypo-thrombinemia, bleeding
ALLERGIC EFFECTS: urticaria
DERMATOLOGIC EFFECTS: rash, loss of hair, pruritus, pigmentation
MUSCULOSKELETAL EFFECTS: arthralgia, myalgia

CLINICAL GUIDELINES

ADMINISTRATION:
• Monitor prothrombin time during therapy because hypoprothrombinemia has been reported with these drugs.
EFFECTS:
• In untreated hyperthyroidism, about 10 percent of patients have leukopenia, often with relative granulopenia.
• Delayed responses are sometimes noted.
• May cause hypoprothrombinemia and bleeding; monitor prothrombin time.
DRUG INTERACTIONS:
• Concomitantly administered thyroid hormone is not inactivated.
OVERDOSAGE/ANTIDOTE:
• Overdosage is characterized by the signs and symptoms of hypothyroidism.
• Treat hypothyroidism with thyroid hormone preparations as needed.

Sodium Iodide I[131]

PHARMACOLOGY

Sodium iodide inhibits the release of thyroid hormone from the gland immediately. Its effect is only partial and not sustained. It is used to decrease vascularity of the thyroid gland prior to surgery.

SPECIAL PRECAUTIONS, ADVERSE EFFECTS, CLINICAL GUIDELINES

See Chapter 19, page 660 for detailed information.

16

Nutritional agents

INTRODUCTION

Drugs affecting the nutritional status of the patient include those useful in restoring health to debilitated or cachectic patients; in correcting specific nutritional or metabolic deficiencies; to supplement, correct, or relieve a deficiency or diseased state. The patient on specific or prolonged drug therapy or recovering from surgery may require dietary supplements.

SPECIFIC THERAPEUTIC CLASSIFICATION

The nutritional agents are grouped as follows:

1. Dietary supplements for oral or tube feeding
2. Electrolytes, oral solutions
3. Hematinic agents
4. Hyperkalemic agents

5. Phosphorus replacement preparations

6. Salt substitutes
7. Vitamins

Dietary Supplements for Oral or Tube Feeding

GENERAL CLINICAL USES

Dietary supplements are available for oral or tube feeding of patients with specific dietary requirements; nutritionally complete and/or standard diets and reducing diets are also available. Because each diet has a specific use, each is discussed separately.

SPECIFIC DIETS AND TRADE NAMES

DIET	TRADE NAME	DIET	TRADE NAME
high calorie	CONTROLYTE NORMOSOL-M 900 NUTRI-1000	low electrolyte	HYCAL
		low lactose	LOLACTENE
high and moderate nitrogen	PROBANA Powder 4.2% protein SUPPORT 10% protein SYSTAGEN 11% protein	low phenylalanine	LOFENALAC
		low residue	ISOCAL PRECISION-LR
		reducing diet	DIETENE
hydrolyzed/digested protein	A/G PRO AMIGEN 5% C.P.H. 7% HYPROTIGEN 10% P.D.P. Liquid Protein PRO-MIX PROTINEX PROTOLAN STUART AMINO ACIDS STUART AMINO ACIDS with B_{12}	standard diet (nutritionally balanced)	MERITENE SUSTACAL SUSTAGEN VIVONEX

High Caloric Diets

GENERAL CLINICAL USES

A high caloric, nutritionally complete food for oral or tube feeding is useful as total or supplementary nutritional support of patients with anorexia or cachexia, or where an impediment to ingestion of solid food is present. This diet is useful in patients requiring a high caloric intake during convalescence from surgery, injuries, or in geriatric patients with persistent anorexia and malnutrition, and in patients with extensive burns.

SPECIAL PRECAUTIONS

- Oral or gavage feeding is contraindicated in the presence of nausea and vomiting and for a period of 12 hours before general anesthesia because of the danger of aspiration of vomitus.
- Administer with caution to comatose patients until assured that it is unlikely they will vomit.
- Defer postoperative feedings until peristalsis is re-established.
- Consider electrolyte content in patients with special restrictions on electrolyte intake (e.g. those on salt-free diets).
- Additional water may be needed to meet daily requirement.

CONTENTS

Skim milk, corn oil, sucrose, corn syrup solids, sodium caseinate, mono- and diglycerides, lecithin, ethyl vanillen, minerals, and vitamins.

DOSAGE

Two quarts supply 2000 calories, also protein, fat, vitamins, and minerals. It is a nutritionally complete product.

High and Moderate Nitrogen Diets

GENERAL CLINICAL USES

High and moderate nitrogen diets for oral or tube feeding are useful when the patient requires an increased nitrogen intake to maintain weight and nitrogen balance.

SPECIAL PRECAUTIONS

- Do not administer parenterally.
- Because of the high caloric contribution, some depleted patients may manifest elevated blood sugar levels requiring insulin for regulation.
- The diet should not be used by diabetics without their physician's approval.
- Electrolyte content of the diet may be excessive for patients with electrolyte imbalance, since it is based on the requirements of normal individuals.
- Caution patients to drink diet slowly, particularly until the body is adjusted to a liquid diet.
- Certain individuals may be sensitive to volume or osmolality; initiate diet slowly as a dilute solution to avoid diarrhea, gastric dumping or gastrointestinal distress.
- Do not increase volume and concentration in a single 24-hour period.
- Nausea, if encountered, is usually due to feeding speed; stop feeding for 1 hour, then resume feeding at a slower rate.

CONTENTS

HIGH NITROGEN DIET: contents of one packet diluted with water to a volume of 300 ml supply: calories, 300; nitrogen in form of pure amino acids, 2 gm; fat, 0.261 gm; carbohydrate as glucose oligosaccharides, 63.1 gm; electrolytes; and vitamins.
MODERATE NITROGEN DIET: ten servings (10 packets) provide 2000 calories; 65 gm

of highest biological value protein (egg albumin) containing 20 gm of nitrogen and 100% of the U.S. Recommended Daily Allowance for protein, and all known essential vitamins and minerals.

DOSAGE

Nitrogen requirement varies with each individual's metabolic condition. When tube feeding, initiate the diet very slowly as a dilute solution to avoid diarrhea, gastric dumping or gastrointestinal distress.

Hydrolyzed Digested Protein Diets

PHARMACOLOGY

Protein hydrolysate is a sterile, nonpyrogenic solution prepared by acid hydrolysis of animal blood fibrin. Alpha amino nitrogen is approximately 55 percent of the total nitrogen content. It provides approximately 175 calories per liter, 292 nOsm/1. The total nitrogen ranges from 6.5 to 7.0 gm/liter. The pH ranges from 5.0 to 6.0. The recommended optimum daily intake of total daily protein is 1 gm/kg body weight.

SPECIAL PRECAUTIONS

• Do not use in patients with severe liver disease or with symptoms of impending hepatic coma.
• Monitor blood ammonia levels, particularly in premature infants and neonates, and in older patients with liver disease, since free ammonia is present in fibrin or casein hydrolysates.
• Use with caution in patients with acidosis and those with renal impairment or azotemia from any cause.
• Use with caution in patients with severe congestive heart failure.

• Avoid circulatory overload, especially in patients with cardiac or pulmonary disorders.
• Do not use in patients with a history of hypersensitivity to protein (modified fibrin) hydrolysate.

ADVERSE EFFECTS

CNS EFFECTS: convulsions; fever, chills with rapid intravenous infusion
CARDIOVASCULAR EFFECTS: vasodilatation
GASTROINTESTINAL EFFECTS: abdominal pain; nausea and vomiting with rapid intravenous infusion
ALLERGIC EFFECTS: urticarial rash; hypersensitivity reactions
LOCAL EFFECTS: phlebitis, thrombosis at site of venipuncture

CLINICAL GUIDELINES

ADMINISTRATION:
• Only solutions which are clear should be administered intravenously.
• The rate of infusion should be slow initially (not more than 2 ml/min); rate may be increased gradually.
EFFECTS:
• Protein intake alone cannot supply calories and at the same time contribute to protein synthesis; therefore, provide other parenteral sources of calories.
DRUG INTERACTIONS:
• Do not use with hypertonic (hyperosmolar) concentrations of dextrose in the presence of intracranial or intraspinal hemorrhage or in delirium tremens if the patient is already dehydrated.
• Antibiotics or other drugs may be added to the solution provided that they are compatible with fibrin hydrolysate.
OVERDOSAGE/ANTIDOTE:
• With excessive intravenous infusion, circulatory overload may occur.
• Treat symptomatically and supportively.

Low Electrolyte Diet

GENERAL CLINICAL USES

Low electrolyte diet is indicated for patients on restricted diets which may not supply minimal caloric needs.

SPECIAL PRECAUTIONS

• Patients with diabetes should use only as directed by physician.

CONTENTS

Low electrolyte diet contains dimineralized, deionized water; citric acid, benzoic acid, carbohydrates, fat, protein; calories 295 per 4 ounces.

DOSAGE

A diet supplement which supplies carbohydrates with low protein and low electrolyte content is available in 4-ounce bottles. A person drinking four 4-ounce bottles consumes 1180 calories and 292 ml of water, a trace of protein, and low and known electrolyte levels.

Low Lactose Diet

GENERAL CLINICAL USES

A low lactose diet is used as supplemental or total feeding, oral or tube, of individuals who can benefit from a restricted lactose intake. It is a nutritionally balanced nourishment which is 99.6 percent lactose free.

CONTENTS

The low lactose diet contains low lactose nonfat dry milk, corn syrup solids, vegetable oil, sucrose, sodium caseinate, magnesium sulfate, mono- and diglycerides, hydroxylated lecithin, ascorbic acid, ferrous sulfate, zinc sulfate, polyglyceral esters, alpha tocopheryl acetate, niacin, copper glu-conate, manganese sulfate, calcium pantothenate, vitamin A palmitate, pyridoxine hydrochloride, thiamin hydrochloride, folic acid, d-biotin, cyanocobalamin, vitamin D_2.

DOSAGE

Three servings, 2 ounces each, provide 680 calories and 75 percent or more of the U.S. Recommended Daily Allowance for protein and all known essential vitamins and minerals.

Low Phenylalanine Diet

GENERAL CLINICAL USES

A diet low in phenylalanine is used in the management of patients with phenylketonuria. It should be supplemented with other foods to provide all other essential nutrients and sufficient phenylalanine to support growth and development.

SPECIAL PRECAUTIONS

• Do not use in individuals other than those with phenylketonuria.

CONTENTS

Phenylalanine content, average 0.8 percent; other components include corn syrup solids, casein hydrolysate low in phenylalanine, corn oil, sugar, arrow root starch, amino acids, vitamin A, thiamine, riboflavin, pyridoxine, cyanocobalamin, ascorbic acid, vitamins D and F, niacinamide, pantothenate calcium, folic acid, iodine, biotin, choline, copper, zinc.

The nutrient level meets or exceeds the Food and Drug Administration requirements for infant formula, except protein. Each quart of low phenylalanine diet supplies 12 mg iron from ferrous sulfate.

DOSAGE

FORMULA FOR INFANTS: use 7.5 ounces (139 grams); add water to make 1 quart of formula. Adapt this diet and other food intake to individual needs.

Low Residue Diet

GENERAL CLINICAL USES

A low residue diet for oral or tube feeding provides well-balanced nutrition when used as the sole source of nourishment for tube-fed patients.

SPECIAL PRECAUTIONS

• Additional water should be given as needed; note particularly in comatose or unconscious patients and in patients with impaired renal concentrating ability, with extensive breakdown of tissue protein, or with fever.

• Tube feeding preparations should be at room temperature during administration.

• Safe use of PRECISION-LR DIET in pregnant or lactating women has not been established.

• PRECISION-LR DIET does not contain vitamin K; therefore, patients on long-term feeding should be observed for hypoprothrombinemia.

CONTENTS

ISOCAL: water, corn syrup solids, soy oil, calcium and sodium caseinate, MCI oil, soy protein isolate, potassium citrate, calcium citrate, lecithin, magnesium chloride, dibasic magnesium diphosphate, sodium citrate, calcium chloride, dibasic calcium phosphate, potassium chloride, carrageenin, ferrous sulfate, vitamin A palmitate, ergocalciferol, D-alphatocopheryl acetate, sodium ascorbate, folic acid, thiamine hydrochloride, riboflavin, niacinamide, pyridoxine hydrochloride, cyanocobalamin, biotin, calcium pantothenate, phytonadione, choline chloride, zinc sulfate, magnesium sulfate, cupric sulfate, potassium iodide.

PRECISION-LR DIET: maltodextrin, pasteurized egg white solids, sugar, calcium glycerol phosphate, potassium bitartrate, magnesium sulfate, vegetable oil, citric acid, ammonium phosphate, choline bitartrate, mono- and diglycerides, ascorbic acid, ferrous sulfate, alpha tocopheryl acetate, zinc sulfate, niacin, copper gluconate, d-calcium pantothenate, magnesium sulfate, vitamin A palmitate, pyridoxine hydrochloride, thiamin hydrochloride, riboflavin, folic acid, d-biotin, potassium iodide, vitamin D_2, cyanocobalamin.

DOSAGE

Tube feedings may be given by continuous feedings or at intervals. No more than 8 ounces should be given at one time; administer over a period of 30 minutes.

Reducing Diet

GENERAL CLINICAL USES

The reducing diet is used for patients who are on a weight reduction program.

SPECIAL PRECAUTIONS

• Use only when supervised by a physician.

CONTENTS

The reducing diet contains 1000, 1200, or 1400 calories and the US recommended daily allowances of all vitamins and minerals. Also, it provides protein 83 gm, fat 26 gm, and carbohydrate 110 gm.

DOSAGE

Individualize according to physician's directions.

Standard (Nutritionally Balanced) Diet

GENERAL CLINICAL USES

The standard (nutritionally balanced) diet for oral or tube feeding is useful in patients who have undergone surgery, following hyperalimentation, or in patients with impaired absorption due to stress.

SPECIAL PRECAUTIONS

• Caution patients to drink diet slowly, particularly until the body is adjusted to a liquid diet.
• Do not syringe feed.
• Certain individuals may be sensitive to volume or osmolality; initiate diet slowly as a dilute solution to avoid diarrhea, gastric dumping, or gastrointestinal distress.
• Do not increase volume and concentration in a single 24-hour period.
• Nausea, if encountered, is usually due to feeding speed; stop feeding for 1 hour, then resume feeding at a slower rate.
• Because of the high caloric contribution from carbohydrates, some depleted individuals may manifest elevated blood sugar levels requiring insulin for regulation.

CONTENTS

Contents of one packet diluted with water to a total volume of 300 ml supply 300 calories and the following: available nitrogen in the form of pure amino acids, 0.98 gm; fat as purified safflower oil, 4.35 gm; carbohydrate as glucose and glucose oligosaccharides, 67.9 gm. This diet provides all the known mineral and nutrient requirements in 1900-calorie daily allowance.

The electrolyte content of the diet may be excessive for patients with electrolyte imbalance because it is based on requirements of normal individuals. Use in pregnancy and lactation may require supplemental vitamins and minerals.

Do not use the diet in diabetic patients without physician's approval.

DOSAGE

Each packet of 80 grams provides 300 calories. Use as required by patient's status.

Electrolytes, Oral Solutions

GENERAL CLINICAL USES

Oral electrolyte formulation replaces mild to moderate electrolyte losses when food intake is discontinued, in infant diarrhea or vomiting, or other conditions of fluid loss or lack of intake.

For information concerning parenteral administration of electrolytes, see Chapter 5, *Drugs Affecting the Heart, Circulation, Blood Vessels, and Blood —Electrolyte Solutions,* page 266.

SPECIFIC PRODUCTS AND DOSAGES

GENERIC NAME	TRADE NAME	USUAL DOSAGE
oral electrolyte formulation	LYTREN PEDIALYTE	**Infants and young children:** 1500–2400 ml per M^2 of body surface **Children 5 to 10 yrs.:** up to 2 quarts daily **Older children and adults:** up to 2 to 3 quarts daily

PHARMACOLOGY

The essential electrolytes—potassium chloride, salts of sodium, calcium, and magnesium, and dextrose—are provided in aqueous solution to supply water and essential electrolytes in amounts needed for maintenance of body functions.

SPECIAL PRECAUTIONS

• Give only enough to meet patient's fluid requirement.

• Severe, continuing diarrhea or other critical losses of fluid require parenteral therapy.

• Do not use in patients with intractable vomiting, adynamic ileus, intestinal obstruction or perforated bowel; depressed renal function (anuria, oliguria).

CLINICAL GUIDELINES

ADMINISTRATION:

• Always use in recommended dilution.

• Discontinue usual foods and fluids prior to administration.

DRUG INTERACTIONS:

• Do not mix with milk, fruit juice, or other electrolyte-containing fluid.

• If additional fluid is required, give as water.

Hematinic Agents

GENERAL CLINICAL USES

The hematinic agents (iron preparations) are used to treat patients with anemias due to iron deficiency, megaloblastic anemias, and anemias of nutritional origin. The hematinic agents include the iron salts, cyanocobalamin, and folic acid.

The recommended daily allowances for iron are: children 4 to 6 yrs.—10 mg; adult males—10 mg; adult females—18 mg.

SPECIFIC PRODUCTS AND DOSAGES

GENERIC NAME	TRADE NAME	ROUTE OF ADMIN.	USUAL DAILY DOSAGE
ferrocholinate	CHEL-IRON FERROLIP FIRON	po	**Adults:** 150 mg/day in divided doses **Children:** 100–150 mg/day in divided doses
ferrous fumarate*	(G)† CHROMAGEN* ROGENIC* Inj. (G) CHROMAGEN	im po	20 mg/day every 3 to 7 days 100 to 400 mg/day in divided doses
ferrous gluconate*	FERGON FERRALET	po	**Adults:** 435–870 mg/day in 1–2 doses **Children:** 435 mg/day
ferrous sulfate	(G) FEOSOL Elixir, Tablets, Capsules IBERLATE Pediatric	po	660–1320 mg/day in divided doses
ferric pyrophosphate	(G)	po	120 mg/day in divided doses
iron dextran injection	CHROMAGEN-D IMFERON	im iv	**Adults under 110 lb:** 100 mg **Adults over 110 lb:** 250 mg **Infants under 10 lb:** 25 mg **Children under 20 lb:** 50 mg 25–100 mg/day
iron protein complex**	FE-PLUS	po	150 mg/day in divided doses
polysaccharide-iron complex	FERROCOL NIFEREX	po	**Adults:** 100–200 mg bid **Children 2–6 yrs.:** 50–100 mg/day

*Contains more than one active ingredient.
**Available in combination products only.
†(G) designates availability as a generic product.

PHARMACOLOGY

The orally administered iron salts are absorbed from the gastrointestinal tract; absorption is enhanced by administering when the stomach is empty. The iron salts replace iron in deficiency anemias regardless of origin. The hematologic response to orally administered iron usually begins in 5 to 10 days, and in less time with parenterally administered drugs. Various salts of iron are available and provide varying amounts of elemental iron, with ferrous fumarate and ferrous sulfate having the largest amounts.

The iron dextran complex is dissociated by the reticuloendothelial system. The ferric iron is incorporated into hemoglobin.

SPECIAL PRECAUTIONS

- Do not administer to patients with hemochromatosis and/or hemosiderosis.
- Conduct periodic evaluations of the blood picture.
- Discontinue if signs of intolerance appear.
- Oral administration of iron may aggravate peptic ulcer, colitis, or enteritis.
- Do not use in patients with a history of hypersensitivity or idiosyncrasy to iron preparations.
- Administer iron dextran with caution to patients with impaired liver function.
- Safe use of iron dextran in pregnancy has not been established.
- Patients with iron deficiency anemia and rheumatoid arthritis may have an acute exacerbation of joint pain or swelling following intravenous administration of iron dextran.
- Unwarranted therapy with parenteral iron will cause excess storage of iron with the possible consequence of exogenous siderosis.

ADVERSE EFFECTS

CNS EFFECTS: syncope, headache, paresthesias with iron dextran

CARDIOVASCULAR EFFECTS: iron dextran—peripheral vascular flushing with rapid intravenous administration

AUTONOMIC EFFECTS: flushing of face and extremities

GASTROINTESTINAL EFFECTS: nausea, vomiting, diarrhea, constipation

ALLERGIC EFFECTS: iron dextran—urticaria, anaphylactic reactions, arthralgia, and myalgia

DERMATOLOGIC EFFECTS: rash

DENTAL EFFECTS: continued use of liquid preparations of iron may stain the teeth.

LOCAL EFFECTS: iron dextran—soreness, inflammation, brown skin, phlebitis

CLINICAL GUIDELINES

ADMINISTRATION:
- Give tablets between meals for best absorption.
- Give tablets after or with meals to minimize gastrointestinal complaints.
- Teeth stains may be prevented to a large extent by taking liquid medication through a straw with a drink of plain water or juice.

EFFECTS:
- Stools may become darkened.
- As little as 1 gm of elemental iron ingested orally may be toxic.

DRUG INTERACTIONS:
- Iron products interfere with absorption of orally administered tetracyclines; they should not be taken within 2 hours of each other.
- Antacids or milk given concomitantly with iron compounds generally decreases the absorption of iron.

OVERDOSAGE/ANTIDOTE:
- Symptoms of iron intoxication include diarrhea, vomiting, pallor, cyanosis, hematemesis, drowsiness, shock, coma, and melena. Overdosage in children may lead to gastrointestinal hemorrhage. With sustained-release formulations, overdosage may be delayed. In acute iron intoxication, increased capillary permeability, reduced plasma volume, increased cardiac output, weak and rapid pulse, and sudden cardiovascular collapse may occur.
- Treatment of overdosage consists of induction of vomiting followed by gastric and/or rectal lavage, followed with milk or bicarbonate of soda. Administer fluids and electrolytes intravenously; use oxygen if indicated. Exchange transfusions and use of certain chelating agents may be useful.

Hyperkalemic Agents (Potassium-Removing Resins)

GENERAL CLINICAL USES

Sodium polystyrene sulfonate is indicated for the symptomatic treatment of hyperkalemia, particularly that associated with acute renal failure.

SPECIFIC PRODUCTS AND DOSAGES

GENERIC NAME	TRADE NAME	ROUTE OF ADMIN.	USUAL DOSAGE
sodium polystyrene sulfonate	KAYEXALATE	po pr	**Adults:** 15–60 gm daily in divided doses **Small children and infants:** reduce dosage 30 gm once or twice daily in a retention enema; retain for 4 to 10 hr., if possible; follow with cleansing enema

Sodium Polystyrene Sulfonate

PHARMACOLOGY

Sodium polystyrene sulfonate is a cation exchange resin which removes potassium. Sodium ions are partially released by potassium ions. This action occurs primarily in the large intestine, where a greater number of potassium ions are excreted than in the small intestine.

SPECIAL PRECAUTIONS

• Since serious potassium deficiency can occur from therapy with sodium polystyrene sulfonate, it is imperative to determine serum potassium levels at least daily, and at times, more frequently.
• Severe hypokalemia is often associated with a lengthened QT interval, a change in T-wave vector, and an appearance of U waves in the ECG.
• Marked hypokalemia can also be manifested by severe muscle weakness, at times extending into frank paralysis.
• Use with caution in patients who cannot tolerate even a small increase in sodium loads, for example, patients with severe congestive heart failure, severe hypertension or marked edema; compensatory restriction of sodium intake from other sources may be indicated.
• This cation exchange resin is not totally selective for potassium in its actions; small amounts of other cations such as magnesium and calcium can also be lost during treatment.
• Monitor patients for all applicable electrolyte disturbances.

• Effective lowering of serum potassium may take hours to days; if rapid correction of severe hypokalemia is necessary, consider some form of dialysis (peritoneal or hemo).

ADVERSE EFFECTS

GASTROINTESTINAL EFFECTS: irritation, anorexia, nausea, vomiting, diarrhea; fecal impaction with large doses in the elderly

METABOLIC AND ENDOCRINE EFFECTS: hypokalemia, hypocalcemia, significant sodium retention

CLINICAL GUIDELINES

ADMINISTRATION:

• Administer in syrup for greater palatability than in water.

• May be introduced into the stomach through a plastic tube and, if desired, mixed with a diet appropriate for a patient in renal failure.

EFFECTS:

• If constipation occurs, patients should be treated with a mild laxative or sorbitol; this will also reduce any tendency to fecal impaction.

DRUG INTERACTIONS:

• The toxic effects of digitalis may be exaggerated by any decreased serum potassium levels.

• When used concurrently with aluminum hydroxide, intestinal obstruction has occurred.

SIGNS OF OVERDOSAGE/ANTIDOTE:

• Overdosage is characterized by the signs and symptoms of hypokalemia. See Special Precautions.

• Discontinue therapy and supplement potassium.

Phosphorus Replacement Preparations

GENERAL CLINICAL USES

The phosphorus preparations supplement phosphorus where there is dietary restriction, poor absorption, or increased need for this element.

The U.S. recommended daily allowance for children 4 to 6 years and adults is 800 mg and for pregnant or lactating women, 1,200 mg.

SPECIFIC PRODUCTS AND DOSAGES

GENERIC NAME	TRADE NAME	ROUTE OF ADMIN.	USUAL ADULT DOSAGE
phosphorus preparations	K-PHOS Neutral Tablets NEUTRA-PHOS Powder, Capsules NEUTRA-PHOS-K Powder, Capsules	po	250–2000 mg/day divided in 3–4 doses

PHARMACOLOGY

Phosphorus preparations lower urinary calcium levels and increase urinary phosphates and pyrophosphates.

SPECIAL PRECAUTIONS

• Do not use in patients with renal insufficiency, severe hepatic disease, and Addison's disease.
• Do not use combined thiazide and phosphate therapy; renal damage may be produced.
• Acidification of urine is contraindicated in patients with urinary stone disease.

ADVERSE EFFECTS

GASTROINTESTINAL EFFECTS: mild laxative effect

CLINICAL GUIDELINES

ADMINISTRATION:
• Should be accompanied by an adequate fluid intake.
EFFECTS:
• Reduce intake if diarrhea occurs or persists.

Salt Substitutes (Sodium-Free)

GENERAL CLINICAL USES

Patients with congestive heart failure, hypertension, edema of pregnancy, obesity, cirrhosis of the liver, renal disease, or corticosteroid therapy may be required to restrict their dietary intake of sodium. The salt substitutes are used to give food salt flavor while reducing the patient's sodium intake.

SPECIFIC PRODUCTS AND DOSAGES

GENERIC NAME	TRADE NAME
potassium chloride, ammonium chloride, choline bitartrate, silica, lactose	CO-SALT
potassium chloride, glutamic acid, potassium glutamate, calcium silicate, tribasic calcium phosphate, 0.01% potassium iodide	NEOCURTASAL
potassium chloride and glutamic acid	DIASAL

SPECIAL PRECAUTIONS

• Excessive use may cause weakness, nausea, muscle cramps; in severe cases, uremia may supervene.
• Do not use in patients with oliguria and severe kidney disease.
• Do not use in patients who may be required to restrict their potassium intake.

Vitamins

INTRODUCTION

The vitamins, substances essential for normal metabolic functions of the body, are usually derived in adequate quantities from foods when the diet is well balanced. They are also available in synthetic, semisynthetic, or natural forms to supplement the diet. The supplements may be "dietary supplements" or "therapeutic supplements."

The Recommended Daily Dietary Allowance (RDA, RDDA) for individual vitamins provides authoritative information to assist in evaluating the formulas of multivitamin preparations. These values, which represent the amount of each vitamin that will maintain good nutrition, are usually considerably greater than the Minimum Daily Requirement (MDR), a value established by the Food and Drug Administration for labeling purposes.

Therapeutic supplements usually contain several times the Recommended Daily Dietary Allowance, whereas dietary supplements usually contain the RDA or less.

Vitamin A

GENERAL CLINICAL USES

Vitamin A is used to treat deficiencies of vitamin A manifested by symptoms such as nyctalopia, xerophthalmia, keratomalacia, metaplasia of the mucous membranes of the respiratory, alimentary, and urinary tracts, and the associated lowered resistance to infection. Vitamin A may be used in the treatment of hyperkeratotic skin conditions, eczema, and excessively dry skin.

The Recommended Daily Dietary Allowance of vitamin A in the adult is 5,000 IU; in pregnant and lactating women it is 6,000 to 8,000 IU.

SPECIFIC PRODUCTS AND DOSAGES

GENERIC NAME	TRADE NAME	ROUTE OF ADMIN.	USUAL DAILY DOSAGE
vitamin A	(G)† VI-DOM-"A" Capsules	po	**Adults and children over 8 yrs.:** 25,000–50,000 IU/day **Children 4–8 yrs.:** 15,000 IU/day **Children under 4 yrs.:** 10,000 IU/day

†(G) designates availability as a generic product.

(continued overleaf)

GENERIC NAME	TRADE NAME	ROUTE OF ADMIN.	USUAL DAILY DOSAGE
water miscible vitamin A palmitate	(G) AQUASOL A	po im	**Adults:** 50,000–100,000 IU/day **Children 1–8 yrs.:** 17,500–35,000 IU/day **Infants:** 7,500–15,000 IU/day

PHARMACOLOGY

Vitamin A, a fat-soluble vitamin, is available in oil or water miscible forms. The aqueous solution produces a more rapid increase in blood concentration and higher blood concentrations than the oil form. Vitamin A is stored in the liver.

SPECIAL PRECAUTIONS

- Absorption or utilization of fats and fat-soluble vitamins may be impaired in patients with hepatic, pancreatic, biliary disorders; sprue, diarrheal disorders.
- Do not use in patients with hypervitaminosis A or with a history of hypersensitivity to vitamin A.
- In pregnancy, avoid doses exceeding 6,000 IU.
- Avoid overdosage.

CLINICAL GUIDELINES

ADMINISTRATION:
- Prolonged administration of doses over 24,000 IU should be under close medical supervision.
- Vitamin A is unstable in air and light; protect from light.

EFFECTS:
- Women taking oral contraceptive agents have shown a significant increase in plasma vitamin A levels.

OVERDOSAGE/ANTIDOTE:
- The following amounts of vitamin A have been found to be toxic: *Acute toxicity:* infants—350,000 IU; adults:—over 2 million IU. *Chronic toxicity:* infants 3–6 months—18,500 IU water dispersed/day for 1–3 months; adults: 1 million IU for 3 days; 50,000 IU daily for longer than 18 months; 500,000 IU daily for 2 months.
- Overdosage is characterized by the hypervitaminosis A syndrome; fatigue, malaise, lethargy, abdominal discomfort, anorexia, vomiting, irritability, headache, increased intracranial pressure, fissures of lips, dry cracking skin, alopecia, pruritus, scaling, massive desquamation, increased pigmentation, hypomenorrhea, hepatomegaly, splenomegaly, jaundice, leukopenia, periosteal thickening, vitamin A plasma levels over 1200 IU/100 cc.
- There is no specific antidote. Treatment consists of withdrawing vitamin A; use symptomatic and supportive treatment.

Vitamin B Complex

Calcium Pantothenate (Pantothenic Acid)
Niacin (Nicotinic Acid)
Pyridoxine HCl
Riboflavin
Thiamine HCl
Thiamine Monohydrate

GENERAL CLINICAL USES

The vitamin B complex group is used to treat or prevent deficiency of thiamine, riboflavin, pyridoxine, niacin, or pantothenic acid, the major components. Deficiency of one component seldom occurs alone.

The Recommended Daily Dietary Allowance of thiamine (vitamin B_1) in children 4–6 years is 0.9 mg; in adults, 1.0–1.4 mg; and an additional 0.3 mg is required during pregnancy and lactation. The RDDA of riboflavin (vitamin B_2) is 1.2–1.5 mg for adults and 0.3 mg additionally in pregnancy and lactation; in children 4–6 years, 1.1 mg. The RDDA of pyridoxine (vitamin B_6) is 2–2.5 mg in the adult; in pregnancy 2.5 mg. Requirements for niacin in children 4–6 years is 12 mg, in adults, 13–18 mg, plus 2 mg additionally during pregnancy and 4 mg during lactation.

SPECIFIC PRODUCTS AND DOSAGES

GENERIC NAME	TRADE NAME	ROUTE OF ADMIN.	USUAL DAILY DOSAGE
calcium pantothenate (pantothenic acid)	PANTHOLIN	po	10–100 mg
niacin	(G)*	po iv	0.5–3 gm 0.1–3 gm
pyridoxine HCl	(G)	po	2–100 mg
riboflavin	(G)	po	5–50 mg
thiamine HCl	(G)	po iv/im	5–100 mg 10–20 mg tid
thiamine monohydrate	(G)	po	5–100 mg

*(G) designates availability as a generic product.

PHARMACOLOGY

The components of the vitamin B complex are water soluble and are absorbed within the gastrointestinal tract. With the exception of niacin is very large doses, they are essentially devoid of secondary pharmacodynamic actions when given in therapeutic doses. Even large doses have little effect. However, large doses of niacin reduce serum lipids.

Thiamine is essential for carbohydrate metabolism. Deficiency causes beriberi. Riboflavin and pyridoxine act as coenzymes in enzyme systems. Niacin is an essential component of coenzymes necessary for carbohydrate, fat, and protein metabolism.

SPECIAL PRECAUTIONS

- Do not use in patients with a history of hypersensitivity to any of the components.
- If administered to patients receiving levodopa for parkinsonism, the intake of pyridoxine should not exceed the recommended daily allowance to avoid interference with the beneficial effects of levodopa.
- Large doses of niacin may produce an abnormal glucose tolerance curve and impairment of liver function; monitor liver function and blood glucose levels during therapy with large doses.
- Use niacin in large doses cautiously in patients with glaucoma, severe diabetes, impaired liver function, or peptic ulcer.

ADVERSE EFFECTS

- With thiamine and niacin, feeling of warmth, pruritus, urticaria, weakness, sweating, nausea, restlessness, tightness of throat, angioneurotic edema, cyanosis, pulmonary edema, gastrointestinal hemorrhage, collapse, death.

- With niacin, elevated uric acid levels have occurred. With large doses, decreased glucose tolerance, abnormal liver function tests, jaundice, and amblyopia may occur.

CLINICAL GUIDELINES

DRUG INTERACTIONS:

- When pyridoxine is administered concurrently with isoniazid, the development of peripheral neuritis is prevented.
- For drug interactions with large doses of niacin, see the discussion of cholesterol- and lipid-reducing agents in Chapter 15.
- Concurrent administration of anticoagulants (oral) may cause hemorrhage.
- Thiamine is unstable in neutral or alkaline solutions; do not use in combination with materials (e.g., carbamates, citrates, barbiturates) that yield alkaline solutions.
- In patients receiving antihypertensive drugs (sympathetic blocking type), niacin may have an additive vasodilating effect; postural hypotension may result.

OVERDOSAGE/ANTIDOTE:

- Excessive quantities of these vitamins are excreted in the urine.
- There is no known antidote.

Cyanocobalamin
Hydroxocobalamin (Vitamin B$_{12}$)

GENERAL CLINICAL USES

Cyanocobalamin and hydroxocobalamin are indicated for treatment of vitamin B$_{12}$ deficiencies due to malabsorption occurring in pernicious or Addison's anemia, gastrointestinal pathology, dysfunction, or surgery, fish tapeworm infestations, gluten enteropathy, sprue, and concomitant folic acid deficiency. These products are also useful in pregnancy, thyrotoxicosis, hemolytic anemia, and renal disease, when requirements for vitamin B$_{12}$ are increased.

SPECIFIC PRODUCTS AND DOSAGES

GENERIC NAME	TRADE NAME	ROUTE OF ADMIN.	USUAL DAILY DOSAGE
cyanocobalamin	(G)† FOLBESYN* REDISOL RUBRAMIN PC	im po	30 mcg daily for 5–10 days; then 100 mcg monthly 1000 mg daily
hydroxocobalamin	(G) NEO-BETALIN 12 Crystalline	im	30–100 mcg daily for 5–10 days, then 100 mcg monthly

*Contains more than one active ingredient.
†(G) designates availability as a generic product.

PHARMACOLOGY

Vitamin B_{12} is essential for cell reproduction and growth, hematopoiesis, and nucleoprotein and myelin synthesis. Both cyanocobalamin and hydroxocobalamin have equal hematopoietic activity; hydroxocobalamin is as effective in treating vitamin B_{12} deficiencies as cyanocobalamin. Hydroxocobalamin is absorbed more slowly than cyanocobalamin and may be taken up by the liver in larger quantities. A sustained rise in serum cobalamin level occurs.

SPECIAL PRECAUTIONS

• Do not use in patients who are sensitive to cobalt and/or vitamin B_{12}.
• Patients with early hereditary optic nerve atrophy (Leber's disease) have suffered severe and swift optic atrophy when treated with vitamin B_{12}.
• Hypokalemia and sudden death may occur when severe megaloblastic anemia is treated intensively.
• Lack of therapeutic response may be due to infection, uremia, concomitant treatment with chloramphenicol or misdiagnosis.
• Indiscriminate administration of vitamin B_{12} may mask the true diagnosis of pernicious anemia.

ADVERSE EFFECTS

RESPIRATORY EFFECTS: pulmonary edema
CARDIOVASCULAR EFFECTS: peripheral vascular thrombosis, congestive heart failure
GASTROINTESTINAL EFFECTS: transient diarrhea
METABOLIC AND ENDOCRINE EFFECTS: feeling of swelling of entire body
HEMATOLOGIC EFFECTS: polycythemia vera
ALLERGIC EFFECTS: anaphylactic shock, death
DERMATOLOGIC EFFECTS: itching, transitory exanthema
LOCAL EFFECTS: mild pain

CLINICAL GUIDELINES

ADMINISTRATION:
• Protect preparations from sunlight.

- Test patient intradermally for sensitivity to cobalamins before administering.

EFFECTS:

- Doses of vitamin B_{12} exceeding 10 mcg daily may produce a hematologic response in patients who have a folate deficiency.

DRUG INTERACTIONS:

- Most antibiotics, methotrexate, and pyrimethamine invalidate folic acid and vitamin B_{12} diagnostic microbiological blood assays.

- Colchicine, para-aminosalicylic acid, or excessive alcohol intake for longer than 2 weeks may produce malabsorption of vitamin B_{12}.

OVERDOSAGE/ANTIDOTE:

- From 50 to 98 percent of an injected dose of 100 to 1000 mcg of vitamin B_{12} may appear in the urine within 48 hours. The major portion is excreted within the first 8 hours.

Folic Acid

GENERAL CLINICAL USES

Folic acid, pteroylglutamic acid, is useful in treating megaloblastic anemias due to folic acid deficiency and nutritional anemias.

The recommended daily allowance of folic acid is 0.4 mg; this amount increases during pregnancy and lactation.

SPECIFIC PRODUCTS AND DOSAGES

GENERIC NAME	TRADE NAME	ROUTE OF ADMIN.	USUAL DAILY DOSAGE
folic acid*	(G)† FOLVITE	po/im/iv/sc	**Adults and children** **Initial:** 0.8–1.0 mg daily **Maintenance:** **Infants**—0.1 mg **Children under 4 yrs.**—up to 0.3 mg **Adults and children over 4 yrs.**—0.4 mg **Pregnant and lactating women**—0.8 mg

*Folic acid is also available in numerous multivitamin products.
†(G) designates availability as a generic product.

PHARMACOLOGY

Folic acid, a member of the vitamin B complex, acts on the megaloblastic bone marrow to produce a normoblastic marrow. It is absorbed from the gastrointestinal tract almost completely and appears in the blood within 30 minutes.

SPECIAL PRECAUTIONS

- Do not administer folic acid alone in treating pernicious anemia and other meg-

aloblastic anemias in which vitamin B_{12} is deficient.
• Treatment with folic acid alone may obscure pernicious anemia.
• In patients with severe intestinal malabsorption, orally administered folic acid will not be absorbed.

ADVERSE EFFECTS
ALLERGIC EFFECTS: sensitization following both oral and parenteral administration

CLINICAL GUIDELINES
ADMINISTRATION:
• In cases of folic acid deficiency, folic acid alone should be used, not a multivitamin preparation.
EFFECTS:
• In the presence of alcoholism, hemolytic anemia, anticonvulsant therapy, or chronic infection, increases in the maintenance dose may be required.
• Dosages above 1 mg daily may obscure pernicious anemia.

Vitamin D
Vitamin D₂ (Calciferol, Calcitriol, Ergocalciferol)
Vitamin D₃ (Cholecalciferol)

GENERAL CLINICAL USES
Vitamin D is useful in treating and preventing vitamin D deficiencies, which are characterized by rickets, osteomalacia, and inadequate absorption of calcium and phosphate.

The Recommended Daily Dietary Allowance of vitamin D is 400 IU for infants, children, and adults under 22 years of age and for pregnant or lactating women.

SPECIFIC PRODUCTS AND DOSAGES

GENERIC NAME	TRADE NAME	ROUTE OF ADMIN.	USUAL DAILY DOSAGE
vitamin D*	(G)†	po	12,000–500,000 IU daily
Ergocalciferol (D₂)*	(G) CALCIFEROL	po/im	12,000–500,000 IU daily
calcitriol*	ROCALTROL	po	0.25–1 mcg/day
cholecalciferol (D₃)*	(G)	po	12,000–500,000 IU daily

*Available in multivitamin products.
†(G) designates availability as a generic product.

PHARMACOLOGY

Vitamin D, a fat-soluble vitamin, increases the absorption of calcium from the intestines and increases tubular reabsorption of phosphate. It also acts in the mobilization of bone calcium and maintenance of serum calcium levels.

Blood calcium should be maintained between 9 and 10 mg%.

SPECIAL PRECAUTIONS

- Absorption or utilization of fats and fat-soluble vitamins may be impaired in patients with hepatic, pancreatic, and biliary disorders, sprue, or diarrheal disorders.
- Do not use in patients with hypercalcemia, malabsorption syndrome, decreased renal function, or hypersensitivity to vitamin D.
- Treat patients with coronary disease, impaired renal function, and arteriosclerosis, especially in the elderly, with caution.

ADVERSE EFFECTS

- See *Overdosage/Antidote.*

CLINICAL GUIDELINES

ADMINISTRATION:

- Overuse of vitamin D may result in hypervitaminosis D.

EFFECTS:

- Doses of 100,000 units or more per day in adults or 200,000 units per day in children can produce toxic effects; elevated serum levels of calcium and phosphorus, drowsiness, gastrointestinal symptoms, renal failure, metastatic calcifications, and hypertension are manifestations of vitamin D toxicity.

DRUG INTERACTIONS:

- Usually administered with vitamin A.
- Mineral oil interferes with absorption of fat-soluble vitamins.
- Concurrent administration of thiazide diuretics may cause hypercalcemia.

OVERDOSAGE/ANTIDOTE:

- Initial signs and symptoms of overdosage, hypervitaminosis D, consist of weakness, fatigue, lassitude, headache, anorexia, nausea, vomiting, and diarrhea. These are followed by hypercalcemia, ectopic calcifications in soft tissue, polydipsia, polyuria.
- There is no specific antidote. Terminate or reduce vitamin D intake. Consider use of low calcium diet, increased fluid intake, and acidification of urine. Treat symptomatically and supportively. Dialysis may be useful.

Vitamin C

Ascorbic Acid
Calcium Ascorbate
Sodium Ascorbate

GENERAL CLINICAL USES

Vitamin C is indicated for the correction and prevention of scurvy and other forms of vitamin C deficiency.

The Recommended Daily Dietary Allowance for pregnant and lactating women is 60 mg, for other adults 45 mg, for children 40 mg, and for infants 35 mg.

SPECIFIC PRODUCTS AND DOSAGES

GENERIC NAME	TRADE NAME	ROUTE OF ADMIN.	USUAL DAILY DOSAGE
ascorbic acid	ASCOR CETANE CEVI-BID	po sc	50–500 mg daily 0.2–2 gm daily
calcium ascorbate	CALSCORBATE	im/iv	50–500 mg daily
sodium ascorbate*	(G)†	po/im	50–500 mg daily

*Available in combination products.
†(G) designates availability as a generic product.

PHARMACOLOGY

Vitamin C, a water-soluble vitamin, aids in the absorption and, possibly, utilization of iron; it is essential for regeneration of tissue. Vitamin C is excreted by the kidneys.

Vitamin C is available as calcium ascorbate for intramuscular or intravenous administration. It is in a neutral solution which provides a fast and effective form for parenteral administration.

SPECIAL PRECAUTIONS

• Never administer calcium ascorbate subcutaneously.
• Do not use in patients with a history of hypersensitivity to vitamin C.

ADVERSE EFFECTS

SYSTEMIC EFFECTS: diarrhea; precipitation of oxalate or urate renal stones if urine becomes acidic during therapy; with rapid IV administration, temporary faintness or dizziness
LOCAL EFFECTS: necrosis in infants after intramuscular administration; soreness at injection site.

CLINICAL GUIDELINES
ADMINISTRATION:
• In patients with diarrhea, absorption may be limited.
EFFECTS:
• In patients with achlorhydria, ascorbic acid may be destroyed in the gastrointestinal tract.
• Vitamin C requirements may be increased in hyperthyroidism, peptic ulcer, neoplastic disease, pregnancy, lactation, and surgery.
DRUG INTERACTIONS:
• Do not administer calcium ascorbate to patients receiving digitalis; cardiac arrhythmias may be precipitated.
• Doses of 2 gm daily will significantly lower the urinary pH in most adults, and may result in unexpected renal tubular reabsorption of acidic drugs.
• Concurrent administration of sulfonamides may result in crystallization.
• Ascorbic acid is chemically incompatible with potassium penicillin G and should

not be administered in the same syringe or parenteral solution.

OVERDOSAGE/ANTIDOTE:

• The water-soluble vitamins have low toxicity. Ingestion of excessive quantities of vitamin C does little harm to the body. The excess vitamin is excreted in the urine.

Vitamin E

GENERAL CLINICAL USES

Vitamin E is indicated in individuals whose dietary fats are restricted to polyunsaturated sources and in the treatment of vitamin E deficiency states. There is limited evidence that vitamin E is of nutritional significance in humans.

The minimal daily requirement has not been established. The Recommended Daily Dietary Allowance in adults is 10–15 IU; in pregnancy and lactation, 15 IU; in infants 4–5 IU; and in children 10 years or younger, 7–10 IU.

SPECIFIC PRODUCTS AND DOSAGES

GENERIC NAME	TRADE NAME	ROUTE OF ADMIN.	USUAL DAILY DOSAGE
vitamin E aqueous*	(G)† AQUASOL E LETHOPHEROL E-FEROL	po im	30–300 IU one to three times daily; varies with the preparation 50–500 mg daily

*Available in multivitamin preparations.
†(G) designates availability as a generic product.

PHARMACOLOGY

Vitamin E, a fat-soluble vitamin, has antioxidant properties and is an essential nutrient in heme synthesis. The biochemical functions of vitamin E are not completely understood.

SPECIAL PRECAUTIONS

• Absorption or utilization of fats and fat-soluble vitamins may be impaired in patients with hepatic, pancreatic, or biliary disorders, sprue, or diarrheal disorders.

• The requirements for vitamin E increase with the uptake of polyunsaturated fatty acids.

OVERDOSAGE/ANTIDOTE

• Administration of vitamin E, 80 IU/kg for 5 months, produced no toxic effect. However, larger doses administered for prolonged periods have caused skeletal muscle weakness, disturbances of reproductive functions, and gastrointestinal upset. These symptoms disappeared within a few weeks when the excessive vitamin E intake was terminated.

Vitamin K

Menadione Sodium Bisulfate
Menadiol Sodium Diphosphate
Phytonadione

GENERAL CLINICAL USES

Vitamin K is indicated in the treatment of anticoagulant-induced prothrombin deficiency, prophylaxis and therapy of hemorrhagic disease of the newborn, hypoprothrombinemia due to antibacterial therapy, secondary hypoprothrombinemia, and drug-induced hypoprothrombinemia.

The Minimum Daily Requirement has been estimated to be 1–5 mcg/kg for infants and 0.05 mcg/kg for adults.

SPECIFIC PRODUCTS AND DOSAGES

GENERIC NAME	TRADE NAME	ROUTE OF ADMIN.	USUAL DOSAGE
menadione sodium bisulfate	HYKINONE	sc/iv/im	2.5–5 mg daily
menadiol sodium diphosphate	KAPPADIONE SYNKAVITE	im/iv/sc	**Infants:** 5–10 mg/kg od or bid **Adults:** 5–15 mg od or bid
	SYNKAYVITE	po	**Adults:** 5–10 mg daily
phytonadione	AQUAMEPHYTON KONAKION	im/iv/sc	**Adults:** 5–20 mg daily **Infants:** 1–2 mg daily

PHARMACOLOGY

Vitamin K, a water-soluble vitamin, may be administered subcutaneously, intravenously, intramuscularly, or orally. This vitamin is necessary for the production in the liver of active prothrombin (factor II), proconvertin (factor VII), and Stuart factor (factor X).

Following intravenous administration, hemorrhage is usually controlled in 3 to 6 hours; a normal prothrombin level may be obtained in 12 to 14 hours.

The precise mechanism of action is not known.

SPECIAL PRECAUTIONS

• When administered intravenously, severe reactions including fatalities have occurred.
• Do not use in patients with a history of hypersensitivity to vitamin K.
• In patients with hepatic disease, large doses may further depress liver function.
• Do not expect an immediate anticoagulant effect.
• The anticoagulant effect of heparin is not counteracted.
• Vitamin K is not a clotting agent; however, overzealous therapy may restore con-

ditions which permit thromboembolic phenomena.

• In liver disease, repeated large doses of vitamin K are not warranted if the initial use is unsatisfactory.

• Do not administer to mother during last few weeks of pregnancy as a prophylactic measure against physiologic hypoprothrombinemia or hemorrhagic disease of the newborn.

• Safe use in pregnancy has not been established.

ADVERSE EFFECTS

CNS EFFECTS: transient "flushing sensations," "peculiar" sensations of taste; dizziness with rapid intravenous administration

RESPIRATORY EFFECTS: dyspnea, cyanosis

CARDIOVASCULAR EFFECTS: rapid, weak pulse; brief hypotension

AUTONOMIC EFFECTS: profuse sweating

GASTROINTESTINAL EFFECTS: gastrointestinal upset

HEPATIC EFFECTS: hyperbilirubinemia in newborn rarely

ALLERGIC EFFECTS: anaphylactoid reactions, urticaria

DERMATOLOGIC EFFECTS: rash

LOCAL EFFECTS: pain, swelling, tenderness

CLINICAL GUIDELINES

ADMINISTRATION:

• Preferably administer subcutaneously or intramuscularly.

• When administering, inject very slowly, not exceeding 1 mg/min.

• Store in a dark place and protect from light at all times; potency is lost on exposure to light.

EFFECTS:

• In patients with liver disease, paradoxical hypothrombinemia may occasionally occur after administration of large doses of vitamin K.

DRUG INTERACTIONS:

• Temporary resistance to prothrombin-depressing anticoagulants may result, especially when large doses of vitamin K are used.

• BSP retention and prolongation of prothrombin time have been reported after maximal doses of vitamin K analogs.

OVERDOSAGE/ANTIDOTE:

• In infants, whether premature or full-term, very large doses of vitamin K may cause hemolytic reaction and kernicterus.

Antineoplastic/ anticancer agents

17

INTRODUCTION

During the last two decades significant advances have been made in the chemotherapeutic treatment of malignancies. Among these advances are the development of new agents, the scheduling of drug administration during specific stages of cell growth, the use of multiple drugs, and the increasing use of combination drug and radiation therapy. The antineoplastic agents are not, as a rule, administered as primary therapy unless the malignancy is inoperable, such as in acute and chronic leukemias, choriocarcinoma, multiple myeloma, and disseminated multiple site malignancies.

Because of the complexity and toxicity of the antineoplastic agents, it is advisable that these agents be used only by and under the supervision of a physician experienced in cancer chemotherapy. It is essential that adequate laboratory and hospital facilities be available to the patient so that the drug effects may be monitored adequately.

SPECIFIC THERAPEUTIC CLASSIFICATION

The antineoplastic/anticancer agents are grouped as follows:

1. Alkylating agents
2. Antibiotics
3. Antimetabolites
4. Hormones: estrogens, progestogens, corticosteroids, androgens
5. Antiestrogenic agents
6. Miscellaneous drugs including synthetic organic agents and plant alkaloids

Each group of antineoplastic compounds exerts its prime action somewhat differently and consequently may be effective against specific types of malignancies. In combination therapy, a frequent approach to treating malignancies, administration of drugs from different groups concurrently may prove more effective than drugs from the same group.

Alkylating Agents

GENERAL CLINICAL USES

The alkylating agents are effective primarily against the malignancies of the reticuloendothelial system such as chronic leukemias, lymphomas, myelomas, and also carcinoma of the breast and ovary. They are frequently used in combination with other antineoplastic agents.

SPECIFIC PRODUCTS AND DOSAGES

GENERIC NAME	TRADE NAME	ROUTE OF ADMIN.	USUAL DAILY DOSAGE	
			INDUCTION	**MAINTENANCE**
busulfan	MYLERAN	po	4–8 mg daily	1–3 mg daily
carmustine (BCNU)	BI CNU	iv	100–200 mg/M^2 as 1 or 2 daily injections	Adjust according to hematologic response
chlorambucil	LEUKERAN	po	0.1–0.2 mg/kg/day	0.03–0.1 mg/kg/day; do not exceed 0.1 mg/kg/day
cisplatin	PLATINOL	iv	20–100 mg/M^2	

(continued facing page)

GENERIC NAME	TRADE NAME	ROUTE OF ADMIN.	USUAL DAILY DOSAGE	
			INDUCTION	MAINTENANCE
cyclophosphamide	CYTOXAN	po iv	1–5 mg/kg day 40–50 mg/kg in 2–5 days	1–5 mg/kg twice weekly 10–15 mg/kg every 1–2 wk
lomustine (CCNU)	CEE NU	po	100–130 mg/M^2	adjust according to hematologic response
mechlorethamine (nitrogen mustard)	MUSTARGEN	iv	0.4 mg/kg as a single dose or divided into 2–4 doses	Not established
		intrapleural intraperitoneal intrapericardial	Consult package insert	
melphalan (phenylalanine mustard)	ALKERAN PAM L-PAM	po	6 mg/day	2 mg daily
pipobroman	VERCYTE	po	1–3 mg/kg day	0.1–0.2 mg/kg/day
triethylenemelamine	TEM	po	2.5–5 mg twice usually for 4 weeks	1 mg daily for 3 or 4 weeks
triethylene thiophosphoramide	(G)* THIOTEPA	local iv	45–60 mg 0.3–0.4 mg/kg at 1 to 4 week intervals	Depends on blood count Adjust according to hematologic response
uracil mustard	(G)	po	1–2 mg daily until clinical improvement	1 mg daily for 3 or 4 weeks

*(G) designates availability as a generic product.

Busulfan
Carmustine (BCNU)
Chlorambucil
Cisplatin
Cyclophosphamide
Lomustine (CCNU)
Mechlorethamine
Melphalan
Pipobroman
Triethylenemelamine
Triethylenethiophosphoramide
Uracil Mustard

PHARMACOLOGY

The alkylating agents act by inhibiting cell division and by inhibiting synthesis of DNA.

SPECIAL PRECAUTIONS

• May cause irreversible hematopoietic depression.

• If leukocyte count falls below 3000, consider prophylactic administration of antibiotics.

• Avoid concurrent administration of other drugs known to produce bone marrow depression.

• Contraindicated in patients with known hypersensitivity to the drug or related drugs.

• Monitor closely hepatic and renal function, particularly in patients with known impairment of these systems.

• The alkylating agents should not be administered to patients who have recently (about 4 weeks) had a full course of radiotherapy or chemotherapy.

- Safe use in pregnancy has not been established.
- Hypersensitivity reactions have been reported with cisplatin.

ADVERSE EFFECTS

CNS EFFECTS: asthenia, drowsiness, headache, fever, nervousness, irritability, depression, dizziness

RESPIRATORY EFFECTS: interstitial pulmonary fibrosis

RENAL EFFECTS: hemorrhagic cystitis, fibrosis of bladder, hematuria

GASTROINTESTINAL EFFECTS: nausea, vomiting, anorexia, abdominal cramps, hemorrhagic colitis

METABOLIC AND ENDOCRINE EFFECTS: hyperuricemia, uric acid neuropathy, interference with spermatogenesis and ovarian function, gynecomastia, sterility

HEPATIC EFFECTS: jaundice

HEMATOLOGIC EFFECTS: leukopenia, thrombocytopenia, anemia

ALLERGIC EFFECTS: hives, rash, anaphylactic reaction

DERMATOLOGIC EFFECTS: alopecia, dermatitis; with cyclophosphamide, darkening of skin and fingernails

OTIC EFFECTS: tinnitus, deafness

LOCAL EFFECTS: extravasation into subcutaneous tissues results in painful inflammation

CLINICAL GUIDELINES

ADMINISTRATION:
- Do not administer the nitrogen mustards if other similar chemotherapeutic agents of radiation have been administered recently, or if neutrophilic and platelet counts are depressed.
- Do not store cyclophosphamide at temperatures above 90°F.
- Triethylenemelamine should be taken on an empty stomach at least 60 minutes before breakfast with water and at least 2 grams of sodium bicarbonate.

EFFECTS:
- If platelet or leukocyte counts fall significantly, discontinue therapy with any alkylating agent.
- May interfere with normal wound healing.
- Patients receiving cyclophosphamide should be encouraged to drink an ample amount of fluids and to void frequently to avoid development of cystitis.
- With cisplatin, ototoxicity (tinnitus, deafness) is more severe in children than in adults.

DRUG INTERACTIONS:
- Concurrent administration of high doses of phenobarbital may increase rate of metabolism and leukopenic activity of cyclophosphamide.

OVERDOSAGE/ANTIDOTE:
- Overdosage of the alkylating agents may be indicated by an exaggeration of adverse effects; bleeding will be noted frequently.
- No antidote to any alkylating agent is known; treat supportively.

Antibiotics

Bleomycin Sulfate
Dactinomycin
Doxorubicin Hydrochloride

Mitomycin
Mithramycin

GENERAL CLINICAL USES

In general, the antibiotics are used in combination with other antineoplastic agents for inoperable malignancies. The antineoplastic antibiotics should be considered palliative treatment.

SPECIFIC PRODUCTS AND DOSAGES

GENERIC NAME	TRADE NAME	ROUTE OF ADMIN.	USUAL DOSAGE
bleomycin sulfate	BLENOXANE	im/iv/sc	0.25–0.50 units/kg weekly or twice weekly **Maintenance dose:** 1 U/day or 5 U/week
dactinomycin (actinomycin D)	COSMEGEN	iv	**Adults:** 0.5 mg/day for 5 days **Children:** 0.015 mg/kg/day for 5 days
doxorubicin HCl	ADRIAMYCIN	iv	60–75 mg/M^2 body surface as a single injection at 21-day intervals
mitomycin	MUTAMYCIN	iv	20 mg/M^2/day as a single dose or 2 mg/M^2/day for 5 days, then after 2 days repeat 2 mg/M^2 for 5 days (20 mg/M^2 total dose)
mithramycin	MITHRACIN	iv	25–30 mcg/kg for 8–10 days; maximal daily dose 30 mcg/kg

PHARMACOLOGY

The antineoplastic antibiotics disrupt cellular functions of host tissues by interfering with DNA-RNA synthesis. These agents have no significant antibacterial activity. Bleomycin sulfate is excreted in urine as active drug, as are dactinomycin, mitomycin, and mithramycin. Dactinomycin is also excreted unchanged in the bile and does not appear to cross the blood-brain barrier. Doxorubicin hydrochloride administered intravenously is cleared rapidly from the plasma, binds significantly to tissues, and is excreted primarily by the liver. It does not cross the blood-brain barrier.

SPECIAL PRECAUTIONS

• Cardiotoxicity including heart failure has occurred with doxorubicin; failure may occur several weeks after therapy.
• Pneumonitis progressing to pulmonary fibrosis may occur, particularly in elderly patients treated with bleomycin.
• Do not administer to patients with thrombocytopenia, coagulation disorders, or bleeding tendencies; further bone marrow suppression may occur.
• In patients receiving cytotoxic antibiotics, the renal, hematologic, and hepatic functions should be carefully and frequently monitored.

• No drug should be used in patients with known hypersensitivity to that drug or related drugs.

• Safe use in pregnancy has not been established.

• Use doxorubincin with caution in patients with hepatic impairment; this drug is excreted primarily in the bile.

ADVERSE EFFECTS

CNS EFFECTS: fever, chills, headache, confusion, drowsiness, syncope, fatigue, pain

RESPIRATORY EFFECTS: with bleomycin sulfate, dyspnea, pneumonitis, pulmonary fibrosis

CARDIOVASCULAR EFFECTS: with doxorubicin, serious irreversible myocardial toxicity with delayed congestive failure

URINARY TRACT EFFECTS: increased serum creatinine and BUN; proteinuria

GASTROINTESTINAL EFFECTS: nausea, vomiting, stomatitis, esophagitis, anorexia, and diarrhea

METABOLIC AND ENDOCRINE EFFECTS: with mithramycin, hypocalcemia, hypokalemia, hypophosphatemia

HEPATIC EFFECTS: with mithramycin, increased SGOT, SGPT, LDH, alkaline phosphatase, serum bilirubin, ornithine carbamyl transferase, isocitric dehydrogenase; decreased BSP

HEMATOLOGIC EFFECTS: thrombocytopenia, leukopenia

ALLERGIC EFFECTS: fever, chills, urticaria, anaphylaxis

DERMATOLOGIC EFFECTS: alopecia, hyperpigmentation of nailbeds and dermal creases, erythema, rash, striae, vesiculation, hyperpigmentation, tenderness of skin, hyperkeratosis, nail changes, pruritus, stomatitis, alopecia

OPHTHALMIC EFFECTS: with doxorubicin, conjunctivitis, lacrimation; with mitomycin, blurring of vision

LOCAL EFFECTS: pain, stinging, phlebitis, thrombophlebitis, phlebosclerosis, cellulitis at injection site

CLINICAL GUIDELINES

ADMINISTRATION:

• Extravasation may result in severe local tissue reactions including cellulitis and necrosis. Stinging or burning on administration of doxorubicin signifies extravasation; terminate administration immediately.

• Administration of bleomycin may result in idiosyncratic reactions similar to anaphylaxis. These reactions have been reported in 1 percent of lymphoma patients treated with bleomycin.

• Do not administer mitomycin if serum creatinine is greater than 1.7 mg%.

• Epistaxis and hematemesis occurring in patients receiving mithramycin are the initial indicators of toxicity.

EFFECTS:

• Advise patients that doxorubicin imparts a red color to the urine for 1 to 2 days.

• Bleomycin may cause hypothermic reactions 3 to 5 hours after administration.

• In patients receiving bleomycin, watch for occurrence of rales which may predict pulmonary toxicity.

• Observe patients carefully and frequently for signs and symptoms of infection.

• With bleomycin, idiosyncratic reactions resembling anaphylaxis have occurred, usually after the first or second dose.

DRUG INTERACTIONS:

• Cross sensitivity between doxorubicin and lincemycin has been reported.

• Doxorubicin is incompatible with heparin; a precipitate may form.

OVERDOSAGE/ANTIDOTE:

• Overdosage of any of these drugs is potentially fatal. Signs of overdosage consist of exaggerated clinical and adverse effects.

• No specific antidotes are known. Treat supportively.

Antimetabolites

GENERAL CLINICAL USES

The antimetabolites, although used primarily in the treatment of acute leukemias, chronic leukemias, carcinoma of the colon and breast, and choriocarcinoma, have been used to treat the entire spectrum of inoperable malignancies.

Use of these agents should be limited to physicians experienced in antimetabolite chemotherapy. Because of the possibility of fatal or severe toxic reactions, inform patients of the risk involved and keep patients under constant supervision.

SPECIFIC PRODUCTS AND DOSAGES

GENERIC NAME	TRADE NAME	ROUTE OF ADMIN.	USUAL DOSAGE	
			INDUCTION	MAINTENANCE
cytarabine (ARA-C) (cytosine arabinoside)	CYTOSAR-U	iv infusion or injection/sc	3–12.5 mg/kg/12 hr	Depends on patient's response
fluorouracil (5-FU) (5-fluorouracil)	EFUDEX FLUOROPLEX (G)* ADRUCIL	topical	Apply twice weekly for 2–4 wk	———
		iv	12 mg/kg/day for 4 days; do not exceed 800 mg daily; 6 mg/kg/day for next 4 doses	12 mg/kg/day once every 30 days or 10–15 mg/kg/ wk; do not exceed 1 gm/wk
floxuridine	FUDR	intra-arterial infusion	0.1–0.6 mg/kg/day	———
		hepatic	0.4–0.6 mg/kg/day	———
mercaptopurine (6-MP)	PURINETHOL	po	2.5–5.0 mg/kg/day	Establish individually
methotrexate	(G)	po	15–30 mg/day for 5 days; repeat 3–5 times with rest period of 1 week in between	———
		iv/im/ intra-arterial	0.625–2.5 mg/kg/day	———
		intrathecal	15/mg/day for 2–5 days	
thioguanine (TG)	(G)	po	2–3 mg/kg/day for 2–4 wk	2 mg/kg/day

*(G) designates availability as a generic product.

Cytarabine
Fluorouracil
Floxuridine
Mercaptopurine
Methotrexate
Thioguanine

PHARMACOLOGY

The antimetabolites exert their antineoplastic activity by interfering with the various metabolic processes including the synthesis of nucleic acids.

Methotrexate, mercaptopurine, and thioguanine, administered orally, are readily absorbed from the gastrointestinal tract. Peak blood levels are reached in 1 to 2 hours. When the antimetabolites are administered parenterally, peak levels are reached in about one-half hour; excretion is primarily by the kidneys.

SPECIAL PRECAUTIONS

• Do not administer to patients with preexisting drug-induced, radiation-induced, or spontaneous bone marrow depression; potentially serious infections; or poor nutritional state.
• Do not use in patients with impaired renal function.
• Do not administer any drug to patients with known hypersensitivity to that drug or related drugs.
• Advise patient to avoid prolonged exposure to ultraviolet rays when under treatment with fluorouracil.
• Safe use in pregnancy has not been established.
• Marked depression of bone marrow, anemia, leukopenia, thrombocytopenia, and bleeding may occur.

ADVERSE EFFECTS

CNS EFFECTS: fever, facial paresthesia, fatigue, chills, dizziness, headache, drowsiness

RENAL EFFECTS: failure, azotemia, cystitis, hematuria, oliguria

GASTROINTESTINAL EFFECTS: nausea, vomiting, diarrhea, abdominal pain, anorexia, stomatitis, gingivitis, enteritis

METABOLIC AND ENDOCRINE EFFECTS: hyperuricemia, defective oogenesis or spermatogenesis, transient oligospermia, menstrual dysfunction, infertility, abortion, fetal effects

HEPATIC EFFECTS: jaundice, biliary stasis, elevated serum transaminase levels

HEMATOLOGIC EFFECTS: leukopenia, cytopenia, anemia, bone marrow suppression, megaloblastosis, thrombocytopenia

ALLERGIC EFFECTS: urticaria

DERMATOLOGIC EFFECTS: alopecia, facial flushing, pruritus, hyperpigmentation, maculopapular rash, photosensitivity, depigmentation, ecchymosis, telangectasia, acne, furunculosis

MUSCULOSKELETAL EFFECTS: myalgias, flu-like syndrome

OPHTHALMIC EFFECTS: blurred vision

LOCAL EFFECTS: cellulitis at injection site, pain, burning; with intravenous administration, thrombophlebitis; with arterial infusion, arterial aneurysm, arterial ischemia, arterial thrombosis, bleeding at catheter site, embolism

CLINICAL GUIDELINES

ADMINISTRATION:
• Advise patients that side effects, primarily anorexia, nausea, and vomiting, may occur. However, if stomatitis and pharyngitis or signs of infection are observed, notify physician immediately.
• Discoloration of fluorouracil solution does not effect potency and safety.
• With mercaptopurine, use small doses initially in patients with renal and hepatic impairment.
EFFECTS:
• Discontinue therapy if stomatitis or

pharyngitis, intractable vomiting, severe diarrhea, thrombocytopenia, or hemorrhage from any site occurs.
• Note that with mercaptopurine, the depression of bone marrow resulting in leukopenia, thrombocytopenia, and bleeding may be delayed; withdraw drug at first abnormally large decrease in leukocytes.

DRUG INTERACTIONS:
• Methotrexate toxicity may be increased by certain drugs, namely, salicylates, sulfonamides, diphenylhydantoin, tetracyclines, chloramphenicol, and para-aminobenzoic acid.

• Vitamin preparations containing folic acid or its derivatives may later the patient's response to methotrexate.

OVERDOSAGE/ANTIDOTE:
• Methotrexate overdosage is reflected as a toxic effect on the hematopoietic system. LEUCOVORIN (citrovorum factor) administered intravenously by infusion in doses up to 75 mg within 12 hours; followed by 12 mg intramuscularly every 6 hours for 4 doses, appears to be an effective antidote.
• No antidotes have been established for the other drugs in this group. Treat supportively.

Hormones
Androgens
Glucocorticoids
Estrogens
Progestogens

GENERAL CLINICAL USES
The androgens, glucocorticoids, estrogens, and progestogens are used alone and/or in combination with other antineoplastic drugs. They offer palliation primarily. The androgens are used for breast cancer in premenopausal or ovariectomized women and in those less than 5 years past menopause or ovariectomy. The corticosteroids are useful in leukemias, lymphomas, multiple myeloma, and CNS metastases. The progestogens are used for endometrial and breast carcinomas, whereas estrogens are useful for palliation of prostatic carcinoma and palliation in postmenopausal women or post-ovariectomy (more than 5 years) women with breast carcinoma.

The dosages of these drugs, as with many medications, should be individualized on the basis of the patient's response and the toxic effects. Consideration must be given to concomitant medications used by the patient for the malignancy or concurrent diseases.

Androgens
Calusterone
Dromostanolone Propionate

Fluoxymesterone
Methyltestosterone
Testolactone
Testosterone Propionate

PHARMACOLOGY

The androgens have palliatave effects in inoperable cancer of the breast. Formulations are available for oral and intramuscular administration. See Chapter 14, *Drugs Affecting the Reproductive Tract*, page 513, for additional information.

SPECIFIC PRODUCTS AND DOSAGES

GENERIC NAME	TRADE NAME	ROUTE OF ADMIN.	USUAL DOSAGE
calusterone	METHOSARB	po	50 mg qid; 150–300 mg/day for at least 3 months
dromostanolone propionate	DROLBAN	im	100 mg three times/wk for 8–12 weeks
fluoxymesterone	HALOTESTIN ORA-TESTRYL	po	15–30 mg daily in divided doses
methyltestosterone	ORETON METHYL	po buccal	200 mg daily 100 mg daily
testolactone	TESLAC	im po	100 mg three times/wk 250 mg qid
testosterone propionate	ORETON Propionate	buccal	100 mg daily

SPECIAL PRECAUTIONS, ADVERSE EFFECTS

See Chapter 14, page 513, for detailed information.

CLINICAL GUIDELINES

See the end of this section, *Hormones,* for detailed information.

Glucocorticoids

Prednisone
Triamcinolone Diacetate

PHARMACOLOGY

Glucocorticoids exert a lymphocytotoxic effect by suppressing mitosis in lymphocytes. For additional information, see Chapter 15, *Endocrine and Other Drugs Affecting Metabolism*, page 535.

SPECIFIC PRODUCTS AND DOSAGES

GENERIC NAME	TRADE NAME	ROUTE OF ADMIN.	USUAL DOSAGE
prednisone	(G)* METICORTEN	po	60–100 mg daily
triamcinolone diacetate	KENACORT	po	4–40 mg daily

*(G) designates availability as a generic product.

SPECIAL PRECAUTIONS, ADVERSE EFFECTS,
CLINICAL GUIDELINES

See the end of this section, *Hormones*, and also Chapter 15, *Endocrine and Other Drugs Affecting Metabolism*, page 534.

Estrogens

Chlorotrianisone
Diethylstilbestrol
Diethylstilbestrol Diphosphate
Estradiol
Estradiol Valerate
Estrogens, Conjugated
Estrogens, Esterified
Ethinyl Estradiol
Polyestradiol Phosphate

PHARMACOLOGY

The estrogens have been found useful in palliative therapy of breast cancer. The mechanism of action is unclear. These hormones may be administered orally, intramuscularly, intravenously, or subcutaneously. See Chapter 14, *Drugs Affecting the Reproductive Tract*, page 522, for additional information.

SPECIFIC PRODUCTS AND DOSAGES

GENERIC NAME	TRADE NAME	ROUTE OF ADMIN.	USUAL ADULT DOSAGE
chlorotrianisene	TACE	po	12–25 mg daily
estrogens, conjugated	(G)* PREMARIN	po	10 mg tid
diethylstilbestrol	(G) STILPHOSTROL	po	1–5 mg tid
diethylstilbestrol diphosphate	STILPHOSTROL	po iv	50–200 mg tid 0.5–1 gm daily by infusion
estrogens, esterified	(G) AMNESTROGEN	po	1.25–10.0 mg tid
estradiol	PROGYNON	sc	25 mg
estradiol valerate	DELESTROGEN	im	30 mg or more every 1–2 weeks
ethinyl estradiol	(G) ESTINYL	po	0.15–1.0 mg tid
polyestradiol phosphate	ESTRADURIN	im	up to 80 mg every 2–4 weeks

*(G) designates availability as a generic product.

Progestogens

Hydroxyprogesterone Caproate
Medroxyprogesterone
Megestrol Acetate

PHARMACOLOGY
The progestogens have actions similar to those of the corpus luteum hormone, progesterone. They act in malignancies on tissues dependent upon this hormone. See Chapter 14, *Drugs Affecting the Reproductive Tract,* page 522.

SPECIFIC PRODUCTS AND DOSAGES—Refer to table on facing page.

SPECIAL PRECAUTIONS, ADVERSE EFFECTS
See Chapter 14, *Drugs Affecting the Reproductive Tract,* page 523.

CLINICAL GUIDELINES
See the end of this section, *Hormones,* page 524, for detailed information.

GENERIC NAME	TRADE NAME	ROUTE OF ADMIN.	USUAL DOSAGE
hydroxyprogesterone caproate	(G)* DELALUTIN	im	1–7 gm/wk
medroxyprogesterone acetate	AMEN DEPO-PROVERA	im	400–1000 mg/wk, then with improvement 400 mg/month
megestrol acetate	MEGACE	po	40–320 mg/day in divided doses for at least 2 months

*(G) designates availability as a generic product.

Androgens/Glucocorticoids/ Estrogens/Progestogens

CLINICAL GUIDELINES

ADMINISTRATION:

• Advise patients receiving estrogens that the nausea, vomiting, and gastrointestinal discomfort may ease with continued treatment.

• With testolactone, patients may experience pain and inflammation at the injection site.

• Administer testolactone by deep intramuscular injection in the upper outer quadrant of the gluteal area.

• Do not administer corticosteroids to patients with ocular herpes simplex because of possible corneal perforation.

EFFECTS:

• Observe diabetic patients receiving estrogens for possible decrease in glucose tolerance.

• Observe patients receiving estrogens and progestogens for signs and symptoms of thrombotic disorders (thrombophlebitis, cerebrovascular disorders, pulmonary embolism, and retinal disorders).

• Watch patient receiving androgens for signs of virilization.

• In patients receiving androgens monitor plasma calcium levels because of possible hypercalcemia.

• Note that corticosteroids may mask signs of infection; monitor patient carefully.

• Watch patient receiving corticosteroids for weight increase, edema, excessive potassium excretion.

• Sudden termination of long-term corticosteroid therapy may result in adrenal suppression; it is imperative that therapy be withdrawn gradually rather than suddenly.

• The effects of corticosteroids are enhanced in patients with hypothyroidism or cirrhosis.

• Corticosteroids may aggravate diabetes.

DRUG INTERACTIONS:

• Concurrent administration of estrogens and progestogens have been implicated in an increased incidence of thromboembolic disease.

• In patients with hypoproteinemia receiving corticosteroids, aspirin should be used cautiously.

• Calusterone may increase sensitivity to oral anticoagulants.

OVERDOSAGE/ANTIDOTE:

• Overdosage of these hormones causes an exaggeration of the clinical and adverse effects.

• There are no known antidotes for any product. Treat supportively.

Antiestrogenic Agent

Tamoxifen

GENERAL CLINICAL USES
Tamoxifen is useful for palliative treatment of advanced breast cancer in postmenopausal women.

SPECIFIC PRODUCTS AND DOSAGES

GENERIC NAME	TRADE NAME	ROUTE OF ADMIN.	USUAL DOSAGE
tamoxifen	NOLVADEX	po	10–20 mg bid

PHARMACOLOGY
Tamoxifen, a nonsteroidal agent with potent antiestrogenic properties, appears to work by competing with estradiol for estrogen receptor protein.

Following oral administration, peak blood levels are reached in 4 to 7 hours. Excretion is slow and in the feces. Prolonged blood levels may be due to enterohepatic circulation.

SPECIAL PRECAUTIONS
• Safe use in pregnancy has not been established.
• Use with caution in patients with existing leukopenia or thrombocytopenia.

ADVERSE EFFECTS
CNS EFFECTS: depression
GASTROINTESTINAL EFFECTS: nausea, vomiting, distaste for food

METABOLIC AND ENDOCRINE EFFECTS: vaginal bleeding, vaginal discharge, menstrual irregularities, hypercalcemia, peripheral edema, hot flashes
MUSCULOSKELETAL EFFECTS: bone and tumor pain
DERMATOLOGIC EFFECTS: pruritus vulvae, erythema surrounding lesion

CLINICAL GUIDELINES
ADMINISTRATION:
• Monitor hematological parameters, including platelet counts, periodically.
EFFECTS:
• Transient decreases in platelet counts have been reported.
• Adverse effects may be controlled by reducing dosage.
OVERDOSAGE/ANTIDOTE
• Overdosage in humans has not been reported. With doses above 100 mg/M^2 bid

serious adverse effects have occurred.
* No specific treatment for overdosage is known. Treat symptomatically and supportively.

Miscellaneous Agents Including Synthetic Agents and Plant Alkaloids

GENERAL CLINICAL USES

Asparaginase is indicated to treat acute lymphocytic leukemia. It is used primarily in combination with other antineoplastic agents.

Dacarbazine is used to treat metastatic malignant melanoma.

Hydroxyurea is useful primarily for treating melanoma and other inoperable or resistant carcinomas.

Mitotane is indicated for treatment of inoperable adrenal cortical carcinoma (functional and nonfunctional).

Procarbazine hydrochloride and vinblastine sulfate are used primarily for palliative treatment of malignancies resistant to other therapies.

Vinblastine sulfate and vincristine sulfate, plant alkaloids, have been found useful in Hodgkin's disease, choriocarcinoma, testicular carcinoma, and occasionally breast tumors; vincristine sulfate, in combination with other antineoplastic agents, has been used to treat various sarcomas.

SPECIFIC PRODUCTS AND DOSAGES

The dosage of these drugs, as with many medications, should be individualized on the basis of the patient's response and the toxic effects. Consideration must be given to concomitant medications used by the patient for the malignancy or concurrent illnesses.

GENERIC NAME	TRADE NAME	ROUTE OF ADMIN.	USUAL DOSAGE ADULTS	CHILDREN
asparaginase	ELSPAR	iv im	200 IU/kg/day in 3 divided doses 6000 IU/M^2 every 3 days	——— ———
dacarbazine	DTIC-Dome	iv	2–4.5 mg/kg/day for 10 days; repeat at 4 wk intervals	———
hydroxyurea	HYDREA	po	80 mg/kg every 3rd day or 20–30 mg/kg/day	———

GENERIC NAME	TRADE NAME	ROUTE OF ADMIN.	USUAL DOSAGE ADULTS	CHILDREN
mitotane	LYSODREN	po	9–10 gm/day divided in 3–doses; max tolerated dose 2–16 gm/day	———
procarbazine HCl	MATULANE	iv	100–200 mg/day; then 300 mg/day until WBC is below 4000/cu mm	50 mg/day, then 100 mg/M^2
vinblastine sulfate	VELBAN	iv	0.1 mg/kg single dose, increase to max of 0.5 mg/kg q 7 days	———
vincristine sulfate	ONCOVIN	iv	0.5–2.0 mg/M^2 every 1–2 weeks	1.5 mg/M^2; do not exceed 3 mg/dose

Asparaginase

PHARMACOLOGY

Asparaginase depletes the exogenous amino acid L-asparagine on which malignant cells depend for growth and survival.

Plasma asparaginase levels are dose-dependent and show a cumulative effect. Asparaginase has been detected in thoracic and cervical lymph. Small to trace amounts have been found in cerebrospinal fluid and urine.

SPECIAL PRECAUTIONS

• Do not use in patients who have had anaphylactic reactions or in those with pancreatitis or a history of pancreatitis.
• Physician must be prepared to treat anaphylaxis with each administration.
• Safe use in pregnancy has not been established.

ADVERSE EFFECTS

CNS EFFECTS: depression, somnolence, fatigue, coma, confusion, agitation, hallucinations, parkinsonlike syndrome, headache, irritability
URINARY TRACT EFFECTS: azotemia, renal shutdown, renal insufficiency, proteinuria
GASTROINTESTINAL EFFECTS: nausea, vomiting, anorexia, abdominal cramps, weight loss, pancreatitis

HEPATIC EFFECTS: elevated SGOT, SOPT, alkaline phosphatase, bilirubin (direct and indirect); depressed serum albumin, cholesterol (total and esters), plasma fibrinogen
METABOLIC AND ENDOCRINE EFFECTS: peripheral edema, malabsorption syndrome, hyperglycemia, glycosuria, polyuria, fatal hypothermia
AUTONOMIC EFFECTS: chills, fever
HEMATOLOGIC EFFECTS: bleeding, hypofibrinogenimia, depression of other clotting factors, decrease in platelets, leukopenia, bone marrow depression
ALLERGIC EFFECTS: rash, urticaria, arthralgia, respiratory distress, acute anaphylaxis

CLINICAL GUIDELINES

ADMINISTRATION:
• Monitor peripheral blood count and bone marrow frequently.
• Frequent serum amylase determinations should be obtained to detect early evidence of pancreatitis. Stop therapy if this occurs.
• Monitor blood sugar during therapy; hyperglycemia may occur.
EFFECTS:
• Acute hemorrhagic pancreatitis, sometimes fatal, has occurred.
• Allergic reactions are frequent and usually occur early during therapy.
• Low leukocyte counts are noted fre-

quently within several days after initiating therapy.
• Serum uric acid may rise markedly.
• Toxicity is greater for adults than children.

DRUG INTERACTIONS:
• Concurrent administration with vincristine, and prednisone may be associated with increased toxicity.
• May diminish effects of methotrexate.
• May interfere with enzymatic detoxification of other drugs, particularly in the liver.

OVERDOSAGE/ANTIDOTE:
• Not established.

Dacarbazine
Hydroxyurea
Mitotane
Procarbazine HCl
Vinclastine Sulfate
Vincristine Sulfate

PHARMACOLOGY
Dacarbazine may inhibit DNA synthesis or may act as an alkylating agent or interact with SH groups; the exact mechanism of action is unknown.

The mechanism of cytotoxic activity of hydroxyurea is unclear. Hydroxyurea may cause an immediate inhibition of DNA synthesis without interfering with the synthesis of RNA or protein. After oral administration, hydroxyurea is readily absorbed and reaches peak serum concentrations in 2 hours. Excretion is by way of the urine.

The mechanism of action of mitotane is unknown.

Although the mode of antineoplastic activity of procarbazine hydrochloride is unclear, evidence indicates an inhibition of protein, RNA, and DNA synthesis. Cross resistance with other chemotherapeutic agents, radiotherapy, or steroids has not been demonstrated. Following oral administration, procarbazine hydrochloride is absorbed rapidly and is equilibrated rapidly between plasma and cerebrospinal fluid. The majority of the drug is excreted in the urine.

Tissue culture studies with vinblastine sulfate indicate an interference with the metabolic pathways of amino acids leading from glutamic acid to the citric acid cycle and to urea. The mechanism of action in humans remains to be clarified.

Although the precise mechanism of action of vincristine sulfate is unknown, it may arrest mitotic division at the stage of metaphase. Vincristine sulfate does not appear to pass the blood-brain barrier.

SPECIAL PRECAUTIONS
• Assure that patients have adequate bone marrow reserve prior to initiating therapy with procarbazine hydrochloride or hydroxyurea.
• Patients with known renal and/or hepatic dysfunction may experience undue toxicity with procarbazine hydrochloride, hydroxyurea or mitotane.
• Procarbazine hydrochloride inhibits amine oxidase activity; therefore, patients should avoid sympathomimetic drugs, tricyclic antidepressants, and other drugs and foods with high tyramine content.
• Patients receiving hydroxyurea who have received irradiation therapy may experience an exacerbation of postirradiation erythema.
• Hydroxyurea therapy may result in megaloblastic erythropoiesis, delayed plasma urea clearance, and reduced rate of iron utilization by erythrocytes.
• Do not administer vinblastine sulfate in leukopenic patients, or in older persons suffering from cachexia or ulcerated areas of the skin.
• Acute uric acid nephropathy had been reported with vincristine sulfate.
• Do not use in patients hypersensitive to these or related drugs.

- Safe use in pregnancy has not been established.
- Observe patients carefully for signs of infections, since patients treated with chemotherapeutic agents are particularly susceptible to infections.
- Hemopoietic depression may occur.
- If shock or severe trauma occurs, discontinue mitotane; adrenal insufficiency may occur.
- Long-term administration of mitotane may result in brain damage.

ADVERSE EFFECTS

CNS EFFECTS: chills, fever, weakness, fatigue, lethargy, drowsiness, paresthesias, headache, depression, insomnia, nervousness, hallucinations, ataxia, tremor, convulsions, disorientation

CARDIOVASCULAR EFFECTS: tachycardia, hypotension, hypertension with vincristine

URINARY TRACT EFFECTS: dysuria; elevated serum uric acid, BUN, and creatinine; polyuria

GASTROINTESTINAL EFFECTS: nausea, vomiting, anorexia, dysphagia, diarrhea, constipation, hematemesis, melena

HEPATIC EFFECTS: jaundice with procarbazine; abnormal BSP retention with hydroxyurea

HEMATOLOGIC EFFECTS: leukopenia, thrombocytopenia, anemia

DERMATOLOGIC EFFECTS: alopecia, rash, purpura, petechiae, dermatitis, herpes, hyperpigmentation, flushing

OPHTHALMIC EFFECTS: retinal hemorrhage, photophobia, photosensitivity, diplopia, papilledema, blurred vision

CLINICAL GUIDELINES

ADMINISTRATION:
- Caution patients to avoid concurrent use of procarbazine hydrochloride and sympathomimetic drugs, tricyclic antidepressants, and other drugs and foods with known high tyramine content.
- Baseline laboratory data (hematologic, renal, hepatic) should be available prior to therapy and obtained at appropriate intervals.
- Advise patients of possible adverse effects.
- With vinblastine sulfate and vincristine sulfate, avoid extravasation, which may result in local tissue necrosis, phlebitis, and sloughing.
- In all patients receiving vincristine sulfate, use routine prophylactic regimen against constipation.

EFFECTS:
- With procarbazine hydrochloride, bone marrow depression often occurs 2 to 3 weeks after initiating treatment.
- Terminate therapy with procarbazine hydrochloride if paresthesias, neuropathies, or confusion occurs.
- Occurrence of leukopenia, hypersensitivity reactions, stomatitis, and diarrhea may be cause for consideration to terminate therapy.
- With vincristine sulfate, constipation may take the form of upper colon impaction, which may respond to high enemas or laxatives.

DRUG INTERACTIONS:
- With procarbazine and hydroxyurea, CNS depression may be potentiated by the concurrent administration of barbiturates, antihistamines, narcotics, hypotensive agents, or phenothiazines.
- Ethyl alcohol should not be used in patients receiving procarbazine hydrochloride because of its ANTABUSE-like effect.

OVERDOSAGE/ANTIDOTE:
- Overdosage with any of these agents may be fatal.
- There is no specific antidote for any drug in this group. Treat supportively.

Drugs stimulating and suppressing immunity

18

INTRODUCTION

Immunity, the ability an individual acquires to prevent, resist, or overcome an infection, may be produced by a variety of substances commonly referred to as vaccines, toxoids/toxins, antisera, antitoxins, and antigens. Antisera are serums that contain antibody or antibodies. Antitoxins are substances in blood serum which are specific antagonists to some particular toxin. Antigens are substances which when introduced into the body tissues stimulate formation of antibodies. Antibodies are gamma globulins primarily produced in the reticuloendothelial system.

Active immunity is also produced by antigens which are available as antitoxins or toxoids/toxins. Other antigenic materials are vaccines which, when introduced into the body, produce active immunization by production of antibodies. Passive immunity differs from active immunity in that the antibodies are produced in another individual and simply administered to the patient to produce immunity.

Many products which produce or affect immunity are available commercially; many additional products, particularly antigens, are available as special orders from the manufacturer. Only products used relatively frequently and marketed regularly will be included herein.

The drugs which suppress the body's immunologic response have contributed to advances in organ transplantation technology and treatment of other disorders in which immunosuppressive action is useful, such as autoimmune hemolytic anemia, rheumatic diseases, and neoplasms.

SPECIFIC THERAPEUTIC CLASSIFICATION

The agents enhancing or stimulating immunity are grouped as follows: antigens, antisera, antitoxins, toxoids, and vaccines.

The drugs suppressing immunologic response can be divided into two groups: the adrenal steroids, specifically, the glucocorticoids, and the specific immunosuppressive agents.

Information about the adrenal steroids may be found in Chapter 15, page 533, and will not be repeated here. The specific immunosuppressive agents include azathioprine, which is used adjunctively for the prevention of rejection in renal homotransplantation, and $Rh_o(D)$ immune globulin (human), which prevents the postpartum formation of antibodies in $Rh_o(D)$ negative women.

Immunity Stimulating Agents

Antigens

SPECIFIC PRODUCTS AND DOSAGES

GENERIC NAME	TRADE NAME	ROUTE OF ADMIN.	USUAL DOSAGE
insect antigen, (stinging insects, others)	(G)*	sc	Individualize
poison ivy extract	(G) RHUS TOX Antigen	im	**Therapeutic:** 1 ml, 1–2 times/day **Prophylactic:** 1 ml every 4–7 days for 4 injections or more: use 0.25–0.5 ml in very sensitive persons

*(G) designates availability as a generic product.

(continued facing page)

GENERIC NAME	TRADE NAME	ROUTE OF ADMIN.	USUAL DOSAGE
poison ivy, oak, and sumac combined	RHUS-ALL Antigen	im	1 ml/week for 2–3 weeks prior to patient's exposure
ragweed and related pollens	(G)	im/sc	Individualize

Insect Antigen, Stinging and Others

GENERAL CLINICAL USES

Stinging insect antigen is used for hyposensitization against stinging insect reactions.

PHARMACOLOGY

Stinging insect antigen is a combination of antigens from bumble bee, honey bee, wasp, hornet, and yellow jacket. Other antigens are available from mosquito, fire ant, deer fly, inhalant factors, caddis fly, mayfly, moth household insects, and cockroach.

SPECIAL PRECAUTIONS

• Use with extreme caution in patients hypersensitive to stinging insects.
• Epinephrine (1:1000) should be immediately at hand when any vaccine is administered.

Poison Ivy Extract

GENERAL CLINICAL USES

Poison ivy extract is used for prophylaxis and treatment of Rhus dermatitis.

PHARMACOLOGY

Poison ivy extract consists of an extract of the solvent soluble irritating principles from the leaves of poison ivy. It is dissolved in sterile oil.

SPECIAL PRECAUTIONS

• Renal complications may follow extensive dermatitis of various types.
• May have aggravation of symptoms.
• Epinephrine (1:1000) should be immediately at hand when administering any vaccine.

ADVERSE EFFECTS

LOCAL EFFECTS: burning sensation, soreness, dull ache

Poison Ivy, Oak, and Sumac Combined Antigen

GENERAL CLINICAL USES

Poison ivy, oak, and sumac combined antigen is used for hyposensitization in Rhus dermatitis.

PHARMACOLOGY

The triple antigen consists of the active principles of poison ivy, oak, and sumac in an oil vehicle.

SPECIAL PRECAUTIONS

• Do not use for treatment of active Rhus dermatitis.

- Epinephrine (1:1000) should be immediately at hand when any vaccine is administered.

ADVERSE EFFECTS
LOCAL EFFECTS: burning sensation, soreness

Ragweed and Related Pollens

GENERAL CLINICAL USES
Ragweed and related pollens antigen is used for hyposensitization against these materials in patients with hypersensitivity.

PHARMACOLOGY
This antigen contains common ragweed and giant ragweed pollens (4 parts each), western ragweed, rough marsh elder, burweed march elder, and cocklebur pollens (1 part each).

SPECIAL PRECAUTIONS
- Use with extreme caution in patients hypersensitive to these pollens.
- Epinephrine (1:1000) should be immediately available when any vaccine is administered.

Antisera

SPECIFIC PRODUCTS AND DOSAGES

GENERIC NAME	TRADE NAME	ROUTE OF ADMIN.	USUAL DOSAGE
antihemophilic factor, human	HUMAFAC KOATE	iv	Individualize; 20–40 units/kg
Factor IX complex, human	KONYNE PROPLEX	iv	Individualize
immune serum globulin, human (gamma globulin)	GAMASTAN IMMU-G IMMUGLOBIN	im	2–10 ml **Treatment:** 0.02 ml/lb **Prophylaxis:** 0.1–0.14 ml/lb
mumps immune globulin, human	HYPAROTIN	im	**Prophylaxis in children:** 1.5 ml **Adults and children 12 yrs. and older:** 3–4.5 ml **Treatment:** 5 times the minimal prophylactic dose

(continued facing page)

GENERIC NAME	TRADE NAME	ROUTE OF ADMIN.	USUAL DOSAGE
pertussis immune globulin, human	HYPERTUSSIS	im	**Treatment:** 1.25 ml; repeat in 24–48 hr **Prophylaxis:** 1.25 ml; larger children: 2.5 ml; repeat in 1–2 wk
rabies immune globulin, human	HYPERAB	im	20 IU/kg; infiltrate wound with 1/2 dose, administer 1/2 im
$Rh_0(D)$ immune globulin human	(G)* RHOGAM GAMULIN RH	im	1 vial, 15 ml; larger amounts may be necessary
tetanus immune globulin, human	(G) HOMO-TET HYPER-TET IMMU-TETANUS	im	**Prophylaxis: adults:** 250 U; **children:** 4 U/kg **Treatment:** 3000–6000 U

*(G) designates availability as a generic product.

Antihemophilic Factor, Human

GENERAL CLINICAL USES

Antihemophilic factor, human, is used in the therapy of hemophilia A (classical hemophilia), a congenital deficiency characterized by a lifelong tendency to prolonged hemorrhage.

PHARMACOLOGY

Antihemophilic factor consisting of factor VIII, AHF, and AHG is a potent source of antihemophilic factor activity. It is prepared from venous plasma. It accelerates the abnormally slow clotting time in hemophiliacs due to Factor VIII deficiency.

SPECIAL PRECAUTIONS

• There are no known contraindications to use.
• Since antihemophilic factor is prepared from human plasma, the risk of transmitting hepatitis is present.

ADVERSE EFFECTS

SYSTEMIC EFFECTS: mild chill, nausea, hives, fever, backache infrequently
LOCAL EFFECTS: stinging in vein proximal to transfusion

Factor IX Complex

GENERAL CLINICAL USES

Factor IX complex is used to treat patients with deficiency of Factor IX, hemophilia B (Christmas disease).

PHARMACOLOGY

Factor IX complex contains Factors II, VII, IX, and X. It is prepared from pooled human plasma.

SPECIAL PRECAUTIONS

• Do not use in patients with active liver disease.
• Since this product is prepared from human plasma, the risk of transmitting hepatitis is present.

ADVERSE EFFECTS
SYSTEMIC EFFECTS: fever, mild chill, nausea, hives
LOCAL EFFECTS: stinging

Immune Serum Globulin, Human (Gamma Globulin)

GENERAL CLINICAL USES

Immune serum globulin is used for prevention or modification of measles (rubeola), modification of measles vaccination symptoms; prevention of German measles (rubella), chickenpox, infectious (epidemic) hepatitis (hepatitis A); deficiency of gamma globulin or of specific immunoglobulins (agammaglobulinemia, hypogammaglobulinemia, dysgammaglobulinemia).

PHARMACOLOGY

Antibodies, as in immune serum globulin, chiefly gamma globulin, are prepared from pooled normal human plasma. The plasma is collected from persons known to be hepatitis-free.

SPECIAL PRECAUTIONS
• Use with caution in patients with a history of prior systemic allergic reactions to immune serum globulin.
• Do not administer intravenously because of the potential for serious hypersensitivity reactions.
• Epinephrine should be available for possible systemic allergic reactions.

ADVERSE EFFECTS
SYSTEMIC EFFECTS: anaphylactic reactions rarely; other hypersensitivity reactions
LOCAL EFFECTS: pain, tenderness, erythema, muscle stiffness at site of injection, local inflammation

Mumps Immune Globulin, Human

GENERAL CLINICAL USES

Mumps immune globulin, human, is indicated for passive immunization of persons against mumps. Passive immunization is indicated for adult males exposed to mumps virus.

PHARMACOLOGY

Mumps immune globulin is prepared from venous blood of human subjects hyperimmunized with mumps vaccine.

SPECIAL PRECAUTIONS
• Use with caution in patients with a history of prior systemic allergic reactions following administration of gamma globulin preparations.

ADVERSE EFFECTS
SYSTEMIC EFFECTS: fever, malaise
LOCAL EFFECTS: tenderness, erythema

Pertussis Immune Globulin, Human

GENERAL CLINICAL USES

Pertussis immune globulin is indicated for passive immunization against pertussis (whopping cough).

PHARMACOLOGY

Pertussis immune globulin is prepared from venous blood of human subjects hyperimmunized with pertussis vaccine.

SPECIAL PRECAUTIONS
• Use with caution in patients with a history of systemic allergic reactions following administration of gamma globulin preparations.

ADVERSE EFFECTS
SYSTEMIC EFFECTS: fever, malaise
LOCAL EFFECTS: tenderness, erythema

Rabies Immune Globulin

GENERAL CLINICAL USES
Rabies immune globulin is indicated for passive immunization against the rabies virus.

PHARMACOLOGY
Rabies immune globulin is derived from pooled venous human blood from subjects exposed to rabies vaccine.

SPECIAL PRECAUTIONS
• Use with caution in patients with a history of prior systemic allergic reaction following administration of gamma globulin preparations.

ADVERSE EFFECTS
SYSTEMIC EFFECTS: fever, malaise
LOCAL EFFECTS: pain, erythema

Rh$_o$(D) Immune Globulin (Human)

GENERAL CLINICAL USES
Rh$_o$(D) immune globulin (human) is effective in preventing the postpartum formation of antibodies to the Rh$_o$(D) factor in the Rh$_o$(D) negative, D^u negative woman.

If an Rh$_o$(D) negative mother has a miscarriage, an abortion, or an ectopic pregnancy, she should be considered as a candidate for protective treatment with Rh$_o$(D) immune globulin.

After transfusion accidents such as when Rh positive blood has been transfused into an Rh$_o$(D) negative, D^u negative indi-

vidual, Rh$_o$(D) immune globulin can prevent Rh immunization in the recipient.

PHARMACOLOGY
Rh$_o$(D) immune globulin prevents the formation of active antibodies in the Rh$_o$(D) negative, D^u negative individual who has received Rh positive blood as a result of delivering an Rh$_o$(D) positive or D^u positive infant, or as a result of a transfusion accident. When the postpartum mother or the recipient of a transfusion accident receives an injection of passive Rh$_o$(D) immune globulin (antibody), the person's antibody response to the foreign Rh$_o$(D) positive cells is suppressed.

SPECIAL PRECAUTIONS
• Do not administer intravenously or in an infant.
• Reactions are infrequent, of a mild nature, and mostly confined to the area of injection.
• Do not administer to an Rh$_o$(D) positive or D^u positive individual.
• Do not administer to an Rh$_o$(D) negative patient who has inadvertently received an Rh$_o$(D) positive blood transfusion within 3 months of delivery.
• Do not administer to a patient previously immunized to the Rh$_o$(D) blood factor.
• Epinephrine (1:1000) should always be at hand in the event of a hypersensitivity reaction.

ADVERSE EFFECTS
HEMATOLOGIC EFFECTS: splenomegaly (1 subject)
ALLERGIC EFFECTS: fever, malaise, myalgia, lethargy

CLINICAL GUIDELINES

ADMINISTRATION:

- Should be administered within 72 hours of the birth of an $Rh_o(D)$ positive or D^u positive baby, of the spontaneous passage or surgical removal of the products of conception (that is, after miscarriage or abortion), or of transfusion accidents.
- Do not freeze.

Tetanus Immune Globulin (Human)

GENERAL CLINICAL USES

Tetanus immune globulin is indicated for immediate, passive immunization against tetanus. Passive immunization is indicated as an emergency measure in persons sustaining other than clean wounds when the immunization history is uncertain. This product may be useful in the treatment of tetanus in conjunction with standard medical procedures.

PHARMACOLOGY

Tetanus immune globulin is prepared from venous blood of human subjects hyperimmunized with tetanus toxoid. It neutralizes tetanus toxin.

SPECIAL PRECAUTIONS

- Never administer intravenously.
- Use caution in patients with a history of prior systemic allergic reactions following administration of gamma globulin preparations.

ADVERSE EFFECTS

SYSTEMIC EFFECTS: low-grade fever; sensitization very rarely; urticaria, angioedema; anaphylactoid reactions rarely.

LOCAL EFFECTS: tenderness, erythema, pain, muscle stiffness at site of injection, local inflammation

Antitoxins

SPECIFIC PRODUCTS AND DOSAGES

GENERIC NAME	TRADE NAME	ROUTE OF ADMIN.	USUAL DOSAGE
black widow spider antivenin	ANTIVENIN	im	2.5 ml; may repeat in 1–3 hr
botulism antitoxin, bivalent	(G)*	iv	**Adult:** 1 vial (10,000 units each Types A and B); may repeat

*(G) designates availability as a generic product.

(continued facing page)

GENERIC NAME	TRADE NAME	ROUTE OF ADMIN.	USUAL DOSAGE
diphtheria antitoxin	(G)	im iv	1,000–10,000 units 20,000–80,000 units
gas gangrene antitoxin	(G)	im/iv	20,000–50,000 units qid
North American coral snake antivenin	(G)	iv	30–50 ml by slow injection; repeat if necessary; may need 10 or more vials (10 ml each).
North and South American antisnakebite serum	(G)	sc/im iv	**Adult:** 1–5 containers 1–20 vials may be needed; administer by constant drip, 120 drops/min.; the smaller the patient, the larger the initial dose required. **Children:** 2 times adult dose
tetanus antitoxin	(G)	im/iv sc/im	**Treatment:** 50,000–100,000 units **Prophylaxis:** 1,500–5,000 units

Black Widow Spider Antivenin (Equine Origin)

GENERAL CLINICAL USES

Black widow spider antivenin is used to treat patients with symptoms due to bites by the black widow spider.

PHARMACOLOGY

Black widow spider antivenin is prepared from the serum of horses hyperimmunized against the venom of the black widow spider (*Latrodectus mactans*).

SPECIAL PRECAUTIONS

• Early use of the antivenin is emphasized for greatest effectiveness and prompt relief of symptoms.
• Patients with a history of hypersensitivity to horse serum should not be treated with this antivenin; test for hypersensitivity prior to administration.
• Observe patient for an average of 8 to 12 days following administration for serum sickness.
• Epinephrine (1:1000) must be available in case of untoward reactions.
• Use central nervous system depressants with caution since the venom is a neurotoxin that can cause respiratory arrest.

ADVERSE EFFECTS

SYSTEMIC EFFECTS: serum sickness (urticaria, fever, pruritus)

Botulism Antitoxin Bivalent (Equine Origin)

GENERAL CLINICAL USES

Botulism antitoxin, bivalent, Types A and B, is indicated in the treatment of all cases of toxemia in which the toxin is known or suspected to be produced by *Clostridium botulinum*, Types A or B, or in which the type is undetermined.

PHARMACOLOGY

Botulism antitoxin bivalent is produced from the plasma of hyperimmunized horses.

SPECIAL PRECAUTIONS

• Use with extreme caution in patients with a history of hypersensitivity or with asthma, angioneurotic edema, or other allergies.
• Do not use in patients who are hypersensitive to horse serum; test prior to use.
• Desensitize patient only if it is necessary to save life.
• Be aware that serum sickness may occur approximately 5 to 13 days after administration.

ADVERSE EFFECTS

SYSTEMIC EFFECTS: serum sickness (urticaria, fever, pruritus)

Diphtheria Antitoxin

GENERAL CLINICAL USES

Diphtheria antitoxin is used in the treatment of diphtheria or for prophylaxis of nonimmune individuals exposed to diphtheria.

PHARMACOLOGY

Diphtheria antitoxin is a concentrated antitoxin obtained from the blood of horses hyperimmunized against diphtheria toxin.

SPECIAL PRECAUTIONS

• Administer on basis of clinical impression; do not await bacteriologic confirmation.
• Use with extreme caution in patients with a history of asthma or allergy.
• Serum sickness may occur in 7 to 12 days after administration.

• Test for hypersensitivity to horse serum; if necessary to administer diphtheria antitoxin, consult manufacturer's instructions for desensitization.

ADVERSE EFFECTS

SYSTEMIC EFFECTS: serum sickness (urticaria, fever, pruritus, malaise, arthralgia)

Gas Gangrene Antitoxin, Polyvalent

GENERAL CLINICAL USES

Gas gangrene antitoxin, polyvalent, may be used prophylactically after injuries likely to be followed by gas gangrene or therapeutically for treatment of infections due to *Clostridium perfringens, C. septicum,* and *C. novyi.*

PHARMACOLOGY

Gas gangrene antitoxin, polyvalent, is derived from the serum of horses immunized against the toxins of *Clostridium perfringens, C. septicum,* and *C. novyi.*

SPECIAL PRECAUTIONS

Test for hypersensitivity to horse serum prior to use; if hypersensitivity results, consult manufacturer's directions for densitization before use.

ADVERSE EFFECTS

SYSTEMIC EFFECTS: serum sickness (urticaria, fever, pruritus)

North American Coral Snake Antivenin (Equine Origin)

GENERAL CLINICAL USES

North American coral snake antivenin is used in patients bitten by the North American coral snake.

PHARMACOLOGY

North American coral snake antivenin is a lyophilized preparation of serum globulins from horses immunized with the venom of eastern coral snakes (*Micruras fulvius*). This antivenin will also neutralize the venom of coral snakes found in eastern North Carolina through Florida and in the area west of the Mississippi River. It cannot neutralize the venom of *Micruroides euryxanthus* (Arizona or Sonoran coral snakes) found in Arizona and New Mexico.

SPECIAL PRECAUTIONS

• Test patient for hypersensitivity to horse serum before use; if results are positive, it may be dangerous to proceed with administration; risks must be considered and weighed before administration.
• Administer immediately for best results.

ADVERSE EFFECTS

SYSTEMIC EFFECTS: *Immediate effects* (usually occur within 30 minutes)—shock, anaphylaxis including apprehension, itching, urticaria; edema of face, throat, and tongue; dyspnea, cyanosis, vomiting, collapse. *Delayed effects*—serum sickness including malaise, fever, lymphadenopathy, arthralgia, urticaria, meningismus or peripheral neuritis
LOCAL EFFECTS: local delayed serum reaction including edema and erythema with itching; Arthus phenomenon including local necrosis of varying severity even to gangrene with complete slough

North and South American Antisnakebite Serum

GENERAL CLINICAL USES

North and South American antisnakebite serum (crotaline antivenin, polyvalent), is useful against the venoms of all 17 species of Crotalidae in North and South America. It is effective against North American rattlesnakes, water moccasins, and copperheads; it is of no value against vipers (e.g., puff, adder, cobra, mamba), other noncrotalid snakes (e.g., American coral snakes), or any venomous spiders or scorpions.

PHARMACOLOGY

This polyvalent crotaline antivenin is a suspension of antibodies prepared from the serum of horses immunized against the venoms of the pit vipers (*Crotalus adamanteus, C. atrox, C. durissus,* and *Bothrops atrox*).

SPECIAL PRECAUTIONS

• Test for hypersensitivity to horse serum before administration; if positive, weigh risk before administration.
• Type patient's blood as early as possible; homolysins present in the venom soon alter the blood protein structure, preventing accurate cross matching.
• Administration at or around the site of the bite is not recommended.

ADVERSE EFFECTS

SYSTEMIC EFFECTS: *Immediate reaction*—shock, anaphylaxis, hypersensitivity reactions including apprehension, itching, urticaria; edema of face, tongue, and throat; cough, dyspnea, cyanosis, vomiting, and collapse. *Serum sickness* (occurs in 6 to 24 hours)—symptoms include malaise, fever, lymphadenopathy, arthralgia, and urticaria; occasionally meningismus or peripheral neuritis. *Accelerated serum reactions*—similar to but more rapid than serum sickness
LOCAL EFFECTS: local delayed serum reaction manifested by progressive edema and erythema with itching; Arthus phenomenon manifested by local necrosis of varying severity, even to gangrene with complete slough

Tetanus Antitoxin, Equine

GENERAL CLINICAL USES

Tetanus antitoxin is used prophylactically in nonimmunized patients with wounds suspected of tetanus contamination; it is also useful in treating patients with active tetanus.

PHARMACOLOGY

Tetanus antitoxin, a solution of antibodies, is derived from the serum of horses hyperimmunized with tetanus toxin or toxoid.

SPECIAL PRECAUTIONS

• Test for hypersensitivity to horse serum before use; if patient is hypersensitive, desensitize him according to manufacturer's directions.

ADVERSE EFFECTS

SYSTEMIC EFFECTS: serum sickness (arthralgia, urticaria, fever, malaise) anaphylactoid shock

LOCAL EFFECTS: pain

Toxoids

SPECIFIC PRODUCTS AND DOSAGES

GENERIC NAME	TRADE NAME	ROUTE OF ADMIN.	USUAL DOSAGE
diphtheria toxoid, adsorbed	(G)*	im	0.5–1 ml, 2 doses 4–6 weeks apart; reinforcing dose of 0.5 ml 1 yr. later
diphtheria toxoid, fluid	(G)	im	0.5–1 ml, 3 doses
diphtheria and tetanus toxoids, adsorbed	(G)	im	0.5 ml, 2 doses 4–8 weeks apart; 3rd dose (0.5 ml) 6–12 months later
diphtheria and tetanus toxoids, plain	(G)	im	0.5 ml, 3 doses, 4–6 weeks apart
diphtheria, tetanus toxoids, and pertussis vaccine	(G) TRIOGEN	im	**Children:** 0.5 ml, 3 doses 4–8 weeks apart; 4th dose 1 yr. later **Adults:** 0.5 ml, 2 doses 4–8 weeks apart; 3rd dose 6–12 months later

*(G) designates availability as a generic product.

(continued facing page)

GENERIC NAME	TRADE NAME	ROUTE OF ADMIN.	USUAL DOSAGE
tetanus toxoid, adsorbed	(G)	im/sc	0.5 ml, 2 doses 4–8 weeks apart; 3rd dose 6–12 months later
tetanus toxoid, fluid	(G)	im/sc	0.5 ml, 3 doses 3–4 weeks apart; 4th dose 6–12 months later

Diphtheria Toxoid, Adsorbed and Fluid

GENERAL CLINICAL USES

Diphtheria toxoid is used for primary immunization of infants and young children. It may be given alone, but is frequently given in combination with tetanus toxoid and pertussis vaccine.

PHARMACOLOGY

Diphtheria toxoid is a preparation of detoxified growth products of *Corynebacterium diphtheriae*. It is available as either a fluid toxoid or an adsorbed toxoid.

SPECIAL PRECAUTIONS

• Use with caution in patients with a history of allergy, asthma, or allergic reactions.
• Do not use in treatment of actual diphtheria infections.
• Epinephrine (1:1000) and other emergency drugs and equipment should be readily available to combat severe systemic reactions if they develop.

ADVERSE EFFECTS

SYSTEMIC EFFECTS: fever, malaise, myalgia rarely, flushing, generalized urticaria, pruritus, tachycardia, hypotension
LOCAL EFFECTS: tenderness, sterile abscess, redness

CLINICAL GUIDELINES

ADMINISTRATION:
• If local or systemic reactions occur after injection, dosage reduction should be considered for subsequent injections.
EFFECTS:
• To maintain immunity, a routine booster dose of 0.5 ml usually should be given at 5- to 10-year intervals.
DRUG INTERACTIONS:
• Patients receiving therapy with corticosteroids or other immunosuppressive agents, such as antimetabolites, irradiation, or alkylating agents, may not respond optimally to active immunization procedures.

Diphtheria and Tetanus Toxoids, Adsorbed and Plain

GENERAL CLINICAL USES

Diphtheria and tetanus toxoids are indicated to induce a rapid and sustained immune response to *Corynebacterium diphtheriae* and *Clostridium tetani*. Two preparations are available for use: (1) in children up to 6 years of age and (2) in children over 6 years and adults.

PHARMACOLOGY

The product containing diphtheria and tetanus toxoids is a mixture of fluid toxoids produced in semisynthetic culture media, inactiviated with formalin, and purified by ultrafiltration. Aluminum phosphate is used as the mineral carrier of the antigens, which provide effective prophylaxis against both diseases.

SPECIAL PRECAUTIONS
• Defer immunization in the presence of active infection or acute respiratory tract disease.
• Elective immunization with adjuvant-containing antigens should be postponed during an outbreak of poliomyelitis. When possible exposure to tetanus infection or diphtheria occurs simultaneously with a poliomyelitis outbreak, use of the fluid form of the single antigen is recommended.
• A history of CNS damage or convulsions is an indication to postpone primary immunization until the second year of life; use of the single antigen is preferred.

ADVERSE EFFECTS
SYSTEMIC EFFECTS: fever, malaise, and myalgia
LOCAL EFFECTS: stinging sensation, tenderness, pain, induration, nodule formation, redness

CLINICAL GUIDELINES
ADMINISTRATION:
• Only well children or adults should be immunized.
EFFECTS:
• Prolonging the interval between primary immunization doses for as long as 6 months does not interfere with the final immunity.
• Occurrence of fever or other unusual local or systemic reactions following an injection indicates that dosage reduction may be desirable for subsequent injections.
DRUG INTERACTIONS:
• Individuals receiving therapy with corticosteroids or other immunosuppressive agents (antimetabolites, irradiation, alkylating agents) may not respond optimally to active immunization procedures; defer immunization.

Diphtheria, and Tetanus Toxoids and Pertussis Vaccine

GENERAL CLINICAL USES
Pertussis vaccine and diphtheria and tetanus toxoids, in combination, are used for immunization of infants and children against diphtheria, tetanus, and whooping cough. By using a combination product, the number of injections is reduced without impairing the resultant immunity. Primary immunization may start as early as 2 months of age.

PHARMACOLOGY
Diphtheria and tetanus toxoids and pertussis vaccine adsorbed contain toxoids of *Corynebacterium diphtheria* and *Clostridium tetani* and pertussis vaccine adsorbed on aluminum potassium phosphate. Pertussis vaccine is prepared from *Bordetella pertussis.*

SPECIAL PRECAUTIONS
• Not recommended for immunization of persons over 6 years of age.
• Inoculation should be postponed in the presence of acute infection.
• If there is an outbreak of poliomyelitis in the community, injection of depot antigens should be delayed unless the risk of waiting outweighs the slightly increased danger of poliomyelitis.
• In older individuals, hypersensitivity reactions to the proteins of diphtheria and pertussis organisms are more frequent and severe than in younger individuals.
• Immunization of infants with cerebral

damage should be delayed until after 1 year of age, and the single antigens in fractional doses should be employed.

• If a convulsion, thrombocytopenia, or other severe reaction occurs after injection, no further injections of pertussis vaccine should be given, complete immunization with single antigens or toxoids.

ADVERSE EFFECTS

SYSTEMIC EFFECTS: convulsions, encephalitis rarely; fever, restlessness, malaise infrequently; encephalopathic symptoms which may be fatal or result in permanent neurological sequelae.

CLINICAL GUIDELINES

ADMINISTRATION:
• Epinephrine (1:1000) and other emergency drugs and equipment should be readily available to combat severe systemic reactions if they develop.

EFFECTS:
• Corticosteroids should not be administered following exposure to infectious agents (mumps, rabies, tetanus) for which no satisfactory antimicrobial therapy is available.
• Individuals receiving therapy with cortiosteroids or other immunosuppressive agents (antimetabolites, irradiation, alkylating agents) may not respond optimally to active immunization procedures; defer immunization.

Tetanus Toxoid, Adsorbed and Fluid

GENERAL CLINICAL USES

Tetanus toxoid is indicated for primary immunization of adults and children in whom the combination product (diphtheria toxoid, tetanus toxoid, pertussis vaccine) is contraindicated; also, for active immunization against tetanus.

PHARMACOLOGY

Tetanus toxoid is prepared by modifying tetanus toxin produced by growing *Clostridium tetani* on semisynthetic media. The toxoid is adsorbed on aluminum phosphate or refined to produce the fluid. Adsorption on aluminum phosphate prolongs and enhances the antigenic properties by retarding the rate of asorption.

SPECIAL PRECAUTIONS

• Only well individuals should be injected.
• Use with caution in patients with a history of allergic reactions, allergy, or asthma.
• Defer use in patients with acute respiratory infections or other active infections.
• Elective immunization with adjuvant containing antigens should be deferred during an outbreak of poliomyelitis.
• When possible exposure to tetanus infections occurs simultaneously with an outbreak of poliomyelities, use of tetanus toxoid, fluid, is recommended.
• Do not use in patients receiving immunosuppressive therapy (drugs or radiation) or in patients with hypogammaglobulinemia or agammaglobulinemia.
• Epinephrine (1:1000) and other emergency drugs and equipment should be readily available to combat severe systemic reactions if they develop.

ADVERSE EFFECTS

SYSTEMIC EFFECTS: fever, malaise, pains, flushing rarely; incidence greater in those over 25 years of age; axillary lymphadenopathy generalized urticaria or pruritus, hypotension, tachycardia

LOCAL EFFECTS: erythema, pain, boggy edema, induration, tenderness, nodule formation at site of subcutaneous injection; usually disappears in a few weeks.

CLINICAL GUIDELINES

ADMINISTRATION:

• If local or systemic reactions occur after injection, dosage reduction should be considered for subsequent injections.

• Any dose of tetanus toxoid received, even a decade earlier, should be counted as an immunizing injection.

• Take precautions to avoid transmission of homologous serum hepatitis and other infectious agents from one person to another.

EFFECTS:

• Severe systemic reactions are very rare.

• A routine recall (booster) dose should be given at 10-year intervals throughout life to maintain immunity.

DRUG INTERACTIONS:

• Individuals receiving therapy with corticosteroids or other immunosuppressive agents (antimetabolites, irradiation, alkylating agents) may not respond optimally to active immunization procedures.

Vaccines

SPECIFIC PRODUCTS AND DOSAGES

GENERIC NAME	TRADE NAME	ROUTE OF ADMIN.	USUAL DOSAGE	
			ADULTS	CHILDREN
cholera vaccine	(G)†	im/sc	0.5 ml, then 1 ml; booster 0.5 ml	**5–10 yrs.:** 0.3 ml, then 0.5 ml; booster 0.3 ml **Under 5 yrs.:** 0.1 ml, then 0.3 ml; booster 0.1 ml
influenza virus vaccine	(G) FLUOGEN	im	Consult with manufacturer	
measles virus vaccine, live, attenuated	ATTENUVAX M-VAC	sc.	0.5 ml (1 container)	0.5 ml (1 container)
measles, mumps, and rubella virus vaccine	M-M-R-II	sc	1 container	1 container
measles and rubella vaccine, live	M-R-VAX II	sc	1 container	1 container
mumps virus vaccine	MUMPSVAX	sc	1 container	———
pertussis vaccine	TRIOGEN*	sc	———	**2 months–6 yrs.:** 0.25–0.5 ml, 4 doses

*Contains more than one active ingredient.
†(G) designates availability as a generic product.

(continued facing page)

GENERIC NAME	TRADE NAME	ROUTE OF ADMIN.	USUAL DOSAGE	
			ADULTS	**CHILDREN**
plague vaccine	(G)	im	**Adults and children over 10 yrs.:** 0.5–1.0 ml for 2 doses; 3 months later, 0.2 ml	**Under 1 yr.:** 1/5 adult dose **1–4 yrs.:** 2/5 adult dose **5–10 yrs.:** 3/5 adult dose
pneumococcal vaccine, polyvalent	PNEUMOVAX	sc/im	0.5 ml	Not established
poliovirus vaccine live, oral, trivalent	(G) DIPLOVAX ORIMUNE	po	——	**Infants:** 0.5 ml, 3 doses **Children and adolescents:** 0.5 ml, 3 doses
rabies vaccine, dried killed virus	(G)	sc	**Immunization:** 1 ml daily for 14 days **Preimmunization exposure:** 1 ml, 3 times 1 week apart; 4th dose after 7 months	Same as adults
Rocky Mountain spotted fever vaccine	(G)	sc	1 ml every 7 days for 3 doses	**Under 12 yrs.:** 0.5 ml every 7 days for 3 doses
rubella virus vaccine, live	CENDEVAX MERUVAX II RUBELOGEN	sc	1 container	1 container
rubella and mumps virus vaccine	BIAVAX-II	sc	1 container	1 container
smallpox vaccine	(G)	intradermal	1 capillary tube	1 capillary tube
smallpox vaccine, dried	DRYVAX	intradermal	1 capillary tube	1 capillary tube
tuberculosis vaccine (BCG)	(G)	intradermal	0.1 ml	**Newborn infants:** 0.05 ml
typhoid vaccine	(G)	sc	**Adults and children over 10 yrs.:** 0.5 ml, 2 doses, 4 weeks apart	**Under 10 yrs.:** 0.25 ml, 2 doses, 4 weeks apart
typhus vaccine	(G)	sc	2 injections of 0.5 ml 4 weeks apart	**Under 10 yrs:** 2 injections of 0.25 ml 4 weeks apart
yellow fever vaccine	(G)	sc	0.5 ml	0.5 ml

Cholera Vaccine

GENERAL CLINICAL USES

Cholera vaccine is used to immunize persons against cholera who must travel into endemic areas; it should not be given to contacts or used for controlling the spread of infection.

PHARMACOLOGY

Cholera vaccine is a sterile suspension of killed cholera organisms (*vibrio cholerae*, Inaba and Ogawa types). The vibrios are washed off the medium, suspended in buffered sodium chloride injection, and killed with phenol, 0.5%.

SPECIAL PRECAUTIONS

• Do not vaccinate individuals who have had a serious reaction to previous injections.
• Postpone immunization in the presence of an acute infection.
• Epinephrine (1:1000) should be available for immediate use when this vaccine is injected.

ADVERSE EFFECTS

SYSTEMIC EFFECTS: malaise, fever, headache
LOCAL EFFECTS: induration, erythema, swelling, tenderness

Influenza Virus Vaccine

GENERAL CLINICAL USES

Influenza virus vaccine, is indicated for immunization of persons 18 years of age and older with chronic health problems. It is also recommended for older persons, particularly those over age 65 yr. High-risk persons 3 to 18 years of age should also be immunized. Persons 18 through 64 years of age and 6 months to 36 months may also be immunized. Pregnant women may be immunized.

PHARMACOLOGY

Influenza virus vaccine contains influenza virus prepared from the allantoic fluids of chick embryos. The innoculation of these antigens stimulates the production of specific antibodies. Antibiotics are not used in the manufacturing process. Each season the vaccine formulation is established by the Bureau of Biologies of the Food and Drug Administration.

SPECIAL PRECAUTIONS

• Do not administer routinely to persons with a history of hypersenistivity to chicken egg. Skin test persons known to be hypersensitive to egg protein before vaccination; persons with adverse reactions should not be vaccinated.
• This vaccine is not effective against all possible strains of influenza virus.
• Any febrile respiratory illness or other active infection is reason for delaying use of influenza virus vaccine, except when, in the opinion of the physician, withholding the agent entails even greater risk.
• Epinephrine (1:1000) must be immediately available should an acute anaphylactoid reaction occur due to any component of the vaccine.

ADVERSE EFFECTS

SYSTEMIC EFFECTS: fever, malaise, myalgia, encephalopathy, hypersensitivity reactions to egg protein.
LOCAL EFFECTS: stinging, aching, redness, tenderness, flare, wheal

CLINICAL GUIDELINES

ADMINISTRATION:
• Potency of this vaccine is destroyed by freezing; do not use if frozen.
• Do not inject intravenously.

EFFECTS:
• Influenza virus is remarkably capricious antigenically; significant changes may occur from time to time. Confirm that this antigen is the proper one to use.

DRUG INTERACTIONS:
• Persons receiving corticosteroids or other immunosuppressive therapy may not obtain the expected antigenic response.

Measles Virus Vaccine, Live Attenuated

GENERAL CLINICAL USES

Measles virus vaccine, live attenuated, is recommended for active immunization of children 1 year of age or older against measles (rubeola). It does not protect when given after exposure to natural measles.

PHARMACOLOGY

Measles virus vaccine, live attenuated, is prepared from an attenuated strain of measles virus grown in cell cultures of chick embryo and lyophilized. It is highly immunogenic and produces a modified measles infection in susceptible persons.

SPECIAL PRECAUTIONS

• Do not use in persons hypersensitive to egg, chicken, chicken feathers, or neomycin; some vaccines contain neomycin as a bactericidal agent.
• Do not use in persons with any febrile respiratory illness, other active febrile infection or active untreated tuberculosis.
• Do not use in patients receiving therapy with ACTH, corticosteroids, irradiation, alkylating agents or antimetabolites. This does not apply to patients who are receiving corticosteroids as replacement therapy (Addison's disease), or those with blood dyscrasias, leukemia, lymphomas of any type, or other malignant neoplasms affecting the bone marrow or lymphatic systems.
• Do not use in patients with gamma globulin deficiency (agammaglobulinemia, hypogammaglobulinemia, and dysgammaglobulinemia).
• Do not give to pregnant women; the possible effects on the fetus are not known.
• If vaccinating postpubertal women, rule out pregnancy and advise patient to prevent pregnancy for 3 months.
• Do not administer less than 1 month before or after immunization with other live virus vaccines with the exception of monovalent or trivalent poliovirus vaccine, live, oral, which may be administered simultaneously.
• Use with caution in vaccinating children with a history of febrile convulsions, cerebral injury, or any other condition in which stress due to fever should be avoided.
• Vaccination should be deferred for at least 3 months following blood or plasma transfusion, or administration of human immune serum globulin, more than 0.02 ml per pound of body weight.

ADVERSE EFFECTS

SYSTEMIC EFFECTS: fever, febrile convulsions, encephalitis, thrombocytopenia, purpura rarely; rash
LOCAL EFFECTS: marked swelling, redness, vesiculation

CLINICAL GUIDELINES

ADMINISTRATION:
• Do not administer intravenously.
• Epinephrine (1:1000) should be available for immediate use should an anaphylactoid reaction occur.

EFFECTS:
• Watch patient for temperature elevation, which may occur after vaccination.

DRUG INTERACTIONS:
• Attenuated measles vaccine, live, may result in a temporary depression of tuberculin skin sensitivity; if tuberculin test is to be done, it should be administered either before or simultaneously with the measles virus vaccine.

Measles and Rubella Virus Vaccine, Live

GENERAL CLINICAL USES
Measles and rubella virus vaccine is indicated for simultaneous immunization against measles (rubeola) and rubella in children from 1 year of age to puberty.

PHARMACOLOGY
Measles and rubella virus vaccine, live, is derived from an attenuated strain of measles virus grown in cell cultures of chick embryo free from avian leukosis, and from an attenuated strain of rubella virus propagated in duck embryo cell culture. The two viruses are mixed, then lyophilized.

SPECIAL PRECAUTIONS
• Do not administer to pregnant women; the effect on the fetus is not known.
• If it is necessary to vaccinate post-pubertal women, pregnancy must be ruled out at the time of vaccination and prevented during the following 3 months.
• Do not use in patients sensitive to chicken or duck, including eggs and feathers, or to neomycin.
• Do not use in patients with any febrile respiratory illness, active febrile infection, or active untreated tuberculosis.
• Do not vaccinate patients receiving therapy with ACTH, corticosteroids, irradiation, alkylating agents or antimetabolites.

This does not apply to patients who are receiving corticosteroids for replacement therapy (for Addison's disease), individuals with blood dyscrasias, leukemia, lymphomas of any type, or other malignant neoplasms affecting the bone marrow or lymphatic system.
• Do not use in patients with gamma globulin deficiency (agammaglobulinemia, hypogammaglobulinemia, dysgammaglobulinemia).
• Do not administer less than 1 month before or after immunization with other live virus vaccines, with the exception of monovalent or trivalent poliovirus vaccine, live, oral, which may be administered simultaneously.
• Administer with caution to children with a history of febrile convulsions, cerebral injury, or any other condition in which stress due to fever should be avoided.
• Defer vaccination for at least 3 months following blood or plasma transfusion, or administration of human immune serum globulin, more than 0.02 ml per pound body weight.

ADVERSE EFFECTS
SYSTEMIC EFFECTS: fever, febrile convulsions rarely; encephalitis; thrombocytopenia, prupura, urticaria, rash, arthritis, arthralgia, polyneuritis, regional lymphadenopathy
LOCAL EFFECTS: erythema, induration, tenderness, swelling, vesiculation

CLINICAL GUIDELINES
ADMINISTRATION:
• Do not administer intravenously.
• Epinephrine (1:1000) should be available for immediate use in case an anaphylactoid reaction occurs.
EFFECTS:
• Temperature elevation may occur 5 to 12 days after vaccination.

- There are no reports of the transmission of live attenuated measles virus from vaccines to susceptible contacts.

DRUG INTERACTIONS:

- Vaccination with attenuated measles and rubella virus vaccine, live, may result in a temporary depression of tuberculin skin sensitivity; if a tuberculin test is to be done, it should be administered either before or simultaneously with this vaccine.

Measles, Mumps, and Rubella Virus Vaccine, Live

GENERAL CLINICAL USES

Measles, mumps, and rubella virus vaccine, live, is indicated for simultaneous immunization against measles, mumps, and rubella in children from 1 year of age to puberty.

PHARMACOLOGY

Measles, mumps, and rubella virus vaccine, live, is prepared from an attenuated measles virus and a strain of mumps virus, both grown in cell cultures of chick embryos free of avian leukosis; and an attenuated strain of rubella virus propagated in duck embryo cell cultures. The three viruses are mixed, then lyophilized.

SPECIAL PRECAUTIONS

- Do not give to pregnant women; possible effects in the fetus have not been established.
- If it is necessary to vaccinate postpubertal women, pregnancy must be ruled out at the time of vaccination and prevented during the following 3 months.
- Do not use in patients sensitive to chicken or duck, including eggs and feathers or to neomycin.
- Do not use in patients with any febrile respiratory illness, other active febrile infection, or active untreated tuberculosis.
- Do not use in patients receiving therapy with ACTH, corticosteroids, irradiation, alkylating agents, or antimetabolites. This does not apply to patients who are receiving corticosteroids as replacement therapy (Addison's disease), those with blood dyscrasias, leukemia, lymphomas of any type, or other malignant neoplasms affecting the bone marrow or lymphatic system.
- Do not use in patients with gamma globulin deficiency (agammaglobulinemia, hypogammaglobulinemia, and dysgammaglobulinemia).
- Do not give less than 1 month before or after immunization with other live virus vaccines, with the exception of monovalent or trivalent poliovirus vaccine, live, oral, which may be administered simultaneously.
- Use caution when administering to children with a history of febrile convulsions, cerebral injury, or any other condition in which stress due to fever should be avoided.
- Defer vaccination for at least 3 months following blood or plasma transfusions, or administration of human immune serum globulin, more than 0.02 ml per pound body weight.

ADVERSE EFFECTS

SYSTEMIC EFFECTS: fever; febrile convulsions rarely; encephalitis, parotitis, thrombocytopenia, purpura, urticaria, rash, arthritis, arthralgia, polyneuritis, regional lymphadenopathy

LOCAL EFFECTS: erythema, induration, tenderness, vesiculation, swelling

CLINICAL GUIDELINES

ADMINISTRATION:

- Do not give intravenously.

- Epinephrine should be available for immediate use in case an anaphylactoid reaction occurs.

EFFECTS:
- Temperature elevation may occur 5 to 12 days after vaccination.
- There are no reports of transmission of live attenuated measles or mumps virus from vaccine to susceptible contacts.

DRUG INTERACTIONS:
- Attenuated measles, mumps, and rubella virus vaccine, live, given individually, may result in a temporary depression of tuberculin skin sensitivity. If a tuberculin test is to be done, it should be administered either before or simultaneously with this vaccine.

Mumps Virus Vaccine, Live

GENERAL CLINICAL USES
Mumps virus vaccine, live, provides protection against natural mumps in most cases. It is indicated for immunization against mumps in children over 1 year of age and adults.

PHARMACOLOGY
Mumps virus vaccine, live, is prepared from Jeryl Lynn (B Level) strain grown in cell cultures of chick embryos free of avian leukosis.

SPECIAL PRECAUTIONS
- Do not give to pregnant women; effects on the fetus are not established.
- When vaccinating postpubortal women, rule out pregnancy and advise patient to prevent pregnancy for 3 months after vaccination.
- Do not use in patients sensitive to eggs, chicken, chicken feathers, or neomycin.
- Do not use in patients with blood dyscrasias, leukemia, lymphomas of any type,

or other malignant neoplasms affecting the bone marrow or lymphatic system.
- Do not use in patients receiving therapy with ACTH, corticosteroids, irradiation, alkylating agents, or antimetabolites. This does not apply to patients receiving corticosteroids as replacement therapy (Addison's disease), or those with gamma globulin deficiency (agammaglobulinemia, hypogammaglobulinemia, and dysgammaglobulinemia).
- Do not use in patients with any active infection.
- Do not give less than 1 month before or after immunization with other live virus vaccines, with the exception of monovalent or trivalent poliovirus vaccine, live, oral, which may be administered simultaneously.
- Defer vaccination for at least 3 months following blood or plasma transfusion, or administration of human immune serum globulin, more than 0.02 ml per pound body weight.

ADVERSE EFFECTS
SYSTEMIC EFFECTS: mild fever; encephalitis, parotitis, purpura, urticaria very rarely

CLINICAL GUIDELINES
ADMINISTRATION:
- Do not administer intravenously.
DRUG INTERACTIONS:
- May depress temporarily tuberculin skin sensitivity; if a tuberculin test is to be done, it should be administered either before or simultaneously with this vaccine.

Pertussis Vaccine

GENERAL CLINICAL USES
Pertussis vaccine is used for primary immunization of infants when the combination product (diphtheria toxoid, tetanus toxoid, pertussis vaccine) is contraindicated. The combination product may be contra-

indicated in patients who have experienced an adverse reaction, especially infants with neurological disorders.

PHARMACOLOGY

Pertussis vaccine is an unwashed suspension of killed *Bordetella pertussis* organisms suspended in sodium chloride with 1:10,000 thimerosal.

SPECIAL PRECAUTIONS

• Do not vaccinate patients who are acutely ill or suspected of having respiratory tract, skin, or other infections or those with agammaglobulinemia.
• Do not immunize if poliomyelitis is present in the community.

ADVERSE EFFECTS

SYSTEMIC EFFECTS: fever, malaise, restlessness, myalgia; severe CNS reactions rarely
LOCAL EFFECTS: sterile abscess rarely; redness, induration, tenderness, nodule formation

Plague Vaccine

GENERAL CLINICAL USES

Plague vaccine is generally used only in persons traveling to Vietnam, Cambodia, or Laos or those whose work brings them into contact with animals carrying *Yersinia pestis.*

PHARMACOLOGY

Plague vaccine is prepared from *Yersinia pestis* grown on artificial media. It is killed with formaldehyde and preserved with phenol.

SPECIAL PRECAUTIONS

• Do not administer in presence of active illness.

ADVERSE EFFECTS

SYSTEMIC EFFECTS: myalgia, fever, malaise, headache, mild lymphadenopathy
LOCAL EFFECTS: pain, erythema, induration

Pneumococcal Vaccine Polyvalent

GENERAL CLINICAL USES

Pneumococcal vaccine, polyvalent, is indicated for immunization against lobar pneumonia and bacteremia caused by those types of pneumococci included in the vaccine.

PHARMACOLOGY

Pneumococcal vaccine, polyvalent, consists of polysaccharide isolates derived from pneumococci capsules. The vaccine protects against the 14 most prevalent capsular types of pneumococci.

SPECIAL PRECAUTIONS

• Do not use in patients hypersensitive to these materials.
• Safe use in pregnancy and in children under 2 years has not been established.
• Delay immunization in persons with any febrile respiratory illness or other active infection.

ADVERSE EFFECTS

LOCAL EFFECTS: erythema, soreness, local induration
SYSTEMIC EFFECTS: low grade fever

CLINICAL GUIDELINES

ADMINISTRATION:
• Administer im or sc, preferably in the deltoid muscle or lateral midthigh.
• Avoid intravascular administration.
EFFECTS:
• Revaccination should not be considered at less than 3-year intervals. Protective

antibodies persist for substantial periods of time in most persons.

Poliovirus Vaccine, Live Oral, Trivalent

GENERAL CLINICAL USES

Poliovirus vaccine, live, oral, trivalent, is indicated for use in the prevention of poliomyelitis caused by poliovirus types 1, 2, and 3. The candidates for routine prophylaxis are infants starting at 3 to 12 weeks of age, all children, and adolescents through the level of high school. It is also recommended for adults, primarily those who are not immune and are subject to increased risk of exposure, as by travel to or contact with epidemic or endemic areas; also those employed in hospitals, medical laboratories, clinics and sanitation facilities, and those in other special situations where in the judgment of the physician responsible, protection may be needed.

PHARMACOLOGY

Poliovirus vaccine, live, oral, trivalent, is a mixture of attenuated polioviruses which have been propagated in monkey kidney tissue culture (ORIMUNE Poliovirus Vaccine) or in human diploid cells (DIPLOVAX Poliovirus Vaccine). Administration of this vaccine stimulates the body to produce an active immunity by stimulating the natural infection without producing untoward symptoms of the disease. Antibodies to poliovirus types 1, 2, and 3 are produced.

SPECIAL PRECAUTIONS

• Do not administer to patients with altered immune states such as lymphomas, leukemias, and generalized malignancies; also patients receiving therapy with corticosteroids, antimetabolites, antineoplastic drugs, and irradiation.
• Do not administer if patient has diarrhea.
• Other viruses (including enteroviruses and polioviruses) may interfere with the desired response to the administered vaccine.
• The vaccine will not be effective in modifying or preventing cases of existing or incubating poliomyelitis.

ADVERSE EFFECTS

SYSTEMIC EFFECTS: paralytic disease (about 1/1,000,000)

Rabies Vaccine/Rabies Vaccine, Dried Killed Virus

GENERAL CLINICAL USES

Rabies vaccine is indicated for use in patients exposed to a suspected rabid animal, that is, those sustaining single bites on abraded or mucosal surfaces, particularly if the animal has signs indicative of rabies or if exposure was severe, such as multiple bites or single bites on the head, neck, face, or arm.

Vaccination with the rabies vaccine before exposure occurs may be desirable for certain high-risk individuals such as veterinarians, delivery men, meter readers, spelunkers, or laboratory personnel working with rabies virus.

PHARMACOLOGY

Rabies vaccine, dried killed virus, is a suspension of embryonic duck tissue infected with fixed virus to which beta propiolactone has been added as a virucidal agent. This vaccine circumvents the use of brain tissue, which is associated with the "paralytic factor."

Rabies vaccine is also made from a suspension of fixed rabies virus obtained from rabbit brain tissues. The virus is inactivated with phenol or ultraviolet irradiation. The antigenicity of the brain vaccine is higher than that of the duck embryo vaccine.

SPECIAL PRECAUTIONS
- Administer with caution to patients with a history of allergy, especially allergy to chicken or duck eggs or protein; or to rabbits.
- Safe use in pregnancy has not been established; however, when postexposure rabies immunization is indicated, pregnancy has not been considered to be a contraindication to use of the killed virus vaccine.

ADVERSE EFFECTS
CNS EFFECTS: fever, malaise, drowsiness, headache, fatigability, transverse myelitis, cranial or peripheral palsy, encephalitis, chills
RESPIRATORY EFFECTS: dyspnea, bronchospasm
GASTROINTESTINAL EFFECTS: abdominal cramps, nausea, vomiting, diarrhea
ALLERGIC EFFECTS: urticaria, anaphylactic reactions, serum sickness
OPHTHALMIC EFFECTS: photophobia
LOCAL EFFECTS: tenderness, erythema, induration, regional lymphenopathy, inflammation

CLINICAL GUIDELINES
ADMINISTRATION:
- Test for hypersensitivity prior to administration.
- Epinephrine (1:1000) should be available in case an anaphylactoid reaction occurs.

DRUG INTERACTIONS:
- Do not administer adrenocorticotropin or adrenal corticosteroids to persons exposed to infectious agents such as rabies, since they may reduce host resistance.

Rocky Mountain Spotted Fever Vaccine

GENERAL CLINICAL USES
Rocky mountain spotted fever vaccine is used in laboratory personnel working with *Rickettsia rickettsii* and in others whose occupations involve exposure to ticks in endemic areas.

PHARMACOLOGY
Rocky Mountain spotted fever vaccine is prepared in embryonated chick yolk sac infected with *R. rickettsii*. When administered to humans immunity is conferred in a relatively short time; annual recall injections are necessary.

SPECIAL PRECAUTIONS
- Do not use in patients with a history of hypersensitivity to chickens or chicken eggs.
- Do not administer intravenously.

ADVERSE EFFECTS
SYSTEMIC EFFECTS: fever, malaise rarely; urticaria, rash, pruritus, asthma (rarely severe)
LOCAL EFFECTS: pain, tenderness, erythema, swelling

Rubella Virus Vaccine, Live

GENERAL CLINICAL USES
Rubella virus vaccine, live, is indicated for immunization against rubella in (1) children between age 1 and puberty, (2)

postpubertal males, and (3) postpubertal females, not pregnant.

PHARMACOLOGY

Rubella virus vaccine, live, for immunization against rubella (German measles), is prepared from Meyer and Perlman's attenuated strain of rubella virus, which is propagated in duck embryo cell culture (MERUVAX) or rabbit kidney cultures (CENDEVAX).

SPECIAL PRECAUTIONS

• Do not give to pregnant women; effects on the fetus are not known.
• When postpubertal women are to be vaccinated, rule out pregnancy and advise patient to prevent it for 3 months.
• Do not use in patients with a history of sensitivity to chicken or duck, chicken or duck eggs or feathers, neomycin or rabbit.
• Do not use in patients with any febrile illness or other active febrile infection.
• Do not use in patients treated with ACTH, corticosteroids, irradiation, alkylating agents, or antimetabolites. This does not apply to patients receiving corticosteroids for replacement therapy (Addison's disease) or those with blood dyscrasias, leukemia, lymphomas of any type, or other malignant neoplasms affecting the bone marrow or lymphatic system.
• Do not use in patients with gammaglobulin deficiency (agammaglobulinemia, hypogammaglobulinemia, and dysgammaglobulinemia).
• Do not give less than 1 month before or after immunization with other live virus vaccines with the exception of monovalent or trivalent poliovirus vaccine, live, oral, which may be administered simultaneously.
• Defer vaccination for at least 3 months following plasma or blood transfusion, or administration of human immune serum globulin, more than 0.02 ml per pound body weight.

ADVERSE EFFECTS

SYSTEMIC EFFECTS: fever; encephalitis very rarely; rash, urticaria, arthritis, arthralgia, polyneuritis
LOCAL EFFECTS: erythema, induration, tenderness, regional lymphadenopathy

CLINICAL GUIDELINES

ADMINISTRATION:
• Do not administer intravenously.
• Epinephrine should be available for immediate use should an anaphylactoid reaction occur.
EFFECTS:
• There is no evidence that live rubella virus vaccine given after exposure will prevent illness.
• May be administered in immediate postpartum period to those nonimmune women who have received anti-R_O (D) immune globulin (human) without interfering with vaccine effectiveness.
DRUG INTERACTIONS:
• May result in a temporary depression of tuberculin skin sensitivity. If a tuberculin test is to be done, it should be administered either before or simultaneously with this vaccine.

Rubella and Mumps Virus Vaccine

GENERAL CLINICAL USES

Rubella and mumps virus vaccine is indicated for simultaneous immunization against rubella and mumps in children from 1 year of age to puberty.

PHARMACOLOGY

Rubella (German measles) and mumps virus vaccine is prepared from an attenuated strain of rubella virus propagated in duck embryo cell culture and from a strain of mumps virus grown in cell cultures of chick embryos free of avian leukosis. The two viruses are mixed and lyophilized.

SPECIAL PRECAUTIONS
- Do not administer in children less than 1 year old.
- Do not give to pregnant women; the possible effects in the fetus are unknown.
- If it is necessary to vaccinate postpubertal women, pregnancy must be ruled out at the time of vaccination and prevented during the following 3 months.
- Do not use in patients sensitive to chicken or duck, including eggs or feathers, or neomycin. Certain preparations contain neomycin.
- Do not use if patient has any febrile respiratory illness or other active febrile infection.
- Do not vaccinate any patient treated with ACTH, corticosteroids, irradiation, alkylating agents or antimetabolites. This contraindication does not apply to patients receiving corticosteroids as replacement therapy (Addison's disease), individuals with blood dyscrasias, leukemia, lymphomas of any type, or other malignant neoplasms affecting the bone marrow or lymphatic system.
- Do not use in patients with gamma globulin deficiency such as agammaglobulinemia, hypogammaglobulinemia, and dysgammaglobulinemia.
- Do not give less than 1 month before or after immunization with other live virus vaccines, with the exception of monovalent or trivalent poliovirus vaccine, live, oral, which may be administered simultaneously.
- Vaccination should be deferred for at least 3 months following blood or plasma transfusion, or administration of human immune serum globulin, more than 0.02 ml per pound of body weight.

ADVERSE EFFECTS
SYSTEMIC EFFECTS: fever; encephalitis rarely; parotitis, thrombocytopenia, urticaria, rash, purpura, arthritis, arthralgia, polyneuritis, regional lymphadenopathy
LOCAL EFFECTS: erythema, induration, tenderness

CLINICAL GUIDELINES
ADMINISTRATION:
- Never administer intravenously.
- Epinephrine (1:1000) should be available in case an anaphylactoid reaction occurs.

EFFECTS:
- There are no reports of transmission of live attenuated mumps virus from vaccinees to susceptible contacts.
- Adverse effects usually are mild and last no more than 3 days.

DRUG INTERACTIONS:
- Attenuated mumps and rubella virus vaccines, live, given individually may result in a temporary depression of tuberculin skin sensitivity. Therefore, if a tuberculin test is to be done, it should be administered either before or simultaneously with this vaccine.

Smallpox Vaccine
Smallpox Vaccine Dried

GENERAL CLINICAL USES
Smallpox vaccine is used to induce immunity against smallpox (vaccinia) virus.

PHARMACOLOGY
The smallpox vaccine is prepared from calf lymph tissue. It contains remnants of polymyxin B, dihydrostreptomycin sulfate, chlortetracycline, and neomycin sulfate which were used during processing.

Smallpox vaccine is also prepared from virus grown in embryonated chicken eggs.

Administration of either preparation results in the antigen stimulating production of antibodies against this virus.

SPECIAL PRECAUTIONS
• Do not use in patients hypersensitive to calf lymph tissue, eggs, chicken feathers, polymyxin B, dihydrostreptomycin sulfate, chlortetracycline, neomycin sulfate, or related compounds.
• Do not vaccinate patients with eczema or other forms of chronic dermatitis, wounds or burns, or their household contacts.
• Do not use for prophylaxis or treatment of herpes infection or warts.
• Avoid vaccination in patients with febrile illness, defective or altered immune mechanisms, leukemias, lymphomas, skin infection, malignant neoplasms affecting bone marrow or lymphatic systems, and during corticosteroid therapy, immunosuppressive drug therapy, or pregnancy.
• Do not vaccinate infants manifesting failure to thrive.
• Do not vaccinate individuals with known or suspected disorders of gamma globulin synthesis.
• Epinephrine (1:1000) should be available should an anaphylactoid reaction occur.

ADVERSE EFFECTS
SYSTEMIC EFFECTS: encephalitis rarely
LOCAL EFFECTS: vesicular or pustular lesion, area of palpable induration surrounding a central lesion, generalized vaccinia, vaccinia necrosum, eczema vaccinatum

Tuberculosis Vaccine (BCG)

GENERAL CLINICAL USES
Tuberculosis vaccine, although controversial, may confer substantial protection against tuberculosis. It effectively converts individuals with a negative tuberculin skin test to positive reactors.

PHARMACOLOGY
Tuberculosis vaccine is a suspension of an attenuated strain of bovine tubercle bacillus (*Mycobacterium bovis*) commonly referred to as BCG (bacillus Calmette-Guerin) vaccine.

SPECIAL PRECAUTIONS
• Screen patients by tuberculin test and physical and x-ray examinations.
• Active tuberculosis must be ruled out before the vaccination is administered.
• Do not vaccinate patients who are acutely ill or suspected of having respiratory tract, skin, or other infections, in those with agammaglobulinemia, and those with a positive tuberculin test.
• Vaccination is contraindicated in presence of skin infection, allergic dermatitis, burns, a fresh smallpox vaccination, impaired immunity or prolonged use of corticosteroids.
• It is prudent to refrain from vaccination during pregnancy unless there is excessive risk of unavoidable exposure to infectious tuberculosis.

ADVERSE EFFECTS
SYSTEMIC EFFECTS: lymphadenitis; osteomyelitis, disseminated BCG infection, death
LOCAL EFFECTS: severe or prolonged ulceration at vaccination site, abscess, granuloma

CLINICAL GUIDELINES
DRUG INTERACTIONS:
• Not effective if given during isoniazid (INH) administration because INH inhibits multiplication of BCG.

Typhoid Vaccine

GENERAL CLINICAL USES

Typhoid vaccine is recommended for immunization of persons who may be exposed to the typhoid bacilli. It is recommended for persons exposed to a carrier in the household, those living in a community where an outbreak of typhoid fever has occurred, or those traveling to endemic areas.

PHARMACOLOGY

Typhoid vaccine is prepared from killed typhoid bacilli (*Salmonella typhosa*). The bacteria are grown on veal infusion agar, washed off, suspended in buffered sodium chloride injection, and killed by a combination of phenol and heat.

SPECIAL PRECAUTIONS

- Do not vaccinate patients with acute respiratory or other active illnesses or patients with debilitating disease or tuberculosis.
- Take all precautions known for prevention of allergic or any other side effects.
- Epinephrine (1:1000) and other emergency drugs and equipment should be readily available to combat severe systemic reactions if they develop.

ADVERSE EFFECTS

SYSTEMIC EFFECTS: myalgia, malaise, headache, fever, nausea
LOCAL EFFECTS: erythema, tenderness, induration at site of injection

Typhus Vaccine

GENERAL CLINICAL USES

Typhus vaccine is used to immunize patients against typhus rickettsiae, epidemic type. The typhus is louse-borne. Vaccina-tion is necessary only for people traveling to certain areas of the world.

PHARMACOLOGY

Typhus vaccine, epidemic type, is prepared from typhus rickettsiae (*Rickettsia prowazekii*) grown in chick embryo culture.

SPECIAL PRECAUTIONS

- Do not use in the presence of active illness; in patients with debiliating disease, tuberculosis, or agammaglobulinemia; or in those receiving corticosteroid, antineoplastic, or immunosuppressive drugs.
- Vaccination is contraindicated in patients with a history of hypersensitivity to eggs, chicken, or chicken feathers. Test for sensitivity prior to use.
- Epinephrine (1:1000) should be on hand in case an anaphylactoid reaction occurs.

ADVERSE EFFECTS

SYSTEMIC EFFECTS: anaphylactoid reactions
LOCAL EFFECTS: pain

Yellow Fever Vaccine

GENERAL CLINICAL USES

Yellow fever vaccine is recommended for persons traveling to countries in which yellow fever is endemic and for laboratory personnel who might be exposed to the disease.

PHARMACOLOGY

Yellow fever vaccine is a suspension of live, attenuated virus grown in chick embryo. This vaccine may produce immunity lasting up to 10 years.

SPECIAL PRECAUTIONS

- Do not use in patients sensitive to eggs, chickens, or chicken feathers.

• Do not use in patients with febrile illnesses or with agammaglobulinemia.
• Do not use in patients receiving corticosteroids, antineoplastic drugs, or immunosuppressive drugs.

• Epinephrine (1:1000) should be on hand in case an anaphylactoid reaction occurs.

ADVERSE EFFECTS
SYSTEMIC EFFECTS: myalgia, fever, headache, encephalitis rarely

Specific Immunosuppressive Agents

Azathioprine

GENERAL CLINICAL USES
Azathioprine is indicated as adjunctive therapy in the prevention of rejection in renal homotransplantation.

SPECIFIC PRODUCTS AND DOSAGES

GENERIC NAME	TRADE NAME	ROUTE OF ADMIN.	USUAL DOSAGE
azathioprine	IMURAN	po	**Initial:** 3–5 mg/kg/day **Maintenance:** 1–2 mg/kg/day
		iv	**Initial:** 3–5 mg/kg/day **Maintenance:** 1–2 mg/kg/day

PHARMACOLOGY
Azathioprine, following oral administration, is well absorbed from the gastrointestinal tract. It is also available for intravenous administration for use in patients unable to take oral medication. The drug is metabolized to 6-mercaptopurine, which is then further metabolized and excreted in the urine. Maximal immunosuppression occurs when this drug is given either starting with the time of antigenic stimulation or within 2 days thereafter. When administered before or after exposure to the antigen, the drug is usually ineffective.

SPECIAL PRECAUTIONS
- Do not use in patients with a history of hypersensitivity to azathioprine.
- Irreversible depression of the bone marrow may be produced.
- If persistent decrease or rapid fall occurs in leukocyte count, reduce or temporarily discontinue drug.
- Watch for signs of infection; if intercurrent infection develops, consider reducing dosage.
- Although no causal relationship has been established, there have been a few reports of lymphomas developing in patients receiving immunosuppressive therapy.
- If persistent negative nitrogen balance occurs in patients on continuous therapy with azathioprine, reduce dosage.
- If toxic hepatitis or biliary stasis occurs, consider withholding drug.
- This drug has potential teratogenic action; therefore, consider benefits and risks before use in women of childbearing potential.
- Since cadaveric kidneys frequently develop a tubular necrosis with delayed onset of adequate function, the clearance of azathioprine and its metabolites may be impaired; dosage should be reduced appropriately.

ADVERSE EFFECTS
GASTROINTESTINAL EFFECTS: pancreatitis, steatorrhea, nausea, vomiting, diarrhea, anorexia
HEPATIC EFFECTS: jaundice, extremely high alkaline phosphatase level, slightly elevated serum bilirubin
HEMATOLOGIC EFFECTS: leukopenia, anemia, thrombocytopenia, bleeding, pancytopenia
ALLERGIC EFFECTS: drug fever
DERMATOLOGIC EFFECTS: oral lesions, rash, and alopecia

MUSCULOSKELETAL EFFECTS: arthralgia

CLINICAL GUIDELINES
ADMINISTRATION:
- Perform complete blood count, including platelets, at least weekly, and more frequently during initial treatment and with high doses.
EFFECTS:
- This drug may have a delayed action; it is important to reduce dosage or withdraw the medication temporarily at the first sign of an abnormally large fall in the leukocyte count and/or other evidence of persistent depression of the bone marrow.
- Patients with impaired renal function may have a slower elimination of the drug with a consequent greater cumulative effect; dosage should be reduced accordingly.
DRUG INTERACTIONS:
- Azathioprine has been administered concurrently with corticosteroids and other cytotoxic agents.
- In patients receiving allopurinol, the concomitant administration of azathioprine will require a reduction in dose to approximately 1/3 to 1/4 the usual dose of azathioprine; allopurinol inhibits the metabolism of azathioprine.

Adrenal Steroids (Glucocorticoids)

GENERAL CLINICAL USES
In large doses the glucocorticoids produce immunosuppression. They are used to prevent rejection following transplantation.

PHARMACOLOGY, SPECIAL PRECAUTIONS, ADVERSE EFFECTS, CLINICAL GUIDELINES
For detailed information, see Chapter 15, page 539.

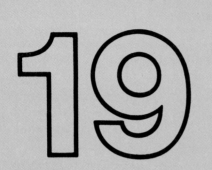

Diagnostic agents

INTRODUCTION

Recent advances have enlarged the spectrum of diagnostic tools available to the physician. Many of the older procedures and techniques have been replaced, or, more commonly, complemented, by the advances in technology.

SPECIFIC THERAPEUTIC CLASSIFICATION

The diagnostic agents comprise three groups based on specific technologies:

1. Radioactive isotopes
2. Radiopaque agents
3. Miscellaneous agents including diagnostic dyes; aminohippuric acid, inulin, mannitol, pentagastrin, betazole hydrochloride, histamine phosphate, metyrapone, sodium dehydrocholate, secretin, neostigmine methylsulfate, edrophonium chloride, and indigotindisulfonate sodium.

Radioactive Isotopes

GENERAL CLINICAL USES
The radioactive isotopes are used to evaluate function, to localize tumors, and to visualize organs. Specific uses of each isotope will be reviewed in this section.

SPECIFIC PRODUCTS AND INDICATIONS
Radiopharmaceuticals should be used only by physicians with specific training in the safe handling of these products.

GENERIC NAME	TRADE NAME	ROUTE OF ADMIN.	IN VIVO DIAGNOSTIC PROCEDURES IN THE FOLLOWING AREAS
chlormerodrin Hg 197	(G)* NEOHYDRIN-197	iv	Kidney, brain
chlormerodrin Hg 203	(G) NEOHYDRIN-203	iv	Brain, kidney
cyanocobalamin Co 57	(G) RACOBALAMIN-57 RUBRATOPE-57	po/im	Gastrointestinal tract, blood
cyanocobalamin Co 60	(G) RUBRATOPE-60	po	Gastrointestinal tract
gold Au 198	(G) AUROTOPE AUROSCAN-198	iv	**Diagnostic use:** liver **Therapeutic use:** neoplastic suppressant
iodinated serum albumin I 125	(G) RISA-125	iv	Blood, plasma volume
iodinated serum albumin I 131 aggregated	(G) ALBUMOTOPE-LS RISA-131	iv	Heart, blood pool, brain, lung
selenomethionine Se 75	(G) SETHOTOPE	iv	Pancreas

*(G) designates availability as a generic product.

(continued overleaf)

GENERIC NAME	TRADE NAME	ROUTE OF ADMIN.	IN VIVO DIAGNOSTIC PROCEDURES IN THE FOLLOWING AREAS
sodium chromate Cr 51	(G) CHROMITOPE	iv	Spleen, placenta, blood pool
sodium iodide I 131	(G) IODOTOPE I 131	po/iv	Thyroid
sodium iodide I 125	(G) IODOTOPE I 125	po/iv	Thyroid
sodium iodohippurate I 131	HIPPURAN I 131	iv	Kidney
sodium phosphate P 32	(G) PHOSPHOTOPE	po/iv	**Diagnostic use:** localization of certain ocular tumors **Therapeutic use:** treatment of polycythemia vera, palliative treatment of chronic myelocytic leukemias and chronic lymphocytic anemia
sodium rose bengal I 131	(G) ROBENGATOPE	iv	Liver
technetium aggregated albumin (human) Tc 99 m	MACROTEC	iv	Lung

Chlormerodrin Hg 203
Chlormerodrin Hg 197

PHARMACOLOGY

Chlormerodrin Hg 203 and Hg 197 are used for scanning the brain for suspected lesions and the kidneys for anatomical and functional abnormalities. In the brain, chlormerodrin concentrates in the neoplastic tissue.

Chlormerodrin, a mercurial diuretic agent, is rapidly cleared by the kidneys.

The half-life of chlormerodrin Hg 197 is 65 hours, and for chlormerodrin Hg, 203, it is 466 days.

SPECIAL PRECAUTIONS
• Do not use in patients with acute nephritis or chronic renal disease.

• Assure minimal radiation exposure to patient and personnel.
• Do not use in patients with a history of hypersensitivity to chlormerodrin.

ADVERSE EFFECTS
ALLERGIC EFFECTS: stomatitis, gastric disturbances, vertigo, febrile reactions, cutaneous eruptions.

Cyanocobalamin Co 57
Cyanocobalamin Co 60

PHARMACOLOGY
Radioactive cyanocobalamin administered orally is handled in the body in the same manner as vitamin B_{12}. If vitamin

B_{12} absorption is impaired or if the intrinsic factor is lacking, the radiocyanocobalamin will be absorbed minimally if at all, and will be excreted in the feces. If intrinsic factor is present and B_{12} absorption is normal the radioactive compound will primarily be absorbed but about one third of the radioactivity will appear in the feces. The absorbed compound will be stored primarily in the liver.

The half-life of Co 57 is 270 days, and it decays to iron 57. The half-life of Co 60 is 5.27 days, and it decays to nickel 60.

SPECIAL PRECAUTIONS

• Use with extreme caution if at all in women who are pregnant or who may become pregnant, during lactation, or in patients under the age of 18 years.

• Postpone tests until after delivery of pregnant women since vitamin B_{12} is taken up by the fetus. It is also excreted in human milk; therefore, substitute formula-feeding for breast-feeding.

• Note that tuberculous patients treated with para aminosalicylic acid (PAS) may have impaired intestinal absorption of vitamin B_{12} which may lead to the development of megaloblastic anemia.

• Assure minimal radiation exposure to patient and personnel.

• Carefully evaluate the need for repeating a test in the same patient, particularly in younger patients.

• Do not conduct radioactive vitamin B_{12} tests until at least 4 days after a flushing dose or therapeutic vitamin B_{12} injection.

• Conduct bone marrow studies, screen B_{12} determination, and reticulocyte response tests before the Schilling test.

• Impaired renal function may require extension of the urine collection to 48 or 72 hours in the Schilling test; the test may be invalid.

ADVERSE EFFECTS

• None noted; very rarely allergiclike reactions and reactions at the site of injection have been reported with parenteral administration.

CLINICAL GUIDELINES

ADMINISTRATION:

• The patient should not receive vitamin B_{12} orally or parenterally for at least 4 days before the Schilling urinary excretion test or the hepatic uptake test, and should fast for 12 hours immediately prior to the test.

• A 12-hour control urine specimen is recommended to confirm interference by gamma-emitting radioisotopes. The patient should fast for 2 more hours.

EFFECTS:

• Factors which may impair absorption of vitamin B_{12} include the following: diseases of the small intestine (diverticulosis, blind loops or strictures, tropical and nontropical sprue, regional enteritis), partial or total gastrectomy, ileal resection, gastric hypo- or anacidity, gastric mucosal atrophy, fish tapeworm, diarrhea and increased intestinal motility, acute infections, inhibitors of gastric secretion, calcium-binding substances (calcium disodium edetate,) sorbose.

• Factors which may increase absorption of vitamin B_{12} include corticosteroids in some cases of pernicious anemia and sprue, calcium in some patients with steatorrhea, tetracycline therapy (but not neomycin or sulfonamides) in some cases of diverticulosis, blind-loop syndrome, or intestinal strictures, antihelmintic therapy is fish tapeworm infection, carbachol and other gastric stimulants in some subjects with low intrinsic factor production, sorbitol in normal subjects (but not in pernicious anemia).

• Factors which may cause impaired absorption to appear normal include fecal contamination of urine specimen.

• Factors which may cause normal absorption to appear impaired include renal dysfunction and incomplete urine collection.

Gold Au 198

PHARMACOLOGY
The half-life or gold Au 198 is 2.7 days.

SPECIAL PRECAUTIONS
• Do not administer intravenously.
• Assure minimal radiation exposure to patient and personnel.
• Do not use in patients with a history of hypersensitivity to gold.

Iodinated (I 125 and I 131) Serum Albumin

PHARMACOLOGY
Following intravenous administration, radioiodinated serum albumin is distributed uniformly throughout the intravascular pool within 10 minutes; at this time labeled albumin can be detected in the lymph and in certain body tissues. Maximal distribution of radioactivity throughout the extravascular space does not occur until 2 to 4 days after administration. This time has been designated "equilibrium time." The radioactivity remaining in the intravascular and extravascular spaces decreases slowly and exponentially. The radioactivity is eliminated almost entirely in the urine with approximately 2 percent eliminated in the feces. The biological half-life in normal individuals appears to be approximately 14 days.

SPECIAL PRECAUTIONS
• Do not administer to pregnant patients, patients who may become pregnant, or lactating patients unless the benefits exceed the risks of the radiation exposure involved.
• Substitute formula-feeding for breast-feeding when it is necessary to administer radioiodinated serum albumin during lactation, since iodine is excreted in milk.
• When examination is required in women of childbearing capability, administer during the first few days following the onset of menses.
• Assure minimal radiation exposure to patient and personnel.
• Do not administer to persons less than 18 years old unless the indications are exceptional.

ADVERSE EFFECTS
• Not established. There is the theoretical possibility of allergic reactions with repeat doses after the initial dose even though the immunological properties of serum albumin are believed to be virtually unaltered by the iodination process.

CLINICAL GUIDELINES
ADMINISTRATION:
• A thyroid-blocking iodine preparation such as Lugol's solution will minimize uptake of radioactive iodine by the thyroid.
• Do not exceed a total dose of 200 μCi in 1 week.

Iodinated (I 131) Serum Albumin Aggregated

PHARMACOLOGY
Iodinated (I 131) serum albumin aggregated, following intravenous administration, is transported rapidly to the lungs where it remains in the pulmonary vasculature. When the pulmonary blood flow is normal, the aggregated radioiodinated (I 131)

albumin is carried throughout the entire lung field; when the lung field is diminished or obstructed by a disease process, the aggregated albumin is prevented from passing through the affected portion. The particles remain in the lung for variable times depending upon their size; the larger particles have longer half-lives, 2 to 8 hours, than the smaller particles. The particles are carried to the liver where they are removed from the bloodstream by Kupffer cells; the particles are phagocytized and metabolized rapidly. I 131 has a half-life of 8.08 days.

SPECIAL PRECAUTIONS

• Do not administer to nursing mothers because iodide is excreted in human milk; if necessary, substitute formula-feeding for breast-feeding.
• Assure minimal radiation exposure to patient and personnel.
• Do not administer to persons under the age of 18 years unless the indications are exceptional.
• Safe use in pregnancy and lactation has not been established.

ADVERSE EFFECTS

• Hypersensitivity reactions are theoretically possible if repeat doses are administered after the initial dose; the immunological properties of serum albumin are virtually unaltered by the iodination process.

CLINICAL GUIDELINES
ADMINISTRATION:
• Administration of a thyroid-blocking iodine preparation such as Lugol's solution will minimize uptake of radioactive iodine by the thyroid.

• Administer by slow intravenous injection.
EFFECTS:
• Neither respiratory distress nor tachycardia is produced in seriously ill patients with pulmonary and/or cardiac disorders.

Selenomethionine Se 75

PHARMACOLOGY

Selenomethionine Se 75 localizes in all organs involved in active protein synthesis. It is incorporated into newly synthesized proteins. In the pancreas, the uptake of selenomethionine Se 75 is relatively high. Significant uptake also occurs in the liver and proximal small intestine, as well as in several other tissues. The half-life of Se 75 is 120 days.

SPECIAL PRECAUTIONS
• Assure minimal radiation exposure to patient and personnel.
• Examinations in women of childbearing capability should be performed during the first few days following onset of menses.
• In pregnant women, transplacental transport and long biologic half-life of selenomethionine Se 75 may result in significant radiation exposure to the fetus.
• Selenomethionine Se 75 may result in significant radiation exposure to the fetus.
• Selenomethionine Se 75 is secreted in milk; therefore substitute formula-feeding for breast-feeding.

CLINICAL GUIDELINES
ADMINISTRATION:
• Pancreatic image quality may degrade in patients fasting prior to administration, which may enhance the hepatic removal of selenomethionine Se 75.

Sodium Chromate (Cr 51) Serum Albumin (Human)

PHARMACOLOGY

Chromium 51 can be firmly bound to albumin; it is not absorbed from the gastrointestinal tract after oral administration. Because the Cr label is not reabsorbed from the gastrointestinal tract, the amount of protein loss can be quantitatively determined. The only route by which intravenously administered Cr 51 can enter the gastrointestinal tract is through abnormal leakage of the labeled protein. Therefore, the site of protein loss can be identified in the same way that bleeding sites are located with Cr 51-tagged erythrocytes.

Localization of the placenta may be accomplished by intravenously administered radiochromated (Cr 51) serum albumin (human). With this agent, radiation risk to mother and fetus is reduced significantly.

The half-life of Cr 51 is 27.8 days.

SPECIAL PRECAUTIONS

- Do not administer during pregnancy and lactation unless the information to be gained outweighs the hazards.
- Assure minimal radiation exposure to the patient and personnel.

ADVERSE EFFECTS

- Although the immunological properties of serum albumin are believed to be virtually unaltered by the tagging process, there is a theoretical possibility that allergic reactions may occur with repeated doses.

CLINICAL GUIDELINES

ADMINISTRATION:

- For detection of gastrointestinal protein loss, a complete cumulative urine-free stool collection is made for 96 hours beginning at time of injection.

Sodium Iodide I 125
Sodium Iodide I 131

PHARMACOLOGY

Ingested iodide is removed from the bloodstream almost exclusively by the thyroid cells and the kidneys.

- It is detected in the thyroid within minutes after ingestion. Iodine is primarily excreted in the urine; small amounts are detectable in feces and sweat; larger amounts are excreted in the milk of lactating women during the first 24 hours after administration.

The half-life of I 131 is 8.08 days, and the final disintegration product is xenon 131. The half-life of I 125 is 60 days.

SPECIAL PRECAUTIONS

- If the drug is administered to the mother during lactation, formula-feeding should be substituted for breast-feeding because iodide is excreted in human milk.
- Do not administer to persons under 18 years of age unless the expected benefit outweighs the hazards.
- Assure minimal radiation exposure to the patient and personnel.
- Interpret test results with caution in patients who have been treated with radioiodine for hyperthyroidism.
- In patients with renal impairment, the urinary excretion of radioiodine may decrease and the levels in plasma, thyroid, and feces increases; the 24-hour uptake studies are usually not affected.

ADVERSE EFFECTS

Adverse effects are rare; nausea, vomiting, and severe throbbing headaches have been reported.

CLINICAL GUIDELINES

ADMINISTRATION:

- Thyroid uptake of radioiodine may be

significantly changed by recent administration of drugs containing iodine in any form and by thyroid and antithyroid drugs.

EFFECTS:

• Thyroid uptake of radioiodine may be markedly increased in patients with chronic cirrhosis.

• Cardiac patients on low sodium diets may show elevated uptake.

• Radioiodine uptake may be decreased in patients with congestive heart failure.

DRUG INTERACTIONS:

• Iodine concentration by the thyroid is prevented by perchlorates or thiocyanates; this may be followed by a "rebound" phenomenon with a period of exaggerated iodine uptake following the initial suppression of uptake.

Sodium Iodohippurate I 131

PHARMACOLOGY

Sodium iodohippurate I 131, administered intravenously, is rapidly removed from the blood and accumulates in the renal tissues. Peak radioactivity is measured within 3 to 6 minutes in normal individuals and in more than 6 minutes in patients with renal impairment. Sodium iosohippurate is primarily excreted by tubular secretion (80 percent) and the remainder by glomerular filtration (20 percent). The half-life of sodium iodohippurate I 131 is 8.08 days.

SPECIAL PRECAUTIONS

• I 131 is excreted in human milk; therefore, formula-feeding should be substituted for breast-feeding if this agent is administered to the mother during lactation.

• Assure minimal radiation exposure to patient and personnel.

• In women with childbearing potential, testing with radiopharmaceuticals should be performed during the first few days following the onset of menses.

• To minimize thyroid uptake of I 131, a saturated solution of potassium iodide may be administered prior to and following the examination.

ADVERSE EFFECTS

• Few have been reported: 2 minor allergic reactions in 1500 renograms; slight sensation of generalized warmth—1 patient; transient vomiting with 30-gm dose; pallor, sweating, fainting; children (including 1-year-old) received 10 gm without ill effects.

CLINICAL GUIDELINES

ADMINISTRATION:

• When administering intravenously, be sure to avoid extravasation or perivascular infiltration.

• Sodium iodihippurate I 131 injection may be diluted with sterile sodium chloride injection USP.

• Adequate hydration of the patient is necessary for an adequate renogram.

Sodium Phosphate P 32

PHARMACOLOGY

Administration of radioactive phosphorus results in rapid distribution to all tissues; with high metabolic and proliferative activity take up more phosphorus than other tissues. After oral administration, 15 to 50 percent is excreted in the urine and feces during the first 4 to 6 days. After intravenous administration, 5 to 10 percent is excreted in the urine in the first 24 hours and about 20 percent is excreted by the end of the first week. The half-life of sodium phosphate P 32 is 14 days.

SPECIAL PRECAUTIONS
- Do not use as part of sequential treatment with an alkylating agent.
- If sodium phosphate P 32 is administered to lactating women, substitute formula-feeding for breast-feeding.
- Assure minimal radiation exposure to patient and personnel.
- Do not administer to pregnant patients or patients less than 16 years of age.
- When used for therapy of polycythelmia vera, it should not be administered when the leukocyte count is below 5000 mm^3 or the platelet count below 150,000 mm^3; in therapy of chronic granulocytic leukemia, do not administer sodium phosphate P 32 when the leukocyte count is below 20,000 mm^3.

ADVERSE EFFECTS
- Not established for diagnostic use; with therapeutic use, bone marrow depression has occurred.

CLINICAL GUIDELINES
ADMINISTRATION:
- Note that orally administered sodium phosphate P 32 is incompletely absorbed; the equivalent intravenous dose is approximately 75 percent of the oral dose.
- The patient should not eat for 2 hours before and 6 hours after oral administration.

DRUG INTERACTION:
- Milk and milk products, iron, bismuth medications, and soft drinks should be avoided during the period of oral radiophosphorus therapy.

OVERDOSAGE/ANTIDOTE:
- Overdosage may produce serious effects on the hematopoietic system including leukemia, thrombocytopenia, and also anemia.
- There is no specific antidote.

Sodium Rose Bengal I 131

PHARMACOLOGY
Following intravenous administration, sodium rose bengal I 131 accumulates in the polygonal cells of the liver; it is excreted by the bile into the intestines. In patients with marked impairment of liver function, sodium rose bengal I 131 is excreted by the kidneys.

In patients with normal livers, the blood clearance half-time is approximately 5 to 15 minutes. Maximal liver uptake occurs approximately 30 minutes after intravenous administration. Therefore, hepatic radioactivity diminishes slowly with about 70 percent cleared in 3 hours.

SPECIAL PRECAUTIONS
- Safe use in pregnancy and lactation has not been established.
- Substitute formula-feeding for breast-feeding in mothers receiving the agent during lactation because I 131 is excreted in human milk.
- Do not administer to patients less than 18 years of age.
- Assure minimal radiation exposure to patient and personnel.
- If sodium rose bengal I 131 is to be administered to patients under 18 years of age, use a suitable thyroid-blocking agent such as Lugol's solution.
- In patients with heart disease, hepatic congestion, or severe shock, liver function testing with sodium rose bengal I 131 may not be reliable.
- Administer to women of childbearing potential a few days after the onset of menstruation.
- Pronounced hepatomegaly may interfere with accurate determination of intestinal entry of I 131 and may invalidate the results of the test.

• Significant renal excretion of the radio-nuclide may occur in patients with intra- and extrahepatic disease. Urinary radioactivity may simulate intestinal radioactivity in the scan.

• Radiation may be minimized by administration of a cholecystogogue and a laxative at appropriate intervals after the test.

CLINICAL GUIDELINES

ADMINISTRATION:

• Inform patients that their stools will be colored red.

EFFECTS:

• Photosensitivity reactions may occur in patients receiving large doses of sodium rose bengal. Keep patient from sunlight or ultraviolet light for 24 hours after administration.

Technetium Aggregated Albumin (Human) (Tc 99m)

PHARMACOLOGY

Technetium (Tc 99m) aggregated albumin administered intravenously has a half time for lung clearance of about 4 hours (range 3.5 to 5 hours). Urinary excretion after 72 hours is approximately 40 percent. The half-life is 5.9 hours.

SPECIAL PRECAUTIONS

• Assure minimal radiation exposure to patient and personnel.

• Safe use in pregnancy has not been established.

• If used in women of childbearing capability, the test should be performed during the first few days following onset of menstruation.

Radiopaque Agents

GENERAL CLINICAL USES

The radiopaque agents are used for visualization of the body cavities, cardio-vascular system, and urinary and respiratory systems, and for evaluation of gallbladder, liver, and gastrointestinal function. They are also used for visualization of joints as in arthrography and diskography.

In the following section, *Specific Products and Uses,* it can be seen that contrast agents have multiple uses.

SPECIFIC PRODUCTS AND USES

Diagnostic procedures using contrast media should be carried out under the direction of personnel with specific training in and knowledge of the procedure to be performed and the medication involved. Appropriate facilities should be available for coping with severe reactions, including hypersensitivity reactions.

For specific dosages, the reader is advised to consult the manufacturer's instructions.

GENERIC NAME	TRADE NAME	PROCEDURE
barium sulfate	(G)* BAROBAG BAROSPERSE BAROTRAST ORATRAST	Upper GI series, lower GI series, barium enema
iodized oil	LIPIODAL	Bronchography, visualization of sinuses and fistulous tracts Hysterosalpingography
iopanoic acid	TELEPAQUE	Cholecystography
iophendylate	PANTOPAQUE	Intraspinal myelography
ipodate calcium	OROGRAFIN CALCIUM	Cholecystography
ipodate sodium	OROGRAFIN SODIUM	Cholecystography
meglumine diatrizoate	CARDIOGRAFIN CYSTOGRAFIN GASTROGRAFIN HYPAQUE RENO-M-30 RENO-M-60 RENO-M-DIP	Angiocardiography, cardiac aortography, cerebral angiography, peripheral arteriography, venography, splenoportography Gastrointestinal tract visualization Operative T-tube or percutaneous transhepatic cholangiography Arthrography Diskography Retrograde cystourethrography, excretory urography, retrograde pyelography, drip infusion pyelography
meglumine iodipamide	CHOLOGRAFIN MEGLUMINE	Cholecystography, cholangiography
meglumine iothalamate	CONRAY CONRAY-30 CYSTO-CONRAY	Peripheral arteriography and venography, cerebral angiography Iv urography, iv infusion urography, retrograde pyelography, cystography, cystourethrography, excretory urography
propyliodone	DIONOSIL OILY	Bronchography
sodium acetrizoate	SALPIX	Hysterosalpingography
sodium diatrizoate	HYPAQUE SODIUM 20% HYPAQUE SODIUM 25% HYPAQUE SODIUM 50%	Cerebral and peripheral aortography, urography, cerebral imaging Drip infusion pyelography, excretory urography, retrograde pyelography Hysterosalpingography
sodium methiodal	SKIODAN SODIUM	Retrograde pyelography
sodium tyropanoate	BILOPAQUE SODIUM	Cholecystography

*(G) designates availability as a generic product.

Barium Sulfate

PHARMACOLOGY

Barium sulfate, a salt insoluble in water, is radiopaque. After oral administration, it is not absorbed but is excreted in the feces. Barium sulfate is also administered rectally as an enema for visualization of the rectum and lower colon.

SPECIAL PRECAUTIONS

• Do not use in patients with a history of hypersensitivity to barium sulfate or related compounds.
• Safe use in pregnancy has not been established.
• Avoid use of barium sulfate in patients with peptic ulcer who are receiving large amounts of calcium carbonate; the combination of calcium carbonate and barium sulfate may result in cementlike fecal impactions.

ADVERSE EFFECTS

LOCAL EFFECTS: after oral administration, constipation, occasionally impaction; after rectal administration, perforation of the bowel wall with peritonitis or formation of a barium granuloma rarely.

CLINICAL GUIDELINES

ADMINISTRATION:
• Administration of a laxative may be necessary following radiography.
OVERDOSAGE/ANTIDOTE:
• Rectal administration of an excessive amount of barium sulfate may result in perforation of the bowel wall with resultant peritonitis. Surgical intervention may be necessary.

Iodized Oil

PHARMACOLOGY

Iodized oil is iodinated poppy seed oil. It is introduced into body cavities for visualization of the uterus, fallopian tubes, sinuses, fistulous tracts, and lungs.

SPECIAL PRECAUTIONS

• Do not use in patients with a history of hypersensitivity to iodized oil or related compounds.
• May interfere with thyroid function tests.
• Use with extreme caution in patients with advanced renal disease or hepatorenal disease.

Iopanoic Acid

PHARMACOLOGY

Iopanoic acid, an organic iodine compound insoluble in water, is administered orally for cholangiography; it is absorbed from the duodenum, excreted by the liver as a glucuronide, and stored and concentrated in the gallbladder. The glucuronide is not reabsorbed; it is visualized in the intestinal tract.

SPECIAL PRECAUTIONS

• Do not administer to patients with severe renal or hepatorenal disease, or with gastrointestinal disorders that prevent absorption of the drug.
• Safe use in pregnancy has not been established; the benefits of cholecystography should be weighed against the possible risk to the fetus.
• In patients with severe advanced liver disease, a greater amount of unchanged material will be diverted for renal excretion, increasing the load on the kidneys.

- Use with caution in patients with coronary disease, especially those with coronary artery disease.
- Patients with pre-existing renal disease should not receive high doses.
- This agent has uricosuric activity.
- In susceptible individuals, renal irritation with reflex vesicular spasm with partial or complete renal shutdown may occur.

ADVERSE EFFECTS
CNS EFFECTS: dizziness, headache
RESPIRATORY EFFECTS: dry throat, burning on swallowing, sore throat
URINARY TRACT EFFECTS: mild stinging sensation during urination
GASTROINTESTINAL EFFECTS: nausea, vomiting, diarrhea, cramps, heartburn
HEMATOLOGIC EFFECTS: thrombocytopenia, petechiae
DERMATOLOGIC EFFECTS: rash, urticaria, pruritus, flushing

CLINICAL GUIDELINES
ADMINISTRATION:
- Patients with renal or hepatic disease should not be dehydrated before test and should drink liberal amounts of fluids after taking the tablets.
- Monitor blood pressure during and after administration of the medium.
- It is unnecessary and undesirable to dehydrate patients, particularly elderly patients.
- Use of large or repeated doses over a number of days is not recommended in elderly patients.
EFFECTS:
- Pseudoalbuminuria may be present for 3 days in response to certain chemical protein precipitation tests. Verify results by other procedures.
- Excretion of uric acid may be increased.

DRUG INTERACTIONS:
- Thyroid function tests, namely, PBI and RAI uptake studies which depend on iodine estimations will not reflect thyroid function for several months after administration of the contrast medium.
- T_3 resin uptake in free thyroxine assays will not be affected since they do not depend on iodine estimations.
- Liver function tests, namely, bilirubin, thymol turbidity, cephalin flocculation, and serum enzyme values are unaffected; BSP clearance may be delayed for up to 2 days.
OVERDOSAGE/ANTIDOTE:
- Cardiovascular collapse and respiratory distress may occur.
- There is no specific antidote; supportive therapy is suggested.

Iophendylate

PHARMACOLOGY
Iophendylate is a mixture of the isomers of ethyl iodophenyl undecanoate. This agent should be removed completely as possible, since complete absorption may take several years.

SPECIAL PRECAUTIONS
- Do not use in patients with a history of hypersensitivity to iodine or related compounds.
- May interfere with thyroid function tests.

ADVERSE EFFECTS
- Severe arachnoiditis causing headache, fever, meningitis, severe back pain, pain in the lower extremities, elevation of leukocyte count and protein content of the cerebrospinal fluid, lipid granuloma, obstruction of the ventricular system, venous intravasation which results in pulmonary embolization.

Ipodate Calcium
Ipodate Sodium

PHARMACOLOGY

The calcium and sodium salts of ipodate are water-soluble organic iodine compounds which are administered orally, absorbed from the gastrointestinal tract, excreted by the liver into the bile, and stored and concentrated in the gallbladder. The calcium salt is absorbed somewhat faster than the sodium salt and may appear in the ducts about 30 minutes after ingestion. Maximal opacification occurs within 10 hours and persists for about 45 minutes. Diagnostically adequate filling may take place within 5 hours or less after ingestion.

SPECIAL PRECAUTIONS

- Do not use in patients with a history of hypersensitivity to ipodate salts or related compounds.
- Patients sensitive to other iodinated compounds should receive these agents with extreme caution.
- Do not administer to patients with renal or hepatorenal disease, or with gastrointestinal disease, which prevents absorption.
- Safe use in pregnancy has not been established.
- Use caution in increasing the dosage above that recommended since the possibility of hypotension increases.
- In patients with combined renal and hepatic disease or severe renal impairment, anuria may occur.
- Renal toxicity has occurred in patients with liver dysfunction.

ADVERSE EFFECTS

CNS EFFECTS: headache
URINARY TRACT EFFECTS: dysuria
GASTROINTESTINAL EFFECTS: nausea, vomiting, diarrhea, abdominal pains

ALLERGIC EFFECTS: urticaria, rash, serum-sicknesslike reactions (fever, rash, arthralgia), anaphylactoid shock

CLINICAL GUIDELINES

ADMINISTRATION:
- Administer to patient with as little water as possible.

EFFECTS:
- Adverse effects are more likely to occur in patients with a history of allergy, asthma, hay fever or urticaria, and in those who have previously demonstrated hypersensitivity to iodine compounds.

DRUG INTERACTIONS:
- May interfere with some chemical determinations made on urine specimens.
- The results of thyroid function tests may be altered.

OVERDOSAGE/ANTIDOTE:
- Cardiovascular collapse and respiratory distress may occur.
- There is no specific antidote; supportive therapy is suggested.

Meglumine Diatrizoate
Sodium Diatrizoate

PHARMACOLOGY

Meglumine diatrizoate and sodium diatrizoate are water-soluble radiopaque agents for direct injection into blood vessels. These materials are transported rapidly through the bloodstream to the kidneys; they are excreted unchanged by glomerular filtration into the urine.

For visualization of the urinary tract, renal accumulation is such that maximal opacification occurs as early as 5 minutes after intravascular administration. After intramuscular administration, the contrast agent is absorbed rapidly and the renal system may be visualized within 20 to 60 minutes.

Intravascular administration provides visualization of the vessels in the path of the flow of the meglumine diatrizoate. Consequently, selective angiography may be performed following administration directly into veins or arteries.

SPECIAL PRECAUTIONS

• Administer with extreme caution to patients with a history of hypersensitivity to salts of diatrizoic acid or related compounds.
• Do not administer to patients with advanced uremia.
• Administration of intravascular contrast agents to patients with multiple myeloma presents a definite risk; anuria, progressive uremia, renal failure, and eventually death have occurred.
• Use extreme caution in patients with known or suspected pheochromocytoma; keep radiopaque material to a minimum; monitor blood pressure throughout the diagnostic procedure.
• Contrast media may promote sickling in individuals who are homozygous for sickle cell disease.
• Iodine-containing contrast agents may alter the results of thyroid function tests.
• Safe use in pregnancy has not been established.
• Hypersensitivity reactions have occurred, particularly in patients with a history of bronchial asthma or allergy or a previous reaction to contrast media.
• Postpone use in patients with known or suspected hepatitis or biliary disorders who have recently taken a cholecystographic contrast agent.
• Use with caution in patients severely debilitated or with marked hypertension or congestive heart failure.
• Use with caution in patients with impaired renal function.
• When used for retrograde cystourethrography, administer with caution to patients with active infections of the urinary tract.

ADVERSE EFFECTS

CNS EFFECTS: headache, dizziness, weakness, tremor, spasm, seizures, hemiparesis
RESPIRATORY EFFECTS: pulmonary edema
CARDIOVASCULAR EFFECTS: increase or decrease in blood pressure, ventricular fibrillation, cardiac arrest, thrombophlebitis
URINARY TRACT EFFECTS: temporary renal shutdown; with retrograde cystography, hematuria, perforation of the urethra or bladder, introduction of infection, oliguria, anuria
AUTONOMIC EFFECTS: flushing, generalized feeling of warmth, chills, fever, and sweating
GASTROINTESTINAL EFFECTS: nausea, vomiting, severe retching and choking, cramps
HEMATOLOGIC EFFECTS: neutropenia
ALLERGIC EFFECTS: wheezing, urticaria, sneezing, lacrimation, anaphylactoid reactions, facial or conjunctival petechiae, and edema
DERMATOLOGIC EFFECTS: pallor, rash, other eruptions, itching
OPHTHALMIC EFFECTS: impairment of vision
LOCAL EFFECTS: burning, stinging, venospasm or venous pain

CLINICAL GUIDELINES

ADMINISTRATION:
• Do not expose solution to strong light.
• In angiocardiography, caution patients that a feeling of bodily warmth in the area injected may be experienced.
• Use sterile technique in retrograde cystourethrography.
EFFECTS:
• Transient nausea and vomiting, tightness of chest or headache may occur.

DRUG INTERACTIONS:
• Meglumine diatrizoate and sodium diatrizoate may interfere with some chemical determinations in urine specimens.

OVERDOSAGE/ANTIDOTE:
• Cardiovascular collapse with hypotension, tachycardia, dyspnea progressing to unconsciousness have occurred. Severe respiratory difficulties including wheezing, bronchial and laryngeal spasms also have occurred.
• There is no specific antidote; supportive therapy is suggested.

Meglumine Iodipamide

PHARMACOLOGY

Meglumine Iodipamide is a radiopaque water-soluble iodine compound for intravenous administration. After intravenous administration, it is carried to the liver and secreted rapidly (10 to 15 minutes) in the bile. It permits visualization of the hepatic and common bile ducts, even in cholecystectomized patients. The gallbladder begins to fill within 1 hour after ingestion; maximal filling takes place in 2 to 2 1/2 hours. Elimination is in the feces. In the presence of severe liver damage, the agent is excreted by the kidneys.

When meglumine iodipamide is used for visualization of the uterus and fallopian tubes, this visualization is achieved immediately.

SPECIAL PRECAUTIONS

• Do not use in patients with a history of hypersensitivity to salts of iodipamide.
• Do not administer to patients with concomitant severe impairments of renal and hepatic function.
• Sickling has occurred in individuals who are homozygous for sickle cell disease.
• Iodine-containing contrast media may alter the results of thyroid function tests.
• Use with extreme caution in patients with a history of sensitivity to iodine or other contrast agents.
• Safe use in pregnancy has not been established.
• Do not use in the presence of acute pelvic inflammatory disease.
• Do not use for visualization of the uterus and tubes within 30 days after curettage or conization.

ADVERSE EFFECTS

CNS EFFECTS: restlessness, sensation of warmth, dizziness, fever, headache, tremors
CARDIOVASCULAR EFFECTS: hypotension, cardiac reactions, cyanosis
URINARY TRACT EFFECTS: alteration of renal function tests, renal failure
AUTONOMIC EFFECTS: perspiration, salivation, flushing, chills
GASTROINTESTINAL EFFECTS: pressure in upper abdomen, nausea, vomiting, abdominal pain and tenderness
ALLERGIC EFFECTS: sneezing, swollen eyelids, laryngospasm, respiratory difficulties, anaphylactoid reaction, urticaria, rashes, arthralgia, circulatory collapse.
DERMATOLOGIC EFFECTS: pallor

CLINICAL GUIDELINES

ADMINISTRATION:
• Administer only by slow intravenous injection.
• The solution may vary from essentially colorless to light amber. Solutions which have become substantially darker should not be used.
• Protect solution from strong light.
• Patient should be prepared by the usual preliminary measures for cholecystography, namely, low residue diet, castor oil the night before, and fasting.

EFFECTS:
• Visualization is rarely achieved in the presence of a serum bilirubin of 3 mg per 100 ml if the elevated bilirubin level is due to mechanical obstruction or hepatocellular damage.

DRUG INTERACTIONS:
• Contrast agents may interfere with some chemical determinations made in urine specimens; therefore, collect urine specimens prior to the administration of the test compound.

OVERDOSAGE/ANTIDOTE:
• Cardiovascular and respiratory collapse may occur.
• There is no specific antidote; supportive therapy is suggested.

Meglumine Iothalamate

PHARMACOLOGY
Meglumine iothalamate is a water-soluble, radiopaque, organic iodine compound which is formulated for intravenous administration. It facilitates visualization of blood vessels and the urinary tract.

SPECIAL PRECAUTIONS
• Do not use in patients with a history of hypersensitivity to iodine or related compounds.
• May interfere with thyroid function tests.
• Do not use in patients with renal impairment or severe cardiovascular disease.
• Safe use in pregnancy has not been established.

ADVERSE EFFECTS
RESPIRATORY EFFECTS: breathing difficulty
CARDIOVASCULAR EFFECTS: cardiovascular collapse

AUTONOMIC EFFECTS: flushing
GASTROINTESTINAL EFFECTS: nausea, vomiting, bitter taste

Propyliodone

PHARMACOLOGY
Propyliodone is a radiopaque agent suspended in peanut oil. Direct instillation into the bronchi results in well defined bronchograms for about 30 minutes. It is usually eliminated from the lungs in 7 to 10 days.

SPECIAL PRECAUTIONS
• Do not use in patients with a history of hypersensitivity to propyliodone or related compounds.
• May interfere with thyroid function tests.
• Do not administer to patients with pulmonary emphysema or bronchiectasis.

Sodium Acetrizoate

PHARMACOLOGY
Sodium acetrizoate is a radiopaque water-soluble organic iodine compound. When used for hysterosalpingography, it leaves no residue and permits adequate visualization of the uterus and fallopian tubes.

SPECIAL PRECAUTIONS
• Do not use in patients with a history of hypersensitivity to sodium acetrizoate or other iodine compounds.
• Administer with caution to patients with advanced renal disease.
• Do not use for hysterosalpingography in the presence of severe vaginal or cervical infection, existing or recent pelvic infec-

tion, marked cervical erosion or endocervicitis, and pregnancy.
• Do not use for hysterosalpingography during the immediate pre-or postmenstrual phase.
• Thyroid function tests may be altered.

Sodium Methiodal

PHARMACOLOGY

Sodium methiodal is a water-soluble radiopaque medium formulated for use in retrograde pyelography.

SPECIAL PRECAUTIONS
• Do not use in patients with a history of hypersensitivity to sodium methiodal or related compounds.
• Because of the possibility of acute renal shutdown, some investigators advise that the study should be done only on one side at a time.
• Safe use in pregnancy has not been established.

ADVERSE EFFECTS
URINARY TRACT EFFECTS: mucosal edema resulting in oliguria or anuria
AUTONOMIC EFFECTS: sweating
GASTROINTESTINAL EFFECTS: nausea, vomiting, excessive salivation
ALLERGIC EFFECTS: sneezing, coughing, nasal stuffiness, rhinitis, conjunctival symptoms, urticaria, pruritus, laryngospasm, angioneurotic edema, bronchospasm, anxiety, dyspnea, dizziness, convulsions, rarely anaphylactoid shock with cardiovascular collapse

CLINICAL GUIDELINES
ADMINISTRATION:
• Warm solution to body temperature before use.

• Solutions made from powder should be sterilized by boiling or autoclaving.
DRUG INTERACTIONS:
• May interfere with thyroid function tests.

Sodium Tyropanoate

PHARMACOLOGY

Sodium tyropanoate is chemically related to iopanoic acid and ipodate sodium. It is an organic iodine compound which after oral administration is absorbed from the duodenum. In the liver it is converted into radiopaque glucuronic acid conjugates which are concentrated by a functioning gallbladder. Upon contraction of the gallbladder, the extrahepatic ducts may be seen. Sodium tyropanoate also has a uricosuric effect.

SPECIAL PRECAUTIONS
• Do not use in patients with a history of hypersensitivity to salts of iopanoic acid.
• Do not use in patients with advanced hepatorenal disease, severe impairment of renal function, or severe gastrointestinal disorders that prevent absorption.
• Safe use in pregnancy has not been established.
• Do not use in children under 12 years of age.
• The uricosuric effect should be considered in patients with impaired renal function.

ADVERSE EFFECTS
CNS EFFECTS: weakness, dizziness, fatigue, light-headedness
RESPIRATORY EFFECTS: dyspnea, laryngotracheal edema rarely
URINARY TRACT EFFECTS: dysuria

AUTONOMIC EFFECTS: perspiration
GASTROINTESTINAL EFFECTS: nausea, vomiting, diarrhea, abdominal cramps and discomfort, difficulty in swallowing
ALLERGIC EFFECTS: rash, pruritus, and urticaria
MUSCULOSKELETAL EFFECTS: pain and cramps in the limbs

CLINICAL GUIDELINES

ADMINISTRATION:
• Administer to patient with as little water as possible.

EFFECTS:
• Excretion of uric acid may be increased.
DRUG INTERACTIONS:
• Elevation of protein bound iodine may last for several months and false positive urine albumin tests for several days.
• May interfere with some chemical determinations made on urine specimens.
OVERDOSAGE/ANTIDOTE:
• Cardiovascular collapse and/or respiratory distress may occur.
• There is no specific antidote; supportive therapy is suggested.

Miscellaneous Agents

GENERAL CLINICAL USES

The group of miscellaneous diagnostic agents includes the dyes, sugars, anticholinesterases, and hormones which are used to evaluate the function of the renal, hepatic, gastrointestinal, and endocrine systems. The specific clinical uses for each of these agents are indicated in the following section.

SPECIFIC PRODUCTS AND USES

USE	GENERIC NAME	TRADE NAME
Circulatory System:		
blood volume	Evans blue	(G)*
circulation time; blood vessel permeability and patency	fluorescein sodium	(G)
cardiac output	indocyanine green	CARDIO-GREEN
Urinary System:		
tubular excretory mass; estimation of effective renal plasma flow	aminohippurate sodium (PAH)	(G)

*(G) designates availability as a generic product.

(continued facing page)

USE	GENERIC NAME	TRADE NAME
renal function; renal plasma flow	aminohippuric acid	(G)
index of relative renal function; localization of ureteral orifices during cystography	indigotindisulfonate sodium	(G)
glomular filtration rate	inulin	(G)
	mannitol	(G)
renal blood flow	phenosulfonphthalein	PHENOL RED
Gastrointestinal Tract: gastric acidity	betazole hydrochloride	HISTALOG
gastric acidity; secretion for gastric analysis	histamine phosphate	(G)
gastric acid secretion	azuresin	(G)
	pentagastrin	PEPTAVALON
gallbladder function	sincalide	(G)
	sodium dehydrocholate	KINEVAC
liver function; liver blood flow	indocyanine green	CARDIO-GREEN
	sulfobromophthalein (BSP)	(G)
Reproductive Tract: Fallopian tube patency	phenolsulfonphthalein	PHENOL RED
Endocrine Disorders: thyroid function	protirelin	THYPINONE
pituitary function; ACTH test	metyrapone	METOPIRONE
parathyroid function	parathyroid hormone	(G)
pancreatic dysfunction	secretin	(G)
Miscellaneous Disorders: myasthenia gravis diagnosis	edrophonium chloride	TENSILON
	neostigmine methylsulfate	PROSTIGMIN METHYLSULFATE
amyloidosis	congo red	(G)

Aminohippuric Acid
Aminohippurate Sodium (PAH)

PHARMACOLOGY

Paraminohippuric acid or sodium aminohippurate, after intravenous administration, is filtered by the renal glomeruli and secreted by the renal tubular epithelium. Consequently, effective renal plasma flow and the functional capacity of the tubular excretory mechanism can then be evaluated.

SPECIAL PRECAUTIONS

• Do not use PAH diagnostic procedures in patients receiving sulfonamides; color re-

actions develop between sulfonamides and PAH-assay reagents.
• Concurrent administration of drugs that share a common excretory pathway with PAH such as penicillin or those that inhibit renal tubular transport such as probenecid or those that have a uricosuric effect such as the salicylates may interfere with PAH clearance.

ADVERSE EFFECTS
CNS EFFECTS: sensation of sudden warmth
GASTROINTESTINAL EFFECTS: nausea, vomiting

CLINICAL GUIDELINES
ADMINISTRATION:
• Infuse drug slowly to avoid nausea, vomiting, and sudden warmth.
DRUG INTERACTIONS:
• Probenecid inhibits tubular secretion of PAH.
• Salicylates which have a uricosuric effect may interfere with PAH clearance.

Azuresin

PHARMACOLOGY
Azuresin, an ion exchange resin linked with the dye, azure A, is displaced by the hydrogen ion. After oral administration the azure A is liberated in the presence of free gastric hydrochloric acid in the stomach. The azure A is then absorbed and excreted in the urine where it can be detected colorimetrically. Visual estimation of the dye content of a urine specimen usually collected 2 hours after administration and compared with a control, will indicate the presence or absence of hydrochloric acid in the stomach. Both false negative and false positive results have occurred.

SPECIAL PRECAUTIONS
• In the presence of pyloric obstruction, severe hepatic or renal disease, impaired intestinal absorption, vomiting, marked dehydration, bladder obstruction, total or subtotal gastrectomy, severe diarrhea, or vomiting, inaccurate results may be obtained.
• Do not use in patients with a history of hypersensitivity to azuresin or related compounds.
• Azuresin cannot be used to demonstrate quantitive variation in the amount of free gastric hydrochloric acid.
• Oral administration of salts containing barium, iron, calcium, magnesium, or aluminum should be discontinued for 48 hours prior to testing.

ADVERSE EFFECTS
• Allergic reactions including urticaria or pruritus rarely.

CLINICAL GUIDELINES
ADMINISTRATION:
• Allow 5 days before repeating the test to allow complete excretion of azure A.
EFFECTS:
• Caution patients that the urine may be colored blue or green for a few days after the test.
DRUG INTERACTIONS:
• Salts of barium, iron, calcium, magnesium, or aluminum will interfere with the test.

Betazole Hydrochloride

PHARMACOLOGY
Betazole hydrochloride, an isomer of histamine, has a pronounced effect on glandular secretions of the gastric mucosa; it stimulates copious flow of highly acidic gastric secretions. It has a slower onset and a

more prolonged duration of action than does histamine. Its effect on blood pressure, gastric acid secretion, and smooth muscle is similar to histamine.

SPECIAL PRECAUTIONS
• Patients with allergic diathesis may react severely to betazole hydrochloride.
• Do not use in patients with a history of hypersensitivity to betazole hydrochloride or related compounds.
• Use great caution in administering betazole hydrochloride to patients with a history of asthma, heart disease, recent gastrointestinal bleeding, or moderate to severe allergic disease.
• Safe use in pregnancy has not been established.

ADVERSE EFFECTS
CNS EFFECTS: headache, syncope, weakness
AUTONOMIC EFFECTS: flushing, hyperhidrosis, sense of warmth
ALLERGIC EFFECTS: urticaria

CLINICAL GUIDELINES
ADMINISTRATION:
• Oral administration is not recommended.
EFFECTS:
• Weakness and syncope may occur.
• The maximum secretory response usually occurs in about 45 minutes and lasts approximately 2 1/2 hours.
DRUG INTERACTIONS:
• Antihistaminic drugs do not affect the stimulation of gastric secretion by betazole hydrochloride.
OVERDOSAGE/ANTIDOTE:
• Hypotension or acute asthma may follow accidental or intentional overdosage. Urticaria also may occur. Administration of epinephrine and antihistamines may be indicated.

• Up to 200 mg have been administered without apparent harm; a higher incidence and severity of side effects has occurred with the high doses. There is no specific antidote.

Congo Red

PHARMACOLOGY
Congo red administered intravenously is retained by the abnormal amyloid deposits. Following congo red staining, amyloid deposits are characterized by a yellow green birefringence when exposed to polarization microscopy.

SPECIAL PRECAUTIONS
• Inject slowly to avoid thrombosis.
• Safe use in pregnancy has not been established.
• Do not use in patients with a history of hypersensitivity to congo red or related compounds.

ADVERSE EFFECTS
• Rare idiosyncratic effects, including death, have occurred.

CLINICAL GUIDELINES
ADMINISTRATION:
• Use water for injection as the carrier since congo red may flocculate in sodium chloride injection.

Edrophonium Chloride

PHARMACOLOGY
Edrophonium chloride is an anticholinesterase agent. It has a short and rapid action which is manifested within 30 to 60 seconds after administration and lasts an average of 10 minutes. It is useful in the differential diagnosis of myasthenia gravis.

An increase in muscle strength is produced.

SPECIAL PRECAUTIONS
• Do not use in patients with a history of hypersensitivity to edrophonium chloride or related compounds or other anticholinesterase agents.
• Do not use in patients with intestinal or urinary obstruction of the mechanical type.
• Use with caution in patients with bronchial asthma or cardiac dysrhythmias.
• Safe use in pregnancy has not been established.
• Patients may develop "anticholinesterase insensitivity" for brief or prolonged periods.

ADVERSE EFFECTS
CNS EFFECTS: convulsions, dysphonia
RESPIRATORY EFFECTS: increased tracheo-bronchial secretions, laryngospasm, bronchiolar constriction, paralysis of muscles of respiration, central respiratory paralysis
CARDIOVASCULAR EFFECTS: bradycardia, cardiac standstill, arrhythmia, fall in cardiac output leading to hypotension
URINARY TRACT EFFECTS: increased frequency, incontinence
AUTONOMIC EFFECTS: diaphoresis
GASTROINTESTINAL EFFECTS: increased salivary, gastric, and intestinal secretion, nausea, vomiting, increased peristalsis, diarrhea, abdominal cramps, dysphagia
OPHTHALMIC EFFECTS: increased lacrimation, pupillary constriction, spasms of accommodation, dyplopia, conjunctival hyperemia
MUSCULOSKELETAL EFFECTS: dysarthria, weakness, fasciculations

CLINICAL GUIDELINES
ADMINISTRATION:
• When administering anticholinergic drugs, a syringe containing atropine should be immediately available.

EFFECTS:
• Watch for signs of cholinergic reactions.
DRUG INTERACTIONS:
• Edrophonium chloride is useful when a curare antagonist is needed to reverse neuromuscular block by curare, tubocurarine, gallamine triethiodate, or dimethyl tubocurarine. It is not effective against decamethonium bromine and succinyl chloride.
OVERDOSAGE/ANTIDOTE:
• Overdosage is characterized by severe cholinergic reactions (exaggerations of the adverse effects).
• Atropine sulfate is the antidote; doses may reach 1.2 mg intravenously initially. Pralidoxime chloride, a cholinesterase reactivator, may be given intravenously. Muscarinelike symptoms, namely, nausea, vomiting, diarrhea, sweating, and increased bronchial and salivary secretions, may occur. The airway may be obstructed by bronchial secretions.

Evans Blue

PHARMACOLOGY
• Evans blue, an azo dye, after intravenous administration, is tightly bound to plasma albumin and remains within the intravascular compartment. Consequently, it may be used for the colorimetric estimation of blood (plasma) volume.

SPECIAL PRECAUTIONS
• Safe use in pregnancy has not been established.
• Do not use in patients with a history of hypersensitivity to Evans blue.

CLINICAL GUIDELINES
ADMINISTRATION:
• Avoid extravsation into the perivascular tissues.

EFFECTS:
• The sclerae and skin may be stained blue; this may persist for several weeks.

Fluorescein Sodium

PHARMACOLOGY

Fluorescein sodium is a negatively charged dye which may be administered intravenously or intra-arterially. The appearance of fluorescence in the lips, eyes, intact skin, or wheal may be taken as the end point. Relative circulation times may be determined as well as the adequacy of circulation to an extremity.

SPECIAL PRECAUTIONS

• Do not use in patients with a history of hypersensitivity to fluorescein sodium or related compounds.
• Use cautiously in patients with a history of allergies, asthma, or hypersensitivity.

ADVERSE EFFECTS

CNS EFFECTS: headache, syncope
RESPIRATORY EFFECTS: transient dyspnea
CARDIOVASCULAR EFFECTS: cardiac arrest, basilar artery ischemia, thrombophlebitis at injection site, severe shock, hypotension
URINARY TRACT EFFECTS: urine is bright yellow and fluoresces for 24 to 36 hours after administration
AUTONOMIC EFFECTS: pyrexia
GASTROINTESTINAL EFFECTS: nausea, vomiting, strange taste, gastrointestinal disturbances
ALLERGIC EFFECTS: urticaria, pruritus, angioneurotic edema
DERMATOLOGIC EFFECTS: temporary yellowish skin discoloration

CLINICAL GUIDELINES

ADMINISTRATION:
• Solutions for injection must be freshly prepared and sterilized.

EFFECTS:
• Fluorescence of the skin may persist for several hours and the dye appears in the urine for a period of 16 to 31 hours.
• Caution patient that the skin may be stained faintly yellow.

OVERDOSAGE/ANTIDOTE:
• Up to 1250 mg have been well tolerated in adults. For emergency use, intravenous epinephrine 1:1000 should be available at the time of administration. An antihistamine should also be accessible.
• There is no specific antidote.

Histamine Phosphate

PHARMACOLOGY

Histamine phosphate stimulates the exocrine glands, smooth muscle, and vascular system principally. It increases the volume and acidity of the gastric juice when administered subcutaneously in the gastric histamine test.

Histamine phosphate administered intravenously may be used for the presumptive diagnosis of pheochromocytoma.

SPECIAL PRECAUTIONS

• Epinephrine must always be available to counteract the effects of histamine.
• Do not use in elderly patients or in those with hypotension, hypertension, heart disease, an unstable vasomotor system, or recent upper gastrointestinal tract hemorrhage.
• Do not administer intravenously for the gastric histamine test.
• Safe use in pregnancy has not been established.

ADVERSE EFFECTS

CNS EFFECTS: dizziness, weakness, headache, nervousness, flushing, syncope, faintness, collapse with convulsions

RESPIRATORY EFFECTS: bronchial constriction, dyspnea, asthma

CARDIOVASCULAR EFFECTS: marked hypertension, hypotension, tachycardia, palpitations

GASTROINTESTINAL EFFECTS: abdominal cramps, symptoms of peptic ulcer, diarrhea, nausea, vomiting, metallic taste

ALLERGIC EFFECTS: urticaria, generalized allergic manifestations

OPHTHALMIC EFFECTS: blurred vision, visual disturbances

LOCAL EFFECTS: erythema, edema

CLINICAL GUIDELINES

ADMINISTRATION:
• Take care not to administer too rapidly or in excessive dosages.
• Monitor blood pressure frequently during intravenous administration.

EFFECTS:
• Attacks of severe asthma or other serious allergic conditions may be precipitated, particularly in patients with bronchial disease.
• Symptoms of peptic ulcer may occur.

DRUG INTERACTIONS:
• Administration of antihistamines prior to testing may diminish or counteract most of the undesirable effects without interfering with stimulation of gastric secretion.

OVERDOSAGE/ANTIDOTE:
• Excessive dosage or overdosage may result in asthma, severe headache, acute circulatory failure, shock, and death. If accidental overdosage is discovered early, temporary application of a tourniquet proximal to the injection site may be tried to slow down the absorption of the drug.
• Antidotes to histamine are epinephrine hydrochloride, 0.1 to 0.5 ml of a 1:1000 aqueous solution given subcutaneously; antihistamines are useful in cases of mild allergic reactions. Phentolamine may be considered to depress any alarming increase in blood pressure.

Indigotindisulfonate Sodium

PHARMACOLOGY

Indigotindisulfonate sodium, an indigo carmine dye, after intravenous administration, is excreted by the kidneys and is visible at the ureteral orifice within 10 minutes. The differential appearance of the dye provides an index of relative renal function.

SPECIAL PRECAUTIONS

• Do not use in patients with a history of hypersensitivity to this agent or related compounds.
• In patients with a history of allergy, test for hypersensitivity before the drug is used diagnostically.
• Safe use in pregnancy has not been established.

ADVERSE EFFECTS

RESPIRATORY EFFECTS: bronchial constriction

DERMATOLOGIC EFFECTS: pruritus, rash

Indocyanine Green

PHARMACOLOGY

Indocyanine green, administered intravenously, is cleared rapidly from the circulation by the hepatic cells and excreted into the bile in an unconjugated form. Excretion is only by the liver. When indocyanine green is used for dye dilution curves, a known amount of dye is injected rapidly as a single bolus into selected sites in the vascular system. The dye-blood mixture is analyzed by an oximeter or densitometer.

SPECIAL PRECAUTIONS

• Do not use in patients with a history of hypersensitivity to indocyanine green, or iodides, or related compounds.

• Thyroid function tests may be inaccurate for at least 1 week following administration of indocyanine green.

• Safe use in pregnancy has not been established.

• Since indocyanine green contains a small amount of sodium iodide, use with extreme caution in patients with a history of allergy to iodides.

ADVERSE EFFECTS

ALLERGIC EFFECTS: anaphylactic shock has occurred in one patient and allergic reactions in uremic patients undergoing hemodialysis.

CLINICAL GUIDELINES

ADMINISTRATION:

• Solutions are unstable; prepare immediately before use.

• Use sterile technique in handling the dye solution.

EFFECTS:

• The dye is stable in whole blood and plasma so that samples may be read hours later.

DRUG INTERACTIONS:

• The absorption peak is reduced by sodium bisulfite, which is frequently a component of heparin preparations.

• Probenecid, in doses from 25 to 100 mg/kg, has been shown to affect the hepatic uptake, storage, and removal of indocyanine green in dogs; this has not been reported in humans but should be considered.

• Do not perform radioactive iodine uptake studies for at least 1 week after use of indocyanine green.

OVERDOSAGE/ANTIDOTE:

• In a group of volunteers who received not less than 6 and as many as 10 consecutive cardiac output determinations, no toxicity was reported.

Inulin

PHARMACOLOGY

Inulin is an inert polysaccharide which is filtered freely at the renal glomeruli. It is neither secreted nor reabsorbed by the renal tubules. Thus, its rate of clearance is equal to the glomerular filtration rate. In the adult male, the inulin clearance is approximately 130 ml/min.

SPECIAL PRECAUTIONS

• Inulin may be used in large quantities to produce an osmotic diuresis and raise serum osmolality significantly.

ADVERSE EFFECTS

• Pyogenic reactions infrequently.

Mannitol

PHARMACOLOGY

Mannitol is a 6-carbon sugar alcohol which is virtually inert metabolically in humans. After intravenous administration, mannitol is filtered by the glomeruli; however, as much as 10 percent may be reabsorbed by the tubules but it is not secreted by the tubular cells. The reabsorption by the tubules introduces an immeasurable variable in the test. Mannitol is an obligatory osmotic diuretic.

SPECIAL PRECAUTIONS

• In large quantities mannitol serves as a diuretic.

• Do not use in patients with edema caused by metabolic abnormalities or cardiac failure.

- Do not use in patients who are not adequately hydrated or whose renal function is known to be severely impaired.
- Do not use in patients with a history of hypersensitivity to mannitol or related compounds.
- Do not use in patients with anuria due to severe renal disease, severe pulmonary congestion or frank pulmonary edema, or active intracranial bleeding except during craniotomy.
- Safe use in pregnancy has not been established.

ADVERSE EFFECTS

CNS EFFECTS: convulsions, fever, slight dizziness, headache
RESPIRATORY EFFECTS: subjective sensations of chest constriction or pain, pulmonary congestion, rhinitis
CARDIOVASCULAR EFFECTS: thrombophlebitis, hypotension, tachycardia, anginalike chest pains
URINARY TRACT EFFECTS: marked diuresis, urinary retention
AUTONOMIC EFFECTS: chills
GASTROINTESTINAL EFFECTS: thirst, nausea, vomiting
METABOLIC AND ENDOCRINE EFFECTS: hypochloremia, electrolyte and fluid imbalance, edema
ALLERGIC EFFECTS: urticaria
DERMATOLOGIC EFFECTS: rash
OPHTHALMIC EFFECTS: blurred vision

CLINICAL GUIDELINES

ADMINISTRATION:
- Inject slowly (approximately 20 ml/minute) to maintain an adequate measurable plasma concentration.

EFFECTS:
- Excretion of sodium and chloride is enhanced.

DRUG INTERACTIONS:
- Electrolyte-free mannitol solution should not be given conjointly with blood.

OVERDOSAGE/ANTIDOTE:
- Overdosage is characterized by marked diuresis.
- There is no specific antidote.

Metyrapone

PHARMACOLOGY

Metyrapone interferes with steroidogenesis in the adrenal cortex. Consequently, it results in reduction of the production of cortisol, corticosterone, and aldosterone. The decreased production of cortisol greatly increases secretion of corticotropin (ACTH) in normal individuals. The response in patients with hypopituitarism is reduced.

SPECIAL PRECAUTIONS

- Do not administer to patients with chronic adrenocortical insufficiency.
- Do not use in patients with a history of hypersensitivity to metyrapone or related compounds.
- Safe use in pregnancy has not been established.
- All corticosteroid therapy must be discontinued prior to and during metyrapone testing.
- Ability of adrenals to respond to exogenous ACTH should be demonstrated before metyrapone is employed as a test.
- The drug may induce acute adrenal insufficiency in patients with reduced adrenal secretory capacity.

ADVERSE EFFECTS

CNS EFFECTS: dizziness, vertigo, headache, drowsiness, sedation
CARDIOVASCULAR EFFECTS: rarely thrombophlebitis with intravenous administration
GASTROINTESTINAL EFFECTS: nausea, abdominal discomfort
ALLERGIC EFFECTS: rash

CLINICAL GUIDELINES
ADMINISTRATION:
• Nausea may be minimized by administering the drug with milk or food.
EFFECTS:
• After oral administration maximal urinary excretion occurs in about 24 hours.
• After intravenous administration maximal urinary excretion occurs the same day.
DRUG INTERACTIONS:
• Erroneous results in pituitary function as determined by the metyrapone test may occur in patients taking diphenylhydantoin for as long as 2 weeks following cessation of therapy.
• A subnormal response may also occur in pregnant women and in patients on estrogen therapy.

Neostigmine Methylsulfate

PHARMACOLOGY
Neostigmine methylsulfate enhances cholinergic action by facilitating the transmission of impulses across the myoneural junction. It inhibits the destruction of acetylcholine at neuromuscular junctions. In normal subjects, neostigmine fasciculations will occur, whereas in patients with myasthenia gravis, they are absent. Neostigmine improves muscle strength in patients with myasthenia gravis.

SPECIAL PRECAUTIONS
• Do not use in patients with mechanical intestinal or urinary obstructions.
• Do not use in patients with a history of hypersensitivity to neostigmine methylsulfate or related compounds.
• Use with caution in patients who have asthma.
• When large doses are administered, prior to simultaneous injection of atropine sulfate may be advisable.

ADVERSE EFFECTS
RESPIRATORY EFFECTS: increased bronchial secretions
AUTONOMIC EFFECTS: diaphoresis
GASTROINTESTINAL EFFECTS: nausea, vomiting, diarrhea, abdominal cramps, increased salivation
OPHTHALMIC EFFECTS: miosis
MUSCULOSKELETAL EFFECTS: muscle cramps, fasciculations, weakness

CLINICAL GUIDELINES
OVERDOSAGE/ANTIDOTE:
• Overdosage may result in cholinergic crisis, which is characterized by increasing muscle weakness which, through involvement of the muscles of respiration, may result in death.
• The antidote for cholinergic agents is atropine. Atropine may abolish or alleviate gastrointestinal side effects or other muscarinic reactions.

Parathyroid Hormone

PHARMACOLOGY, SPECIAL PRECAUTIONS, ADVERSE EFFECTS, CLINICAL GUIDELINES
For detailed information, see Chapter 15, page 563.

Pentagastrin

PHARMACOLOGY
Pentagastrin acts as a physiologic gastric acid secretagogue. After subcutaneous administration it stimulates gastric acid secretion in approximately 10 minutes with a peak response occurring in 20 to 30 minutes. The effect usually lasts 60 to 80 minutes.

SPECIAL PRECAUTIONS
• Do not use in patients with a history of hypersensitivity to pentagastrin.

- Safe use in pregnancy has not been established.
- Use with caution in patients with biliary, hepatic, or gastric disease.

ADVERSE EFFECTS

CNS EFFECTS: dizziness, faintness, lightheadedness, drowsiness, sinking feeling, tiredness, headache
RESPIRATORY EFFECTS: shortness of breath
CARDIOVASCULAR EFFECTS: flushing, tachycardia
AUTONOMIC EFFECTS: generalized burning sensation
GASTROINTESTINAL EFFECTS: abdominal pain, desire to defecate, nausea, bile collected in specimen, vomiting, borborygmi, blood-tinged mucus
ALLERGIC EFFECTS: hypersensitivity reactions
OPHTHALMIC EFFECTS: blurred vision
LOCAL EFFECTS: pain at site of injection
MUSCULOSKELETAL EFFECTS: heavy sensation in arms and legs, tingling in fingers

CLINICAL GUIDELINES

ADMINISTRATION:
- Effect begins in about 10 minutes; peak is in about 20 to 30 minutes.

EFFECTS:
- There are insufficient data to establish a dose in children.

OVERDOSAGE/ANTIDOTE:
- Overdosage is characterized by an exaggeration of the adverse effects. Gastric acid secretion may be inhibited.
- There is no specific antidote.

Phenolsulfonphthalein (Phenol Red, PSP)

PHARMACOLOGY

After intramuscular or intravenous administration, phenolsulfonphthalein is bound almost entirely to the plasma proteins. The drug is excreted partially by glomerular filtration and primarily by tubular secretion. The dye appears at the ureteral orifice within about 2 minutes after intravenous administration. Since some of the dye is excreted in the bile, supranormal values are suggestive of hepatic insufficiency. The PSP test is not a renal clearance procedure but is based on the observation that about 30 percent of an intramuscular dose is excreted by adults within 20 minutes and 30 to 70 percent within 2 hours.

SPECIAL PRECAUTIONS
- Administer with extreme caution to patients with a history of allergy.
- Idiosyncratic reactions requiring treatment with an antihistamine and/or epinephrine may occur.
- Avoid concurrent administration of any medication which might discolor the urine for 24 hours before performing a PSP test.
- Safe use in pregnancy has not been established.
- Excretion of PSP is diminished in the presence of cardiac failure, particularly after intramuscular administration.

ADVERSE EFFECTS
- Idiosyncratic reactions have occurred occasionally.

CLINICAL GUIDELINES

ADMINISTRATION:
- Patients should empty bladder prior to administration of drug and force fluids 1 to 1 1/2 hours before test.
- The solution must be made isotonic and alkaline with sodium bicarbonate prior to use.
- Intravenous administration is usually preferred since absorption after intramuscular administration may be somewhat erratic.

EFFECTS:
• The urine will be colored red.

DRUG INTERACTIONS:
• Patients with gout or those receiving acidic drugs may show false impairment of renal function owing to competitive inhibition of transport.
• Synthetic weakly acidic compounds—pyridone N-acetic acid, PAH, certain glucuronides, ethereal sulfates, and penicillins—compete for this secretory mechanism.

Protirelin

PHARMACOLOGY

Protirelin, a synthetic tripeptide structurally similar to naturally occurring thyrotropin-releasing hormone, increases the release of thyroid-stimulating hormone (TSH) from the anterior pituitary. Following intravenous administration, the plasma half-life is approximately 5 minutes. TSH levels reach a peak in 20 to 30 minutes. The decline is slow, reaching baseline levels after approximately 3 hours.

SPECIAL PRECAUTIONS

• Transient changes in blood pressure occur frequently.
• Thyroid hormone reduces the TSH response to protirelin; patients should be taken off thyroid medications containing levothyroxine (T_4) at least 14 days before testing.
• It is not advisable to withdraw maintenance doses of adrenocortical drugs used in therapy of known hypopituitarism.
• Safe use in pregnancy has not been established.

ADVERSE EFFECTS

CNS EFFECTS: light-headedness, headache, anxiety, tingling sensation, drowsiness

RESPIRATORY EFFECTS: tightness in throat, pressure in chest

CARDIOVASCULAR EFFECTS: increased systolic pressure (usually less than 30 mm Hg) and/or increased diastolic pressure (usually less than 20 mm Hg)

URINARY TRACT EFFECTS: urge to urinate

AUTONOMIC EFFECTS: flushed sensation, dry mouth, sweating

GASTROINTESTINAL EFFECTS: nausea, bad taste, abdominal discomfort

METABOLIC AND ENDOCRINE EFFECTS: breast engorgement and leakage in lactating women

CLINICAL GUIDELINES

ADMINISTRATION:
• The patient should be supine when the drug is administered and blood pressure should be monitored during the first 15 minutes.

DRUG INTERACTIONS:
• Chronic administration of levodopa may inhibit TSH response to protirelin.
• Prolonged treatment with the glucocorticoids at physiological doses has no significant effect on the TSH response to thyrotropin-releasing hormone, but the administration of pharmacological doses of the steroids reduces the TSH response.
• Elevated serum lipids may interfere with the TSH assay.

Secretin

PHARMACOLOGY

Secretin, a hormone obtained from porcine duodenal mucosa, after intravenous administration, increases the bicarbonate content and volume of pancreatic secretion. Reduced bicarbonate content and volume are indicative of pancreatic insufficiency.

SPECIAL PRECAUTIONS

• Do not use in patients with a history of atopic asthma, a history of allergy, or a positive skin test.
• Conduct skin test in patients with a history of hypersensitivity, allergy, or asthma.
• Use with caution if at all in patients with acute pancreatitis.
• Special precautions should be used in patients who are sensitive to penicillin.

ADVERSE EFFECTS

CARDIOVASCULAR EFFECTS: vasomotor reactions

CLINICAL GUIDELINES

ADMINISTRATION:
• The solution should be freshly prepared before each administration.
• Administer intravenously slowly.
EFFECTS:
• Volume reductions are indicative of pancreatic duct obstruction.

Sincalide

PHARMACOLOGY

Sincalide, administered intravenously, produces a substantial reduction in gallbladder size by causing this organ to contract. The gallbladder contracts maximally in 5 to 15 minutes, in comparison to a fatty meal which causes progressive contraction in about 40 minutes. A 40 percent reduction in radiographic area of the gallbladder is considered satisfactory contraction.

SPECIAL PRECAUTIONS

• Safe use in pregnancy or in children has not been established.
• Stimulation of gallbladder contraction in patients with small gallbladder stones could lead to the evacuation of the stones from the gallbladder, resulting in their lodging in the cystic duct or in the common bile duct.

ADVERSE EFFECTS

CNS EFFECTS: dizziness
AUTONOMIC EFFECTS: flushing
GASTROINTESTINAL EFFECTS: abdominal discomfort or pain, urge to defecate, nausea

CLINICAL GUIDELINES

DRUG INTERACTIONS:
• Concurrent administration with secretin stimulates pancreatic secretion and increases the volume of pancreatic secretion and the output of bicarbonate and protein (enzymes) by the gland.

Sodium Dehydrocholate

PHARMACOLOGY

Sodium dehydrocholate administered intravenously results in an increase in the volume of bile excreted; the increase is 100 to 200 percent above the normal flow.

SPECIAL PRECAUTIONS

• The use of sodium dehydrocholate for determining circulation time as part of a routine cardiovascular diagnostic study is not recommended because of the severe adverse reactions which have occurred with this drug.
• Safe use in pregnancy has not been established.
• Do not administer in patients with biliary tract obstruction, acute hepatitis, or a history of previous adverse reactions to the drug.
• Use with caution in patients with a history of allergy.
• Avoid doing circulation time determinations in patients in an obviously critical or terminal state.

ADVERSE EFFECTS

CNS EFFECTS: headache, faintness
RESPIRATORY EFFECTS: dyspnea
CARDIOVASCULAR EFFECTS: tachycardia, hypotension

AUTONOMIC EFFECTS: sweating, chills, and fever

GASTROINTESTINAL EFFECTS: nausea, vomiting, diarrhea, abdominal discomfort

ALLERGIC EFFECTS: anaphylactoid reactions, urticaria

DERMATOLOGIC EFFECTS: erythema, pruritus

CLINICAL GUIDELINES

ADMINISTRATION:
* Avoid extravasation into the perivascular tissues; a moderate local reaction, consisting of a mild fleeting pain which subsides without inflammation, or a more severe reaction, with pain, redness, and swelling, lasting for several hours or days, may occur.

Sulfobromophthalein Sodium (BSP)

PHARMACOLOGY
Sulfobromophthalein sodium, after intravenous administration, is bound to plasma proteins and released in liver cells. In the liver approximately 80 percent is conjugated; the conjugated compounds are excreted in bile. Clearance depends upon the ability of the hepatic cells to absorb, conjugate, and excrete sulfobromophthalein sodium. In the normal liver the dye is excreted within 30 minutes.

SPECIAL PRECAUTIONS
* Do not use in patients with a history of hypersensitivity to sulfobromophthalein or related compounds.
* Note that allergic reactions usually occur in patients who have previously received sulfobromophthalein sodium.
* Do not use in newborn and premature infants since they do not possess the enzymes for conjugating BSP.
* Administer with extreme caution, if at all, in patients in whom a previous perivascular infiltration has occurred, in known asthmatic patients, and in patients with a history of any allergic disease.
* Never inject into an artery.

ADVERSE EFFECTS
CNS EFFECTS: vertigo, fever, chills, malaise

CARDIOVASCULAR EFFECTS: hypotension, tachycardia

GASTROINTESTINAL EFFECTS: nausea, vomiting

ALLERGIC EFFECTS: urticaria, pruritus, anaphylactic reactions rarely

CLINICAL GUIDELINES
ADMINISTRATION:
* Patients should be fasting and resting.
* Avoid extravasation during administration; cellular destruction will occur; avoid intra-arterial injection.
* Never administer until the crystals are completely dissolved.
* Advise patient that the urine and stool may be red.

EFFECTS:
* Extravasation may result in the tissues becoming indurated, painful, and occasionally photosensitive. If it occurs, elevate the extremity and apply ice packs immediately.

DRUG INTERACTIONS:
* Anabolic steroids, certain estrogens, androgens, B vitamins, and oral contraceptive agents interfere with BSP excretion in nearly all patients.
* Morphine, meperidine, amidine and amine oxidase inhibitors occasionally give slightly elevated readings.
* Patients almost invariably experience thrombophlebitis if BSP is injected into the same arm a few days after injection of a radiopaque substance.
* Contrast agents used in gallbladder studies interfere with BSP clearance and excretion; allow 1 week between tests.

OVERDOSAGE/ANTIDOTE:
* Preparations to deal with an acute anaphylactoid reaction should be on hand when the BSP is administered.
* There is no specific antidote.

20

Drug overdosage, intoxication, abuse

Drug overdosage or intoxication or abuse is caused by administration of a drug dose exceeding the recognized maximal therapeutic dose or administration of consecutive doses within a time less than recommended by established therapeutic guidelines. Essentially it is the result of improper or incorrect drug use, regardless of the route of administration. Overdosage or intoxication may be intentional or accidental.

The results of overdosage may be partial or complete loss of consciousness, depression, impairment of vital functions, or enhancement of adverse or pharmacologic drug effects. Regardless of the drug ingested, certain emergency actions must be taken immediately:

1. Establish an airway to assure adequate pulmonary ventilation.
2. Support circulation by administration of intravenous fluids.

3. Empty stomach by inducing vomiting or by gastric lavage. Gastric lavage is indicated within 3 hours of ingestion of the product. However, induction of vomiting is the preferred treatment since it has been found that the stomach is emptied more completely following vomiting than by gastric lavage. Specimens of vomitus should be preserved for analysis.

4. Monitor vital signs at least every 15 minutes.

5. Maintain homeostasis—measure electrolytes and urine output, use indwelling urethral catheter, monitor electrocardiogram.

6. Ascertain by diagnostic testing type or types of drugs ingested, timing of ingestion, existing illnesses, drug addiction, history of overdosing.

7. Initiate specific antidotal therapy.

Specific antidotal therapy varies with the drug involved in the overdose. Drug not removed by emesis or lavage may be moved rapidly through the intestines, and its absorption minimized, by administration of castor oil. Overtreatment should be avoided. Intensive supportive therapy may reduce the need for antidotal medication. In the preceding chapters, specific antidotes, if any, for each drug are indicated under the heading *Overdosage/Antidote*.

Dialysis may be considered in the patient with compromised renal function and particularly for overdosage of barbiturates and salicylates. Prior to instituting dialysis, assure that the drug involved in the overdose is amenable to removal by dialysis. Dialysis is particularly useful when retention of the drug may result in hepatic, renal, auditory, or neurological damage.

Institution of procedures to enhance the excretion of the drug should be considered. Alkalinization of the urine will increase the removal of intermediate- or long-acting barbiturates and also salicylates. Alkalinization increases the ionized form of barbiturates and salicylates; tubular reabsorption is subsequently decreased, which results in a rapid clearance of the drug.

Drug overdosage, acute intoxication, or acute abuse are always medical emergencies and should be treated accordingly.

DRUG ANTAGONISTS AND ANTIDOTES

The drug antagonists and antidotes are divided into the following groups: (1) anticholinesterase antidotes, (2) chelating agents, (3) miscellaneous antidotal products reviewed in detail elsewhere but included herein and cross referenced, and (4) the narcotic antagonists.

Anticholinesterase Antidotes

SPECIFIC PRODUCTS, USES, AND DOSAGES—Refer to table on overleaf.

GENERIC NAME	TRADE NAME	USE	ROUTE OF ADMIN.	USUAL DOSAGE	
				ADULTS	CHILDREN
atropine sulfate	(G)*	Poisoning with organophosphates, anticholinesterases, neostigmine, pyridostigmine, ambenonium	im/iv/sc	1–4 mg, repeat in 5–30 min. until symptoms controlled **maximum:** 50 mg/day	Consult package insert
pralidoxime chloride	PROTOPAM Chloride	Poisoning with organophosphates, anticholinesterases, neostigmine, pyridostigmine, ambenonium	im/iv/sc	Infuse 1–2 gm in 100 ml saline over 15–30 min.; may repeat in 1 hr.	20–40 mg/kg in 100 ml saline over 15–30 min.; may repeat in 1 hr.
			iv	**Anticholinesterase overdosage:** 1–2 gm iv then 250 mg every 5 min. as needed	Consult manufacturer

*(G) designates availability as a generic product.

Atropine Sulfate

GENERAL CLINICAL USES

In addition to the therapeutic adjunctive uses in treating peptic ulcer and other gastrointestinal disorders and urinary tract disorders, atropine sulfate is an important antidotal drug. It is used to treat overdosage or intoxication caused by cholinesterase inhibitors such as the organophosphorus insecticides.

For detailed information, see Chapter 8, page 390.

Pralidoxime Chloride

GENERAL CLINICAL USES

Pralidoxime chloride is indicated as an antidote in (1) the treatment of poisoning due to those pesticides and chemicals of the organophosphate class which have anticholinesterase activity and (2) the control of overdosage of anticholinesterase drugs (neostigmine, pyridostigmine, ambenonium) used in the treatment of myasthenia gravis.

PHARMACOLOGY

Pralidoxime, an anticholinesterase antagonist, acts to reactivate cholinesterase (mainly outside the central nervous system) which has been inactivated by phosphorylation due to an organophosphate insecticide or related compound. The destruction of the accumulated acetylcholine can then proceed and neuromuscular junctions will again function normally. It relieves paralysis of the muscles of respiration.

Pralidoxime antagonizes the effects in the neuromuscular junction of the carbamate anticholinesterases, neostigmine, pyridostigmine, and ambenonium, used in the treatment of myasthenia gravis. It is not, however, as effective as an antidote for these drugs as it is for the organophosphates.

Pralidoxime is relatively short-acting, and repeated doses may be necessary. It is excreted rapidly in the urine partly unchanged and partly as a metabolite produced by the liver.

SPECIAL PRECAUTIONS
• Not effective in the treatment of poisoning due to phosphorus, inorganic phosphates or organophosphates not having anticholinesterase activity.
• A decrease in renal function will result in increased blood levels of the drug.
• Use with great caution in treating organophosphate overdosage in cases of myasthenia gravis, since it may precipitate a myasthenic crisis.

ADVERSE EFFECTS
CNS EFFECTS: dizziness, drowsiness
RESPIRATORY EFFECTS: hyperventilation
CARDIOVASCULAR EFFECTS: tachycardia
GASTROINTESTINAL EFFECTS: nausea
MUSCULOSKELETAL EFFECTS: muscular weakness

OPHTHALMIC EFFECTS: blurred vision, diplopia, impaired accommodation

CLINICAL GUIDELINES
ADMINISTRATION:
• Intravenous administration should be carried out slowly, preferably by infusion, since certain side effects, such as tachycardia, laryngospasm, and muscle rigidity, have been attributed in a few cases to a too rapid rate of administration.
• Reduce dosage in patients with renal insufficiency.
EFFECTS:
• Pralidoxime has been used in the treatment of poisonings in humans by the following: Azodren, Diazinon, Dichlorvos (DDVP) with chlordaze, Disulfoton, EPN, Isoflurophate, Malathion, Metasystox I and Fenthion, methyl dimeton, methyl parathion, Mevinphos, parathion, parathion and Mevinphos, Phophamidon, Sirin, Systox, TEPP.

Chelating Agents

SPECIFIC PRODUCTS, USES, AND DOSAGES

GENERIC NAME	TRADE NAME	USE	ROUTE OF ADMIN.	USUAL DOSAGE	
				ADULTS	**CHILDREN**
calcium disodium edetate	CALCIUM DISODIUM VERSONATE	Lead intoxication	im	0.5 gm/30 lb/day; repeat if necessary	0.5 gm/30 lb bid, repeat if necessary
			iv	200 mg diluted bid	Not established
			po	4 gm/day in divided doses	1 gm/35 lb/day in divided doses
					(continued overleaf)

GENERIC NAME	TRADE NAME	USE	ROUTE OF ADMIN.	USUAL DOSAGE ADULTS	USUAL DOSAGE CHILDREN
deferoxamine mesylate	DESFERAL Mesylate	Iron intoxication	im	1 gm, then 0.5–1.0 gm every 4 hr for 2 doses; do not exceed 6 gm in 24 hr.	Not established
			iv	0.5–2 gm at rate not exceeding 15 mg/kg/hr. Do not exceed 6 gm in 24 hr.	Not established
dimercaprol	BAL in Oil	Intoxication with arsenic, gold, mercury, lead	im	2.5–5.0 mg/kg qid then bid	Not established
disodium edetate	ENDRATE SODIUM VERSENATE	Intoxication with calcium, digitalis (to treat heart block and ventricular arrhythmia)	iv infusion over 3–4 hrs.	15–60 mg/kg/day; **maximum:** 3 gm/day	40 mg/kg/day; **maximum:** 70 mg/kg/day
penicillamine	CUPRIMINE	Overdosage with copper (Wilson's disease)	po	250–500 mg qid; **maximum:** 2 gm/day	**Young children and infants over 6 mos.:** 250–500 mg qid; **maximum:** 2 gm/day

Calcium Disodium Edetate

GENERAL CLINICAL USES

Calcium disodium edetate is indicated for the reduction of blood levels and depot stores of lead in lead poisoning (acute and chronic) and lead encephalopathy. It may be of use in chelation of radioactive and nuclear fission products such as plutonium and yttrium.

PHARMACOLOGY

The calcium in calcium disodium edetate is readily displaced by heavy metals such as lead to form stable complexes. Following parenteral administration, the chelate is formed and excreted in the urine; 50 percent appears in the first hour.

SPECIAL PRECAUTIONS

• Do not give during period of anuria.

• May produce toxic and potentially fatal effects.

• Avoid rapid intravenous infusion in lead encephalopathy; intramuscular administration is preferred.

• Safe use in pregnancy has not been established.

• May produce the same signs of renal damage as severe lead poisoning, that is, proteinuria, microscopic hematuria.

• The presence of large renal epithelial cells or increasing numbers of erythrocytes in the urinary sediment, or greater proteinuria, calls for immediate termination of calcium disodium edetate.

• Monitor renal function, cardiac rhythm periodically.

- Avoid (by avoiding rapid intravenous administration) increasing intracranial pressure suddenly, particularly in patients with cerebral edema.

ADVERSE EFFECTS

CNS EFFECTS: chills, fever
CARDIOVASCULAR EFFECTS: hypotension
URINARY TRACT EFFECTS: with parenteral administration, renal tubular necrosis; with oral administration, erythrocytes and albumin in urine
GASTROINTESTINAL EFFECTS: diarrhea, abdominal cramps, vomiting
HEMATOLOGIC EFFECTS: transient bone marrow depression
ALLERGIC EFFECTS: sneezing, nasal congestion, lacrimation
DERMATOLOGIC EFFECTS: cheilosis
MUSCULOSKELETAL EFFECTS: leg and other muscle cramps

CLINICAL GUIDELINES

ADMINISTRATION:
- When drug is to be administered intramuscularly, prepare the solution with procaine 0.5% to 1.5% since intramuscular injection is extremely painful.
- Therapy is most effective when initiated immediately after toxic exposure.
EFFECTS:
- Use in poisoning by copper, cadmium, chromium, manganese, gold, and nickel is questionable or of unproved value; it is not effective in mercury or arsenic poisoning.
- Will not produce negative calcium balance because the drug is fully saturated with calcium.
DRUG INTERACTIONS:
- Hemosiderin, hemoglobin, ferritin, various enzymes, and nucleic acids will interfere with the action of chelating agents.
OVERDOSAGE/ANTIDOTE:
- Overdosage produces renal toxicity, namely, proteinuria, hematuria, etc.

- There is no specific antidote. Treat supportively.

Deferoxamine Mesylate

GENERAL CLINICAL USES

Deferoxamine mesylate is used to facilitate the removal of iron in the treatment of acute iron intoxication. It is also used as an adjunct, and not a substitute, for standard measures generally used in treating chronic iron intoxication.

PHARMACOLOGY

Deferoxamine readily complexes with the ferric ion to form ferrioxamine, a colored, stable, water-soluble chelate; it also has some affinity for the ferrous ion. It can also remove iron from transferrin, ferritin, and hemosiderin without significantly affecting the body levels of other metals or trace elements.

SPECIAL PRECAUTIONS

- Do not use in patients with severe renal disease or anuria, since the drug and the chelate which it forms with iron are excreted primarily by the kidneys.
- Long-term administration has produced cataracts; conduct periodic ophthalmic examinations.
- Do not administer to women of childbearing potential, particularly during early pregnancy, except when in the judgment of the physician, the potential benefits outweigh the possible hazards.
- Do not give large doses to patients with severe renal insufficiency.

ADVERSE EFFECTS

CNS EFFECTS: fever
CARDIOVASCULAR EFFECTS: hypotension, tachycardia

GASTROINTESTINAL   EFFECTS: abdominal discomfort, diarrhea

ALLERGIC EFFECTS: urticaria, anaphylactic reaction

DERMATOLOGIC EFFECTS: erythema; also wheal formation, rash, pruritus

MUSCULOSKELETAL EFFECTS: leg cramps

LOCAL EFFECTS: pain, induration; with intramuscular administration, severe transient pain

CLINICAL GUIDELINES

ADMINISTRATION:

• Administer by slow intravenous infusion or intramuscularly; avoid rapid intravenous administration.

• Use intramuscular administration for all patients not in shock.

• Use intravenous infusion only for patients in cardiovascular collapse; do not exceed 15 mg/kg/hr.

EFFECTS:

• Urine is colored a reddish-brown after parenteral administration.

Dimercaprol

GENERAL CLINICAL USES

Dimercaprol in oil is indicated in the treatment of arsenic, gold, and mercury poisonings. It has proven an effective drug for acute mercury poisoning, if therapy is begun within 1 to 2 hours after ingestion. It has not been effective for chronic mercury poisoning.

PHARMACOLOGY

Dimercaprol promotes the excretion of arsenic, gold, and mercury in poisonings. It forms a chelate with the heavy metal, thereby protecting the sulfhydryl-dependent enzyme systems from heavy metal inhibition. Following parenteral administration, the highest systemic concentration is reached within 30 minutes.

SPECIAL PRECAUTIONS

• Do not use in instances of hepatic insufficiency, with the exception of post-arsenical jaundice.

• Discontinue or use only with extreme caution if acute renal insufficiency develops during therapy.

• Pain may occur at site of injection; a fever which may persist during therapy may occur in approximately 30 percent of children.

• A transient reduction in the percentage of polymorphonuclear leukocytes may also be observed.

• Because the dimercaprol-metal complex breaks down easily in an acid medium, production of an alkaline urine affords protection of the kidneys during therapy.

ADVERSE EFFECTS

CNS EFFECTS: headache, weakness, unrest, anxiety

RESPIRATORY EFFECTS: a feeling of constriction, even pain, in the throat, chest or hands; rhinorrhea

CARDIOVASCULAR EFFECTS: hypertension, tachycardia

GASTROINTESTINAL EFFECTS: nausea, vomiting, burning sensation of lips, mouth, and throat, salivation, abdominal pain

MUSCULOSKELETAL EFFECTS: tingling of hands

OPHTHALMIC EFFECTS: conjunctivitis, lacrimation, blepharal spasm

URINARY TRACT EFFECTS: burning sensation in the penis

AUTONOMIC EFFECTS: sweating of the forehead, hands, and other areas

LOCAL EFFECTS: pain at injection site, particularly in children

Disodium Edetate

GENERAL CLINICAL USES
Disodium edetate is used as a chelating agent in the treatment of pathologic states secondary to hypercalcemia; do not use this drug for treating heavy metal poisoning because of its high affinity for calcium. It may be used for emergency treatment of hypercalcemia and of ventricular arrhythmias that are associated with digitalis toxicity.

PHARMACOLOGY, SPECIAL PRECAUTIONS, ADVERSE EFFECTS, CLINICAL GUIDELINES
For detailed information, see Chapter 15, page 568.

Penicillamine

GENERAL CLINICAL USES
Penicillamine is indicated for the removal of copper, mercury, or lead from the body in disorders such as Wilson's disease and lead or mercury poisoning.

PHARMACOLOGY
Penicillamine, a degradation product of penicillin, chelates effectively with copper, mercury, and lead. It facilitates excretion of these metals in the urine. Penicillamine, following oral administration, is absorbed rapidly from the gastrointestinal tract and is excreted rapidly in the urine.

SPECIAL PRECAUTIONS
• Do not use in patients with a history of hypersensitivity to penicillamine and related drugs.
• Use with caution in patients with impaired renal function.
• Safe use in pregnancy has not been established.

ADVERSE EFFECTS
CNS EFFECTS: fever
CARDIOVASCULAR EFFECTS: thrombophlebitis
URINARY TRACT EFFECTS: nephrosis
GASTROINTESTINAL EFFECTS: nausea, vomiting, anorexia
HEMATOLOGICAL EFFECTS: leukopenia, thrombocytopenia, eosinophilia, lymphadenopathy, agranulocytosis (1 case)
ALLERGIC EFFECTS: urticaria
DERMATOLOGIC EFFECTS: maculopapular or erythematous rash, cheilosis
MUSCULOSKELETAL EFFECTS: arthralgia
OPHTHALMIC EFFECTS: optic neuritis

CLINICAL GUIDELINES
ADMINISTRATION:
• Administer on an empty stomach.
• Adverse effects are most likely to occur shortly after therapy is begun.

Miscellaneous Antidotes

SPECIFIC PRODUCTS, USES, AND DOSAGES — Refer to table on overleaf.

GENERIC NAME	TRADE NAME	USE	ROUTE OF ADMIN.	USUAL DOSAGE
amyl nitrite	(G)*	Cyanide poisoning	inhal.	See Chapter 5, page 285.
atropine sulfate	(G)	Overdosage of parasympathomimetics (cholinergics)	im/iv	See Chapter 8, page 390.
glucagon	(G)	Insulin overdosage	iv/sc/im	See Chapter 15, page 559.
leucovorin calcium	(G)	Reverses the effects of folic acid antagonists (i.e., methotrexate)	im	Give in equal amounts to the weight of the antagonists given
protamine sulfate	(G)	Heparin overdosage	iv	Total dosage is determined by the amount of heparin given over the previous 3–4 hours; **maximal single dose:** 50 mg
vitamin K	(G)	Overdosage of oral anticoagulants	im/iv/sc	See Chapter 16, page 603.

*(G) designates availability as a generic product.

Leucovorin Calcium

PHARMACOLOGY

Leucovorin calcium, the calcium salt of folinic acid, circumvents the action of folate reductase. Leucovorin is an antidote for the toxic effects of folic acid antagonists, such as methotrexate. An intramuscular dose greater than 1 mg does not appear to be more effective than a dose of 1 mg.

SPECIAL PRECAUTIONS
- Improper therapy for pernicious anemia and other megaloblastic anemias secondary to lack of vitamin B_{12}.

ADVERSE EFFECTS
ALLERGIC EFFECTS: sensitization

CLINICAL GUIDELINES
ADMINISTRATION:
- Administer within 1 hour if possible in the treatment of overdosage of folic acid antagonists; it is usually ineffective if administered after 4 hours.

Protamine Sulfate

GENERAL CLINICAL USES
Protamine sulfate is indicated in the treatment of heparin overdosage.

PHARMACOLOGY
Protamine sulfate is a true antithromboplastin. When administered alone, protamine sulfate has an anticoagulant effect. However, when given in the presence of heparin, a stable salt is formed which results in the loss of anticoagulant activity of both drugs. It is a heparin antagonist. Each mg neutralizes 80–100 USP units of heparin activity. The effect is almost immediate and lasts about 2 hours.

SPECIAL PRECAUTIONS

• Keep patient under close observation since hyperheparinemia or bleeding has occurred 30 minutes to 18 hours after cardiac surgery in spite of complete neutralization of heparin by adequate doses of protamine sulfate.
• Safe use in pregnancy has not been established.
• Because of the anticoagulant effect, it is unwise to administer more than 100 mg over a short period unless there is certain knowledge of a larger requirement.

ADVERSE EFFECTS

CNS EFFECTS: feeling of warmth
RESPIRATORY EFFECTS: dyspnea
CARDIOVASCULAR EFFECTS: hypotension, bradycardia

DERMATOLOGIC EFFECTS: transitory flushing

CLINICAL GUIDELINES

ADMINISTRATION:
• Give by slow intravenous injection in 1 to 3 minutes in doses not exceeding 5 mg in any 10 minute period.
• Facilities to treat shock should be available.
EFFECTS:
• Each mg of protamine sulfate neutralizes approximately 90 USP units of heparin derived from lung tissue and about 115 USP units derived from intestinal mucosa.
DRUG INTERACTIONS:
• Protamine sulfate 1% solution neutralizes heparin sodium.

Narcotic Antagonists

SPECIFIC PRODUCTS AND DOSAGES

GENERIC NAME	TRADE NAME	USE	ROUTE OF ADMIN.	USUAL DOSAGE	
				ADULTS	CHILDREN
levallorphan tartrate	LORFAN	Narcotic overdose	iv	Initially 1 mg, then 0.5 mg twice at 5 to 10-min. intervals; **maximum:** 3 mg/day	0.02 mg/kg; then 0.01–0.02 mg/kg in 10–15 min. **Neonates:** 0.05–0.1 mg into umbilical vein
			im/sc	———	**Neonates:** 0.05–0.1 mg
naloxone HCl	NARCAN	Narcotic overdose	im/iv/sc	0.1–0.4 mg; repeat in 2–3 minutes	Not established
	NARCAN Neonatal		im/iv/sc	———	0.01 mg/kg; repeat in 2–3 min.

Levallorphan Tartrate

GENERAL CLINICAL USES

Levallorphan tartrate is indicated in the treatment of significant narcotic-induced respiratory depression.

PHARMACOLOGY

Levallorphan tartrate, administered intravenously, acts as a narcotic antagonist in the presence of a strong narcotic effect. If used in the absence of such an effect, it may cause respiratory depression and other problems. The drug is indicated only in narcotic-induced respiratory depression.

SPECIAL PRECAUTIONS

• Do not use in patients with mild respiratory depression.
• Do not use in narcotic addicts, in whom it may produce withdrawal symptoms.
• This drug is ineffective against respiratory depression due to barbiturates, anesthetics, other non-narcotic agents or pathologic causes, and may increase it.
• In the absence of a narcotic, it may cause respiratory depression.
• Also use other supportive measures such as artificial respiration and oxygen in treatment of significant narcotic-induced respiratory depression.
• Repeated doses may result in decreasing effectiveness and may eventually produce respiratory depression equal to or greater than that produced by narcotics.

ADVERSE EFFECTS

CNS EFFECTS: lethargy, dizziness, drowsiness, dysphoria
AUTONOMIC EFFECTS: sweating
GASTROINTESTINAL EFFECTS: nausea, vomiting
DERMATOLOGIC EFFECTS: pallor
MUSCULOSKELETAL EFFECTS: heaviness in limbs

OPHTHALMIC EFFECTS: miosis, and pseudoptosis

CLINICAL GUIDELINES

OVERDOSAGE/ANTIDOTE:
• With high doses, psychomimetric manifestations such as vivid dreams, visual hallucinations, disorientation, feelings of unreality; and increased crying in asphyxia neonatorum.
• There is no specific antidote. Use supportive therapy.

Naloxone Hydrochloride

GENERAL CLINICAL USES

Naloxone hydrochloride is indicated for partial or complete reversal of narcotic depression, including respiratory depression, induced by natural or synthetic narcotics, prophoxyphene, and the narcotic-antagonist analgesic, pentazocine. It is also indicated for the diagnosis of suspected acute opiate overdosage. It is the only narcotic antagonist effective for pentazocine overdosage.

PHARMACOLOGY

Naloxone hydrochloride is essentially a pure narcotic antagonist which may be administered intramuscularly, intravenously, or subcutaneously. It does not possess the "agonistic" or morphinelike properties characteristic of other narcotic antagonists. It does not produce respiratory depression, psychomimetric effects, or pupillary constriction. In the absence of narcotics or agonistic effects of other narcotic antagonists, it exhibits essentially no pharmacologic activity.

Naloxone hydrochloride will produce withdrawal symptoms in patients physically dependent on narcotics.

When naloxone hydrochloride is administered intravenously, the effects appear within 2 minutes; effects are only slightly less rapid after subcutaneous or intramuscular administration. Intramuscular administration produces a more prolonged effect than intravenous administration.

SPECIAL PRECAUTIONS
• Do not use in patients with a history of hypersensitivity to this drug or related drugs.
• Use cautiously in persons who are known or suspected to be physically dependent on opiates, including newborns of drug-addicted mothers; abrupt and complete reversal of narcotic effects may precipitate an acute abstinence syndrome.
• Keep patient under continued surveillance; administer repeated doses as necessary.
• Not effective against respiratory dependence due to nonopiate drugs.
• Safe use in pregnancy has not been established.
• Other resuscitative measures, such as maintenance of a free airway, artificial ventilation, cardiac massage, and vasopressor agents, may be required.

ADVERSE EFFECTS
GASTROINTESTINAL EFFECTS: nausea and vomiting rarely in postoperative patients

Glossary

Acetonuria: occurrence of excess acetone bodies in the urine.

Achalasia: failure to relax in the part of a bodily opening, such as a sphincter or the esophagus; cardiospasm.

Achlorhydria: absence of hydrochloric acid in the gastric juice.

Acidosis: a condition in which the pH of the blood is low (acidic) due to loss of base or accumulation of acid.

Acneiform rash: skin eruption resembling acne, which may be related to drug ingestion.

Adenoma: benign epithelial tumor with a glandlike structure.

Adjuvant: a substance assisting other remedies.

Adynamic ileus: flaccid condition characterized by paralysis and obstruction of the bowel, producing severe colic.

Agammaglobulinemia: decreased concentration or absence of gamma globulin from the blood.

Agranulocytosis: marked decrease in circulating neutrophilic leukocytes.

Akathisia: inability to sit still.

Albuminuria: occurrence of albumin (protein) in the urine.

Alopecia: loss of hair from the body or scalp.

Amblyopia: dimness of vision without detectable organic lesions of the eye.

Amnesia: loss of memory.

Analeptic: referring to stimulation of the central nervous system, particularly respiration and wakefulness.

Anaphylactoid: resembling anaphylaxis.

Anaphylaxis: allergic reaction which develops suddenly and requires immediate medical attention; symptoms include itching, hives, nasal congestion, nausea, abdominal cramping and/or diarrhea; more severe symptoms may follow, including choking, shortness of breath, loss of consciousness (anaphylactic shock).

Angioneurotic edema: disorder of the vasomotor system resulting in a temporary accumulation of fluid in the skin and/or mucous membranes.

Anorexia: decreased appetite for food.

Antigenicity: potency as an antigen.

Antiseptic: agent which inhibits or prevents growth of organisms without killing them.

Anuria: total suppression of urine secretion by the kidneys.

Aphasia: defect or loss of the power of expression by speech, writing, or signs of comprehending spoken or written language due to injury of the brain centers.

Apnea: cessation of breathing.

Arachnoiditis: inflammation of the membranes interposed between the pia mater and the dura mater, the protective membranes covering the brain.

Asphyxia: suffocation; anoxia and increased carbon dioxide in the blood and tissues.

Ataxia: muscle incoordination resulting in irregular movements.

Atelectasis: incomplete expansion or collapse of the lungs.

Azotemia: elevated blood level of nitrogenous materials.

Bactericidal: having the ability to kill bacteria; in contrast to bacteriostatic, which refers to suppression of growth of bacteria.

Benign: not malignant.

Bradycardia: abnormally slow heart beat; pulse is usually 60 per minute or less.

Bronchospasm: sudden involuntary contraction of the muscles of the bronchi.

Bruits (vascular): abnormal sounds or murmurs heard in ascultation.

Bruxism: grinding or gnashing of the teeth in other than chewing movements of the mandible.

Cachexia: profound and marked state of constitutional disorder; general ill health and malnutrition.

Carpopedal spasm: contractions occurring in the hands and feet.

Catatonia: form of schizophrenia characterized by stupor, negativism, and lack of contact with reality.

Caudal block: type of anesthesia in which the anesthetic solution is introduced into the sacral canal through the sacral hiatus.

Cellulitis: inflammation of subcutaneous tissue.

Cephalgia: headache, pain in the head.

Cheilosis: condition marked by fissuring and dry scaling of the red surface of the lips and angles of the mouth.

Cholestasis: suppression of bile flow.

Citrovorum factor: leucovorin, folinic acid; a term used to designate 5-formyl tetrahydrofolic acid, which is used in treatment of metablastic anemia and in anemia due to methotrexate.

Climacteric: change of life; cessation of fertility in either male or female (menopause).

Clonic movements: spasms resulting in convulsive movements usually of the extremities.

Coombs' test: test to detect antibodies in the blood, particularly sensitized erythrocytes in erythroblastosis fetalis and other hemolytic syndromes.

Coryza: acute catarrhal condition; headcold.

Crystalluria: presence of crystals in urine.

Cystitis: inflammation of the bladder.

Delirium: a syndrome characterized by trembling, hallucinations, excitement, anxiety, and exhaustion.

Dependence: the physical or psychological state in which the usual or increasing doses of a drug are required to prevent the onset of abstinence symptoms.

Depilation: process of removing hair.

Dermatitis (exfoliative, contact): inflammation of the skin; contact dermatitis is caused by contact with a foreign material; exfoliative dermatitis is a skin inflammation in which there is extensive scaling, itching, abnormal redness, and hair loss.

Dialysis: the diffusion of solution across a permeable membrane in the direction of the concentration gradient for each specific solute.

Diaphoresis: profuse perspiration.

Diplopia: perception of two images of a single object.

Disorientation: loss of sense of time, place, or identity; confusion.

Disulfiram reaction: symptoms that result from the interaction of alcohol and any drug that is capable of provoking the syndrome of intense flushing and warming of the face, severe throbbing headaches, shortness of breath, chest pains, nausea, repeated vomiting, sweating, and weakness. Severe reactions may lead to hypotension, vertigo, unconsciousness, convulsions, and death.

Diuresis: increased secretion of urine.

Dysarthria: imperfect articulation in speech.

Dyscrasia: term denoting abnormal cellular composition of the blood.

Dyskinesia: abnormal movement.

Dyspepsia: impairment of digestion.

Dysphagia: difficulty in swallowing.

Dysphoria: restlessness, malaise, disquiet.

Dyspnea: difficulty in breathing.

Dystonia: disordered tonicity of muscle.

Dystonic reactions/Dystonia: involuntary, irregular clonic contractions of the muscles, particularly those of the face and mouth, resulting in slurred speech, dysphagia, oculogyric crisis, trismus, torticollis, retrocollis, and muscle weakness.

Dysuria: painful or difficult urination.

Ecchymosis: discoloration of the skin caused by extravasation of blood; bruise.

Eczematous eruption: an inflammatory skin disorder resembling eczema which is characterized by vesiculation, infiltration, watery discharge, and the development of scales and crusts.

Endemic: pertaining to a particular region, such as a disease which has a low incidence but which is constantly present in a given community.

Enterocolitis: inflammation of the small intestine and colon.

Enuresis: involuntary urination, particularly at night (nocturnal).

Eosinophilia: marked increase in circulating eosinophils.

Epidural block: type of anesthesia produced by injection of an anesthetic agent into the epidural space.

Epileptiform: resembling epilepsy, such as recurring severe and sudden paroxysms.

Epistaxis: nosebleed; hemorrhage from the nose.

Erythema: red coloration of the skin due to congestion of the capillaries.

Erythema multiforme: acute skin disease with papules and discolored spots which last for several days and are accompanied by slight burning and itching.

Escharotic: corrosive or caustic agent capable of producing sloughing of the skin.

Euphoria: sense of well-being and buoyancy.

Euthyroid: having a normally functioning thyroid gland.

Exanthema: skin eruption.

Exfoliative dermatitis: *see* dermatitis.

Expectorant: a medicine promoting the ejection by spitting of mucus or other fluids from the lungs and trachea.

Extracorporeal hemodialysis: application of the dialysis principle to blood flowing outside the body on one side of a permeable membrane.

Extrapyramidal disorder: disorder outside the pyramidal system of the central nervous system.

Extrasystole: premature contraction of the heart which is independent of the normal rhythm and arises in response to an impulse in some part of the heart other than the sinoauricular node.

Extravasation: escape of blood from a vessel into the tissues.

Fasciculation: involuntary contraction or twitching of a group of muscle fibers.

Febrile: feverish.

Fibrillation: muscular tremor especially of the heart in which the individual fibers take up their own independent action.

Flaccid (paralysis): a totally relaxed state of the muscle.

Flatus: gas or air in the gastrointestinal tract.

Folliculitis: inflammation of the hair follicle(s).

Formication: a sensation like that produced by ants and other insects crawling over the skin.

Galactorrhea: excessive or spontaneous lactation.

Gastralgia: pain in the stomach.

Glaucoma: disease of the eye characterized by increased intraocular pressure, resulting in atrophy of the retina, cupping of the optic disc, and eventual blindness.

Globus hystericus: subjective sensation of choking; lump in the throat.

Glossitis: inflammation of the tongue.

Glycosuria: presence of glucose (sugar) in the urine.

Gonioscopy: an examination of the angle of the anterior chamber of the eye with a special ophthalmoscope.

Grand mal seizure: a type of epilepsy characterized by severe convulsions and loss of consciousness.

Gynecomastia: excessive enlargement of the breast in the male.

Habituation: gradual adaptation to a stimulus or to the environment.

Hemiparesis: muscular weakness or paralysis affecting one side of the body.

Hemodialysis: application of the dialysis principle to an artificial kidney on one side of the membrane while dialysis bath is circulated on the other.

Hemorrhagic diathesis: condition caused by bleeding in which the tissues react in special ways to the stimulus; the person is more than usually susceptible to certain diseases.

Hemostasis: stopping of bleeding.

Hirsutism: abnormal hairiness, especially in women.

Horner's syndrome: a complex of symptoms characterized by sinking in of the eyeball, ptosis of the upper eyelid, constriction of the pupil, narrowing of the palpebral fissures, and anhidrosis caused by paralysis of the cervical sympathetic nerves.

Hyper: over, above, in excess of.

Hypercapnia: excess carbon dioxide in the blood.

Hyperemia: excess of blood to any part of the body.

Hyperesthesia: excessive sensitiveness of the skin or of a special sense.

Hyperglycemia: blood glucose level above the normal limit.

Hyperkalemia: increased serum potassium levels manifested by weakness, cramps, and cardiac dysrhythmias.

Hyperpigmentation: extremely marked discoloration or pigmentation.

Hyperpyrexia: excessively high body temperature.

Hyperreflexia: exaggeration of the reflexes.

Hypersensitivity: an allergic state characterized by intolerance to even small doses of a drug or other material; intolerance may be expressed as a rash, nasal congestion, breathing difficulty, or gastrointestinal upset.

Hyperthermia: excessively high body temperature.

Hypertrichosis: abnormal growth of hair.

Hyperuricemia: elevated concentration of uric acid in the blood.

Hyperventilation: increased respirations; both rate and depth of respiration may be increased.

Hyphema: hemorrhage into the anterior chamber of the eye.

Hypo: below, under, deficient.

Hypodermoclysis: introduction of fluids into the subcutaneous tissues, especially physiological sodium chloride solution, in a large quantity.

Hypoglycemia: blood glucose level below the normal limit.

Hypokalemia: abnormally low potassium concentration in the blood.

Hypolipidemia: decreased or absence of lipids (fats) in the blood.

Hyponatremia: lowered serum sodium levels manifested by dry mouth, thirst, lethargy, and drowsiness.

Hypothermia: abnormally low body temperature.

Hypovolemia: decreased blood volume.

Hypoxia: low oxygen content or tension; deficient oxygenation of the blood.

Icterus: jaundice; a syndrome characterized by hyperbilirubinemia and deposition of bile pigment in the skin and mucous membranes, with resulting yellow appearance of the patient.

Idiosyncrasy: abnormal mechanism of drug response that occurs in individuals who have a particular defect in the body chemistry which produces an effect totally unrelated to the drug's normal pharmacologic reaction; it is not a form of allergy.

Incontinence: inability to control a natural discharge such as urine or feces.

Induration: abnormally hard spot or place.

Infiltration (administration): accumulation in a tissue of a substance being injected (administered).

Iso: the same, equal to.

Jaundice: a yellow coloration of the skin and the sclera of the eyes which occurs when excessive bile pigments accumulate in the blood as a result of impaired liver function. It may be caused by disease or drugs.

Keratitis: horny growth of the skin; callosity.

Keratomalacia: softening of the cornea.

Keratosis nigrans: any horny growth such as a wart or callosity with hyperpigmentation.

Kernicterus: severe cerebral form of icterus neonatorum associated with ervthroblastosis fetalis in which there are degrading changes and pigmentation of the nuclear masses of the brain and spinal cord with bile pigments.

Laryngospasm: involuntary sudden closure of the larynx.

Lavage: irrigation or washing out of an organ, such as the stomach.

L. E. phenomenon: lupus erythematosus, a disease of unknown origin, primarily involving the body's immune system, which is characterized by enlarged lymph nodes, low-grade fever, skin rashes, aching muscles, multiple joint pains, and pleuritic chest pains.

Leukopenia: marked decrease in leukocytes.

Libido: sexual desire.

Livedo reticularis: a peripheral vascular condition characterized by a reddish blue netlike mottling of the skin of the extremities.

Loffler's syndrome: eosinophilic pneumonopathy; a condition characterized by transient infiltration of the lungs associated with an increase of the eosinophilic leukocytes in the blood and with only slight systemic manifestations.

Lupus erythematosus: a disease of the body's immune system, limited to the skin or involving several other body systems. The disease is characterized by chronic progressive inflammation and destruction of the connective tissues of the skin, blood vessels, joints, brain, heart muscle, lungs, and kidneys.

Lymphadenopathy: disease of the lymph nodes, usually accompanied by enlargement of the nodes in various parts of the body.

Maculopapular rash: skin eruption characterized by spotted or blotched papules; skin elevations.

Malaise: vague feeling of bodily discomfort.

Mastalgia: pain in the mammary gland.

Medullated nerves: nerves covered by myelin sheaths.

Megaloblastic anemia: deficient production of erythrocytes, characterized by megaloblasts in the blood.

Melena: passage of dark, patchy stools stained with blood pigments or with altered blood.

Metaplasia: changes in the type of adult cells in a tissue to a form which is not normal for that tissue.

Metapyrone test: a test for anterior pituitary function. In the hypopituitary patient, the adrenal cortex responds normally to stimulation by pyrogen, subnormally to metapyrone.

Methemoglobinemia: presence of methemoglobin, a modified form of oxyhemoglobin.

MIC: minimal inhibitory concentration of an antibiotic; that amount which will inhibit growth of a microorganism.

Miosis: contraction of the pupil.

Morbilliform rash: measleslike rash.

Myalgia: pain in a muscle or muscles.

Mydriasis: extreme dilatation of the pupil.

Myopia: nearsightedness.

Myxedema: form of hypothyroidism occurring in adults.

Natriuresis: excretion of excessive amounts of sodium.

Nephrosis: disease of the kidney characterized by degenerative lesions of the renal tubules and marked by edema, albuminuria, and decreased serum albumin.

Neuromuscular interference by a drug with the myoneural transmission of impulses at the skeletal neuromuscular junction.

Neuropathy, peripheral: any disease, particularly degenerative processes, of the peripheral nerves.

Neutropenia: decreased number of neutrophilic leukocytes.

Nocturia: excessive urination at night.

Nonmedullated nerves: nerves not covered by myelin sheaths.

Nyctalopia: night blindness.

Nystagmus: involuntary rapid movement of the eyeball.

Oculogyration: involuntary movements of the eye.

Oliguria: reduced daily output of urine.

Opisthotonus: form of tetanic spasm in which the head and heels are bent backward and the body bowed forward.

Orthostatic hypotension: decrease in blood pressure caused by standing erect or by other changes in position.

Osteoarthritis: degenerative joint disease usually involving multiple joints, particularly those concerned with weight-bearing.

Osteomalacia: disease of the bones in which softening occurs; bones become brittle and/or flexible, leading to deformities.

Osteoporosis: abnormal porosity and rarefaction of bones by the enlargement of their canals and the formation of abnormal spaces.

Ototoxicity: the quality of being poisonous or damaging to the ear (affecting hearing or balance).

Overdosage: administration, either accidental or intentional, of a dose greater than that recommended for therapeutic effect.

Palpitation: unduly rapid action of the heart which is felt by the patient.

Pancytopenia: a decrease in all blood cells.

Papilledema: edema of the optic papilla (optic disc); choked disc.

Paradoxical excitement: a response opposite or contradictory to that expected.

Paralytic ileus: *see* Adynamic ileus.

Paresthesias: abnormal sensations such as burning, prickling, formication.

Parkinson's syndrome: a group of symptoms including myoclonia, hyperreflexia, fasciculation, tremor, muscular rigidity, immobile facies, salivation, cramps, resulting from a lesion of the globus pallidus.

Parotitis: inflammation of the parotid gland; mumps.

Paroxysm: sudden recurrence or intensification of symptoms; also, a spasm or seizure.

Pericarditis: inflammation of the pericardium, the membrane surrounding the heart.

Perimembranous colitis: inflammation of the colon characterized by the formation of mucouslike membranes.

Peritoneal dialysis: the diffusion of solutes through the epithelium of the peritoneum; the peritoneal cavity is distended with 2 or 3 liters of warmed, sterile solution which is allowed to equilibrate, then is drained by gravity.

Petechiae: small red spots in the skin caused by effusion of blood.

Pheochromocytoma: chromaffin cell tumor of the adrenal medulla and other tissues; its tissue contains epinephrine and its presence is associated with symptoms of paroxysmal hypertension.

Phlebitis: inflammation of a vein.

Photophobia: abnormal intolerance of light.

Photosensitivity: skin reaction, usually drug-induced, characterized by development of a rash or exaggerated sunburn on exposure to the sun or another source of ultraviolet rays. The reaction is usually confined to uncovered areas of skin.

Pollinosis: allergic reaction in the body to the airborne pollen of plants.

Polyarthralgia: pain in several joints.

Polyuria: excessive increase in the daily output of urine.

Porphyria: disease of metabolism in which porphyrins (iron-free or magnesium-free derivatives involved in respiration) are retained in the body.

Potentiation: when two drugs are administered the resultant action is greater than the sum of the actions of each drug used alone.

Precordial: pertaining to the region over the heart.

Priapism: persistent abnormal erection of the penis, usually without sexual desire.

Prophylaxis: prevention of disease; preventive treatment.

Pruritus: itching, usually intense.

Pseudolactation: secretion of milk not related to the postpartum state.

Pseudoparkinsonism: a false, usually drug-related condition resembling Parkinson's syndrome and characterized by muscular rigidity, immobile facies, tremor of intent, salivation, and cramps.

Purgative: cathartic; causing evacuation from the bowels.

Purpura: disease characterized by the formation of red to purple patches on the skin or mucous membranes, due to subcutaneous extravasation of blood.

Pyelitis: inflammation of the renal pelvis.

Pyelonephritis: inflammation of the kidney and its pelvis.

Pyrexia: fever; febrile condition; abnormal elevation of body temperature.

Pyrosis: heartburn; a burning sensation in the esophagus and stomach with sour eructation.

Rebound congestion: congestion, usually of the mucous membranes, recurring following withdrawal of a stimulus.

Retrocollis: spasmodic wryneck in which the head is drawn directly backward.

Rhinorrhea: free nasal discharge, usually thin.

Rouleau formation: roll of erythrocytes, like a pile of coins.

Scotomata: appearance of dark, moving, vanishing, cloudy patches in the visual field.

Scurvy: condition due to deficiency of vitamin C in the diet; it is marked by weakness, anemia, spongy gums, and tendency toward musculocutaneous hemorrhage.

Semisynthetic: referring to products, in particular drugs, which are in part a natural product and in part produced in the laboratory by chemical means.

Septicemia: presence of pathogenic bacteria and their associated poisons (toxins) in the blood.

Sialadenitis: inflammation of a salivary gland.

Sialorrhea: excessive secretion of saliva.

Sideroblastic anemia: peculiar form of bone marrow failure in which the erythrocytes may be hypochromic or normally filled with hemoglobin; there is a high percentage of sideroblasts (enucleated erythrocytes) with nonheme granules in the cytoplasm.

Status asthmaticus: the most extreme form of asthma, a condition manifested by recurrent paroxysms of dyspnea of a wheezing type.

Stevens-Johnson syndrome: complex of symptoms consisting of extreme inflammatory eruption of skin and mucosa of the mouth, pharynx, anogenital region, and conjunctiva.

Superinfection: development of a secondary infection that is superimposed on an initial infection currently being treated.

Susceptibility: vulnerability of bacteria to suppression or killing by a drug.

Syncope: fainting; a temporary suspension of consciousness due to cerebral anemia.

Synergism: more profound effect resulting from the combined action of two or more items, for example drugs, than is caused by each item individually.

Synthetic: in reference to drugs, those which are produced in the laboratory by chemical means.

Tachycardia: excessively rapid heartbeat; a pulse rate above 100 per minute.

Tachyphylaxis: tolerance to a drug that develops after administration of a few doses.

Tardive dyskinesia: drug-induced disorder of the nervous system characterized by involuntary bizarre movements of the jaws, lips, and tongue. It occurs after long-term treatment with certain psychotherapeutic agents.

Tetany: syndrome manifested by sharp flexion of the wrist and ankle joints (carpopedal spasm), muscle twitching, cramps, and convulsions.

Thrombocytopenia: decrease in the number of blood platelets.

Thrombocytopenic purpura: condition in which the blood platelets (thrombocytes) are markedly decreased, resulting in bruising and hemorrhaging due to decreased clotting ability of the blood.

Tinnitus: a noise, usually described as ringing, buzzing, or roaring, in the ears.

Tolerance: ability to endure the continued or increasing use of a drug.

Torticollis: wryneck; contraction of the cervical muscles producing twitching of the neck and an unnatural position of the head.

Trismus: motor disturbance of the trigeminal nerve, especially spasm of the masticatory muscles, with difficulty in opening the mouth.

Tyramine: chemical component of many foods and beverages. Tyramine can increase blood pressure, but enzymes normally present in the body neutralize its effects. Certain drugs, including monoamine oxidase inhibitors (MAO-inhibitors), block the neutralizing enzymes, and extreme hypertension may occur. Foods containing tyramine include aged cheeses, beef liver, chicken liver, salted dried fish, pickled herring, yeast extracts, broad bean pods, banana skins, raspberries, avocados, Chianti wines, vermouth, beer (unpasteurized), sour cream.

Urethritis: inflammation of the urethra.

Uricosuria: increased elevation of uric acid in urine.

Urticaria: hives; smooth elevated patches of skin which itch severely.

Uveitis: inflammation of the uvea, the pigmentary layer of the eye.

Vaccinia: virus disease of cattle; communicated to humans, usually by vaccination, it confers a greater or lesser degree of immunity against smallpox.

Varicella: chickenpox.

Vertigo: usually considered dizziness; patient experiences a sensation that he is revolving in space or that the external world is revolving around him.

Vesicular: composed of or related to small, sacklike bodies.

Vital signs: signs pertaining to life, such as, pulse, heart rate, respiratory rate, temperature.

Wilson's disease: progressive hepatolenticular degeneration.

Withdrawal reactions: stereotyped symptom complex occurring after abrupt discontinuance of a drug; it is characteristic for the particular drug.

Xanthopsia: form of colored vision in which objects looked at appear yellow.

Xeroderma: skin disease resembling ichthyosis and marked by a dry, rough, discolored state of the skin with the formation of a scaly desquamation.

Xerophthalmia: conjunctivitis with atrophy and no liquid discharge. The eye is abnormally dry and lusterless.

References

Guide to I.V. Admixture Compatibility. Oradell, NJ, Medical Economics Co. by arrangement with New England Deaconess Hospital, Boston, 1975.

Apelgren, Scott E., and Brandt, Rowles: *Clinical Pharmacy Handbook for Patient Counseling.* Hamilton, IL, Drug Intelligence Publications, Inc., 1975.

Conn, Howard F. (ed.): *Current Therapy 1978.* Philadelphia, W.B. Saunders Co., 1978.

DiPalma, J. R. (ed.): *Drill's Pharmacology in Medicine,* ed. 4. New York, McGraw-Hill Book Co., 1971.

Drug Interactions. Oradell, NJ, Medical Economics Co.

Drugs Used with Neonates and During Pregnancy. Oradell, NJ, Medical Economics Co., 1976.

Goodman, L. S., and Gilman, A.: *The Pharmacological Basis of Therapeutics,* ed. 5. New York, The Macmillan Co., 1975.

Kastrup, E. K. (ed.): *Facts and Comparisons.* St. Louis, Facts and Comparisons, Inc. (published yearly, with monthly supplements).

Meyers, F. H., Jawetz, E., and Goldfiend, A.: *A Review of Medical Pharmacology,* ed. 6. Los Altos, CA, Lange Medical Publications, 1978.

Physicians' Desk Reference Oradell, NJ, Medical Economics Co. (published yearly, with periodic supplements).

Physicians' Desk Reference for Ophthalmology, 1978–79. Oradell, NJ, Medical Economics Co., 1979.

Drug directory

Location of Primary Information in Italic Type

DRUG NAME
ABBOKINASE, 277
acenocoumarol, 220, *222**
acetaminophen, 128, *129**†
acetazolamide, 169, *174, 253,* 451,
*454**†
acetazolamide sodium, *253**
acetic acid, 464, *465, 468**†
acetohexamide, *556**
acetophenazine, 112, *116**
acetophenetidin, *129**†
acetosulfone sodium, 76, *77**
acetylcholine chloride, 451, *452**
acetylsalicylic acid, 129, *130**†
ACHROMYCIN, 12, 62, 347, 376,
444
ACHROMYCIN V, 62
acidulated phosphate fluoride, *435**
ACIDULIN, 405
ACNEDERM, 413‡
ACNE-DOME, 413
ACNOMEL, 413
acrisorcin, 68, *69,* 418*
ACTH, *543**

ACTHAR, 543
ACTIDIL, 304
actinomycin D, *608,* 609*
ACTOL, 312‡
ADAPIN, 107
ADIPEX, 362
ADPHEN, 362
ADRENALIN, 292, 317, 330
ADRIAMYCIN, 609
ADRUCIL, 611
ADSORBOCARPINE, 451
AEROSEB-DEX, 421, 537‡
AEROSPORIN, 53, 347, 443, 464
A-FIL, 431
AFRIN, 331
AGORAL, 394
A/G PRO, 581
AIRET, 317
AKINETON, 184
AKRINOL, 68, 418
ALBAMYCIN CALCIUM, 42
ALBAMYCIN SODIUM, 42
albumin, normal serum (human), 279,
*280**†

ALBUMOTOPE-LS, 655
ALBUSPAN 5%, 279
ALBUSPAN 25%, 279
ALCAINE, 440
alcohol, 424, *425**†
ALDACTONE, 257
ALDOMET, 227
ALKA-SELTZER, 368‡
ALKA-2, 368‡
alkalinizing agents, 343
ALKERAN, 607
alkylamines, *302,* 303, *305*
ALLEREST, 330
ALLERTOC, 304‡
allopurinol, 485, *486**
ALPEN, 49
ALPHA CHYMAR, 460
alphaprodine hydrochloride, 133,
*134**
alseroxylon, 226, 227, *228**
ALUDROX, 368‡
aluminum acetate solution, *468**
aluminum hydroxide, *368**†
aluminum silicate, 359, *360**

*Generic Name
†Available as a generic product
‡More than one active ingredient

707

*Generic Name
†Available as a generic product
‡More than one active ingredient

*Generic Name
†Available as a generic product
‡More than one active ingredient

*Generic Name
†Available as a generic product
‡More than one active ingredient

METHOSARB, 614
methotrexate, 611, *612**†
methotrimeprazine, 134, *143**
methoxamine hydrochloride, 293, *299**
methoxsalen, 429, *430**
methoxyflurane, 154, *159**
methsuximide, 169, *173**
methyclothiazide, 251*
methylbenzethonium chloride, 436, *437**
methylcellulose, 395, *399,* 438*†
methyldopa, 226, 227, *237**
methyldopate hydrochloride, 226, 227, *237**
methylene blue, 340, *341, 353**
methylergonovine maleate, *530**
methylphenidate HCL, 123, *126**
methylprednisolone, 535, 538, *539**†
methylprednisolone acetate, *377,* 421, *422, 491,* 538, *539**†
methylprednisolone sodium succinate, 538, *539**
methylprednisolone acetate, *377,* 421, *422, 491,* 538, *539**
methylrosaniline chloride, *75**
methyl salicylate, 411, *413**
methyltestosterone, 513, 614*†
methyprylon, 192, *200**
methysergide maleate, 181, *183**
METICORTELONE ACETATE, 421, 539
METICORTEN, 538, 615
METI-DERM, 421, 538
METI-DERM WITH NEOMYCIN, 538‡
METIMYD, 57, 443, 447, 539‡
metoclopramide hydrochloride, *406**
metocurine iodide, 495, *504**
metolazone, *250**
METOPIRONE, 673
metoprolol tartrate, 226, 227, *239**
METRETON, 447, 539‡
metronidazole, 12, 13, 97, *98,* 376, 515, 516*
METUBINE IODIDE, 495
METYCAINE, 163
metyrapone, 654, 673, 680*
MICATIN, 69, 74, 419
MICOFUR, 74
miconazole nitrate, 65, 69, *72,* 74, *75,* 419, 516*
MICRONEFRIN, 317
MICRONOR, 518
MIDICEL, 58
milk of magnesia, 395, *399**†
MILONTIN, 169

MILTOWN, 102
MILTOWN INTRAMUSCULAR, 494
MILTRATE, 284‡
mineral oil, 394, *396**†
MINIPRESS, 228
MINOCIN, 62
minocycline hydrochloride, 62, *63**
MINTEZOL, 15
MIOCEL, 451‡
MIOCHOL, 451
MI-PILO, 451
MIRADON, 220
MISTURA P, 451
MITHRACIN, 568, 609
mithramycin, 568, 569, 608, *609**
mitomycin, 608, *609**
mitotane, 620, *621**
M-M-R, 638‡
MOBAN, 116
MOBIDIN, 129, 492
MODANE, 394
MODANE BULK, 395
MODERIL, 228
molindone hydrochloride, *116**
MONISTAT, 7, 9, 74, 516
morphine sulfate, 134, *137,* 342*†
morrhuate sodium, *282**†
MOTRIN, 129, 472
6-MP, *611, 612**
M-R-VAX, 638‡
MUDRANE, 327‡
mumps immune globulin, human, 626, *628**
mumps virus vaccine, 638, *644**
MUMPSVAX, 638
MURIPSIN, 402, 405‡
MUSTARGEN, 607
MUTAMYCIN, 609
M-VAC, 638
MYAMBUTOL, 86
MYCELEX, 68
MYCIFRADIN SULFATE, 21, 376
MYCIGUENT, 21
MYCOLOG, 42, 418, 539‡
MYCOSTATIN, 74, 419, 516
MYDRIACYL, 458
MYLAXEN, 495
MYLERAN, 606
MYLICON, 373
MYOCHRYSINE, 472
MYOFLEX, 411
MYOTONACHOL, 356
MYRINGACAINE, 462‡
MYSOLINE, 168
MYTELASE, 506
MYTRATE, 451

NAFCIL, 50
nafcillin sodium, *50**
NALDECON, 330‡
NALFON, 129, 472
nalidixic acid, 347, *348**
naloxone hydrochloride, 333, 334, 335, 695, *696**
nandrolone decanoate, 540, *541**
nandrolone phenpropionate, 540, 541*
naphazoline hydrochloride, 330, *332**†
NAPROSYN, 472
naproxen, 129, 472, *478**
NAQUA, 251
NARCAN, 334, 695
NARCAN NEONATAL, 334, 695
NARDIL, 108
natamycin, *444**
NATURETIN, 250
NAVANE, 116
NEBCIN, 21
NEGATAN, 269
negatol, 269, *272**
NEG GRAM, 347
NEMA, 15
NEMBUTAL, 168, 204
NEO-BETALIN, 12, 597
NEOBIOTIC, 21‡
NEO-CALGLUCON, 565
NEO-COROVAS, 284
NEO-CORTEF, 464, 466‡
NEOCURTASAL, 592‡
NEO-DELTA-CORTEF, 418, 421, 466, 539
NEO-HOMBREOL, 513
NEOHYDRIN-197, 655
NEOHYDRIN-203, 655
NEOLOID, 394
NEO-MEDROL, 418, 421, 464‡
neomycin, 418, 465*†
neomycin palmitate, 418*
neomycin sulfate, 21, *26,* 376, 418, 443, 444, *464**†
NEO-POLYCIN, 41, 53, 443†
NEOSPORIN, 41, 418, 442, 443‡
NEOSPORIN-G, 42‡
neostigmine bromide, 356, *357,* 506, *507**†
neostigmine methylsulfate, 356, *357, 507, 654,* 673, *681**†
NEO-SYNALAR, 418, 421‡
NEO-SYNEPHRINE, 330
NEPTAZANE, 253, 451‡
NESACAINE, 163
NEUTRALOX, 368‡

*Generic Name
†Available as a generic product
‡More than one active ingredient

paregoric, 370, *371**†
PAREPECTOLIN, 359, 370‡
PAREST, 192
pargyline hydrochloride, 226, 227, *241**
PARNATE, 108
paromomycin sulfate, 12, *14, 376**
PARSIDOL, 184
PAS, 86
PATHIBAMATE, 389‡
PATHILON, 389
PATHOCIL, 49
PAVATRAN, 285, 389
PAVERIL PHOSPHATE, 285, 389
PAVULON, 495
PBZ, 426
p-diisobutyphenoxy-polyethyoxyethanol, *521**
P D P LIQUID PROTEIN, 581
pectin, 359, *360,* 438*†
PECTO-KALIN, 359‡
PEDAMETH, 340
PEDIAFLOR, 435
PEDIALYTE, 587
PEDIAMYCIN, 40
PEGANONE, 168
PENBRITIN, 49
penicillamine, 472, *483,* 690, *693**
penicillin G, *50**†
penicillin G benzathine, *50**
penicillin G procaine, *50**†
penicillin V potassium, *50**†
penicillins, 20, 48, *50,* 346
pentaerythritol tetranitrate, 284, *288**†
pentagastrin, 654, 673, *681**
pentazocine hydrochloride, 134, *144**
pentazocine lactate, 134, *144**
PENTAZYME, 402‡
PENTHRANE, 154
pentobarbital, 168, *170,* 204, *207**†
PENTOTHAL, 148, 168
PENTRAX, 414‡
PENTRITOL, 284
pentyl p-(dimethylamino)-benzoate, 431, *432**
pepsin, *402**
PEPTAVALON, 673
PERCORTEN ACETATE PELLETS, 533
PERCORTEN PIVALATE, 533
PERGONAL, 527
PERIACTIN, 304
PERI-COLACE, 394‡
PERIFOAM, 374‡
PERITRATE, 284
PERMATIL, 112
perphenazine, 112, *116,* 381, *384**

perphenazine-amitriptyline, 112, *116*‡
PERSADOX, 413
PERSANTINE, 284
PERTOFRANE, 107
pertussis immune globulin, human, 627, *628**
pertussis vaccine, 638, *644**
peruvian balsam, 374*
PETN, 284, *288**
PFIKLOR, 572‡
PFIZERPEN G, 50
PHAZYME, 373, 402‡
phenacemide, 169, *178**
phenacetin, *129**†
phenazopyridine hydrochloride, 342*
phendimetrazine tartrate, 362, *363**†
phenelzine sulfate, 108, *109**
PHENERGAN, 304, 327, 381‡
PHENERGAN V.C., 327
phenindione, 220, *224**
PHENMETRAZINE HCl, 362, *363*
phenobarbital, 168, 203, *204**†
phenobarbital sodium, 168, *170,* 204*†
phenol, 436, *437**
phenolphthalein, white, 394, *398**†
phenolphthalein, yellow, 394, *398**†
PHENOL RED, 673
phenol sodium phenolate, 436, *437**
phenolsulfophthalein, 673, *682**†
phenothiazines, 112, *116, 302,* 304, *306, 380, 384*
PHENOXENE, 184
phenoxybenzamine hydrochloride, 226, 227, *243**
phenprocoumon, 220, *222**
phensuximide, 169, *173**
phentermine hydrochloride, 362, *363**†
phentolamine, 226, 227, *243**
PHENURONE, 169
phenylalanine mustard, 607*
phenylbutazone, 129, 472, *481,* 485, 488*
phenylephrine, 330, *331**
phenylmercuric acetate, 520, *521**
phenylpropanolamine, 330, *331,* 362, *367**†
phenytoin, 168, *171**
PHISOAC, 413
PHISODERM, 428
PHISO-HEX, 424, 428
PHOS-FLUR, 435
PHOSPHOLINE, 451
phosphorus preparations, 591, *592**
PHOSPHO-SODA, 395‡

PHOSPHOTOPE, 656
phthalylsulfathiazole, 57, *58**†
physostigmine, 451, *452**
physostigmine salicylate, 356, *357, 406**†
phytonadione, 270, *276,* 603*
pilocarpine hydrochloride, 451, *452**†
pilocarpine nitrate, 451, *452**
pilocarpine ocular therapeutic system, 451, *452**
PILOFRIN, 451
PIMA, 327
piperacetazine, 114, *116**
piperazine, 14, 15, *17**†
piperazine estrone sulfate, *522**
piperocaine hydrochloride, 163, *164**
PIPIZAN, 15
pipobroman, *607**
PITOCIN, 530
pitocin citrate, *530**
PITRESSIN, 570
PITRESSIN TANNATE, 570
PLACIDYL, 192
plague vaccine, 639, *645**†
plantago seed husks, 395, *399**
PLAQUENIL, 472
PLASMANATE 5%, 279
PLASMANATE 25%, 279
PLASMATEIN 5%, 279
PLATINOL, 606
PLEGINE, 362
pneumococcal vaccine, polyvalent, 639, *645**
PNEUMOVAX, 639
poison ivy extract, 624, *625**†
poison ivy, oak, sumac combined antigen, *625**
POLARAMINE, 303
polio virus vaccine, live, oral, trivalent, 639, *646**
POLYCILLIN, 346
POLYCILLIN-N, 49
POLYCITRA, 343
polyestradiol phosphate, *522, 615,* 616*
polyethylene glycol, 374*
POLYMOX, 49
polymyxin B sulfate, 52, 53, *55, 180,* 347, 418, 443, *444,* 464, *465,* 516, 517*
polymyxins, 20, *52,* 347
polysaccharide-iron complex, *588**
POLYSPORIN, 41, 442‡
polythiazide, *250**
POLY-VI-FLOR, 435‡
PONDIMIN, 362

*Generic Name
†Available as a generic product
‡More than one active ingredient

*Generic Name
†Available as a generic product
‡More than one active ingredient

SOMA, 493
SOMA COMPOUND, 493‡
somatropin, 542, 543, *544**
SOMBULEX, 204
SOMOPHYLLIN, 317
SONILYN, 57
SOPOR, 192
sorbitol irrigant, *355*†*
SOTRADECOL INJECTION, 282
SOXOMIDE, 58, 346
SOY-DOME, 424
SPECTROCIN, 42
spironolactone, 249, 257, *260**
STADOL, 134
standard diet, 581, *586**
stanozolol, *541**
STAPHCILLIN, 50, 346
STATROL, 53, 443‡
STELAZINE, 114
STERANE, 491, 538
STILPHOSTROL, 522, 616
STIMULAX, 394‡
stinging insect antigen, 624, *625*†*
STOXIL, 95, 444
STREPTASE, 277
streptokinase, *277**
streptokinase-streptodornase, 421, *423**
streptomycin sulfate, 21, *27,* 87, 94*†
STUART AMINO ACIDS, 581
STUART AMINO ACIDS with B₁₂, 581
SUBLIMAZE, 133
succinimides, 169, *173*
succinylcholine chloride, 495, *503*†*
SUCCUS CINERARIA MARITIMA, 448
SUCOSTRIN, 495
SUDABID, 330
SUDAFED, 330
SULCOLON, 58
SULF-10, 57
sulfabenzamide, 57, *59,* 516, 517*
SULFACEL-15, 443
sulfacetamide sodium, 57, 59, 418, 443, *444,* 517*
sulfachlorpyridazine, 57, *59**
sulfacytine, 57, *59,* 345*
sulfadiazine, 57, *59*†*
SULFAMAL, 58, 516
sulfameter, 57, *59**
sulfamethizole, 58, *59**
sulfamethoxazole, 58, *59,* 346*
sulfamethoxypyridazine, 58, *59**
SULFAMYLON, 57, 418
sulfanilamide, 58, *59,* 516, 517*†
sulfasalazine, 58, *59,* 376*
SULFATHALIDINE, 57
sulfathiazole, 58, *59,* 516, *517**
sulfinpyrazone, 58, *59,* 485, 489*

sulfisoxazole, 58, *59,* 346, *444,* 516, 517*†
sulfisoxazole acetyl, 58, *59**
sulfisoxazole diolamine, 58, *59,* 346*
sulfobromophthalein, 673, *685*†*
sulfonamides, 20, 56, *59,* 345
sulfoxone sodium, *77**
SULFOXYL, 413, 414
sulfur colloidal, 413, 414, *416**
sulindac, 472, *479**
sulisobenzone, 431, *433**
SULLA, 57
SULTRIN, 57, 516‡
SULTRIN TRIPLE SULFA, 58‡
SUMYCIN, 12, 62, 347
SUNDARE, 431
SUNDOWN SUNSCREEN, 431
SUNSTICK, 431
SUPPORT, 581
SURFACAINE, 411
SURFADIL, 304, 426‡
SURITAL, 148
SUSTACAL, 581
SUSTAGEN, 581
SYLLAMALT, 395
SYMMETREL, 94, 185
SYNALAR, 421
SYNCURINE, 494
SYNEMOL, 421
SYNKAYVITE, 270, 603
SYNTHROID, 575
SYNTOCINON, 530

T₃, 576
T₄, 575
TACARYL, 304
TACE, 522, 616
TAGAMET, 392
talbutal, 204, 207*
TALWIN, 134
tamoxifen, *618**
TANDEARIL, 129, 472, 485
TAO, 42
TAPAZOLE, 578
TARACTAN, 114
tar extract, 414, *416**
TAVIST, 304
technetium aggregated albumin (human), Tc 99m, 656, 663*
TEGOPEN, 49
TEGRETOL, 169
TELDRIN, 303
TELEPAQUE, 664
TEM, 607
TEMARIL, 304
TENSILON, 506, 673
TENUATE, 361
terbutaline sulfate, 318, *325**
TERRA-CORTRIL, 62, 418‡
TERRAMYCIN, 12, 15, 62, 418, 516

TERRAMYCIN CALCIUM, 62
TERRAMYCIN IM, 62
TERRAMCYIN IV, 62
TERRAMYCIN WITH POLYMYXIN B, 62, 443
TERRASTATIN, 62‡
TESLAC, 614
TESSALON, 312‡
testolactone, 614*
testosterone, *513,* 574*†
testosterone cypionate, *513*†*
testosterone enanthate, *513*†*
testosterone propionate, *513,* 614*†
tetanus antitoxin, 631, *634*†*
tetanus immune globulin (human), 627, *630**
tetanus toxoid, adsorbed, 635, *637*†*
tetanus toxoid, fluid, 635, *637*†*
tetracaine hydrochloride, 163, 164, 411, *412,* 440, *441*†*
tetrachloroethylene, 14, 15, *19*†*
tetracycline, 12, 14, 62, *63,* 347, 376*†
tetracycline hydrochloride, 62, *63,* 347, *444**
tetracycline phosphate complex, 62, *63**
tetracyclines, 20, 61, *63,* 347
TETRACYN, 12, 62, 347
tetrahydrozoline hydrochloride, 331, *332**
TETREX, 62
TETREX-S, 347
TG, 611, *612*
THEOBID, 317
THEO-NAR, 312‡
theophylline, 317, *318*†*
theophylline monethanolamine, 317, *318*†*
theophylline sodium glycinate, 317, *318**
THERA-FLUR, 435
THERIODIDE-131, 578
thiabendazole, 14, 15, *19**
thiamine hydrochloride, 594, *595*†*
thiamine monohydrate, 594, *595*†*
thiamylal sodium, 148, *151**
thiazides, *249*
thiethylperazine, 381, *384**
thimerosal, 424, *425**
thioguanine, 611, *612*†*
THIOMERIN, 256
thiopental sodium, 148, *151,* 168, *170**
thioridazine hydrochloride, 114, *116**
THIOSULFIL, 58
THIOSULFIL FORTE, 58
THIOTEPA, 607
thiothixene, *116**
thiphenamil, 389, *390*

*Generic Name
†Available as a generic product
‡More than one active ingredient

Index